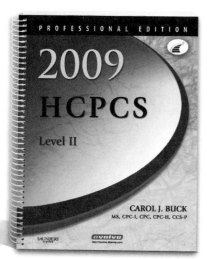
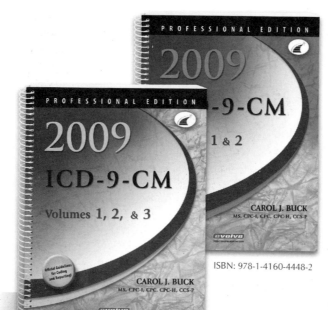
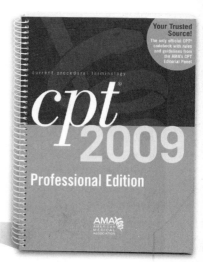

30341

Need more ICD-9 study resources?

This clear, easy-to-use textbook is **your key to ICD-9-CM coding success,** offering **everything you need to understand and apply the official codes of the ICD-9-CM.** You'll find **detailed background information** on the evolution and importance of medical coding, as well as **reliable, straightforward guidelines** for each of the coding classifications you'll use in practice.

Master the ICD-9-CM concepts needed to ensure proper reimbursement with features like...

- **ICD-9-CM guidelines** that open each coding chapter, with examples that clearly demonstrate their real-world applications.

- A **full-color design** that makes anatomy and physiology stand out and provides visual reinforcement of key content.

- **Illustrations and overviews of anatomy, physiology, and related disease conditions** in each coding chapter that help you better visualize and understand what the codes represent.

- **Problem-solving exercises** throughout each chapter that provide valuable practice using key coding principles as you learn them.

- **Also available as a paperless eBook!** Visit http://evolveebookstore.elsevier.com to find out more!

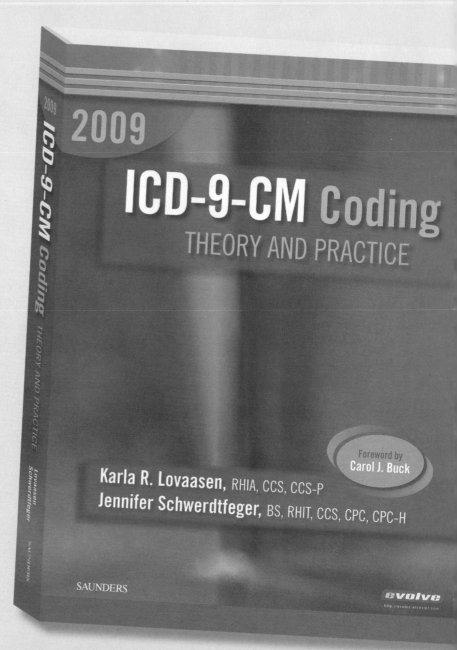

2009

ICD-9-CM Coding
THEORY AND PRACTICE

Karla R. Lovaasen, RHIA, CCS, CCS-P
Jennifer Schwerdtfeger, BS, RHIT, CCS, CPC, CPC-H

Foreword by
Carol J. Buck

SAUNDERS

evolve
http://evolve.elsevier.com

ICD-9-CM Coding: Theory and Practice, 2009 Edition
Karla R. Lovaasen, RHIA, CCS, CCS-P and Jennifer Schwerdtfeger, BS, RHIT, CCS, CPC, CPC-H
2009 • 768 pp., 400 illus. • ISBN: 978-1-4160-5881-6

STANDARD EDITION

2009 HCPCS

Level II

CAROL J. BUCK

MS, CPC-I, CPC, CPC-H, CCS-P
Program Director, Retired
Medical Secretary Programs
Northwest Technical College
East Grand Forks, Minnesota

SAUNDERS

ELSEVIER

SAUNDERS

ELSEVIER

11830 Westline Industrial Drive
St. Louis, Missouri 63146

2009 HCPCS LEVEL II STANDARD EDITION   ISBN: 978-1-4160-5204-3

Notice

Knowledge and best practice in this field are constantly changing. As new research and experience broaden our knowledge, changes in practice, treatment, and drug therapy may become necessary or appropriate. Readers are advised to check the most current information provided (i) on procedures featured or (ii) by the manufacturer of each product to be administered, to verify the recommended dose or formula, the method and duration of administration, and contraindications. It is the responsibility of the practitioner, relying on his or her own experience and knowledge of the patient, to make diagnoses, to determine dosages and the best treatment for each individual patient, and to take all appropriate safety precautions. To the fullest extent of the law, neither the Publisher nor the Author assumes any liability for any injury and/or damage to persons or property arising out of or related to any use of the material contained in this book.

The Publisher

NOTE: *Current Procedural Terminology, 2009* was used in updating this text.

2009 Current Procedural Terminology (CPT) is copyright 2008 American Medical Association. All Rights Reserved. No fee schedules, basic units, relative values, or related listings are included in CPT. The AMA assumes no liability for the data contained herein. Applicable FARS/DFARS restrictions apply to government use.

Library of Congress Cataloging-in-Publication Data

Buck, Carol J.
  2009 HCPCS : level II / Carol J. Buck. — Standard ed.
    p. ; cm.
  Includes index.
  ISBN 978-1-4160-5204-3 (pbk. : alk. paper) 1. Medicine—Terminology—Code numbers. I. Title.
    [DNLM: 1. Health Services—classification. 2. Equipment and Supplies—classification. 3. Forms and Records Control—methods. 4. Therapeutics—classification. WB 15 B992z 2009]
  R123. B83 2009b
  610.1′4—dc22
                                        2008047716

Publisher: Michael S. Ledbetter
Associate Developmental Editor: Jenna Johnson
Publishing Services Managers: Melissa Lastarria, Pat Joiner-Myers
Senior Designer: Amy Buxton

Printed in the United States of America

Last digit is the print number: 9 8 7 6 5 4 3 2

CONTENTS

Select IOMs are displayed in the appendix of this text, but are not a substitute for checking the Centers for Medicare and Medicaid Services (http://www.cms.hhs.gov/Manuals/IOM/list.asp) website for any updates since publication of this text.

Medical coding has long been a part of the health care profession. Through the years medical coding systems have become more complex and extensive. Today, medical coding is an intricate and immense process that is present in every health care setting. The increased use of electronic submissions for health care services only increases the need for coders who understand the coding process.

2009 HCPCS Level II was developed to help meet the needs of students preparing for a career in medical coding.

All material adheres to the latest government versions available at the time of printing.

Annotated

Throughout this text, revisions and additions are indicated by the following symbols:

◀▶ **New:** Additions to the previous edition are indicated by the color triangle.

←→ **Revised:** Revisions within the line or code from the previous edition are indicated by the color arrow.

✔ **Reinstated** indicates a code that was previously deleted and has now been reactivated.

✖ deleted words have been removed from this year's edition.

HCPCS Symbols

✪ **Special coverage instructions** apply to these codes. Usually these special coverage instructions are included in the Internet Only Manuals (IOM) select references in the Appendix.

◆ **Not covered or valid by Medicare** is indicated by the diamond. Usually the reason for the exclusion is included in the Internet Only Manuals (IOM) select references in the Appendix.

✳ **Carrier discretion** is an indication that you must contact the individual third-party payers to find out the coverage available for codes identified by this symbol.

▶ **ASC** (Ambulatory Surgical Center) ancillary services are paid separately or at a special rate when provided integral to a surgical procedure on the ASC list.

NDC Drugs approved for Medicare Part B are listed as NDC (National Drug Code). All other FDA-approved drugs are listed as Other.

Color typeface terms are terms added by the publisher and do not appear in the official code set.

SYMBOLS AND CONVENTIONS

HCPCS Symbols

Special coverage instructions apply to these codes. Usually these instructions are included in the Internet Only Manuals (IOM) select references in the Appendix of this text.

⊛ L3540   Miscellaneous shoe additions, sole, full
IOM: 100-2, 15, 290

The Internet Only Manuals (IOM) give instructions regarding use of the code. IOM select references are located in the Appendix of this text.

Not covered or valid by Medicare is indicated by the diamond. Usually the reason for the exclusion is included in the IOM references in the Appendix of this text.

◆ A6533   Gradient compression stocking, thigh length, 18–30 mm Hg, each
IOM: 100-02, 15, 130; 100-03, 4, 280.1

Carrier discretion is an indication that you must contact the individual third-party payers for the coverage for these codes.

✻ A6154   Wound pouch, each

The ❱ symbol appears by codes approved for separate payment of ancillary services in ambulatory surgical centers (ASC).

⊛ C9239❱ Injection, temsirolimus, 1 mg

Codes shown are for illustration purposes only and may not be current codes.

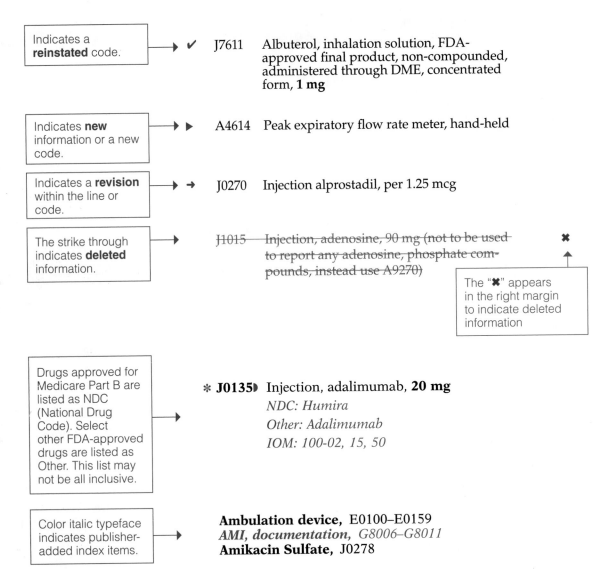

| Indicates a **reinstated** code. | → ✔ | J7611 | Albuterol, inhalation solution, FDA-approved final product, non-compounded, administered through DME, concentrated form, **1 mg** |

| Indicates **new** information or a new code. | → ▶ | A4614 | Peak expiratory flow rate meter, hand-held |

| Indicates a **revision** within the line or code. | → → | J0270 | Injection alprostadil, per 1.25 mcg |

The strike through indicates **deleted** information.

~~J1015   Injection, adenosine, 90 mg (not to be used to report any adenosine, phosphate compounds, instead use A9270)~~   ✖

The "✖" appears in the right margin to indicate deleted information

Drugs approved for Medicare Part B are listed as NDC (National Drug Code). Select other FDA-approved drugs are listed as Other. This list may not be all inclusive.

✳ **J0135▶** Injection, adalimumab, **20 mg**
NDC: Humira
Other: Adalimumab
IOM: 100-02, 15, 50

Color italic typeface indicates publisher-added index items.

Ambulation device, E0100–E0159
AMI, documentation, G8006–G8011
Amikacin Sulfate, J0278

Codes shown are for illustration purposes only and may not be current codes.

2009 HCPCS UPDATES

HCPCS 2009 New/Revised/Deleted Codes and Modifiers

2009 HCPCS quarterly updates will be posted on the companion website
(http://evolve.elsevier.com/Buck/HCPCS) when available.

NEW CODES/MODIFIERS

CG	C9359	G0403	G8486	G8504	G8522	G8540	J9207	Q4107
JC	C9898	G0404	G8487	G8505	G8523	G8541	J9330	Q4108
JD	C9899	G0405	G8488	G8506	G8524	G8542	K0672	Q4109
KE	E0487	G0406	G8489	G8507	G8525	G8543	L0113	Q4110
RA	E0656	G0407	G8490	G8508	G8526	G8544	L6711	Q4111
RB	E0657	G0408	G8491	G8509	G8527	J0641	L6712	Q4112
RE	E0770	G0409	G8492	G8510	G8528	J1267	L6713	Q4113
A6545	E1354	G0410	G8493	G8511	G8529	J1453	L6714	Q4114
A9284	E1356	G0411	G8494	G8512	G8530	J1459	L6721	S2118
A9580	E1357	G0412	G8495	G8513	G8531	J1930	L6722	S2270
C8929	E1358	G0413	G8496	G8514	G8532	J1953	L8604	S3628
C8930	E2230	G0414	G8497	G8515	G8533	J2785	Q4100	S3711
C9245	E2231	G0415	G8498	G8516	G8534	J3101	Q4101	S3860
C9246	E2295	G0416	G8499	G8517	G8535	J3300	Q4102	S3861
C9247	G0398	G0417	G8500	G8518	G8536	J7186	Q4103	S3862
C9248	G0399	G0418	G8501	G8519	G8537	J7606	Q4104	S9433
C9356	G0400	G0419	G8502	G8520	G8538	J8705	Q4105	
C9358	G0402	G8485	G8503	G8521	G8539	J9033	Q4106	

REINSTATED CODES

J1750	J7611	J7612	J7613	J7614

REVISED CODES/MODIFIERS

Administrative and Long Description Change
C8921
C8922
C8923
C8924
C8925
C8926
C8927
C8928

Administrative Data Field Change
A6200
A6201
A6202

Change In Both Administrative Data And Long Description
C8921
C8922
C8923
C8924
C8925
C8926
C8927
C8928

Long Description Change
KT
A6010
A6011
A6021
A6022
A6023
A6024
A6196
A6197
A6198
A6199
A6203
A6204
A6205
A6206
A6207
A6208
A6209
A6210
A6211
A6212
A6213
A6214
A6215
A6219
A6220
A6221
A6222
A6223

A6224
A6228
A6229
A6230
A6231
A6232
A6233
A6234
A6235
A6236
A6237
A6238
A6239
A6240
A6241
A6242
A6243
A6244
A6245
A6246
A6247
A6248
A6251
A6252
A6253
A6254
A6255
A6256
A6257
A6258

A6259
A6260
A6261
A6262
A6266
A6407
A9502
G0129
G0248
G0249
G0250
G8417
G8418
G8419
G8420
G8427
G8428
G8429
G8430
G8431
G8433
G8437
G8438
G8439
G8440
G8446
G8447
G8448
G8457
J0348

J1572
J2788
J2790
J3301
J7639
J9000
J9001
J9010
J9015
J9017
J9020
J9040
J9045
J9050
J9098
J9100
J9110
J9120
J9150
J9151
J9160
J9165
J9170
J9181
J9185
J9190
J9200
J9201
J9206
J9208

J9209
J9211
J9212
J9213
J9214
J9215
J9216
J9230
J9265
J9266
J9268
J9270
J9300
J9310
J9320
J9340
J9350
J9355
J9357
J9360
J9390
J9600
K0669
K0899
L4360
L8681
L8689
L8695
S0088

Miscellaneous Change
KL
Q0512

Payment Change
A4608
A4615
A4616
A4617
A4620
E1231
E1232
E1233
E1234
E1235
E1236
E1237
E1238
E1353
E1355
E2301

Short Description Change
J0395
J1571
J1573
J1626
J2469
J2724
Q0166
Q0179

DELETED CODES/MODIFIERS

RP
C9003
C9237
C9238
C9239
C9240
C9241
C9242
C9243

C9244
C9357
C9723
G0297
G0300
G0308
G0309
G0310
G0311

G0312
G0313
G0314
G0315
G0316
G0317
G0318
G0319
G0320

G0321
G0322
G0323
G0324
G0325
G0326
G0327
G0332
G0344

G0366
G0367
G0368
G0377
J1751
J1752
J3100
J7340
J7341

J7342
J7343
J7344
J7346
J7347
J7348
J7349
J7602
J7603

J9182
L2860
L3890
L5993
L5994
L5995
L7611
L7612
L7613

L7614
L7621
L7622
Q4096
Q4097
Q4098
Q4099
S0141
S0143

S2075
S2076
S2077
S2135
S9092

AMBULATORY SURGICAL CENTERS (ASC) ANCILLARY SERVICES

D5 Designation, Deleted/ Discontinued Code; No Payment Made		K2 Designation, Drugs and Biological Paid Separately When Provided Integral to a Surgical Procedure on ASC List; Payment Based on OPPS Rate			N1 Designation, Packaged Service/ Item; No Separate Payment Made
C9003	J3100	C9245	J1212	J9033	A9580
C9237	J7340	C9246	J1267	J9165	C1821
C9238	J7341	C9248	J1453	J9207	C9247
C9239	J7342	J0132	J1455	J9330	C9352
C9240	J7343	J0470	J1459	Q4101	C9353
C9241	J7344	J0550	J1750	Q4102	J0190
C9242	J7346	J0630	J1930	Q4103	J0350
C9243	J7347	J0641	J1953	Q4104	J0400
C9244	J7348		J2460	Q4105	J1324
C9357	J7349		J2515	Q4106	J2170
J1751	J9182		J2785	Q4107	J3300
J1752	Q4096		J2805	Q4108	J7197
	Q4097		J3101	Q4110	J8600
	Q4098		J3400	Q4111	J9040
			J7186	Q4112	J9045
			J7191	Q4113	J9212
			J7516	Q4114	L8604
			J8705		L8690
					Q2009
					Q4100
					Q4109

HCPCS 2009 INDEX

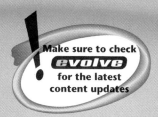

Make sure to check **evolve** for the latest content updates

A

Abarelix, J0128
Abatacept, J0129
Abciximab, J0130
Abdomen
   dressing holder/binder, A4462
   pad, low profile, L1270
Abduction control, each, L2624
Abduction rotation bar, foot, L3140–L3170
Absorption dressing, A6251–A6256
Access, site, occlusive, device, G0269
Access system, A4301
Accessories
   ambulation devices, E0153–E0159
   artificial kidney and machine (*see also* ESRD),
     E1510–E1699
   beds, E0271-E0280, E0300–E0326
   wheelchairs, E0950–E1030, E1050–E1298,
     E2201–E2399, E2300–E2399, K0001–K0109
ACE/ARB therapy, G8468–G8481
Acetazolamide sodium, J1120
Acetylcysteine, inhalation solution, J7604, J7608
Acetylcysteine, injection, J0132
Activity, therapy, G0176
Acyclovir, J0133
Adalimumab, J0135
Adenosine, J0150, J0152
Adhesive, A4364
   bandage, A6413
   disc or foam pad, A5126
   remover, A4365, A4455
   support, breast prosthesis, A4280
   wound, closure, G0168
Administration, Part D
   supply, tositumomab, G3001
   vaccine, hepatitis B, G0010
   vaccine, influenza, G0008
   vaccine, pneumococcal, G0009
Admission, observation, G0379
Administrative, Miscellaneous and
   Investigational, A9000–A9999
Adrenalin, J0170
Advanced life support, A0390, A0426, A0427,
   A0433
Aerosol
   compressor, E0571, E0572
   compressor filter, K0178–K0179
   mask, K0180
AFO, E1815, E1830, L1900–L1990, L4392, L4396
Agalsidase beta, J0180
Aggrastat, J3245
A-hydroCort, J1710
Aide, home, health, G0156, S9122, T1021
   bath/toilet, E0160–E0162, E0235, E0240–E0249
   services, G0151–G0156, G0179–G0181, S5180,
     S5181, S9122, T1021, T1022

Air bubble detector, dialysis, E1530
Air fluidized bed, E0194
Air pressure pad/mattress, E0186, E0197
Air travel and nonemergency transportation,
   A0140
Alarm,
   not otherwise classified, A9280
   pressure, dialysis, E1540
   symptom, documentation, G8248, G8274
Alatrofloxacin mesylate, J0200
Albumin, human, P9041, P9042
Albuterol, all formulations, inhalation solution,
   concentrated, ~~J7602,~~ J7610, J7611 ←
Albuterol, all formulations, inhalation solution,
   unit dose, ~~J7603,~~ J7609, J7613 ←
Albuterol, all formulations, inhalation
   solution, J7620
Alcohol/substance, assessment, G0396, G0397,
   H0001, H0003, H0049
Alcohol, A4244
Alcohol wipes, A4245
Aldesleukin (IL2), J9015
Alefacept, J0215
Alemtuzumab, J9010
Alert device, A9280
Alginate dressing, A6196–A6199
Alglucerase, J0205
Alglucosidase, J0220
Alphanate, J7186 ◄
Alpha-1-proteinase inhibitor, human, J0256
Alprostadil, injection, J0270
Alprostadil, urethral suppository, J0275
ALS mileage, A0390
Alteplase recombinant, J2997
Alternating pressure mattress/pad, A4640, E0180,
   E0181, E0277
Ambulance, A0021–A0999
   air, A0430, A0431, A0435, A0436
   disposable supplies, A0382–A0398
   oxygen, A0422
Ambulation device, E0100–E0159
AMI, documentation, G8006–G8011
Amikacin Sulfate, J0278
Aminolevulinic acid HCl, J7308
Aminophylline, J0280
Amiodarone Hcl, J0282
Amitriptyline HCI, J1320
Ammonia N-13, A9526
Ammonia test paper, A4774
Amniotic membrane, V2790
Amobarbital, J0300
Amphotericin B, J0285
Amphotericin B Lipid Complex, J0287–J0289
Ampicillin sodium, J0290
Ampicillin sodium/sulbactam sodium, J0295
Amputee
   adapter, wheelchair, E0959
   prosthesis, L5000–L7510, L7520, L7900, L8400–
     L8465

◄▶ New   ←→ Revised   ✔ Reinstated   ✖ Deleted

B

◀▶ New   ←→ Revised   ✔ Reinstated   ✖ Deleted

Belt
- extremity, E0945
- ostomy, A4367
- pelvic, E0944
- safety, K0031
- wheelchair, E0978, E0979

Bench, bathtub (*see also* **Bathtub**), E0245
Bendamustine HCl, J9033 ◄
Benesch boot, L3212–L3214
Benztropine, J0515
Betadine, A4246, A4247
Betameth, J0704
Betamethasone inhalation solution, J7624
Betamethasone acetate and betamethasone sodium phosphate, J0702
Betamethasone sodium phosphate, J0704
Bethanechol chloride, J0520
Bevacizumab, J9035
Bifocal, glass or plastic, V2200–V2299
Bilirubin (phototherapy) light, E0202
Binder, A4465
Biofeedback device, E0746
Bioimpedance, electrical, cardiac output, M0302
Biopsy, esophageal, documentation, G8251
Biperiden lactate, J0190
Bitolterol mesylate, inhalation solution, concentrated, J7628
Bitolterol mesylate, inhalation solution, unit dose, J7629
Bivalirudin, J0583
Bladder calculi irrigation solution, Q2004
Bleomycin sulfate, J9040
Blood
- *count, G0306, G0307, S3630*
- fresh frozen plasma, P9017
- glucose monitor, E0607, E2100, E2101, S1030, S1031
- glucose test, A4253
- granulocytes, pheresis, P9050
- ketone test, A4252
- leak detector, dialysis, E1560
- leukocyte poor, P9016
- mucoprotein, P2038
- occult, G0394
- platelets, P9019
- platelets, irradiated, P9032
- platelets, leukocytes reduced, P9031
- platelets, leukocytes reduced, irradiated, P9033
- platelets, pheresis, P9034
- platelets, pheresis, irradiated, P9036
- platelets, pheresis, leukocytes reduced, P9035
- platelets, pheresis, leukocytes reduced, irradiated, P9037
- *pressure, documentation, G8476–G8478*
- pressure monitor, A4660, A4663, A4670
- pump, dialysis, E1620
- red blood cells, deglycerolized, P9039
- red blood cells, irradiated, P9038

Blood *(Continued)*
- red blood cells, leukocytes reduced, P9016
- red blood cells, leukocytes reduced, irradiated, P9040
- red blood cells, washed, P9022
- strips, A4253
- supply, P9010 P9022
- testing supplies, A4770
- tubing, A4750, A4755

Blood collection devices accessory, A4257, E0620
BMI, G8417–G8422
Body jacket
- scoliosis, L1300, L1310

Body sock, L0984
Body, mass, index, G8417–G8422
Bond or adhesive, ostomy skin, A4364
Bone,
- *density, study, G0130*
- *marrow, aspiration, G0364*

Boot
- pelvic, E0944
- surgical, ambulatory, L3260

Bortezomib, J9041
Botulinum toxin type A, J0585
Botulinum toxin type B, J0587
Brachytherapy radioelements, Q3001
Breast prosthesis, L8000–L8035, L8600
Breast prosthesis, adhesive skin support, A4280
Breast pump
- accessories, A4281–A4286
- electric, any type, E0603
- heavy duty, hospital grade, E0604
- manual, any type, E0602

Breathing circuit, A4618
Brompheniramine maleate, J0945
Budesonide inhalation solution, J7626, J7627, J7633, J7634
Bulking agent, L8604 ◄
Buprenorphine hydrochloride, J0592
Bus, nonemergency transportation, A0110
Busulfan, J0594, J8510
Butorphanol tartrate, J0595
Bypass, graft, coronary, artery
- *documentation, G8034–G8041, G8159–G8172*
- *surgery, S2205–S2209*

C

Cabergoline, oral, J8515
Caffeine citrate, J0706
CABG, documentation, G8034–G8041, G8159–G8172
Cabinet/System, ultraviolet, E0691–E0694
CAD documentation, G8036–G8041
Calcitriol, J0636
Calcitonin-salmon, J0630
Calcium disodium edetate, J0600
Calcium, documentation, G8099–G8100, G8289

◄ ▶ New   ← → Revised   ✔ Reinstated   ✖ Deleted

Calcium gluconate, J0610
Calcium glycerophosphate and calcium lactate, J0620
Calcium lactate and calcium glycerophosphate, J0620
Calcium leucovorin, J0640
Calibrator solution, A4256
Cancer, screening
  cervical or vaginal, G0101
  colorectal, G0104–G0106, G0120–G0122, G0328, S3890
  prostate, G0102, G0103
Cane, E0100, E0105
  accessory, A4636, A4637
Canister, disposable, used with suction pump, A7000
Canister, non-disposable, used with suction pump, A7001
Cannula, nasal, A4615
Capecitabine, oral, J8520, J8521
Carbon filter, A4680
Carboplatin, J9045
Cardia Event, recorder, implantable, E0616
Cardiokymography, Q0035
Cardiovascular services, M0300–M0301
Carmustine, J9050
Care, coordinated, G9001–G9011, H1002
Case management, T1016, T1017
Caspofungin acetate, J0637
Cast
  hand restoration, L6900–L6915
  materials, special, A4590
  supplies, A4580, A4590, Q4001–Q4051
  thermoplastic, L2106, L2126
Caster, front, for power wheelchair, K0099
Caster, wheelchair, E0997, E0998
Catheter, A4300–A4355
  anchoring device, A5200, A4333, A4334
  cap, disposable (dialysis), A4860
  external collection device, A4327–A4330, A4347
  implanted, A7042, A7043
  indwelling, A4338–A4346
  insertion tray, A4354
  intermittent with insertion supplies, A4353
  irrigation supplies, A4355
  male external, A4324, A4325, A4348
  oropharyngeal suction, A4628
  starter set, A4329
  trachea (suction), A4609, A4610, A4624
  transtracheal oxygen, A4608
  vascular, A4300, A4301
Catheterization, specimen collection, P9612, P9615
CBC, G0306, G0307
Cefazolin sodium, J0690
Cefepime HCl, J0692
Cefotaxime sodium, J0698
Ceftazidime, J0713

Ceftizoxime sodium, J0715
Ceftriaxone sodium, J0696
Cefuroxime sodium, J0697
CellCept, K0412
Cellular therapy, M0075
Cement, ostomy, A4364
Centrifuge, A4650
Cephalin Floculation, blood, P2028
Cephalothin sodium, J1890
Cephapirin sodium, J0710
Certification, physician, home, health, G0179–G0182
Cerumen, removal, G0268
Cervical
  cancer, screening, G0101
  cap contraceptive, A4261
  cytopathology, G0123, G0124, G0141–G0148
  halo, L0810–L0830
  head harness/halter, E0942
  orthosis, L0100–L0200
  traction, E0855, E0856
Cervical-thoracic-lumbar-sacral orthosis (CTLSO), L0700, L0710
Cetuximab, J9055
Chair
  adjustable, dialysis, E1570
  lift, E0627
  rollabout, E1031
  sitz bath, E0160–E0162
  transport, E1035–E1039
Chelation therapy, M0300
Chemical endarterectomy, M0300
Chemistry and toxicology tests, P2028–P3001
Chemotherapy
  administration, Q0083–Q0085 (hospital reporting only)
  documentation G8371–G8374
  drug, oral, not otherwise classified, J8999
  drugs (*see also* drug by name), J9000–J9999
Chest shell (cuirass), E0457
Chest Wall Oscillation System, E0483
  hose, replacement, A7026
  vest, replacement, A7025
Chest wrap, E0459
Chin cup, cervical, L0150
Chloramphenicol sodium succinate, J0720
Chlordiazepoxide HCl, J1990
Chloromycetin Sodium Succinate, J0720
Chloroprocaine HCl, J2400
Chloroquine HCl, J0390
Chlorothiazide sodium, J1205
Chlorpromazine HCl, J3230
Choroid, lesion, destruction, G0186
Chorionic gonadotropin, J0725
Chromic phosphate P32 suspension, A9564
Chromium CR-51 sodium chromate, A9553
Cidofovir, J0740
Cilastatin sodium, imipenem, J0743

◀▶ New   ←→ Revised   ✔ Reinstated   ✖ Deleted

Ciprofloxacin, for intravenous infusion, J0744
Cisplatin, J9060, J9062
Cladribine, J9065
Clamp
   dialysis, A4910, A4918, A4920
   external urethral, A4356
Cleanser, wound, A6260
Cleansing agent, dialysis equipment, A4790
Clofarabine, J9027
Clonidine, J0735
Closure, wound, adhesive, tissue, G0168
Clotting time tube, A4771
Clubfoot wedge, L3380
Cochlear prosthetic implant, L8614
   accessories, L8615–L8617
   batteries, L8621–L8624
   replacement, L8619
Codeine phosphate, J0745
Colchicine, J0760
Cold/Heat, application, E0200–E0240
Colistimethate sodium, J0770
Collagen
   skin test, G0025
   urinary tract implant, L8603
   wound dressing, A6020–A6024
Collar, cervical
   multiple post, L0180–L0200
   nonadjust (foam), L0120
Colorectal, screening, cancer, G0104–G0106, G0120–
   G0122, G0328, S3890
Coly-Mycin M, J0770
Comfort items, A9190
Complete, blood, count, G0306, G0307
Commode, E0160–E0175
   chair, E0170–E0171
   lift, E0625, E0172
   pail, E0167
   seat, wheelchair, E0968
Composite dressing, A6200–A6205
Compressed gas system, E0424–E0480
Compressor
   aerosol, E0571, E0572, E0575
   air, E0565
   nebulizer, E0570–E0585
   pneumatic, E0650–E0676
Compression bandage, A4460
Compression burn garment, A6501–A6512
Compression stockings, A6530–A6549
Compressor, E0565, E0570, E0571, E0572, E0650–
   E0652
Conductive gel/paste, A4558
Conductivity meter, bath, dialysis, E1550
Conference, team, G0175, G9007, S0220, S0221
Congo red, blood, P2029
Contact layer, A6206–A6208
Contact lens, V2500–V2599
Continent device, A5081, A5082, A5083

Continuous glucose monitoring system
   receiver, A9278
   sensor, A9276
   transmitter, A9277
Continuous passive motion exercise device, E0936
Continuous positive airway pressure (CPAP)
   device, E0601
   compressor, K0269
Contraceptive
   cervical cap, A4261
   condoms, A4267, A4268
   diaphragm, A4266
   intrauterine, copper, J7300
   intrauterine, levonorgestrel releasing, J7302
   levonorgestrel, implants and supplies, A4260
   patch, J7304
   spermicide, A4269
   supply, A4267–A4269
   vaginal ring, J7303
Contracts, maintenance, ESRD, A4890
Contrast material
   injection during MRI, A4643
   low osmolar, A4644–A4646
Coordinated, care, G9001–G9011
COPD, documentation, G8093, G8094, G8293,G8296
Corneal tissue processing, V2785
Corset, spinal orthosis, L0970–L0976
Corticorelin ovine triflutate, J0795
Corticotropin, J0800
Corvert, *see* **Ibutilide fumarate**
Cosyntropin, J0835
Cough stimulating device, E0482
Count, blood, G0306, G0307, S3636
Counterpulsation, external, G0166
Cover, wound
   alginate dressing, A6196–A6198
   foam dressing, A6209–A6214
   hydrogel dressing, A6242–A6248
   non-contact wound warming cover, and accessory,
     A6000, E0231, E0232
   specialty absorptive dressing, A6251–A6256
CPAP (continuous positive airway pressure)
   device, E0601
   headgear, K0185
   humidifier, A7046
   intermittent assist, E0452
Cradle, bed, E0280
Crib, E0300
Cromolyn sodium, inhalation solution, unit
   dose, J7631, J7632
Crutches, E0110–E0118
   accessories, A4635–A4637, K0102
Cryoprecipitate, each unit, P9012
CT/MRI, documentation, G8243
CTLSO, L1000–L1120, L0700, L0710
Cuirass, E0457
Culture sensitivity study, P7001
Cushion, wheelchair, E0977

◀▶ New   ←→ Revised   ✔ Reinstated   ✖ Deleted

Cyanocobalamin Cobalt C057, A9559
Cycler dialysis machine, E1594
Cyclophosphamide, J9070–J9092
Cyclophosphamide, lyophilized, J9093–J9097
Cyclophosphamide, oral, J8530
Cyclosporine, J7502, J7515, J7516
Cytarabine, J9110
Cytarabine liposome, J9098
Cytomegalovirus immune globulin (human), J0850
Cytopathology, cervical or vaginal, G0123, G0124, G0141–G0148

D

Dacarbazine, J9130, J9140
Daclizumab, J7513
Dactinomycin, J9120
Dalalone, J1100
Dalteparin sodium, J1645
Daptomycin, J0878
Darbepoetin Alfa, J0881–J0882
Daunorubicin Citrate, J9151
Daunorubicin HCl, J9150
DaunoXome, *see* Daunorubicin citrate
Decitabine, J0894
Decubitus care equipment, E0180–E0199
Deferoxamine mesylate, J0895
Defibrillator, external, E0617, K0606
    battery, K0607
    electrode, K0609
    garment, K0608
Deionizer, water purification system, E1615
Delivery/set-up/dispensing, A9901
Denileukin diftitox, J9160
Density, bone, study, G0130
Depo-estradiol cypionate, J1000
Desmopressin acetate, J2597
Destruction, lesion, choroid, G0186
Detector, blood leak, dialysis, E1560
DEXA, documentation, G8341, G8345
Dexamethasone acetate, J1094
Dexamethasone, inhalation solution, concentrated, J7637
Dexamethasone, inhalation solution, unit dose, J7638
Dexamethasone, oral, J8540
Dexamethasone sodium phosphate, J1100
Dextran, J7100
Dextrose
    saline (normal), J7042
    water, J7060, J7070
Dextrostick, A4772
Diabetes
    evaluation, G0245, G0246
    patient, documentation, G8015–G8026
    shoes, A5500–A5508
    training, outpatient, G0108, G0109

Diagnostic
    radiology services, R0070–R0076
Dialysate concentrate additives, A4765
Dialysate solution, A4728
Dialysate testing solution, A4760
Dialysis
    air bubble detector, E1530
    bath conductivity, meter, E1550
    chemicals/antiseptics solution, A4674
    disposable cycler set, A4671
    documentation, G8075–G8085
    emergency, G0257
    equipment, E1510–E1702
    extension line, A4672–A4673
    filter, A4680
    fluid barrier, E1575
    forceps, A4910
    home, S9335, S9339
    kit, A4820
    pressure alarm, E1540
    shunt, A4740
    supplies, A4650–A4927
    thermometer, A4910
    tourniquet, A4910
    unipuncture control system, E1580
    unscheduled, G0257
    venous pressure clamp, A4918
Dialyzer, A4690
Diaper, T1500, T4521–T4540
Diaper, adult incontinence garment, A4520
Diazepam, J3360
Diazoxide, J1730
Dicyclomine HCl, J0500
Diethylstilbestrol diphosphate, J9165
Digoxin, J1160
Digoxin immune fab (ovine), J1162
Dihydroergotamine mesylate, J1110
Dimenhydrinate, J1240
Dimercaprol, J0470
Dimethyl sulfoxide (DMSO), J1212
Diphenhydramine HCl, J1200
Dipyridamole, J1245
Disarticulation
    lower extremities, prosthesis, L5000–L5999
    upper extremities, prosthesis, L6000–L6692
Discharge medications, documentation, G8257
Disease
    chronic, obstructive, pulmonary, documentation, G8093, G8094, G8293, G8296
    coronary, artery, documentation G8036–G8041
    end-stage, renal, documentation, G8075–G8082
    status, oncology, G9063–G9139
Disposable supplies, ambulance, A0382, A0384, A0392–A0398
Dispensing, fee, pharmacy, G0333, Q0510–Q0514, S9430

◀▶ New   ←→ Revised   ✔ Reinstated   ✖ Deleted

DME
  miscellaneous, A9900–A9999
  repair, E1340
DMSO, J1212
Dobutamine HCl, J1250
Docetaxel, J9170
Documentation
  alarm symptom, G8248, G8274
  AMI, G8006–G8011
  antibiotic, prophylaxis, G8152–G8154, G8193,
    G8196, G8204, G8209
  antidepressant, G8126–G8131
  antimicrobial, G8200
  antiplatelet, therapy, G8036–G8038, G8172, G8223
  aspirin, G8006–G8008, G8170–G8171, G8354
  asthma, G8370
  barium swallow, G8254
  biopsy, esophageal, G8251
  blood pressure, G8476–G8478
  bypass, graft, coronary, artery, documentation,
    G8034–G8041, G8159–G8172
  CABG, G8034–G8041, G8159-G8172
  CAD, G8036-G8041
  calcium, G8099–G8100, G8289
  chemotherapy, G8371–G8374
  COPD, G8093, G8094, G8293, G8296
  CT/MRI, G8243
  DEXA, G8341, G8345
  diabetic, patient, G8015–G8026
  dialysis, G8075–G8085
  discharge medications, G8257
  disease, coronary, artery, G8036–G8041
  disease, end-stage, renal, G8075–G8082
  dysphagia, G8231–G8234
  dysphagia, screening, G8231–G8234, V5364
  ECG, G8351, G8357
  ESRD, G8075–G8082
  eye, functions, G8314–G8334
  falls, G8054–G8056, G8271
  fracture, osteoporosis, G8338
  glaucoma, G8305–G8308
  heart, failure, G8027–G8032
  influenza, immunization, G8482–G8484
  influenza, vaccination, G8108–G8110
  intraocular pressure, G8302–G8308
  mammogram, G8111–G8114
  mental status, G8365
  moles, G8246, G8276
  optic nerve head, evaluation, G8298, G8299
  osteoarthritis, G8185, G8186
  osteoporosis, G8051–G8053, G8338, G8401
  oxygen saturation, G8362
  pharmacologic, therapy, G8285, G8341
  pneumonia, G8012–G8014
  prior, myocardial infarction, G8033–G8035
  prophylaxis, antimicrobial, G8200
  prophylaxis, DVT, G8217–G8221

Documentation (Continued)
  prophylaxis, thromboembolism, venous, G8155–
    G8157, G8214
  prophylaxis, thrombosis, deep, vein, G8217–G8221
  prophylaxis, VTE, G8214
  rehabilitation, services, G8238
  self-exam, G8282
  skin, exam, G8279
  stenosis, internal carotid, G8240
  surrogate, G8260
  T-PA, G8231
  urinary, incontinence, G8060–G8063, G8266–G8268
  vaccine, pneumococcal, G8115–G8117
  vital signs, G8360
  vitamin D, G8289
  warfarin, G8183, G8184
Dolasetron mesylate, J1260
Dome and mouthpiece (for nebulizer), A7016
Dopamine HCl, J1265
Doripenem, J1267 ◄
Dornase alpha, inhalation solution, unit dose
  form, J7639
Doxercalciferol, J1270
Doxil, J9001
Doxorubicin HCl, J9000, J9001
Drainage
  bag, A4357, A4358
  board, postural, E0606
  bottle, A5102
Dressing (*see also* **Bandage),** A6020–A6406
  alginate, A6196–A6199
  collagen, A6020–A6024
  composite, A6200–A6205
  contact layer, A6206–A6208
  foam, A6209–A6215
  gauze, A6216–A6230, A6402–A6406
  holder/binder, A4462
  hydrocolloid, A6234–A6241
  hydrogel, A6242–A6248
  specialty absorptive, A6251–A6256
  transparent film, A6257–A6259
  tubular, A6457
Droperidol, J1790
  and fentanyl citrate, J1810
Dropper, A4649
Drugs (*see also* **Table of Drugs)**
  administered through a metered dose inhaler, J3535
  antiemetic, J8489, J8597, Q0163–Q0181
  chemotherapy, J8500–J9999
  disposable delivery system, 5 ml or less per hour,
    A4306
  disposable delivery system, 50 ml or greater per
    hour, A4305
  immunosuppressive, J7500–J7599
  infusion supplies, A4230–A4232, A4221, A4222
  inhalation solutions, J7608–J7699
  non-prescription, A9150

◄ ▶ New   ← → Revised   ✔ Reinstated   ✖ Deleted

Drugs (*see also* **Table of Drugs**) (*Continued*)
  not otherwise classified, J3490, J7599, J7699, J7799, J8499, J8999, J9999
  oral, NOS, J8499
  prescription, oral, J8499, J8999
Dry pressure pad/mattress, E0179, E0184, E0199
Durable medical equipment (DME), E0100–E1830, K Codes
Duraclon, *see* Clonidine
Dyphylline, J1180
Dysphagia, screening, documentation, G8231–G8234, V5364
Dystrophic, nails, trimming, G0127

E

Ear mold, V5264
ECG, documentation, G8351, G8357
Echocardiography injectable contrast material, A9700
Eculizumab, J1300
ED, visit, G0380–G0384
Edetate calcium disodium, J0600
Edetate disodium, J3520
Eggcrate dry pressure pad/mattress, E0184, E0199
Elbow
  disarticulation, endoskeletal, L6450
  orthosis (EO), E1800, L3700–L3740, L3760
  protector, E0191
Electric, nerve, stimulator, transcutaneous, A4595, E0720–E0749
Electrical work, dialysis equipment, A4870
Electrocardiogram, G8351, G8357
Electromagnetic, therapy, G0295, G0329
Electrodes, per pair, A4556
Elevating leg rest, K0195
Elliotts b solution, J9175
Emergency department, visit, G0380–G0384
EMG, E0746
Eminase, J0350
Endarterectomy, chemical, M0300
Endoscope sheath, A4270
Endoskeletal system, addition, L5848, L5856–L5857, L5925
End-stage renal disease
  documentation, G8075–G8082
Enfuvirtide, J1324
Enoxaparin sodium, J1650
Enema, bag, A4458
Enteral
  feeding supply kit (syringe) (pump) (gravity), B4034–B4036
  formulae, B4149–B4156
  nutrition infusion pump (with alarm) (without), B9000, B9002
  therapy, supplies, B4000–B9999

Epinephrine, J0170
Epirubicin HCl, J9178
Epoetin alpha, J0885–J0886, Q4081
Epoprostenol, J1325
Equipment
  decubitus, E0181–E0199
  exercise, A9300, E0935, E0936
  orthopedic, E0910–E0948, E1800–E8002
  oxygen, E0424–E0486, E1353–E1406
  pump, E0781, E0784, E0791
  respiratory, E0424–E0601
  safety, E0700, E0705
  traction, E0830–E0900
  transfer, E0705
  trapeze, E0910–E0912, E0940
  whirlpool, E1300, E1310
Ergonovine maleate, J1330
Ertapenem sodium, J1335
Erythromycin lactobionate, J1364
ESRD (End-Stage Renal Disease; *see also* **Dialysis)**
  documentation, G8075–G8085
  machines and accessories, E1500–E1699
  plumbing, A4870
  supplies, A4651–A4929
Estrogen conjugated, J1410
Estrone (5, Aqueous), J1435
Ethanolamine oleate, J1430
Etidronate disodium, J1436
Etonogestrel implant system, J7307
Etoposide, J9181, ~~J9182~~ ←
Etoposide, oral, J8560
Euflexxa, J7323
Evaluation,
  conformity, V5020
  contact lens, S0592
  diabetic, G0245, G0246
  footwear, G8410–G8416
  fundus, G8325–G8328
  hearing, G8057–G8059, S0618, V5008, V5010
  hospice, G0337
  multidisciplinary, H2000
  nursing, T1001
  ocularist, S9150
  optic nerve head, G8298, G8299
  performance measurement, S3005
  resident, T2011
  speech, S9152
  team, T1024
  treatment response, G0254
Examination,
  gynecological, S0610–S0613
  ophthalmological, S0620, S0621
  pinworm, Q0113
  rectal, S0605
  ringworm, S0605
Exercise
  class, S9451
  equipment, A9300, E0935, E0936

◄► New   ←→ Revised   ✔ Reinstated   ✖ Deleted

External
  ambulatory infusion pump, E0781, E0784
  ambulatory insulin delivery system, A9274
  power, battery components, L7360–L7368
  power, elbow, L7160–L7191
  urinary supplies, A4356-A4359
Extremity
  belt/harness, E0945
  traction, E0870–E0880
Eye
  case, V2756
  functions, documentation, G8314–G8334
  lens (contact) (spectacle), V2100–V2615
  prosthetic, V2623, V2629
  service (miscellaneous), V2700–V2799

F

Faceplate, ostomy, A4361
Face tent, oxygen, A4619
Factor VIIA coagulation factor, recombinant, J7189
Factor VIII, anti-hemophilic factor, J7190–J7192
Factor IX, J7193, J7194, J7195
Falls, documentation, G8054–G8056, G8271
Family Planning Education, H1010
Fee
  coordinated care, G9001–G9011
  dispensing, pharmacy, G0333, Q0510–Q0514, S9430
Fentanyl citrate, J3010
Fentanyl citrate and droperidol, J1810
Fern test, Q0114
Filgrastim (G-CSF), J1440, J1441
Filler, wound
  alginate dressing, A6199
  foam dressing, A6215
  hydrocolloid dressing, A6240, A6241
  hydrogel dressing, A6248
  not elsewhere classified, A6261, A6262
Film, transparent (for dressing), A6257–A6259
Filter
  aerosol compressor, A7014
  dialysis carbon, A4680
  ostomy, A4368
  tracheostoma, A4481
  ultrasonic generator, A7014
Fistula cannulation set, A4730
Flebogamma, J1572
Flowmeter, E0440, E0555, E0580
Floxuridine, J9200
Fluconazole, injection, J1450
Fludarabine phosphate, J9185
Fluid barrier, dialysis, E1575
Flunisolide inhalation solution, J7641
Fluocinolone, J7311
Fluorodeoxyglucose F-18 FDG, A9552
Fluorouracil, J9190

Foam dressing, A6209–A6215
Foam pad adhesive, A5126
Folding walker, E0135, E0143
Foley catheter, A4312–A4316, A4338–A4346
Fomepizole, J1451
Fomivirsen sodium intraocular, J1452
Fondaparinux sodium, J1652
Footdrop splint, L4398
Footplate, E0175, E0970, L3031
Footwear, orthopedic, L3201–L3265
Forearm crutches, E0110, E0111
Formoterol, J7640
Formoterol fumarate, J7606 ◀
Fosaprepitant, J1453 ◀
Foscarnet sodium, J1455
Fosphenytoin, Q2009
Fracture
  bedpan, E0276
  documentation, osteoporosis, G8338
  frame, E0920, E0930, E0946–E0948
  orthosis, L2106–L2136, L3980–L3986
  orthotic additions, L2180–L2192, L3995
Fragmin, *see* **Dalteparin sodium**
Frames (spectacles), V2020, V2025
Fulvestrant, J9395
Furosemide, J1940

G

Gait trainer, E8000–E8002
Gallium Ga67, A9556
Gallium nitrate, J1457
Galsulfase, J1458
Gammagard liquid, J1569
Gamma globulin, J1460–J1561
Gamonex, J1561
Ganciclovir, implant, J7310
Ganciclovir sodium, J1570
Garamycin, J1580
Gas system
  compressed, E0424, E0425
  gaseous, E0430, E0431, E0441, E0443
  liquid, E0434–E0440, E0442, E0444
Gatifloxacin, J1590
Gauze (*see also* **Bandage**)
  impregnated, A6222–A6233, A6266
  non-impregnated, A6402–A6404
Gefitinib, J8565
Gel
  conductive, A4558
  pressure pad, E0185, E0196
Gemcitabine HCl, J9201
Gemtuzumab ozogamicin, J9300
Generator
  ultrasonic with nebulizer, E0574
Gentamicin (Sulfate), J1580

◀▶ New   ←→ Revised   ✓ Reinstated   ✖ Deleted

Glasses
 air conduction, V5070
 binaural, V5120–V5150
 bone conduction, V5080
 frames, V2020, V2025
 hearing aid, V5230
Glaucoma
 documentation, G8305–G8308
 screening, G0117, G0118
Gloves, A4927
Glucagon HCl, J1610
Glucose monitor with integrated lancing/blood sample collection, E2101
Glucose monitor with integrated voice synthesizer, E2100
Glucose test strips, A4253, A4772
Gluteal pad, L2650
Glycopyrrolate, inhalation solution, concentrated, J7642
Glycopyrrolate, inhalation solution, unit dose, J7643
Gold sodium thiomalate, J1600
Gomco drain bottle, A4912
Gonadorelin HCl, J1620
Goserelin acetate implant (*see also* **Implant),** J9202
Grab bar, trapeze, E0910, E0940
Gradient, compression stockings, A6530–A6549
Grade-aid, wheelchair, E0974
Granisetron HCl, J1626
Gravity traction device, E0941
Gravlee jet washer, A4470
Guaiac, stool, G0394
Guidelines, practice, oncology, G9056–G9062

H

Hair analysis (excluding arsenic), P2031
Hallus-Valgus dynamic splint, L3100
Hallux prosthetic implant, L8642
Haloperidol, J1630
 decanoate, J1631
Halo procedures, L0810–L0860
Halter, cervical head, E0942
Hand finger orthosis, prefabricated, L3923
Hand restoration, L6900–L6915
 partial prosthesis, L6000–L6020
 orthosis (WHFO), E1805, E1825, L3800–L3805, L3900-L3954
 rims, wheelchair, E0967
Handgrip (cane, crutch, walker), A4636
Harness, E0942, E0944, E0945
Headgear (for positive airway pressure device), K0185
Hearing
 assessment, G8057–G8059, S0618, V5008, V5010
 devices, V5000–V5299, L8614
 services, V5000–V5999

Heart, failure, documentation, G8027–G8032
Heat
 application, E0200–E0239
 lamp, E0200, E0205
 infrared heating pad system, A4639, E0221
 pad, E0210, E0215, E0237, E0238, E0249
Heater (nebulizer), E1372
Heavy duty, wheelchair, E1280–E1298, K0006, K0007, K0801–K0886
Heel
 elevator, air, E0370
 protector, E0191
 shoe, L3430–L3485
 stabilizer, L3170
Helicopter, ambulance (*see also* **Ambulance)**
Helmet, cervical, L0100, L0110
Helmet, head, A8000–A8004
Hemin, J1640
Hemi-wheelchair, E1083–E1086
Hemipelvectomy prosthesis, L5280
Hemodialysis machine, E1590
Hemodialyzer, portable, E1635
Hemofil M, J7190
Hemophilia clotting factor, J7190–J7198
Hemophilia clotting factor, NOC, J7199
Hemostats, A4850
Hemostix, A4773
Hepagam B IM, J1571, J1573 ←
Hepagam B IV, J1573 ◀
Heparin infusion pump, dialysis, E1520
Heparin lock flush, J1642
Heparin sodium, J1644
Hepatitis B, vaccine, administration, G0010
Hep-Lock (U/P), J1642
Hexalite, A4590
High osmolar contrast material, Q9958–Q9964
Hip
 disarticulation prosthesis, L5250, L5270
 orthosis (HO), L1600–L1690
Hip-knee-ankle-foot orthosis (HKAFO), L2040–L2090
Histrelin acetate, J1675
Histrelin implant, J9225
HKAFO, L2040–L2090
Home
 glucose, monitor, E0607, E2100, E2101, S1030, S1031
 health, aide, G0156, S9122, T1021
 health, clinical, social worker, G0155
 health, nursing, skilled, G0154
 health, occupational, therapist, G0152
 health, physical therapist, G0151
 health, physician, certification, G0179–G0182
 health, respiratory therapy, S5180, S5181
 therapist, speech, S9128
Home Health Agency Services, T0221
HOPPS, C1000–C9999

Hospital
  bed, E0250–E0304, E0328, E0329
  observation, G0378, G0379
Hospital Outpatient Payment System, *C1000–C9999*
Hot water bottle, E0220
Humidifier, A7046, E0550–E0563
Hyalgan, J7321
Hyaluronate, sodium, J7317
Hyaluronidase, J3470
Hyaluronidase, ovine, J3471–J3473
Hydralazine HCl, J0360
Hydraulic patient lift, E0630
Hydrocollator, E0225, E0239
Hydrocolloid dressing, A6234–A6241
Hydrocortisone
  acetate, J1700
  sodium phosphate, J1710
  sodium succinate, J1720
Hydrogel dressing, A6242–A6248, A6231–A6233
Hydromorphone, J1170
Hydroxyzine HCl, J3410
Hylan G-F 20, J7322
Hyoscyamine Sulfate, J1980
Hyperbaric oxygen chamber, topical, A4575
Hypertonic saline solution, J7130

I

Ibandronate sodium, J1740
Ibutilide Fumarate, J1742
Ice
  cap, E0230
  collar, E0230
Idarubicin HCl, J9211
Idursulfase, J1743
Ifosfamide, J9208
Iliac, artery, angiography, G0278
Imiglucerase, J1785
Immune globulin
  Flebogamma, J1572
  Gammagard liquid, J1569
  Gamunex, J1561
  HepaGam B, J1571
  NOS, J1566
  Octagam, J1568
  Privigen, J1459 ◄
  Rho(D), J2788, J2790 ◄
  Rhophylac, J2791
  Subcutaneous, J1562
Immunosuppressive drug, not otherwise classified, J7599
Implant
  access system, A4301
  aqueous shunt, L8612
  breast, L8600
  cochlear, L8614, L8619
  collagen, urinary tract, L8603
  dextranomer/hyaluronic acid copolymer, L8604 ◄

Implant *(Continued)*
  ganciclovir, J7310
  hallux, L8642
  urinary tract, L8603, L8606
  infusion pump, programmable, E0783, E0786
  joint, L8630, L8641, L8658
  lacrimal duct, A4262, A4263
  metacarpophalangeal joint, L8630
  metatarsal joint, L8641
  neurostimulator pulse generator, L8681–L8688
  not otherwise specified, L8699
  ocular, L8610
  ossicular, L8613
  osteogenesis stimulator, E0749
  percutaneous access system, A4301
  replacement implantable intraspinal catheter, E0785
  synthetic, urinary, L8606
  vascular graft, L8670
Implantable radiation dosimeter, A4650
Impregnated gauze dressing, A6222–A6230
Incontinence
  appliances and supplies, A4310, A4360, A5071–A5075, A5102–A5114, K0280, K0281
  garmet, A4520, T4521–T4543
  supply, A4335, A4356–A4358
  treatment system, E0740
  urinary, documentation, G8060–G8063, G8266–G8268
Indium IN-111 carpromab pendetide, A9507
Indium IN-111 ibritumomab tiuxetan, A9542
Indium IN-111 labeled autologous white blood cells, A9570
Indium IN-111 labeled autologous platelets, A9571
Indium IN-111 oxyquinoline, A9547
Indium IN-111 pentetate, A9548
Indium IN-111 pentetreotide, A9572
Indium IN-111 satumomab, A4642
Infarction, myocardial, acute, documentation, G8006–G8011
Infliximab injection, J1745
Influenza
  immunization, documentation, G8482–G8484
  vaccination, documentation, G8108–G8110
  vaccine, administration, G0008
Infusion
  pump, ambulatory, with administrative equipment, E0781
  pump, heparin, dialysis, E1520
  pump, implantable, E0782, E0783
  pump, implantable, refill kit, A4220
  pump, insulin, E0784
  pump, mechanical, reusable, E0779, E0780
  pump, uninterrupted infusion of Epiprostenol, K0455
  saline, J7030–J7060
  supplies, A4219, A4221, A4222, A4230–A4232, E0776–E0791 ←

◄► New   ←→ Revised   ✔ Reinstated   ✖ Deleted

Infusion *(Continued)*
therapy, other than chemotherapeutic drugs, Q0081
Inhalation solution *(see also* **drug name),** J7608–J7699
Injection device, needle-free, A4210
Injections *(see also* **drug name),** J0120–J7320
arthrography, sacroiliac, joint, G0259, G0260
supplies for self-administered, A4211
INR, monitoring, G0248–G0250
Insertion tray, A4310–A4316
Insulin, J1815, J1817, S5550–S5571
ambulatory, external, system, A9274
Interferon
Alpha, J9212–J9215
Beta-1 a, J1825, Q3025–Q3026
Beta- 1 b, J1830
Gamma, J9216
Intermittent
assist device with continuous positive airway pressure device, E0470–E0472
limb compression device, E0676
peritoneal dialysis system, E1592
positive pressure breathing (IPPB) machine, E0500
Interphalangeal joint, prosthetic implant, L8658, L8659
Interscapular thoracic prosthesis
endoskeletal, L6570
upper limb, L6350–L6370
Intervention, tobacco, G8402, G8403, G8453, G8454, G9016
Intraconazole, J1835
Intraocular
lenses, V2630–V2632
pressure, documentation, G8302–G8308
Intrapulmonary percussive ventilation system, E0481
Intrauterine copper contraceptive, J7300
Iodine Iobenguane sulfate I-131, A9508
Iodine I-123 sodium iodide, A9509, A9516
Iodine I-125 serum albumin, A9532
Iodine I-125 sodium iodide, A9527
Iodine I-125 sodium iothalamate, A9554
Iodine I-131 iodinated serum albumin, A9524
Iodine I-131 sodium iodide capsule, A9517, A9528
Iodine I-131 sodium iodide solution, A9529–A9531
Iodine I-131 tositumomab, A9544–A9545
Iodine swabs/wipes, A4247
IPD
system, E1592
IPPB machine, E0500
Ipratropium bromide, inhalation solution, unit dose, J7644, J7645
Irinotecan, J9206
Iron Dextran, J1750, ~~J1751, J1752~~ ←
Iron sucrose, J1756

Irrigation/evacuation system, bowel
control unit, E0350
disposable supplies for, E0352
Irrigation solution for bladder calculi, Q2004
Irrigation supplies, A4320–A4322, A4355, A4397–A4400
Islet, transplant, G0341–G0343, S2102
Isoetharine HCL, inhalation solution, concentrated, J7647, J7648
Isoetharine HCL, inhalation solution, unit dose, J7649, J7650
Isolates, B4150, B4152
Isoproterenol HCL, inhalation solution, concentrated, J7657, J7658
Isoproterenol HCL, inhalation solution, unit dose, J7659, J7660
Item, non-covered, A9270
IUD, J7300, S4989
IV pole, each, E0776, K0105
Ixabepilone, J9207 ◄

J

Jacket
scoliosis, L1300, L1310
Jaw, motion, rehabilitation system, E1700–E1702
Jenamicin, J1580

K

Kanamycin sulfate, J1840, J1850
Kartop patient lift, toilet or bathroom *(see also* **Lift),** E0625
Ketorolac thomethamine, J1885
Kidney
ESRD supply, A4650–A4927
machine, accessories, E1500–E1699
machine, E1500–E1699
system, E1510
wearable artificial, E1632
Kits
enteral feeding supply (syringe) (pump) (gravity), B4034–B4036
fistula cannulation (set), A4730
parenteral nutrition, B4220–B4224
surgical dressing (tray), A4550
tracheostomy, A4625
Knee
arthroscopy, surgical, G0289, S2112, S2300
disarticulation, prosthesis, L5150, L5160
joint, miniature, L5826
orthosis (KO), E1810, L1800–L1885
Knee-ankle-foot orthosis (KAFO), L2000–L2039, L2126–L2136
Knee-ankle-foot orthosis (KAFO) addition, high strength, lightweight material, L2755
Kyphosis pad, L1020, L1025

◄► New   ←→ Revised   ✔ Reinstated   ✖ Deleted

L

Laboratory
services, P0000–P9999
Laboratory tests
  chemistry, P2028–P2038
  microbiology, P7001
  miscellaneous, P9010–P9615, Q0111–Q0115
  toxicology, P3000–P3001, Q0091
Lacrimal duct implant
  permanent, A4263
  temporary, A4262
Lactated Ringer's infusion, J7120
Laetrile, J3570
Lancet, A4258, A4259
Lanreotide, J1930 ◄
Laronidase, J1931
Larynx, artificial, L8500
Laser blood collection device and accessory, E0620, A4257
Lead investigation, T1029
Lead wires, per pair, A4557
Leg
  bag, A4358, A5105, A5112
  extensions for walker, E0158
  rest, elevating, K0195
  rest, wheelchair, E0990
  strap, replacement, A5113–A5114
Legg Perthes orthosis, L1700–L1755
Lens
  aniseikonic, V2118, V2318
  contact, V2500–V2599
  eye, V2100–V2615, V2700–V2799
  intraocular, V2630–V2632
  low vision, V2600–V2615
  progressive, V2781
Lepirudin, J1945
Lesion, destruction, choroid, G0186
Leucovorin calcium, J0640
Leukocyte poor blood, each unit, P9016
Leuprolide acetate, J9217, J9218, J9219, J1950
Levalbuterol, all formulations, inhalation solution, concentrated, J7602, J7607, J7612 ←
Levalbuterol, all formulations, inhalation solution, unit dose, J7603, J7614, J7615 ←
Levetiracetam, J1953 ◄
Levocarnitine, J1955
Levofloxacin, J1956
Levoleucovorin, J0641 ◄
Levonorgestrel, (contraceptive), implants and supplies, J7306
Levorphanol tartrate, J1960
Lidocaine HCl, J2001
Lift
  patient (includes seat lift), E0621–E0635
  shoe, L3300–L3334
Lightweight, wheelchair, E1087–E1090, E1240–E1270, E2618

Lincomycin HCl, J2010
Linezolid, J2020
Liquid barrier, ostomy, A4363
Lodging, recipient, escort nonemergency transport, A0180, A0200
LOPS, G0245–G0247
Lorazepam, J2060
Loss of protective sensation, G0245–G0247
Low osmolar contrast material, Q9965–Q9967
LSO, L0621–L0640
Lubricant, A4402, A4332
Lumbar flexion, L0540
Lumbar-sacral orthosis (LSO), L0621–L0640
LVRS, services, G0302–G0305
Lymphocyte immune globulin, J7504, J7511

M

Machine
  IPPB, E0500
  kidney, E1500–E1699
Magnesium sulphate, J3475
Maintenance contract, ESRD, A4890
Mammogram, documentation, G8111–G8114
Mammography, screening, G0202
Mannitol, J2150
Mapping, vessel, for hemodialysis access, G0365
Marker, tissue, A4648
Mask
  aerosol, K0180
  oxygen, A4620
Mastectomy
  bra, L8000
  form, L8020
  prosthesis, L8030, L8600
  sleeve, L8010
Mattress
  air pressure, E0186
  alternating pressure, E0277
  dry pressure, E0184
  gel pressure, E0196
  hospital bed, E0271, E0272
  non-powered, pressure reducing, E0373
  overlay, E0371–E0372
  powered, pressure reducing, E0277
  water pressure, E0187
Mecasermin, J2170
Mechlorethamine HCl, J9230
Medicaid, codes, T1000–T9999
Medical and surgical supplies, A4206–A8999
Medical nutritional therapy, G0270, G0271
Medical services, other, M0000–M9999
Medroxyprogesterone acetate, J1051, J1055
Medroxyprogesterone acetate/estradiol cypionate, J1056
Melphalan HCl, J9245

◄▶ New   ←→ Revised   ✔ Reinstated   ✖ Deleted

Melphalan, oral, J8600
Mental, health, training services, G0177
Mental status, documentation, G8365
Meperidine, J2175
Meperidine and promethazine, J2180
Mepivacaine HCl, J0670
Meropenem, J2185
Mesna, J9209
Metacarpophalangeal joint, prosthetic implant, L8630, L8631
Metaproterenol sulfate, inhalation solution, concentrated, J7667, J7668
Metaproterenol sulfate, inhalation solution, unit dose, J7669, J7670
Metaraminol bitartrate, J0380
Metatarsal joint, prosthetic implant, L8641
Meter, bath conductivity, dialysis, E1550
Methacholine chloride, J7674
Methadone HCl, J1230
Methocarbamol, J2800
Methotrexate, oral, J8610
Methotrexate sodium, J9250, J9260
Methyldopa HCl, J0210
Methylene blue, A9535
Methylprednisolone
    acetate, J1020–J1040
    oral, J7509
    sodium succinate, J2920, J2930
Metoclopramide HCl, J2765
Micafungin sodium, J2248
Microbiology test, P7001
Midazolam HCl, J2250
Mileage, ALS, A0390
Mileage, ambulance, A0380, A0390
Milrinone lactate, J2260
Mini-bus, nonemergency transportation, A0120
Mitomycin, J9280–J9291
Mitoxantrone HCl, J9293
MNT, G0270, G0271
Mobility device, physician, service, G0372
Modalities, with office visit, M0005–M0008
Moisture exchanger for use with invasive mechanical ventilation, A4483
Moisturizer, skin, A6250
Moles, documentation, G8246, G8276
Monitor
    blood glucose, E0607
    blood pressure, A4670
    pacemaker, E0610, E0615
Monitoring feature/device, A9279
Monitoring, INR, G0248–G0250
Monoclonal antibodies, J7505
Morphine sulfate, J2270, J2271
    sterile, preservative-free, J2275
Motion, jaw, rehabilitation system, E1700–E1702
Mouthpiece (for respiratory equipment), A4617
Moxifloxacin, J2280
MRI/CT, documentation, G8243

Mucoprotein, blood, P2038
Multiaxial ankle, L5986
Multidisciplinary services, H2000–H2001, T1023–T1028
Multiple post collar, cervical, L0180–L0200
Multi-Podus type AFO, L4396
Muromonab-CD3, J7505
Mycophenolate mofetil, J7517
Mycophenolic acid, J7518
Myocardial infarction, documentation
    acute, G8006–G8011
    prior, G8033–G8035

N

Nabilone, J8650
Nails, trimming, dystrophic, G0127
Nalbuphine HCl, J2300
Naloxone HCl, J2310
Naltrexone, J2315
Nandrolone
    decanoate, J2320–J2322
    Narrowing device, wheelchair, E0969
Nasal application device, K0183
Nasal pillows/seals (for nasal application device), K0184
Nasal vaccine inhalation, J3530
Nasogastric tubing, B4081, B4082
Natalizumab, J2323
Nebulizer, E0570–E0585
    aerosol compressor, E0571
    aerosol mask, A7015
    corrugated tubing, disposable, A7010
    corrugated tubing, non-disposable, A7011
    filter, disposable, A7013
    filter, non-disposable, A7014
    heater, E1372
    large volume, disposable, prefilled, A7008
    large volume, disposable, unfilled, A7007
    not used with oxygen, durable, glass, A7017
    pneumatic, administration set, A7003, A7005, A7006
    pneumatic, nonfiltered, A7004
    portable, E0570
    small volume, A7003–A7005
    ultrasonic, E0575
    ultrasonic, dome and mouthpiece, A7016
    ultrasonic, reservoir bottle, non-disposable, A7009
    water collection device, large volume nebulizer, A7012
Needle, A4215
    non-coring, A4212
    with syringe, A4206–A4209
Negative pressure wound therapy pump, E2402
    accessories, A6550
Nelarabine, J9261
Neonatal transport, ambulance, base rate, A0225
Neostigmine methylsulfate, J2710
Nerve, conduction, sensory, test, G0255

◄▶ New   ←→ Revised   ✔ Reinstated   ✖ Deleted

Nerve stimulator with batteries, E0765
Nesiritide injection, J2324
Neuromuscular stimulator, E0745
Neurostimulator
    battery recharging system, L8695
    pulse generator, L8681–L8688
Nitrogen N-13 ammonia, A9526
NMES, E0720–E0749
Nonchemotherapy drug, oral, NOS, J8499
Noncovered services, A9270
Nonemergency transportation, A0080–A0210
Nonimpregnated gauze dressing, A6216–A6221,
    A6402–A6404
Nonprescription drug, A9150
Not otherwise classified drug, J3490, J7599, J7699,
    J7799, J8499, J8999, J9999, Q0181
NPH, J1820
NPWT, pump, E2402
NTIOL category 1, Q1001
NTIOL category 2, Q1002
NTIOL category 3, Q1003
NTIOL category 4, Q1004
NTIOL category 5, Q1005
Nursing care, T1030–T1031
Nursing service, direct, skilled, outpatient,
    G0128
Nursing, skilled, home, health, G0154
Nutrition
    enteral infusion pump, B9000, B9002
    parenteral infusion pump, B9004, B9006
    parenteral solution, B4164–B5200
    therapy, medical, G0270, G0271

O

Observation
    admission, G0379
    hospital, G0378
Occipital/mandibular support, cervical, L0160
Occult, blood, G0394
Occupational, therapy, G0129, S9129
Octafluoropropane, Q9956
Octagam, J1568
Octreotide acetate, J2353, J2354
Ocular prosthetic implant, L8610
Omalizumab, J2357
Ondansetron HCl, J2405
Oncology
    disease status, G9063–G9139
    practice guidelines, G9056–G9062
    visit, G9050–G9055
One arm, drive attachment, K0101
Oprelvekin, J2355
Optic nerve head, evaluation documentation,
    G8298, G8299
O & P supply/accessory/service, L9900
Oral device/appliance, E0485–E0486

Oral/nasal mask, A7027
    nasal pillows, A7029
    oral cushion, A7028
Oral, NOS, drug, J8499
Oropharyngeal suction catheter, A4628
Orphenadrine, J2360
Orthopedic shoes
    arch support, L3040–L3100
    footwear, L3201–L3265, *L3000–L3649*
    insert, L3000–L3030
    lift, L3300–L3334
    miscellaneous additions, L3500–L3595
    positioning device, L3140–L3170
    transfer, L3600–L3649
    wedge, L3340–L3420
Orthotic additions
    carbon graphite lamination, L2755
    fracture, L2180–L2192, L3995
    halo, L0860
    lower extremity, L2200–L2999, L4320
    ratchet lock, L2430
    scoliosis, L1010–L1120, L1210–L1290
    shoe, L3300–L3595, L3649
    spinal, L0970–L0984
    upper limb, *L3900, L3901,* L3970–L3974, L3995
Orthotic devices
    ankle-foot (AFO; *see also* Orthopedic shoes), E1815,
        E1816, E1830, L1900–L1990, L2102–L2116,
        L3160
    anterior-posterior-lateral, L0700, L0710
    cervical, L0100–L0200
    cervical-thoracic-lumbar-sacral (CTLSO), L0700,
        L0710
    elbow (EO), E1800, E1801, L3700–L3740
    fracture, L2102–L2136, L3980–L3986
    halo, L0810–L0830
    hand, finger, prefabricated, L3923
    hand, (WHFO), E1805, E1825, L3807, L3900–L3954
    hip (HO), L1600–L1690
    hip-knee-ankle-foot (HKAFO), L2040–L2090
    interface material, E1820
    knee (KO), E1810, E1811, L1800–L1885
    knee-ankle-foot (KAFO; *see also* Orthopedic shoes),
        L2000–L2038, L2126–L2136
    Legg Perthes, L1700–L1755
    lumbar, L0625–L0640
    multiple post collar, L0180–L0200
    not otherwise specified, L0999, L1499, L2999,
        L3999, L5999, L7499, L8039, L8239
    pneumatic splint, L4350–L4380
    pronation/supination, E1818
    repair or replacement, L4000–L4210
    replace soft interface material, L4390–L4394
    sacroiliac, L0600–L0620
    scoliosis, L1000–L1499
    shoe, *see* Orthopedic shoes
    shoulder (SO), L1840, L3650–L3677
    shoulder-elbow-wrist-hand (SEWHO), L3960–L3978

◄► New   ←→ Revised   ✔ Reinstated   ✖ Deleted

Orthotic devices *(Continued)*
side bar disconnect, L2768
spinal, cervical, L0100–L0200
spinal, DME, K0112–K0116
thoracic, L0210
thoracic-hip-knee-ankle (THKO), L1500–L1520
toe, E1830
wrist-hand-finger (WHFO), E1805, E1806, E1825, L3900–L3954
Orthovisc, J7324
Ossicula prosthetic implant, L8613
Osteoarthritis, G8185, G8186
Osteogenesis stimulator, E0747–E0749, E0760
Osteoporosis
assessment, G8051–G8053
documentation, G8099–G8107, G8338, G8401
Ostomy
accessories, A5093
belt, A4396
pouches, A4416–A4434
skin barrier, A4401–A4449
supplies, A4361–A4421, A5051–A5149
Overdoor, traction, E0860
Oxacillin sodium, J2700
Oxaliplatin, J9263
Oxygen
ambulance, A0422
battery charger, E1357 ◄
battery pack/cartridge, E1356 ◄
catheter, transtracheal, A7018
chamber, hyperbaric, topical, A4575
concentrator, E1390–E1391
DC power adapter, E1358 ◄
equipment, E0424–E0486, E1353–E1406
mask, A4620
medication supplies, A4611–A4627
rack/stand, E1355
regulator, E1353
respiratory equipment/supplies, A4611–A4627, E0424–E0480
saturation, documentation, G8362
supplies and equipment, E0425–E0444, E0455
tent, E0455
tubing, A4616
water vapor enriching system, E1405, E1406
wheeled cart, E1354 ◄
Oxymorphone HCl, J2410
Oxytetracycline HCl, J2460
Oxytocin, J2590

P

Pacemaker monitor, E0610, E0615
Paclitaxel, J9265
Paclitaxel protein-bound particles, J9264
Pad
correction, CTLSO, L1020–L1060

Pad *(Continued)*
gel pressure, E0185, E0196
heat, E0210, E0215, E0217, E0238, E0249
orthotic device interface, E1820
sheepskin, E0188, E0189
water circulating cold with pump, E0218
water circulating heat with pump, E0217
water circulating heat unit, E0249
Pail, for use with commode chair, E0167
Palate, prosthetic implant, L8618
Palifermin, J2425
Palonosetron HCl, J2469
Pamidronate disodium, J2430
Pan, for use with commode chair, E0167
Panitumumab, J9303
Papanicolaou (Pap) screening smear, P3000, P3001, Q0091
Papaverine HCl, J2440
Paraffin, A4265
Paraffin bath unit, E0235
Parenteral nutrition
administration kit, B4224
pump, B9004, B9006
solution, B4164–B5200
supply kit, B4220, B4222
Paricalcitol, J2501
Parking fee, nonemergency transport, A0170
Paste, conductive, A4558
Pathology and laboratory tests, miscellaneous, P9010–P9615
Patient support system, E0636
Pediculosis (lice) treatment, A9180
PEFR, peak expiratory flow rate meter, A4614
Pegademase bovine, J2504
Pegaptanib, J2503
Pegaspargase, J9266
Pegfilgrastim, J2505
Pelvic belt/harness/boot, E0944
Pelvic, traction, E0890, E0900, E0947
Pemetrexed, J9305
Penicillin
G benzathine/G benzathine and penicillin G procaine, J0530–J0580
G potassium, J2540
G procaine, aqueous, J2510
Pentamidine isethionate, J2545, J7676
Pentastarch, 10% solution, J2513
Pentazocine HCl, J3070
Pentobarbital sodium, J2515
Pentostatin, J9268
Percussor, E0480
Percutaneous access system, A4301
Perflexane lipid microspheres, Q9955
Perflutren lipid microspheres, Q9957
Peroneal strap, L0980
Peroxide, A4244
Perphenazine, J3310

◄▶ New   ←→ Revised   ✔ Reinstated   ✖ Deleted

◄▶ New   ←→ Revised   ✔ Reinstated   ✖ Deleted

Prosthesis *(Continued)*
 tracheo-esophageal, L8507–L8509
 upper extremity, L6000–L6999
 vacuum erection system, L7900
Prosthetic additions
 lower extremity, L5610–L5999
 upper extremity, L6600–L7405
Protamine sulfate, J2720
Protectant, skin, A6250
Protector, heel or elbow, E0191
Protein C Concentrate, J2724
Protirelin, J2725
Pulse generator, E2120
Pump
 alternating pressure pad, E0182
 ambulatory infusion, E0781
 ambulatory insulin, E0784
 blood, dialysis, E1620
 breast, E0602–E0604
 enteral infusion, B9000, B9002
 external infusion, E0779
 heparin infusion, E1520
 implantable infusion, E0782, E0783
 implantable infusion, refill kit, A4220
 infusion, supplies, A4230, A4232
 negative pressure wound therapy, K0538
 parenteral infusion, B9004, B9006
 suction, portable, E0600
 water circulating pad, E0236
 wound, negative, pressure, E2402
Purification system, E1610, E1615
Pyridoxine HCl, J3415

Q

Quad cane, E0105
Quinupristin/dalfopristin, J2770

R

Rack/stand, oxygen, E1355
Radioelements for brachytherapy, Q3001
Radiology service, R0070–R0076
Radiological, supplies, A4641, A4642
Radiopharmaceutical diagnostic imaging agent, A4641, A4642, A9500, A9532
Radiopharmaceutical, therapeutic, A9600, A9605
Radiosurgery, stereotactic, G0173, G0251, G0339, G0340
Rail
 bathtub, E0241, E0242, E0246
 bed, E0305, E0310
 toilet, E0243
Ranibizumab, J2778
Rasburicase, J2783
Reaching/grabbing device, A9281

Reagent strip, A4252
Reciprocating peritoneal dialysis system, E1630
Reclast, J3488
Reclining, wheelchair, E1014, E1050–E1070, E1100–E1110
Reconstruction, angiography, G0288
Red blood cells, P9021, P9022
Regadenoson, J2785 ◄
Regular insulin, J1820
Regulator, oxygen, E1353
Rehabilitation
 cardiac, S9472, S9473
 documentation, G8238
 low vision, G9041–G9044
 program, H2001
 psychosocial, H2017, H2018
 services, vision, G9041–G9044
 system, jaw, motion, E1700–E1702
 vestibular, S9476
Removal, cerumen, G0268
Renal, artery, angiography, G0275
Repair
 contract, ESRD, A4890
 durable medical equipment, E1340
 maxillofacial prosthesis, L8049
 orthosis, L4000–L4130
 prosthetic, L7500, L7510
Replacement
 battery, A4630
 pad (alternating pressure), A4640
 tanks, dialysis, A4880
 tip for cane, crutches, walker, A4637
 underarm pad for crutches, A4635
RespiGam, *see* **Respiratory syncytial virus immune globulin**
Respiratory
 DME, A7000–A7527
 equipment, E0424–E0601
 function, therapeutic, procedure, G0237–G0239, S5180, S5181
 supplies, A4604–A4629
Respiratory syncytial virus immune globulin, J1565
Restraint, any type, E0710
Reteplase, J2993
Rho(D) immune globulin, human, J2788, J2790, J2791, J2792
Rib belt, thoracic, A4572, L0210, L0220
Ringers lactate infusion, J7120
Ring, ostomy, A4404
Risperidone, J2794
Rituximab, J9310
Robin-Aids, L6000, L6010, L6020, L6855, L6860
Rocking bed, E0462
Rollabout chair, E1031
Ropivacaine HCl, J2795
Rubidium Rb-82, A9555

◄▶ New ←→ Revised ✔ Reinstated ✖ Deleted

S

Sacral nerve stimulation test lead, A4290
Safety equipment, E0700
    vest, wheelchair, E0980
Saline
    hypertonic, J7130
    infusion, J7030–J7060
    solution, J7030–J7050, A4216–A4218
Saliva, artificial, A9155
Samarium SM 153 Lexidronamm, A9605
Sargramostim (GM-CSF), J2820
Scoliosis, L1000–L1499
    additions, L1010–L1120, L1210–L1290
Screening
    cancer, cervical or vaginal, G0101
    colorectal, cancer, G0104–G0106, G0120–G0122,
        G0328, S3890
    cytopathology cervical or vaginal, G0123, G0124,
        G0141–G0148
    dysphagia, documentation, G8231–G8234, V5364
    glaucoma, G0117, G0118
    language, V5363
    prostate, cancer, G0102, G0103
    speech, V5362
Self-exam, documentation, G8282
Sealant
    skin, A6250
Seat
    attachment, walker, E0156
    insert, wheelchair, E0992
    lift (patient), E0621, E0627–E0629
    upholstery, wheelchair, E0975
Secretin, J2850
Semen analysis, G0027
Semi-reclining, wheelchair, E1100, E1110
Sensitivity study, P7001
Sensory nerve conduction test, G0255
Sermorelin acetate, Q0515
Serum clotting time tube, A4771
Service
    hearing, V5000–V5999
    laboratory, P0000–P9999
    mental, health, training, G0177
    non-covered, A9270
    physician, for mobility device, G0372
    pulmonary, for LVRS, G0302–G0305
    speech-language, V5336–V5364
    vision, V2020–V2799
    vision, rehabilitation, G9041–G9044
SEWHO, L3960–L3974
SEXA, G0130
Sheepskin pad, E0188, E0189
Shoes
    arch support, L3040–L3100
    for diabetics, A5500–A5508
    insert, L3000–L3030

Shoes *(Continued)*
    lift, L3300–L3334
    miscellaneous additions, L3500–L3595
    orthopedic, L3201–L3265
    positioning device, L3140–L3170
    transfer, L3600–L3649
    wedge, L3340–L3485
Shoulder
    disarticulation, prosthetic, L6300–L6320, L6550
    orthosis (SO), L3650–L3675
    spinal, cervical, L0100–L0200
Shoulder-elbow-wrist-hand orthosis (SEWHO),
    L3960–L3969
Shunt accessory for dialysis, A4740
    aqueous, L8612
Sigmoidoscopy, cancer screening, G0104, G0106
Sincalide, J2805
Sirolimus, J7520
Sitz bath, E0160–E0162
Skin
    barrier, ostomy, A4362, A4363, A4369–A4373,
        A4385, A5120
    bond or cement, ostomy, A4364
    exam, documentation, G8279
    sealant, protectant, moisturizer, A6250
Sling, A4565
    patient lift, E0621, E0630, E0635
Smear, Papanicolaou, screening, P3000, P3001, Q0091
SNCT, G0255
Social worker, clinical, home, health, G0155
Social worker, nonemergency transport, A0160
Sock
    body sock, L0984
    prosthetic sock, L8420–L8435, L8470, L8480,
        L8485
    stump sock, L8470–L8485
Sodium
    chloride injection, J2912
    ferric gluconate complex in sucrose, J2916
    fluoride F-18, A9580 ◀
    hyaluronate
        Euflexxa, J7323
        Hyalgan, J7321
        Orthovisc, J7324
        Supartz, J7321
    phosphate P32, A9563
    succinate, J1720
Solution
    calibrator, A4256
    dialysate, A4760
    elliotts b, J9175
    enteral formulae, B4149–B4156
    parenteral nutrition, B4164–B5200
Solvent, adhesive remover, A4365, A4455
Somatrem, J2940
Somatropin, J2941
Sorbent cartridge, ESRD, E1636
Special size, wheelchair, E1220–E1239

◀▶ New   ←→ Revised   ✔ Reinstated   ✖ Deleted

Specialty absorptive dressing, A6251–A6256
Spectinomycin HCl, J3320
Speech assessment, V5362–V5364
Speech generating device, E2500–E2599
Speech-Language, services, V5336–V5364
Speech, pathologist, G0153
Spinal orthosis
   cervical, L0100 L0200
   cervical-thoracic-lumbar-sacral (CTLSO), L0700,
     L0710
   DME, K0112–K0116
   halo, L0810–L0830
   multiple post collar, L0180–L0200
   scoliosis, L1000–L1499
   torso supports, L0960
Splint, A4570, L3100, L4350–L4380
   ankle, L4390–L4398
   dynamic, E1800, E1805, E1810, E1815, E1825,
     E1830, E1840
   footdrop, L4398
   supplies, miscellaneous, Q4051
Standard, wheelchair, E1130, K0001
Static progressive stretch, E1801, E1806, E1811,
     E1816, E1818, E1821
Status
   current, tobacco, G8455–G8457
   disease, oncology, G9063–G9139
Stenosis, internal carotid, documentation, G8240
Stent, transcatheter, placement, G0290, G0291,
   S2211
Sterile cefuroxime sodium, J0697
Sterile water, A4216–A4217
Stereotactic, radiosurgery, G0173, G0251, G0339,
   G0340
Stimulators
   neuromuscular, E0744, E0745
   osteogenesis, electrical, E0747–E0749
   ultrasound, E0760
   salivary reflex, E0755
   stoma absorptive cover, A5083
   transcutaneous, electric, nerve, A4595, E0720–E0749
Stockings, gradient, compression, A6530–A6549
Stockings, surgical, A4490–A4510
Stomach tube, B4083
Stool, guaiac, G0394
Streptokinase, J2995
Streptomycin, J3000
Streptozocin, J9320
Strip, blood glucose test, A4253, A4772
   urine reagent, A4250
Strontium-89 chloride, supply of, A9600
Study, bone density, G0130
Stump sock, L8470–L8485
Stylet, A4212
Substance/Alcohol, assessment, G0396, G0397,
   H0001, H0003, H0049
Succinylcholine chloride, J0330

Suction pump
   gastric, home model, E2000
   portable, E0600
   respiratory, home model, E0600
Sumatriptan succinate, J3030
Supartz, J7321
Supply/accessory/service, A9900
Supplies
   cast, A4580, A4590, Q4001–Q4051
   contraceptive, A4267–A4269
   dialysis, A4650–A4927
   DME, other, A4630–A4640
   enteral, therapy, B4000–B9999
   infusion, A4221, A4222, A4230–A4232, E0776–
     E0791
   ostomy, A4361–A4434, A5051–A5093, A5120–A5200
   parenteral, therapy, B4000–B9999
   radiological, A4641, A4642
   respiratory, A4604–A4629
   splint, Q4051
   surgical, miscellaneous, A4649
   urinary, external, A4356–A4358
Support
   arch, L3040–L3090
   cervical, L0100–L0200
   spinal, L0960
   stockings, L8100–L8239
Surgical
   arthroscopy, knee, G0289, S2112, S2113
   boot, L3208–L3211
   brush, dialysis, A4910
   dressing, A6196–A6406
   procedure, noncovered, G0293, G0294
   stocking, A4490–A4510
   supplies, A4649
   tray, A4550
Surrogate, documentation, G8260
Swabs, betadine or iodine, A4247
Syringe, A4213
   with needle, A4206–A4209
Synvisc, J7322
System
   external, ambulatory insulin, A9274
   rehabilitation, jaw, motion, E1700–E1702
   transport, E1035–E1039

T

Tables, bed, E0274, E0315
Tacrolimus, oral, J7507
Tacrolimus, parenteral, J7525
Tape, A4450–A4452
Taxi, non emergency transportation, A0100
Team, conference, G0175, G9007, S0220, S0221
Technetium TC 99M Arcitumomab, A9568
Technetium TC 99M Bicisate, A9557
Technetium TC 99M Depreotide, A9536

◄▶ New   ←→ Revised   ✔ Reinstated   ✘ Deleted

Technetium TC 99M Disofenin, A9510
Technetium TC 99M Exametazine, A9521
Technetium TC 99M Exametazine labeled autologous white blood cells, A9569
Technetium TC 99M Fanolesomab, A9566
Technetium TC 99M Glucepatate, A9550
Technetium TC 99M - Labeled red blood cells, A9560
Technetium TC 99M Macroaggregated albumin, A9540
Technetium TC 99M Mebrofenin, A9537
Technetium TC 99M Mertiatide, A9562
Technetium TC 99M Oxidronate, A9561
Technetium TC 99M Pentetate, A9539, A9567
Technetium TC 99M Pertechnetate, A9512
Technetium TC 99M Pyrophosphate, A9538
Technetium TC 99M Sestamibi, A9500
Technetium TC 99M Succimer, A9551
Technetium TC 99M Sulfur colloid, A9541
Technetium TC 99M Teboroxime, A9501
Technetium TC 99M Tetrofosmin, A9502
TEEV, J0900
Telehealth, Q3014
Telehealth transmission, T1014
Temozolmide, oral, J8700
Temporary codes, Q0000–Q9999, S0009–S9999
Temsirolimus, J9330 ◀
Tenecteplase, J3100, J3101 ←
Teniposide, Q2017
TENS, A4595, E0720–E0749
Tent, oxygen, E0455
Terbutaline sulfate, J3105
Terbutaline sulfate, inhalation solution, concentrated, J7680
Terbutaline sulfate, inhalation solution, unit dose, J7681
Teriparatide, J3110
Terminal devices, L6700–L6895
Test
  occult, blood, G0394
  sensory, nerve, conduction, G0255
Testosterone
  aqueous, J3140
  cypionate and estradiol cypionate, J1060
  enanthate, J3120, J3130
  enanthate and estradiol valerate, J0900
  propionate, J3150
  suspension, J3140
Tetanus immune globulin, human, J1670
Tetracycline, J0120
Thallous Chloride TL 201, A9505
Theophylline, J2810
Therapeutic lightbox, A4634, E0203
Therapy
  ACE/ARB, G8468–G8481
  activity, G0176
  electromagnetic, G0295, G0329
  enteral, supplies, B4000–B9999

Therapy *(Continued)*
  medical, nutritional, G0270, G0271
  occupational, G0129, S9129
  occupational, health, G0152
  respiratory, function, procedure, G0237–G0239, S5180, S5181
  parenteral, supplies, B4000–B9999
  pharmacologic, documentation, G8285, G8341
  speech, home, G0153, S9128
  wound, negative, pressure, pump, E2402
Thermometer, A4931–A4932
Thermometer, dialysis, A4910
Thiamine HCl, J3411
Thiethylperazine maleate, J3280
Thiotepa, J9340
Thoracic-hip-knee-ankle (THKAO), L1500–L1520
Thoracic-lumbar-sacral orthosis (TLSO)
  scoliosis, L1200–L1290
  spinal, L0430–L0492
Thoracic orthosis, L0210
Thymol turbidity, blood, P2033
Thyrotropin Alfa, J3240
Tigecycline, J3243
Tinzarparin sodium, J1655
Tip (cane, crutch, walker) replacement, A4637
Tire, wheelchair, E0999
Tirofiban, J3246
Tissue marker, A4648
Tissue of human origin, J7340, J7342, J7346, J7350 ←
Tissue of non-human origin, J7343, J7345 ←
TLSO, L0430–L0492, L1200–L1290
Tobacco
  intervention, G8402, G8403, G8453, G8454, G9016
  status, current, G8455–G8457
Tobramycin, inhalation solution, unit dose, J7682, J7685
Tobramycin sulfate, J3260
Toilet accessories, E0167–E0179, E0243, E0244, E0625
Tolazoline HCl, J2670
Toll, non emergency transport, A0170
Topical hyperbaric oxygen chamber, A4575
Topotecan, J8705, J9350 ←
Torsemide, J3265
Tositumomab, administration and supply, G3001
T-PA, documentation, G8231
Tracheostoma heat moisture exchange system, A7501–A7509
Tracheostomy
  care kit, A4629
  filter, A4481
  speaking valve, L8501
  supplies, A4623, A4629, A7523–A7524
  tube, A7520–A7522
Tracheotomy mask or collar, A7525–A7526

◀▶ New   ←→ Revised   ✔ Reinstated   ✖ Deleted

Traction
  cervical, E0855, E0856
  extremity, E0870–E0880
  device, ambulatory, E0830
  equipment, E0840–E0948
  pelvic, E0890, E0900, E0947
Training
  diabetes, outpatient, G0108, G0109
  services, mental, health, G0177
Transcatheter, placement, stent, G0290, G0291,
    S2211
Transcutaneous electrical nerve stimulator
    (TENS), E0720–~~E0749~~ E0770 ←
Transducer protector, dialysis, E1575
Transfer (shoe orthosis), L3600–L3640
Transfer system with seat, E1035
Transluminal, angioplasty, G0392, G0393
Transplant
  islet, G0341–G0343, S2102
Transparent film (for dressing), A6257–A6259
Transport
  chair, E1035–E1039
  system, E1035–E1039
  x-ray, R0070–R0076
Transportation
  ambulance, A0021–A0999, Q3019, Q3020
  corneal tissue, V2785
  EKG (portable), R0076
  handicapped, A0130
  non emergency, A0080–A0210, T2001–T2005
  service, including ambulance, A0021–A0999,
    T2006
  taxi, non emergency, A0100
  toll, non emergency, A0170
  volunteer, non emergency, A0080, A0090
  x-ray (portable), R0070, R0075
Transtracheal oxygen catheter, A7018
Trapeze bar, E0910–E0912, E0940
Trauma, response, team, G0390
Tray
  insertion, A4310–A4316
  irrigation, A4320
  surgical (*see also* kits), A4550
  wheelchair, E0950
Treatment
  pediculosis (lice), A9180
  services, behavioral health, H0002–H2037
Treprostinil, J3285
Triamcinolone, J3301–J3303
  acetonide, J3300, J3301 ←
  diacetate, J3302
  hexacetonide, J3303
  inhalation solution, concentrated, J7683
  inhalation solution, unit dose, J7684
Triflupromazine HCl, J3400
Trifocal, glass or plastic, V2300–V2399
Trimethobenzamide HCl, J3250

Trimetrexate glucuoronate, J3305
Trimming, nails, dystrophic, G0127
Triptorelin pamoate, J3315
Truss, L8300–L8330
Tube/Tubing
  anchoring device, A5200
  blood, A4750, A4755
  drainage extension, A4331
  gastrostomy, B4087, B4088
  irrigation, A4355
  larynectomy, A4622
  nasogastric, B4081, B4082
  oxygen, A4616
  serum clotting time, A4771
  stomach, B4083
  suction pump, each, A7002
  tire, K0091, K0093, K0095, K0097
  tracheostomy, A4622
  urinary drainage, K0280

U

Ultrasonic nebulizer, E0575
Ultrasound, G0389, S8055, S9024
Ultraviolet, cabinet/system, E0691–E0694
Ultraviolet light therapy system, A4633, E0691–
    E0694
Unclassified drug, J3490
Underpads, disposable, A4554
Unipuncture control system, dialysis, E1580
Upper extremity addition, locking elbow, L6693
Upper extremity fracture orthosis, L3980–
    L3999
Upper limb prosthesis, L6000–L7499
Urea, J3350
Ureterostomy supplies, A4454–A4590
Urethral suppository, Alprostadil, J0275
Urinal, E0325, E0326
Urinary
  catheter, A4338–A4346, A4351–A4353
  collection and retention (supplies), A4310–
    A4359
  incontinence, documentation, G8060–G8063,
    G8266–G8268
  supplies, external, A4335, A4356–A4358
  tract implant, collagen, L8603
  tract implant, snythetic, L8606
Urine
  sensitivity study, P7001
  tests, A4250
Urofollitropin, J3355
Urokinase, J3364, J3365
U-V lens, V2755

◀▶ New   ←→ Revised   ✔ Reinstated   ✖ Deleted

V

Vabra aspirator, A4480
Vaccination, administration
documentation, influenza, G8108–G8110
documentation, pneumococcal, G8115–G8117
hepatitis B, G0010
influenza virus, G0008
pneumococcal, G0009
Vaccine
administration, influenza, G0008
administration, pneumococcal, G0009
hepatitis B, administration, G0010
Vaginal
cancer, screening, G0101
cytopathology, G0123, G0124, G0141–G0148
Vancomycin HCl, J3370
Vaporizer, E0605
Vascular
catheter (appliances and supplies), A4300–A4306
graft material, synthetic, L8670
Vasoxyl, J3390
Venous pressure clamp, dialysis, A4918
Ventilator
battery, A4611–A4613
moisture exchanger, disposable, A4483
negative pressure, E0460
volume, stationary or portable, E0450, E0461–E0464
Ventricular assist device, Q0480–Q0505
Verteporfin, J3396
Vest, safety, wheelchair, E0980
Vinblastine sulfate, J9360
Vincristine sulfate, J9370–J9380
Vinorelbine tartrate, J9390
Vision service, V2020–V2799
Visit, emergency department, G0380–G0384
Vital signs, documentation, G8360
Vitamin B-12 cyanocobalamin, J3420
Vitamin D, documentation, G8289
Vitamin K, J3430
Voice amplifier, L8510
Voice prosthesis, L8511–L8514
Von Willebrand Factor Complex, human, J7187
Voriconazole, J3465

W

Waiver, T2012–T2050
Walker, E0130–E0149
accessories, A4636, A4637
attachments, E0153–E0159
Walking splint, L4386
Warfarin, documentation, G8183, G8184
Washer, Gravlee jet, A4470

Water
dextrose, J7042, J7060, J7070
distilled (for nebulizer), A7018
pressure pad/mattress, E0187, E0198
purification system (ESRD), E1610, E1615
softening system (ESRD), E1625
sterile, A4714
WBC/CBC, G0306
Wedges, shoe, L3340–L3420
Wet mount, Q0111
Wheel attachment, rigid pickup walker, E0155
Wheelchair, E0950–E1298, K0001–K0108, K0801–K0886
accessories, E0192, E0950–E1030, E1065–E1069, E2211–E2230, E2300–E2399
amputee, E1170–E1200
back, fully reclining, manual, E1226
component or accessory, not otherwise specified, K0108
cushions, E2601–E2619
heavy duty, E1280–E1298, K0006, K0007, K0801–K0886
lightweight, E1087–E1090, E1240–E1270, E2618
narrowing device, E0969
power add-on, E0983–E0984
reclining, fully, E1014, E1050–E1070, E1100–E1110
semi-reclining, E1100, E1110
shock absorber, E1015–E1018
specially sized, E1220, E1230
standard, E1130, K0001
stump support system, K0551
tire, E0999
transfer board or device, E0705
tray, K0107
van, non-emergency, A0130
youth, E1091
WHFO with inflatable air chamber, L3807
WHO, wrist extension, L3914
Whirlpool equipment, E1300–E1310
Wig, A9282
Wipes, A4245, A4247
Wound cleanser, A6260
Wound, closure, adhesive, G0168
Wound cover
alginate dressing, A6196–A6198
collagen dressing, A6020–A6024
foam dressing, A6209–A6214
hydrocolloid dressing, A6234–A6239
hydrogel dressing, A6242–A6247
non-contact wound warming cover, and accessory, E0231, E0232
specialty absorptive dressing, A6251–A6256

◄► New   ←→ Revised   ✔ Reinstated   ✖ Deleted

Wound filler
alginate dressing, A6199
collagen based, A6010
foam dressing, A6215
hydrocolloid dressing, A6240, A6241
hydrogel dressing, A6248
not elsewhere classified, A6261, A6262
Wound pouch, A6154
Wound, therapy, negative, pressure, pump,
E2402
Wrist
disarticulation prosthesis, L6050, L6055
hand/finger orthosis (WHFO), E1805, E1825,
L3800–L3954

X

Xenon Xe 133, A9558
Xylocaine HCl, J2000
X-ray
equipment, portable, Q0092, R0070, R0075
single, energy, absorptiometry (SEXA), G0130
transport, R0070–R0076

Y

Yttrium Y-90 ibritumomab, A9543

Z

Ziconotide, J2278
Zidovudine, J3485
Ziprasidone mesylate, J3486
Zoledronic acid, J3487
Zometa, J3487

2009
TABLE OF DRUGS

IA	Intra-arterial administration	
IV	Intravenous administration	
IM	Intramuscular administration	
IT	Intrathecal	
SC	Subcutaneous administration	
INH	Administration by inhaled solution	
VAR	Various routes of administration	
OTH	Other routes of administration	
ORAL	Administered orally	

Intravenous administration includes all methods, such as gravity infusion, injections, and timed pushes. The "VAR" posting denotes various routes of administration and is used for drugs that are commonly administered into joints, cavities, tissues, or topical applications, in addition to other parenteral administrations. Listings posted with "OTH" indicate other administration methods, such as suppositories or catheter injections.

DRUG NAME	DOSAGE	METHOD OF ADMINISTRATION	HCPCS CODE
A			
Abarelix	10 mg		**J0128**
Abatacept	10 mg		**J0129**
Abbokinase	5,000 IU vial	IV	J3364
	250,000 IU vial	IV	J3365
Abbokinase, Open Cath	5,000 IU vial	IV	J3364
Abciximab	10 mg	IV	J0130
Abelcet	10 mg	IV	J0287
	50 mg		J0285
Abilify	0.25 mg		J0400
ABLC	50 mg	IV	J0285
Abraxane	1 mg		J9264
Acetadote	100 mg		J0132
	per gram		J7608
Acetazolamide sodium	up to 500 mg	IM, IV	**J1120**
Acetylcysteine			
inhalation			J7699
injection	100 mg		**J0132**
unit dose form	per gram	INH	**J7604, J7608**
Achromycin	up to 250 mg	IM, IV	J0120
ACTH	up to 40 units	IV, IM, SC	J0800
Acthar	up to 40 units	IV, IM, SC	J0800
Acthib			J3490
Acthrel	1 mcg		J0795
Actimmune	0.25 mg	SC	J1830
	3 million units	SC	J9216
Actinomycin D	0.5 mg		J9120
Activase	1 mg	IV	J2997
Acutect	up to 20 millicuries		A9504
Acyclovir			J8499
Acyclovir Sodium	5 mg		J0133

◀▶ New   ←→ Revised   ✔ Reinstated   ✖ Deleted

TABLE OF DRUGS

DRUG NAME	DOSAGE	METHOD OF ADMINISTRATION	HCPCS CODE
Acyclovir	5 mg		**J0133**
Adagen	*25 IU*		*J2504*
Adalimumab	20 mg		**J0135**
Adenocard	*6 mg*	*IV*	*J0150*
	30 mg	*IV*	*J0152*
Adenoscan	*6 mg*	*IV*	*J0150*
	30 mg	IV	**J0152**
Adenosine	6 mg	IV	**J0150**
	30 mg	IV	**J0152**
Adrenalin	*up to 1 ml*	*SC, IM*	*J0170*
Adrenalin Chloride	*up to 1 ml ampule*	*SC, IM*	*J0170*
Adrenalin, epinephrine	up to 1 ml ampule	SC, IM	**J0170**
Adrenocort	*1 mg*		*J1100*
Adriamycin, PFS, RDF	*10 mg*	*IV*	*J9000*
Adrucil	*500 mg*	*IV*	*J9190*
Advate	*per IU*		*J7192*
AeroBid	*per mg*		*J7641*
AeroBid-M	*per mg*		*J7641*
Agalsidase beta	1 mg	*IV*	**J0180**
Aggrastat	*0.25 mg*	*IM, IV*	*J3246*
Aglucosidase alfa	*10 mg*	*IV*	*J0220*
A-hydroCort	*up to 50 mg*	*IV, IM, SC*	*J1710*
	up to 100 m		*J1720*
Akineton	*per 5 mg*	*IM, IV*	*J0190*
Ala-Tet	*up to 250 mg*	*IM, IV*	*J0120*
Alatrofloxacin mesylate, injection	100 mg	IV	**J0200**
Albuterol	0.5 mg	INH	**J7620**
concentrated form	1 mg	INH	~~J7602,~~ **J7610, J7611** ←
unit dose form	1 mg	INH	~~J7603,~~ **J7609, J7613** ←
Aldesleukin	per single use vial	IM, IV	**J9015**
Aldomet	*up to 250 mg*	*IV*	*J0210*
Aldurazyme	*0.1 mg*		*J1931*
Alefacept	0.5 mg		**J0215**
Alemtuzumab	10 mg		**J9010**
Alferon N	*250,000 IU*	*IM*	*J9215*
Alglucerase	per 10 units	IV	**J0205**
Alglucosidase	10 mg	IV	**J0220**
Alimta	*10 mg*		*J9305*
Alkaban-AQ	*1 mg*	*IV*	*J9360*

◄▶ New   ←→ Revised   ✔ Reinstated   ✖ Deleted

DRUG NAME	DOSAGE	METHOD OF ADMINISTRATION	HCPCS CODE
Alkeran	2 mg	ORAL	J8600
	50 mg	IV	J9245
Allopurinol Sodium			J9999
Aloprim			J9999
Aloxi	25 mcg		J2469
Alpha 1-proteinase inhibitor, human	10 mg	IV	J0256
Alphanate			J7186 ◀
Alphanate	per IU		J7190
AlphaNine SD	per IU		J7193, J7194
Alprostadil			
injection	1.25 mcg	OTH injection	J0270
urethral suppository	EA	OTH	J0275
Alteplase recombinant	1 mg	IV	J2997
Altima			J3490
Alupent	per 10 mg	INH	J7667, J7668
noncompounded, unit dose	10 mg	INH	J7669
AmBisome	10 mg	IV	J0289
Amcort	per 5 mg	IM	J3302
A-methaPred	up to 40 mg	IM, IV	J2920
	up to 125 mg	IM, IV	J2930
Amevive	0.5 mg		J0215
Amgen	1 mcg	SC	J9212
Amicar	5 gm		S0017
Amifostine	500 mg	IV	J0207
Amikin	100 mg	IM, IV	J0278
Amikin Pediatric	100 mg	IM, IV	J0278
Amikacin sulfate	100 mg	IM, IV	J0278
Aminaid	1 unit		B4154
Aminocaproic Acid			J3490
Aminolevalinic acid Hcl	unit dose (354 mg)	OTH	J7308
Aminophylline	up to 250 mg	IV	J0280
Aminophylline	up to 250 mg	IV	J0280
Amiodarone HCl	30 mg	IV	J0282
Amirosyn-RF	premix		B5000
Amitriptyline HCl	up to 20 mg	IM	J1320
Amobarbital	up to 125 mg	IM, IV	J0300
Amphadase	up to 150 units		J3470
Amphocin	50 mg	IV	J0285
Amphotec	10 mg	IV	J0288
Amphotericin B	50 mg	IV	J0285
Amphotericin B, lipid complex	10 mg	IV	J0287-J0289

◀ ▶ New   ← → Revised   ✔ Reinstated   ✖ Deleted

DRUG NAME	DOSAGE	METHOD OF ADMINISTRATION	HCPCS CODE
Ampicillin			
sodium	up to 500 mg	IM, IV	**J0290**
sodium/sulbactam sodium	per 1.5 gm	IM, IV	**J0295**
Amygdalin			*J3570*
Amytal	*up to 125 mg*	*IM, IV*	*J0300*
Anabolin LA 100	*up to 50 mg*	*IM*	*J2320*
Anadulafungin	1 mg	*IV*	**J0348**
Ancef	*500 mg*	*IV, IM*	*J0690*
Andrest 90-4	*up to 1 cc*	*IM*	*J0900*
Andro-Cyp	*up to 100 mg*	*IM*	*J1070*
	1 cc, 200 mg	*IM*	*J1080*
Andro-Cyp 200	*up to 100 mg*	*IM*	*J1070*
	1 cc, 200 mg	*IM*	*J1080*
Andro L.A. 200	*up to 100 mg*	*IM*	*J3120*
	up to 200 mg	*IM*	*J3130*
Andro-Estro 90-4	*up to 1 cc*	*IM*	*J0900*
Andro/Fem	*up to 1 ml*	*IM*	*J1060*
Androgyn L.A	*up to 1 cc*	*IM*	*J0900*
Andronate 200	*200 mg*		*J1080*
Androlone-50, see Nandrolone phenpropionate			
Androlone-D 100	*up to 50 mg*	*IM*	*J2320*
Andronaq-50	*up to 50 mg*	*IM*	*J3140*
Andronaq-LA	*up to 100 mg*	*IM*	*J1070*
	1 cc, 200 mg	*IM*	*J1080*
Andronate-200	*up to 100 mg*	*IM*	*J1070*
	1 cc, 200 mg	*IM*	*J1080*
Andronate-100	*up to 100 mg*	*IM*	*J1070*
	1 cc, 200 mg	*IM*	*J1080*
Andropository 100	*up to 100 mg*	*IM*	*J3120*
	up to 200 mg	*IM*	*J3130*
Andryl 200	*up to 100 mg*	*IM*	*J3120*
	up to 200 mg	*IM*	*J3130*
AN-DTPA	*up to 25 millicurie*		*A9539*
	up to 75 millicurie		*A9567*
Anectine	*up to 20 mg*	*IM, IV*	*J0330*
Anergan 25	*up to 50 mg*	*IM, IV*	*J2550*
	12.5 mg	*ORAL*	*Q0169*
	25 mg	*ORAL*	*Q0170*
Anergan 50	*up to 50 mg*	*IM, IV*	*J2550*
	12.5 mg	*ORAL*	*Q0169*
	25 mg	*ORAL*	*Q0170*

◀▶ New   ←→ Revised   ✔ Reinstated   ✖ Deleted

DRUG NAME	DOSAGE	METHOD OF ADMINISTRATION	HCPCS CODE
Angiomax	*1 mg*		*J0583*
Anistreplase	30 units	IV	**J0350**
Antagon	*250 mcg*		*S0132*
Anti-Inhibitor	per IU	IV	**J7198**
Antispas	*up to 20 mg*	*IM*	*J0500*
Antithrombin III (human)	per IU	IV	**J7197**
Antizol	*15 mg*		*J1451*
Anzemet	*10 mg*	*IV*	*J1260*
	50 mg	*ORAL*	*S0174*
	100 mg	*ORAL*	*Q0180*
Apidra	*per 50 units*		*J1815, J1817*
A.P.L.	*per 1,000 USP units*	*IM*	*J0725*
Apokyn	*1 mg*		*J0364*
Apomorphine Hydrochloride	1 mg		**J0364**
Apresoline	*up to 20 mg*	*IV, IM*	*J0360*
Aprotinin	10,000 kiu		**J0365**
AquaMEPHYTON	*per 1 mg*	*IM, SC, IV*	*J3430*
Ara-C	*100 mg*		*J9100*
Aralast	*10 mg*	*IV*	*J0256*
Aralen	*up to 250 mg*	*IM*	*J0390*
Aramine	*per 10 mg*	*IV, IM, SC*	*J0380*
Aranesp			
ESRD use	*1 mcg*		*J0882*
Non-ESRD use	*1 mcg*		*J0881*
Arbutamine	1 mg	IV	**J0395**
Aredia	*per 30 mg*	*IV*	*J2430*
Arfonad, see Trimethaphan camsylate			
Arformoterol tartrate	15 mcg		**J7605**
Arimidex			*J8999*
Aripiprazole	0.25 mg		**J0400**
Aristocort	*5 mg*	*IM*	*J3302*
Aristocort Forte	*per 5 mg*	*IM*	*J3302*
Aristocort Intralesional	*per 5 mg*	*IM*	*J3302*
Aristospan Intra-Articular	*per 5 mg*	*VAR*	*J3303*
Aristospan Intralesional	*per 5 mg*	*VAR*	*J3303*
Arixtra	*per 0.5 m*		*J1652*
Aromasin			*J8999*
Arranon	*50 mg*		*J9261*
Arrestin	*up to 200 mg*	*IM*	*J3250*
	250 mg	*ORAL*	*Q0173*
Arsenic trioxide	1 mg	IV	**J9017**

◀▶ New   ←→ Revised   ✔ Reinstated   ✖ Deleted

DRUG NAME	DOSAGE	METHOD OF ADMINISTRATION	HCPCS CODE
Asparaginase	10,000 units	IV, IM	J9020
Astramorph PF	up to 10 mg	IM, IV, SC	J2270
	100 mg	IM, IV, SC	J2271
Atgam	250 mg	IV	J7504
Ativan	2 mg	IM, IV	J2060
ATnativ	per IU		J7197
AtroPen	up to 0.3 mg		J0460
Atropine			
concentrated form	per mg	INH	J7635
unit dose form	per mg	INH	J7636
sulfate	up to 0.3 mg	IV, IM, SC	J0460
Atrovent	per mg	INH	J7644, J7645
Aurothioglucose	up to 50 mg	IM	J2910
Autologous cultured chondrocytes implant			J7330
Autoplex T	per IU	IV	J7198, J7199
Avastin	10 mg		J9035
Avelox	100 mg		J2280
Avonex	11 mcg	IM	Q3025
	11 mcg	SC	Q3026
	33 mcg	IM	J1825
Azacitidine	1 mg		J9025
Azactam			J3490
Azasan	50 mg		J7500
Azathioprine	50 mg	ORAL	J7500
Azathioprine			
parenteral	100 mg	IV	J7501
dihydrate	1 gm	ORAL	Q0144
injection	500 mg	IV	J0456
Azmacort			
concentrated form	per mg		J7683
unit dose	per mg		J7684
B			
Baci-RX			J3490
Baciim			J3490
Bacitracin			J3490
Baclofen	10 mg	IT	J0475
Baclofen for intrathecal trial	50 mcg	OTH	J0476
Bactocill	up to 250 mg	IM, IV	J2700
Bactrim IV	10 ml		S0039
BAL in oil	per 100 mg	IM	J0470
Banflex	up to 60 mg	IV, IM	J2360

◀▶ New   ←→ Revised   ✔ Reinstated   ✖ Deleted

DRUG NAME	DOSAGE	METHOD OF ADMINISTRATION	HCPCS CODE
Basiliximab	20 mg	IV	**J0480**
Baygam	*1 cc*	*IM*	*J1460*
	2 cc		*J1470*
	3 cc		*J1480*
	4 cc		*J1490*
	5 cc		*J1500*
	6 cc		*J1600*
	7 cc		*J1520*
	8 cc		*J1530*
	9 cc		*J1540*
	10 cc		*J1550*
	over 10 cc		*J1560*
Bayhep			*J3490*
Bayhep B			*J3490*
BayRHo-D	*50 mcg*		*J2788*
	300 mc		*J2790*
	100 IU		*J2792*
BayTet	*up to 250 units*		*J1670*
BCG (Bacillus Calmette and Guérin), live	per vial	IV	**J9031**
BD Posiflush	*10 ml*		*A4216*
Bebulin VH	*per IU*		*J7194*
Beclomethasone inhalation solution, unit dose form	per mg	INH	**J7622**
Beclovent	*per mg*		*J7622*
Beconase	*per mg*		*J7622*
Bena-D 10	up to 50 mg	IV, IM	J1200
Bena-D 50	up to 50 mg	IV, IM	J1200
Benadryl	up to 50 mg	IV, IM	J1200
Benahist 10	up to 50 mg	IV, IM	J1200
Benahist 50	up to 50 mg	IV, IM	J1200
Ben-Allergin-50	up to 50 mg	IV, IM	J1200
	50 mg	*ORAL*	*Q0163*
Bendamustine HCl	1 mg		**J9033** ◀
Benefix	*per IU*	*IV*	*J7195*
Benoject-10	up to 50 mg	IV, IM	J1200
Benoject-50	up to 50 mg	IV, IM	J1200
Bentyl	up to 20 mg	IM	J0500
Benzacot	*up to 200 mg*		*J3250*
Benztropine mesylate	per 1 mg	IM, IV	**J0515**
Berubigen	up to 1,000 mcg	IM, SC	J3420
Beta-2	*per mg*		*J7648*
Betalin 12	up to 1,000 mcg	IM, SC	J3420

◀▶ New   ←→ Revised   ✔ Reinstated   ✖ Deleted

DRUG NAME	DOSAGE	METHOD OF ADMINISTRATION	HCPCS CODE
Betameth	per 4 mg	IM, IV	J0704
Betamethasone acetate & betamethasone sodium phosphate	per 3 mg	IM	J0702
Betamethasone inhalation solution, unit dose form	per mg	INH	J7624
Betamethasone sodium phosphate	per 4 mg	IM, IV	J0704
Betaseron	0.25 mg	SC	J1830
Bethanechol chloride	up to 5 mg	SC	J0520
Bevacizumab	10 mg		J9035
Bexxar	per treatment dose		A9545
Bicclate	per IU		J7192
Bicillin C-R	up to 600,000 units	IM	J0530
	up to 1,200,000 units	IM	J0540
	up to 2,400,000 units	IM	J0550
Bicillin C-R 900/300	up to 600,000 units	IM	J0530
	up to 1,200,000 units	IM	J0540
	up to 2,400,000 units	IM	J0550
Bicillin L-A	up to 600,000 units	IM	J0560
	up to 1,200,000 units	IM	J0570
	up to 2,400,000 units	INJ	J0580
BiCNU	100 mg	IV	J9050
Bioclate	per IU		J7192
Biperiden lactate	per 5 mg	IM, IV	J0190
Bitolterol mesylate			
concentrated form	per mg	INH	J7628
unit dose form	per mg	INH	J7629
Bivalirudin	1 mg		J0583
Blenoxane	15 units	IM, IV, SC	J9040
Bleomycin sulfate	15 units	IM, IV, SC	J9040
B Lodrane	per 10 mg		J0945
Boniva	1 mg		J1740
Bortezomib	0.1 mg		J9041
Botox	per unit		J0585
Botulinum toxin			
type A	per unit	IM	J0585
type B	per 100 units	IM	J0587
Bravelle	75 IU		J3355
Brethine			
concentrated form	per 1 mg	INH	J7680
unit dose	per 1 mg	INH	J7681
	up to 1 mg	SC, IV	J3105
Bretylium			J3490
Brevital Sodium			J3490

 New   Revised   ✔ Reinstated   ✖ Deleted

DRUG NAME	DOSAGE	METHOD OF ADMINISTRATION	HCPCS CODE
Bricanyl	*per mg*		*J7680*
Bricanyl Subcutaneous	*up to 1 mg*	SC, IV	*J3105*
Brodspec	*up to 250 mg*	IM, IV	*J0120*
Brom-a-cot	*per 10 mg*		*J0945*
Brompheniramine maleate	*per 10 mg*	IM, SC, IV	**J0945**
Broncho Saline	*10 ml*		*A4216*
Bronkephrine, see Ethylnorepinephrine HCl			
Bronkosol			
concentrated form	*per mg*	*INH*	*J7647, J7648*
unit dose form	*per mg*	*INH*	*J7649, J7650*
Brovana			*J7699*
BroveX	*per 10 mg*		*J0945*
Budesonide inhalation solution			
concentrated form	0.25 mg	INH	**J7633, J7634**
unit dose form	0.5 mg	INH	**J7626, J7627**
Bumetanide			*J3490*
Bumex	*0.5 mg*		*S0171*
Bupivacaine			*J3490*
Buprenex	*0.1 mg*		*J0592*
Buprenorphine Hydrochloride	0.1 mg		**J0592**
Busulfan	1 mg		**J0594**
Busulfan	2 mg	ORAL	**J8510**
Busulfex	*1 mg*		*J0594*
	2 mg		*J8510*
Butorphanol tartrate	1 mg		**J0595**
C			
Cabergoline	0.25 mg	ORAL	**J8515**
Cafcit	*5 mg*	*IV*	*J0706*
Caffeine citrate	5 mg	IV	**J0706**
Cefobid	*1 gm*		*S0021*
Cefotan			*J3490*
Caine-1	*10 mg*	*IV*	*J2001*
Caine-2	*10 mg*	*IV*	*J2001*
Calcijex	*0.1 mcg*	*IM*	*J0636*
Calcimar	*up to 400 units*	*SC, IM*	*J0630*
Calcitonin-salmon	up to 400 units	SC, IM	**J0630**
Calcitriol	0.1 mcg	IM	**J0636**
Calcium Disodium Versenate	*up to 1,000 mg*	*IV, SC, IM*	*J0600*
Calcium EDTA	*up to 1,000 mg*		*J0600*
Calcium gluconate	per 10 ml	IV	**J0610**
Calcium glycerophosphate & calcium lactate	per 10 ml	IM, SC	**J0620**

◀▶ New   ←→ Revised   ✔ Reinstated   ✖ Deleted

DRUG NAME	DOSAGE	METHOD OF ADMINISTRATION	HCPCS CODE
Calcium glycerophosphate and calcium lactate	10 ml	IM, SC	J0620
Calphosan	per 10 ml	IM, SC	J0620
Campath	10 mg		J9010
Camptosar	20 mg	IV	J9206
Cancidas	5 mg		J0637
Capecitabine	150 mg	ORAL	J8520
	500 mg	ORAL	J8521
Carbocaine with Neo-Cobefrin	per 10 ml	VAR	J0670
Carbocaine	per 10 ml	VAR	J0670
Carboplatin	50 mg	IV	J9045
Cardiogen 82	up to 60 millicurie		A9555
Cardiolite	40 millicuries		A9500
Carimune	500 mg		J1566
Carimune Classic			J1566
Carimune NF			J1566
Carmustine	100 mg	IV	J9050
Carnitor	per 1 g	IV	J1955
Carticel			J7330
Casec	1 unit		B4155
Caspofungin acetate	5 mg	IV	J0637
Catapres	1 mg		J0735
Cathflo Activase	1 mg		J2997
Caverject injection	1.25 mcg		J0270
CEAScan	up to 45 millicuries		A9568
Ceenu			J8999
Cefadyl	up to 1 g	IV, IM	J0710
Cefazolin sodium	500 mg	IV, IM	J0690
Cefepime hydrochloride	500 mg	IV	J0692
Cefizox	per 500 mg	IM, IV	J0715
Cefotaxime sodium	per 1 g	IV, IM	J0698
Cefoxitin sodium	1 g	IV, IM	J0694
Ceftazidime	per 500 mg	IM, IV	J0713
Ceftizoxime sodium	per 500 mg	IV, IM	J0715
	per 250 mg	IV, IM	J0696
Cefuroxime sodium, sterile	per 750 mg	IM, IV	J0697
Celestone Phosphate	per 4 mg	IM, IV	J0704, J7624
Celestone Soluspan	per 3 mg	IM	J0702
Celestone Syrup	3 mg		J0702
CellCept	250 mg	ORAL	J7517
Cel-U-Jec	per 4 mg	IM, IV	J0704
Cenacort A-40	per 10 mg	IM	J3301

◀▶ New   ←→ Revised   ✔ Reinstated   ✖ Deleted

DRUG NAME	DOSAGE	METHOD OF ADMINISTRATION	HCPCS CODE
Cenacort Forte	per 5 mg	IM	J3302
Centran 40	500 ml		J7100
Cephalothin sodium	up to 1 g	IM, IV	J1890
Cephapirin sodium	up to 1 g	IV, IM	J0710
Ceptaz	per 500 mg		J0713
Cerebyx	50 mg		Q2009
	750 mg		S0078
Ceredase	per 10 units	IV	J0205
Ceretec	up to 25 millicurie		A9521
	Per study dose		A9569
Cerezyme	per unit	IV	J1785
Cerubidine	10 mg	IV	J9150
Cesamet	1 mg	ORAL	J8650
Cetuximab	10 mg		J9055
Chealamide	per 150 mg	IV	J3520
Chloramphenicol sodium succinate	up to 1 g	IV	J0720
Chlordiazepoxide HCl	up to 100 mg	IM, IV	J1990
Chloromycetin Sodium Succinate	up to 1 g	IV	J0720
Chloroprocaine HCl	per 30 ml	VAR	J2400
	10 mg	ORAL	Q0171
	25 mg	ORAL	Q0172
	up to 50 mg	IM, IV	J3230
Chloroquine HCl	up to 250 mg	IM	J0390
Chlorothiazide sodium	per 500 mg	IV	J1205
Chlorpromazine HCl	up to 50 mg	IM, IV	J3230
Chlolografin Meglumine	per ml		Q9961
Chorex-5	per 1,000 USP units	IM	J0725
Chorex-10	per 1,000 USP units	IM	J0725
Chorignon	per 1,000 USP units	IM	J0725
Chorionic gonadotropin	per 1,000 USP units	IM	J0725
Chromitope Sodium	up to 10 millicurie		A9553
Choron 10	per 1,000 USP units	IM	J0725
Cidofovir	375 mg	IV	J0740
Cilastatin sodium, imipenem	per 250 mg	IV, IM	J0743
Cimetidine HCL			J3490
Cinolene	per 5 mg		J3302
Cipro IV	200 mg	IV	J0706
Ciprofloxacin	200 mg	IV	J0706
CIS-MDP	up to 30 millicuries		A9503
Cisplatin, powder or solution	per 10 mg	IV	J9060
Cisplatin	50 mg	IV	J9062

◀ ▶ New   ← → Revised   ✔ Reinstated   ✖ Deleted

DRUG NAME	DOSAGE	METHOD OF ADMINISTRATION	HCPCS CODE
CIS-PYRO	up to 25 millicurie		A9538
Cladribine	per mg	IV	J9065
Claforan	per 1 gm	IM, IV	J0698
Cleocin Phosphate			J3490
Clinagen LA	up to 40 mg		J0970
Clincacort	per 5 mg		J3302
Clindamycin Phosphate			J3490
Clofarabine	1 mg		J9027
Clolar	1 mg		J9027
Clonidine Hydrochloride	1 mg	epidural	J0735
Clorpres	1 mg		J0735
Clozaril	25 mg		S0136
Cobal-1000	up to 1,000 mcg		J3420
Cobex	up to 1,000 mcg	IM, SC	J3420
Codeine phosphate	per 30 mg	IM, IV, SC	J0745
Codimal-A	per 10 mg	IM, SC, IV	J0945
Cogentin	per 1 mg	IM, IV	J0515
Colchicine	per 1 mg	IV	J0760
Colhist	per 10 mg		J0945
Colistimethate sodium	up to 150 mg	IM, IV	J0770, S0142
Coly-Mycin M	up to 150 mg	IM, IV	J0770
Combivent			
albuterol	up to 2.5 mg		J7620
ipratropium	up to 0.5 mg		J7620
Compa-Z	up to 10 mg	IM, IV	J0780
Compazine	up to 10 mg	IM, IV	J0780, J8498
	5 mg	ORAL	Q0164, S0183
	10 mg	ORAL	Q0165
Compoz	50 mg		Q0163
Compro			J8498
Comptosar	20 mg		J9206
Conray	per ml		Q9961
Conray 30	per ml		Q9958
Conray 400	per ml		Q9964
Conray 43	per ml		Q9960
Controlyte	1 unit		B4155
Copaxone	20 m		J1595
Cophene-B	per 10 mg	IM, SC, IV	J0945
Copper contraceptive, intrauterine		OTH	J7300
Cordarone	30 mg	IV	J0282
Corgonject-5	per 1,000 USP units	IM	J0725

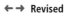 ◀▶ New   ←→ Revised   ✔ Reinstated   ✖ Deleted

DRUG NAME	DOSAGE	METHOD OF ADMINISTRATION	HCPCS CODE
Cortastat	*1 mg*		**J1094, J1100**
Cortef Acetate	*up to 25 mg*		**J1700**
Corticorelin ovine triflutate	1 mcg		**J0795**
Corticotropin	up to 40 units	IV, IM, SC	**J0800**
Cortimed	*80 mg*		**J1040**
Cortisone Acetate			**J3490**
Cortrosyn	*per 0.25 mg*	*IM, IV*	**J0835**
Corvert	*1 mg*		**J1742**
Cosmegen	*0.5 mg*	*IV*	**J9120**
Cosyntropin	per 0.25 mg	IM, IV	**J0835**
Cotolone	*up to 1 ml*		**J2650**
	Per 5 mg		**J7510**
Cotranzine	*up to 10 mg*	*IM, IV*	**J0780**
Criticare HN	*1 unit*		**B4153**
Cromolyn sodium, unit dose form	per 10 mg	INH	**J7631, J7632**
Cromolyn Sodium, inhalation solution			**J7699**
Crystal B-12	*up to 1,000 mcg*		**J3420**
Crysticillin 300 A.S.	*up to 600,000 Units*	*IM, IV*	**J2510**
Crysticillin 600 A.S.	*up to 600,000 Units*	*IM, IV*	**J2510**
Cubicin	*1 mg*		**J0878**
Curity Sterile Saline	*500 ml*		**A4217**
Curity Sterile Water	*500 ml*		**A4217**
Cyano	*up to 1,000 mcg*		**J3420**
Cyanocobalamin	*up to 1,000 mcg*		**J3420**
Cyclophosphamide	100 mg	IV	**J9070**
	200 mg	IV	**J9080**
	500 mg	IV	**J9090**
	1 g	IV	**J9091**
	2 g	IV	**J9092**
lyophilized	100 mg	IV	**J9093**
	200 mg	IV	**J9094**
	500 mg	IV	**J9095**
	1 g	IV	**J9096**
	2 g	IV	**J9097**
oral	25 mg	ORAL	**J8530**
Cyclosporine	25 mg	ORAL	**J7515**
	100 mg	ORAL	**J7502**
parenteral	250 mg	IV	**J7516**
Cymetra	*1 cc*		**Q4112**
Cyomin	*up to 1,000 mcg*		**J3420**

◄▶ New   ←→ Revised   ✔ Reinstated   ✘ Deleted

DRUG NAME	DOSAGE	METHOD OF ADMINISTRATION	HCPCS CODE
Cysto-Cornray LI	*per ml*		*Q9958*
Cystografin	*per ml*		*Q9958*
Cystografin-Dilute	*per ml*		*Q9958*
Cytarabine	100 mg	SC, IV	**J9100**
Cytarabine	500 mg	SC, IV	**J9110**
Cytarabine liposome	10 mg		**J9098**
CytoGam	*per vial*		*J0850*
Cytomegalovirus immune globulin intravenous (human)	per vial	IV	**J0850**
Cytosar-U	*100 mg*	*SC, IV*	*J9100*
	500 mg	*SC, IV*	*J9110*
Cytovene	*500 mg*	*IV*	*J1570*
Cytoxan	*100 mg*	*IV*	*J9070*
	200 mg	*IV*	*J9080*
	500 mg	*IV*	*J9090*
	1 gm	*IV*	*J9091*
	2 gm	*IV*	*J9092*
lyophilized	*100 mg*	*IV*	*J9093*
	200 mg	*IV*	*J9094*
	500 mg	*IV*	*J9095*
	1 g	*IV*	*J9096*
	2 g	*IV*	*J9097*
oral	*25 mg*	*ORAL*	*J8530*
D			
D-5-W, infusion	1000 cc	IV	**J7070**
Dacarbazine	100 mg	IV	**J9130**
	200 mg	IV	**J9140**
Daclizumab	25 mg	IV	**J7513**
Dacogen			*J0894*
Dactinomycin	0.5 mg	IV	**J9120**
Dalalone	*1 mg*	*IM, IV, OTH*	*J1100*
Dalalone L.A	*1 mg*	*IM*	*J1094, J1094*
Dalteparin sodium	per 2500 IU	SC	**J1645**
Daptomycin	1 mg		**J0878**
Darbepoetin Alfa	1 mcg		**J0881, J0882**
Daunomycin	*10 mg*		*J9150*
Daunorubicin citrate, liposomal formulation	10 mg	IV	**J9151**
Daunorubicin HCl	10 mg	IV	**J9150**
Daunoxome	*10 mg*	*IV*	*J9151*
DDAVP	*1 mcg*	*IV, SC*	*J2597*
Debioclip Kit	*3.75 mg*		*J3310*

◄▶ New   ←→ Revised   ✔ Reinstated   ✖ Deleted

DRUG NAME	DOSAGE	METHOD OF ADMINISTRATION	HCPCS CODE
Decadron Phosphate	1 mg	IM, IV, OTH	J1100
			J1094
Decadron	1 mg	IM, IV, OTH	J1100
	0.25 mg		J8540
Decadrone-L.A.	1 mg	IM	J1094
Deca-Durabolin	up to 50 mg	IM	J2320
	up to 100 mg	IM	J2321
	up to 200 mg	IM	J2322
Decaject	1 mg	IM, IV, OTH	J1100
Decaject-L.A.	1 mg	IM	J1094
Decitabine	1 mg		J0894
Decolone-50	up to 50 mg	IM	J2320
Decolone-100	up to 50 mg	IM	J2320
De-Comberol	up to 1 ml	IM	J1060
Decongest	per 10 mg		J0945, Q0163
Deferoxamine mesylate	500 mg	IM, SC, IV	J0895
Definity	per ml		Q9957
Dehist	per 10 mg	IM, SC, IV	J0945
Dekasol	1 mg		J1100
Dekasol-10	1 mg		J1100
Dekasol LA	1 mg		J1094
Delacone D.P.	1 mg		J1094
Deladumone OB	up to 1 cc	IM	J0900
Deladumone	up to 1 cc	IM	J0900
Delatest	up to 100 mg	IM	J3120
	up to 200 mg	IM	J3130
Delatestadiol	up to 1 cc	IM	J0900
Delatestryl	up to 100 mg	IM	J3120
	up to 200 mg	IM	J3130
Delta-Cortef	5 mg	ORAL	J7510
Deltasone	5 mg		J7506
Delestrogen	up to 10 mg	IM	J1380
	up to 20 mg	IM	J1390
	up to 40 mg	IM	J0970
Demadex	10 mg/ml	IV	J3265
Demerol HCl	per 100 mg	IM, IV, SC	J2175
Denileukin diftitox	300 mcg		J9160
DepAndro 100	up to 100 mg	IM	J1070
	1 cc, 200 mg	IM	J1080
	up to 100 mg		J3150

◀▶ New   ←→ Revised   ✔ Reinstated   ✘ Deleted

DRUG NAME	DOSAGE	METHOD OF ADMINISTRATION	HCPCS CODE
DepAndro 200	up to 100 mg	IM	J1070
	1 cc, 200 mg	IM	J1080
DepAndrogyn	up to 1 ml	IM	J1060
DepGynogen	up to 5 mg	IM	J1000
DepoCyt	10 mg		J9098
DepMedalone 40	20 mg	IM	J1020
	40 mg	IM	J1030
	80 mg	IM	J1040
DepMedalone 80	20 mg	IM	J1020
	40 mg	IM	J1030
	80 mg	IM	J1040
DepoAndro	up to 100 mg		J1070
Depo-Cobolin	up to 1,000 mcg		J3420
Depodur	up to 10 mg		J2270
	100 mg		J2271
Depo-estradiol cypionate	up to 5 mg	IM	**J1000**
Depogen	up to 5 mg	IM	J1000
Depoject	20 mg	IM	J1020
	40 mg	IM	J1030
	80 mg	IM	J1040
Depo-Medrol	20 mg	IM	J1020
	40 mg	IM	J1030
	80 mg	IM	J1040
Depopred-40	20 mg	IM	J1020
	40 mg	IM	J1030
	80 mg	IM	J1040
Depopred-80	20 mg	IM	J1020
	40 mg	IM	J1030
	80 mg	IM	J1040
Depo-Provera	50 mg	IM	J1051
	150 mg	IM	J1055
Depo-Subq Provera 104	50 mg		J1051
Depotest	up to 100 mg	IM	J1070
	1 cc, 200 mg	IM	J1080
Depo-Testadiol	up to 1 ml	IM	J1060
Depotestadiol	200 mg		J1080

◄► New   ←→ Revised   ✔ Reinstated   ✖ Deleted

DRUG NAME	DOSAGE	METHOD OF ADMINISTRATION	HCPCS CODE
Depotestrogen	up to 1 ml	IM	J1060
Depo-Testosterone	1 cc, 200 mg	IM	J1080
	up to 100 mg	IM	J1070, J3120
Dermagraft	per square centimeter		Q4106
Desferal Mesylate	500 mg	IM, SC, IV	J0895
Desmopressin acetate	1 mcg	IV, SC	J2597
Dexacen LA-8	1 mg	IM	J1094
Dexacen-4	1 mg	IM, IV, OTH	J1100
Dexamethasone			
concentrated form	per mg	INH	J7637
unit form	per mg	INH	J7638
oral	0.25 mg	ORAL	J8540
	1 mg		J1100
Dexamethasone acetate	1 mg	IM	J1094
Dexamethasone sodium phosphate	1 mg	IM, IV, OTH	J1100
Dexasone	1 mg	IM, IV, OTH	J1100
Dexasone L.A.	1 mg	IM	J1094
Dexferrum	50 mg		J1750
Dexim	1 mg		J1100
Dexone	0.25 mg	ORAL	J8540
	1 mg	IM, IV, OTH	J1100
Dexone LA	1 mg	IM	J1094
Dexpak JR Taperpak	0.25 mg	ORAL	J8540
Dexrazoxane hydrochloride	250 mg	IV	J1190
Dextran 40	500 ml	IV	J7100
Dextran 70	500 ml		J7110
Dextran 75	500 ml	IV	J7110
Dextrose	1,000 cc		J7070
Dextrose, other			J7799
Dextrose 5%/normal saline solution	500 ml = 1 unit	IV	J7042
Dextrose/Dobutamine	per 250 mg		J1250
Dextrose/Heparin Sodium	per 1,000 mg		J1644
Dextrose Hypertonic			J7799
Dextrose/Lidocaine HCL	10 mg		J2001
Dextrose/Milrinone Lactate	5 mcg		J2260
Dextrose/Morphine Sulfate	up to 10 mg		J2270
Dextrose-NACL	500 ml = 1 unit		J7042
Dextrose/Sodium Chloride	500 ml = 1 unit		J7042
Dextrose/Sodium Chloride, other			J7799
Dextrose/Theophylline	per 40 mg		J2810
Dextrose/water (5%)	500 ml = 1 unit	IV	J7060
D.H.E. 45	per 1 mg		J1110

◀▶ New   ←→ Revised   ✔ Reinstated   ✖ Deleted

DRUG NAME	DOSAGE	METHOD OF ADMINISTRATION	HCPCS CODE
Diamox	up to 500 mg	IM, IV	J1120
Diastat	up to 5 mg		J3360
Diazepam	up to 5 mg	IM, IV	J3360
Diazoxide	up to 300 mg	IV	J1730
Dibent	up to 20 mg	IM	J0500
Dicyclocot	up to 20 mg	IM	J0500
Dicyclomine HCl	up to 20 mg	IM	J0500
Didronel	per 300 mg	IV	J1436
Diethylstilbestrol diphosphate	250 mg	IV	J9165
Diflucan	200 mg	IV	J1450
Digibind	per vial		J1162
DigiFab	per vial		J1162
Digoxin	up to 0.5 mg	IM, IV	J1160
Digoxin immune fab (ovine)	per vial		J1162
Dihydrex	up to 50 mg	IV, IM	J1200
	50 mg	ORAL	Q0163
Dihydroergotamine mesylate	per 1 mg	IM, IV	J1110
Dilantin	per 50 mg	IM, IV	J1165
Dilaudid	up to 4 mg	SC, IM, IV	J1170
	250 mg	OTH	S0092
Dilocaine	10 mg	IV	J2001
Dilomine	up to 20 mg	IM	J0500
Dilor	up to 500 mg	IM	J1180
Dimenhydrinate	up to 50 mg	IM, IV	J1240
Dimercaprol	per 100 mg	IM	J0470
Dimethyl sulfoxide	50%, 50 ml	OTH	J1212
Dinate	up to 50 mg	IM, IV	J1240
Dioval	up to 10 mg	IM	J1380
	up to 20 mg	IM	J1390
	up to 40 mg	IM	J0970
Dioval 40	up to 10 mg	IM	J1380
	up to 20 mg	IM	J1390
	up to 40 mg	IM	J0970
Dioval XX	up to 10 mg	IM	J1380
	up to 20 mg	IM	J1390
	up to 40 mg	IM	J0970
Diphenacen-50	up to 50 mg	IV, IM	J1200
	50 mg	ORAL	Q0163
Diphenhydramine HCl			
injection	up to 50 mg	IV, IM	J1200
oral	50 mg	ORAL	Q0163

◄► New   ←→ Revised   ✔ Reinstated   ✖ Deleted

DRUG NAME	DOSAGE	METHOD OF ADMINISTRATION	HCPCS CODE
Diprivan			*J3490*
Dipyridamole	per 10 mg	IV	**J1245**
Disotate	*per 150 mg*	*IV*	*J3520*
Di-Spaz	*up to 20 mg*	*IM*	*J0500*
Ditate-DS	*up to 1 cc*	*IM*	*J0900*
Diruril	*per 500 mg*	*IV*	*J1205*
Diuril Sodium	*per 500 mg*	*IV*	*J1205*
Dizac	*up to 5 mg*		*J3360*
D-Med 80	*20 mg*	*IM*	*J1020*
	40 mg	*IM*	*J1030*
	80 mg	*IM*	*J1040*
DMSO, Dimethyl sulfoxide 50%	50 ml	OTH	**J1212**
Dobutamine HCl	per 250 mg	IV	**J1250**
Dobutrex	*per 250 mg*	*IV*	*J1250*
Docetaxel	20 mg	IV	**J9170**
Dolasetron mesylate			
injection	10 mg	IV	**J1260**
tablets	100 mg	ORAL	**Q0180**
Dolophine	*5 mg*		*S0109*
Dolophine HCl	*up to 10 mg*	*IM, SC*	*J1230*
Dommanate	*up to 50 mg*	*IM, IV*	*J1240*
Donbax	*10 mg*		*J1267*
Dopamine	40 mg		**J1265**
Dopamine in D5W	*40 mg*		*J1265*
Dopamine HCl	40 mg		**J1265**
Doripenem	10 mg		**J1267** ◄
Dornase alpha, unit dose form	per mg	INH	**J7639**
Dostinex	*0.25 mg*	*ORAL*	*J8515*
Doxercalciferol	1 mcg	IV	**J1270**
Doxil	*10 mg*	*IV*	*J9001*
Doxorubicin			
HCL	10 mg	IV	**J9000**
HCL, all lipid	10 mg	IV	**J9001**
Dramamine	*up to 50 mg*	*IM, IV*	*J1240*
Dramanate	*up to 50 mg*	*IM, IV*	*J1240*
Dramilin	*up to 50 mg*	*IM, IV*	*J1240*
Dramocen	*up to 50 mg*	*IM, IV*	*J1240*
Dramoject	*up to 50 mg*	*IM, IV*	*J1240*
Draximage MDP-10	*up to 30 millicuries*		*A9503*
Draximage MDP-25	*up to 30 millicuries*		*A9503*

◄ ▶ New   ← → Revised   ✔ Reinstated   ✖ Deleted

DRUG NAME	DOSAGE	METHOD OF ADMINISTRATION	HCPCS CODE
Dronabinol	2.5 mg	ORAL	**Q0167**
	5 mg	ORAL	**Q0168**
Droperidol	up to 5 mg	IM, IV	**J1790**
Droxia			*J8999*
Drug administered through a metered dose inhaler		INH	**J3535**
Droperidol and fentanyl citrate	up to 2 ml ampule	IM, IV	**J1810**
DTIC-Dome	100 mg	IV	J9130
	200 mg	IV	J9140
DTPA	*up to 25 millicurie*		*A9539*
	Up to 75 millicurie		*A9567*
Dua-Gen L.A., see Testosterone enanthate, estradiol valerate cypionate			*J0900*
DuoNeb, albuterol	*up to 2.5 mg*		*J7620*
DuoNeb, inpratropium	*up to 0.5 mg*		*J7620*
Duospan	*up to 1 ml*		*J1060*
Duoval P.A.	*up to 1 cc*	*IM*	*J0900*
Durabolin, see Nandrolone phenpropionate			
Duraclon	*1 mg*	*epidural*	*J0735*
Dura-Estrin	*up to 5 mg*	*IM*	*J1000*
Duracillin A.S.	*up to 600,000 units*	*IM, IV*	*J2510*
Duragen-10	*up to 10 mg*	*IM*	*J1380*
	up to 20 mg	*IM*	*J1390*
	up to 40 mg	*IM*	*J0970*
Duragen-20	*up to 10 mg*	*IM*	*J1380*
	up to 20 mg	*IM*	*J1390*
	up to 40 mg	*IM*	*J0970*
Duragen-40	*up to 10 mg*	*IM*	*J1380*
	up to 20 mg	*IM*	*J1390*
	up to 40 mg	*IM*	*J0970*
Duralone-40	*20 mg*	*IM*	*J1020*
	40 mg	*IM*	*J1030*
	80 mg	*IM*	*J1040*
Duralone-80	*20 mg*	*IM*	*J1020*
	40 mg	*IM*	*J1030*
	80 mg	*IM*	*J1040*
Duralutin, see Hydroxyprogesterone Caproate			
Duramorph	*10 mg*	*IM, IV, SC*	*J2271*
	up to 10 mg	*IM, IV, SC*	*J2270*
	500 mg	*OTH*	*S0093*
Duratest-100	*up to 100 mg*	*IM*	*J1070*
	1 cc, 200 mg	*IM*	*J1080*

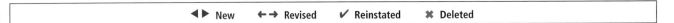

◄► New   ←→ Revised   ✔ Reinstated   ✘ Deleted

DRUG NAME	DOSAGE	METHOD OF ADMINISTRATION	HCPCS CODE
Duratest-200	up to 100 mg	IM	J1070
	1 cc, 200 mg	IM	J1080
Duratestin	up to 1 ml		J1060
Duratestrin	up to 1 ml	IM	J1060
Durathate-200	up to 100 mg	IM	J3120
	up to 200 mg	IM	J3130
Duro Cort	80 mg		J1040
Dymenate	up to 50 mg	IM, IV	J1240
Dyphylline	up to 500 mg	IM	J1180
Dytuss	50 mg		Q0163
E			
Eculizumab	10 mg		J1300
Edetate calcium disodium	up to 1000 mg	IV, SC, IM	J0600
Edetate disodium	per 150 mg	IV	J3520
Edex	per 1.25 millicurie		J0270
Edisylate	up to 10 mg		J0780
Elavil	up to 20 mg	IM	J1320
Elitek	0.5 mg		J2783
Eliuard	per 3.75 mg		J1950
Ellence	2 mg		J9178
Elliotts b solution	1 ml	OTH	J9175
Eloxatin	0.5 mg		J9263
Elspar	10,000 units	IV, IM	J9020
Emend	1 mg		J1453
Ememd	5 mg	ORAL	J8501
Emend Tri-Fold	5 mg	ORAL	J8501
Emete-Con, see Benzquinamide			
Eminase	30 units	IV	J0350
Enbrel	25 mg	IM, IV	J1438
Endrate ethylenediamine-tetra-acetic acid	per 150 mg	IV	J3520
Endoxan-Asta	100 mg		J9070
Enfuvirtide	1 mg		J1324
Engerix-B			J3490
Enovil	up to 20 mg	IM	J1320
Enoxaparin sodium	10 mg	SC	J1650
Enrich	1 unit		B4150
Ensure	1 unit		B4150
Ensure HN	1 unit		B4150, B4152
Ensure Plus HN	1 unit		B4152
Ensure Powder	1 unit		B4150

◀▶ New   ←→ Revised   ✔ Reinstated   ✖ Deleted

DRUG NAME	DOSAGE	METHOD OF ADMINISTRATION	HCPCS CODE
Epinephrine, adrenalin	up to 1 ml amp	SC, IM	**J0170**
Epinephrine HCL			*J7799*
Epinephrine, other			*J7799*
EpiPen	*up to 1 ml*	*SC, IM*	*J0170*
Epirubicin hydrochloride	2 mg		**J9178**
Epoetin alfa	1000 units		**Q4055**
Epogen	*1,000 units*		*J0885*
			J0886
			Q4081
Epoprostenol	0.5 mg	IV	**J1325**
Epsom Salt	*per 500 mg*		*J3475*
Eptifibatide, injection	5 mg	IM, IV	**J1327**
Eraxis	*1 mg*	*IV*	*J0348*
Erbitux	*10 mg*		*J9055*
Ergamisol	*50 mg*	*ORAL*	*S0177*
Ergonovine maleate	up to 0.2 mg	IM, IV	**J1330**
Ergotrate	*0.2 mg*		*J1330*
Ertapenem sodium	500 mg		**J1335**
Erthrocin	*500 mg*		*J1364*
Erythromycin lactobionate	500 mg	IV	**J1364**
Estra-D	*up to 5 mg*	*IM*	*J1000*
Estra-L 20	*up to 10 mg*	*IM*	*J1380*
	up to 20 mg	*IM*	*J1390*
	up to 40 mg	*IM*	*J1370*
Estra-L 40	*up to 10 mg*	*IM*	*J1380*
	up to 20 mg	*IM*	*J1390*
	up to 40 mg	*IM*	*J1370*
Estra-Testrin	*up to 1 cc*	*IM*	*J0900*
Estradiol Cypionate	*up to 5 mg*	*IM*	*J1000, J1056, J1060*
Estradiol			
L.A.	*up to 10 mg*	*IM*	*J1380*
	up to 20 mg	*IM*	*J1390*
	up to 40 mg	*IM*	*J1370*
L.A. 20	*up to 10 mg*	*IM*	*J1380*
	up to 20 mg	*IM*	*J1390*
	up to 40 mg	*IM*	*J1370*
L.A. 40	*up to 10 mg*	*IM*	*J1380*
	up to 20 mg	*IM*	*J1390*
	up to 40 mg	*IM*	*J1370*

◄► New   ←→ Revised   ✔ Reinstated   ✖ Deleted

DRUG NAME	DOSAGE	METHOD OF ADMINISTRATION	HCPCS CODE
Estradiol valerate	up to 10 mg	IM	J1380
	up to 20 mg	IM	J1390
	up to 40 mg	IM	J0970
Estragyn 5	per 1 mg		J1435
Estrin	up to 5 mg		J1000
Estring Vaginal Ring			S4989
Estro-A	per 1 mg		J1435
Estro-Cyp	up to 5 mg	IM	J1000
Estrogen, conjugated	per 25 mg	IV, IM	J1410
Estroject L.A	up to 5 mg	IM	J1000
Estro-LA	up to 5 mg		J1000
Estrone	per 1 mg	IM	J1435
Estrone 5	per 1 mg	IM	J1435
Estrone Aqueous	per 1 mg	IM	J1435
Estronol	per 1 mg	IM	J1435
Estronol-L.A.	up to 5 mg	IM	J1000
Etanercept, injection	25 mg	IM, IV	J1438
Ethamolin	100 mg		J1430
Ethanolamine	100 mg		J1430
Ethyol	500 mg	IV	J0207
Etidronate disodium	per 300 mg	IV	J1436
Etonogestrel implant			J7307
Etopophos	10 mg	IV	J9181
Etoposide	10 mg	IV	J9181
	100 mg	IV	J9182	✖
oral	50 mg	ORAL	J8560
Euflexxa			J7323
Eulexin	125 mg	ORAL	S0175
Everone	up to 100 mg	IM	J3120
	up to 200 mg	IM	J3130
F			
Fabrazyme	1 mg	IV	J0180
Factor IX Complex	per IU		J7194
Factor VIIa (coagulation factor, recombinant)	1 mcg	IV	J7189
Factor VIII (anti-hemophilic factor)			
human	per IU	IV	J7190
porcine	per IU	IV	J7191
recombinant	per IU	IV	J7192
Factor IX			
anti-hemophilic factor, purified, non-recombinant	per IU	IV	J7193

◀▶ New   ←→ Revised   ✔ Reinstated   ✖ Deleted

DRUG NAME	DOSAGE	METHOD OF ADMINISTRATION	HCPCS CODE
Factor IX—cont'd			
anti-hemophilic factor, recombinant	per IU	IV	J7195
complex	per IU	IV	J7194
Factors, other hemophilia clotting	per IU	IV	J7196
Factrel	per 100 mcg	SC, IV	J1620
Famotidine			J3490
Faslodex	25 mg		J9395
Feiba VH Immuno	per IU	IV	J7196
Fentanyl citrate	0.1 mg	IM, IV	J3010
FerAmine HBC	premix		B5100
Feridex IV	per ml		Q9953
Ferrlecit	12.5 mg		J2916
Fertinex	75 IU		J3355
Filgrastim (G-CSF)	300 mcg	SC, IV	J1440
	480 mcg	SC, IV	J1441
Flagyl I.V. RTU	500 mg		S0030
Flebogamma	500 mg	IV	J1572
	1 cc		J1460
Flexoject	up to 60 mg	IV, IM	J2360
Flexon	up to 60 mg	IV, IM	J2360
Flolan	0.5 mg	IV	J1325
Floxin IV	400 mg		S0034
Floxuridine	500 mg	IV	J9200
Fluconazole	200 mg	IV	J1450
Fludara	50 mg	IV	J9185
Fludarabine phosphate	50 mg	IV	J9185
Flunisolide inhalation solution, unit dose form	per mg	INH	J7641
Fluocinolone			J7311
Fluorouracil	500 mg	IV	J9190
Flutamide			J8999
Flutamide Citrate			J8999
Folex	5 mg	IA, IM, IT, IV	J9250
	50 mg	IA, IM, IT, IV	J9260
Folex PFS	5 mg	IA, IM, IT, IV	J9250
	50 mg	IA, IM, IT, IV	J9260
Follutein	per 1,000 USP units	IM	J0725
Fomepizole	15 mg		J1451
Fomivirsen sodium	1.65 mg	Intraocular	J1452
Fondaparinux sodium	0.5 mg		J1652
Foradil Aerolizer	12 mcg		J7640
Formoterol	12 mcg	INH	J7640
Formoterol fumarate	20 mcg		J7606

◀▶ New ←→ Revised ✔ Reinstated ✖ Deleted

DRUG NAME	DOSAGE	METHOD OF ADMINISTRATION	HCPCS CODE
Fortaz	per 500 mg	IM, IV	J0713
Fosaprepitant	1 mg		J1453 ◄
Forteo	10 mcg		J3110
Fortovase	200 mg	ORAL	S0140
Foscarnet sodium	per 1,000 mg	IV	J1455
Foscavir	per 1,000 mg	IV	J1455
Fosphenytoin	50 mg		Q2009
Fragmin	per 2,500 IU		J1645
FUDR	500 mg	IV	J9200
Fulvestrant	25 mg		J9395
Fungizone intravenous	50 mg	IV	J0285
Fungizone for Tissue Culture	50 mg	IV	J0285
Furomide M.D.	up to 20 mg	IM, IV	J1940
Furosemide	up to 20 mg	IM, IV	J1940
Fuzeon	1 mg		J1324
G			
Gallium nitrate	1 mg		J1457
Galsulfase	1 mg		J1458
Gamastan	1 cc	IM	J1460
	2 cc	IM	J1470
	3 cc	IM	J1480
	4 cc	IM	J1490
	5 cc	IM	J1500
	6 cc	IM	J1510
	7 cc	IM	J1520
	8 cc	IM	J1530
	9 cc	IM	J1540
	10 cc	IM	J1550
	over 10 cc	IM	J1560
Gammagard Liquid	500 mg		J1569
Gammagard S/D			J1566
Gamma globulin	1 cc	IM	J1460
	2 cc	IM	J1470
	3 cc	IM	J1480
	4 cc	IM	J1490
	5 cc	IM	J1500
	6 cc	IM	J1510
	7 cc	IM	J1520
	8 cc	IM	J1530
	9 cc	IM	J1540
	10 cc	IM	J1550
	over 10 cc	IM	J1560

◄▶ New   ←→ Revised   ✔ Reinstated   ✘ Deleted

DRUG NAME	DOSAGE	METHOD OF ADMINISTRATION	HCPCS CODE
GammaGraft	*per square centimeter*		*Q4111*
Gammar	*1 cc*	*IM*	*J1460*
	2 cc	*IM*	*J1470*
	3 cc	*IM*	*J1480*
	4 cc	*IM*	*J1490*
	5 cc	*IM*	*J1500*
	6 cc	*IM*	*J1510*
	7 cc	*IM*	*J1520*
	8 cc	*IM*	*J1530*
	9 cc	*IM*	*J1540*
	10 cc	*IM*	*J1550*
	over 10 cc	*IM*	*J1560*
Gammar-P IV	*500 m*		*J1566*
Gammar-IV, see Immune globin intravenous (human)			
Gamulin RH			
immune globulin			*J2791*
immune globulin, human	*1 dose package, 300 mcg*	*IM*	*J2790*
immune globulin, human, solvent detergent	*100 IU*	*IV*	*J2792*
RhoGAM	*1 dose package, 300 mcg*	*IM*	*J2790*
	50 mg		*J2788*
Gamunex	*500 mg*		**J1561**
Ganciclovir, implant	*4.5 mg*	*OTH*	**J7310**
Ganciclovir sodium	*500 mg*	*IV*	**J1570**
Ganirelix Acetate			*J3490*
Ganite	*1 mg*		*J1457*
	Per millicurie		*A9556*
Garamycin, gentamicin	*up to 80 mg*	*IM, IV*	**J1580**
Gastrocrom	*per 10 mg*		*J7631*
Gastrografin	*per ml*		*Q9963*
Gastromark	*per 100 ml*		*Q9954*
Gatifloxacin	*10 mg*	*IV*	**J1590**
Gefitinib	*250 mg*		**J8565**
Gemcitabine HCl	*200 mg*	*IV*	**J9201**
Gemsar	*200 mg*	*IV*	*J9201*
Gemtuzumab ozogamicin	*5 mg*	*IV*	**J9300**
Genarc	*per IU*		*J7192*
Gendex 75	*500 ml*		*J7110*
GenESA	*1 mg*		*J0395*

◄▶ New	←→ Revised	✔ Reinstated	✖ Deleted

DRUG NAME	DOSAGE	METHOD OF ADMINISTRATION	HCPCS CODE
Gengraf	*100 mg*		*J7502*
	25 mg	*ORAL*	*J7515*
	250 mg		*J7516*
Genotropin	*1 mg*		*J2941*
Gentamicin Sulfate	*up to 80 mg*	*IM, IV*	*J1580*
inhalation solution			*J7699*
Gentran	*500 ml*	*IV*	*J7100*
Gentran 75	*500 ml*	*IV*	*J7110*
Geodon	*10 mg*		*J3486*
Geref Diagnostic	*1 mcg*		*Q0515*
Gerval Protein	*1 unit*		*B4155*
Gesterol 50	*per 50 mg*		*J2675*
Gesterone	*per 50 mg*		*J2675*
Gestrin	*per 50 m*		*J2675*
Glatiramer Acetate	20 mg		**J1595**
Gleevec	*100 mg*		*S0088*
Glofil-125			*J3490*
GlucaGen	*per 1 mg*		*J1610*
GlucaGen Hypokit	*per 1 mg*		*J1610*
Glucagon Diagnositc	*per 1 mg*		*J1610*
Glucagon Emergency	*per 1 mg*		*J1610*
Glucagon Hcl	per 1 mg	SC, IM, IV	**J1610**
Glukor	*per 1,000 USP units*	*IM*	*J0725*
Glycopyrrolate			
concentrated form	per 1 mg	INH	**J7642**
unit dose form	per 1 mg	INH	**J7643**
Gold sodium thiomalate	up to 50 mg	IM	**J1600**
Golkil-125	*up to 10 microcuries*		*A9554*
Gonadorelin HCl	per 100 mcg	SC, IV	**J1620**
Gonal-F			*J3490*
Gonic	*per 1,000 USP units*	*IM*	*J0725*
Goserelin acetate implant	per 3.6 mg	SC	**J9202**
Graftjacket	*per square centimeter*		*Q4106*
Graftjacket express	*1 cc*		*Q4113*
Granisetron HCl			
injection	100 mcg	IV	**J1626**
oral	1 mg	ORAL	**Q0166**
Granite			*J3490*
Gynogen L.A. A10	*up to 10 mg*	*IM*	*J1380*
	up to 20 mg	*IM*	*J1390*
	up to 40 mg	*IM*	*J0970*

◄► New   ←→ Revised   ✔ Reinstated   ✘ Deleted

DRUG NAME	DOSAGE	METHOD OF ADMINISTRATION	HCPCS CODE
Gynogen L.A. A20	up to 10 mg	IM	J1380
	up to 20 mg	IM	J1390
	up to 40 mg	IM	J0970
Gynogen L.A. A40	up to 10 mg	IM	J1380
	up to 20 mg	IM	J1390
	up to 40 mg	IM	J0970
H			
Haldol	up to 5 mg	IM, IV	J1630
Haloperidol	up to 5 mg	IM, IV	J1630
Haloperidol decanoate	per 50 mg	IM	J1631
Haloperidol Lactate	up to 5 mg		J1630
Hectoral	1 mcg	IV	J1270
Helixate FS	per IU		J7192
Hemin	1 mg		J1640
Hemofil M	per IU	IV	J7190
Hemophilia clotting factors (e.g., anti-inhibitors)	per IU	IV	J7198
NOC	per IU	IV	J7199
Hepagam B	0.5 ml	IM	J1571
	0.5 ml	IV	J1573
Hepatolite	up to 15 millicuries		A9510
Hep Flush-10	per 10 units		J1642
Hep-Lock	10 units	IV	J1642
Hep-Lock 100	per 10 units		J1642
Hep-Lock Flush	per 10 units		J1642
Hep-Lock PF	per 10 units		J1642
Hep-Lock U/P	10 units	IV	J1642
Heparin Combination	per 10 units		J1642
Heparin Lock Flush	per 10 units		J1642
Heparin Lock Flush/Saline Flush	per 10 units		J1642
Heparin (Procine) In D5W	per 1,000 units		J1644
Heparin (Procine) In Nacl	per 10 units		J1642
	Per 1,000 units		J1644
Heparin (Procine) Lock Flush	per 10 units		J1642
Heparin sodium	1,000 units	IV, SC	J1644
Heparin Sodium (Bovine)	per 1,000 units		J1644
Heparin Sodium Flush	per 10 units		J1642
Heparin sodium (heparin lock flush)	10 units	IV	J1642
Heparin Sodium (Procine)	per 1,000 units		J1644
Heparin Sodium/Sodium Chloride	per 1,000 units		J1644
HepatAmine	premix		B5100

◄▶ New   ←→ Revised   ✔ Reinstated   ✖ Deleted

DRUG NAME	DOSAGE	METHOD OF ADMINISTRATION	HCPCS CODE
Hepatic-acid	1 unit		B4154
Hep-Pak	per 10 units		J1642
	Per 1,000 units		J1644
Herceptin	10 mg	IV	J9355
Hexabrix 320	per ml		Q9967
Hexadrol Phosphate	1 mg	IM, IV, OTH	J1100
			J1094
Hibtiter			J3490
Histaject	per 10 mg	IM, SC, IV	J0945
Histerone 50	up to 50 mg	IM	J3140
Histerone 100	up to 50 mg	IM	J3140
Histine B	per 10 mg		J0945
Histrelin			
acetate	10 mcg		J1675
implant	50 mg		J9225
HSA Sterile Diluent	10 ml		A4216
Humalog	per 5 units		J1815
	per 50 units		J1817
Humate-P	per IU		J7187
Humatrope	1 mg		J2941
Humegon	75 IU		S0122
Humira	20 mg		J0135
Humulin	per 5 units		J1815
	per 50 units		J1817
Hyalgan			J7321
Hyaluronic Acid			J3490
Hyaluronidase	up to 150 units	SC, IV	J3470
Hyaluronidase			
ovine	up to 999 units		J3471
ovine	per 1000 units		J3472
recombinant	1 usp		J3473
Hylutin			J3490
Hyate:C	per IU	IV	J7191
Hybolin Improved, see Nandrolone phenpropionate			
Hybolin Decanoate	up to 50 mg	IM	J2320
	up to 100 mg	IM	J2321
	up to 200 mg	IM	J2322
Hycamtin	0.25 mg	ORAL	J8705
	4 mg	IV	J9350
Hydase	up to 150 units		J3470
Hydralazine HCl	up to 20 mg	IV, IM	J0360
Hydrate	up to 50 mg	IM, IV	J1240

◀▶ New   ←→ Revised   ✔ Reinstated   ✖ Deleted

DRUG NAME	DOSAGE	METHOD OF ADMINISTRATION	HCPCS CODE
Hydrea			*J8999*
Hydrocortisone acetate	up to 25 mg	IV, IM, SC	**J1700**
Hydrocortisone sodium phosphate	up to 50 mg	IV, IM, SC	**J1710**
Hydrocortisone succinate sodium	up to 100 mg	IV, IM, SC	**J1720**
Hydrocortone Acetate	*up to 25 mg*	*IV, IM, SC*	*J1700*
Hydrocortone Phosphate	*up to 50 mg*	*IM, IV, SC*	*J1710*
Hydromorphone HCl	up to 4 mg	SC, IM, IV	**J1170**
Hydroxocobalamin	*up to 1,000 mcg*		*J3420*
Hydroxyurea			*J8999*
Hydroxyzine HCl	up to 25 mg	IM	**J3410**
Hydroxyzine Pamoate	25 mg	ORAL	**Q0177**
	50 mg	ORAL	**Q0178**
Hylan G-F 20			**J7322**
Hylenex	*up to 150 units*		*J3470*
	1 USP unit		*J3473*
Hyoscyamine sulfate	up to 0.25 mg	SC, IM, IV	**J1980**
Hypaque	*per ml*		*Q9961, Q9963*
Hypaque Sodium Oral	*per ml*		*Q9958*
Hyperhep B			*J3490*
Hyperrho S/D	*300 mc*		*J2790*
	100 IU		*J2792*
Hyperstat IV	*up to 300 mg*	*IV*	*J1730*
Hyper-Tet	*up to 250 units*	*IM*	*J1670*
HypRho-D	*300 mcg*	*IM*	*J2790*
			J2791
	50 mcg		*J2788*
Hyrexin-50	*up to 50 mg*	*IV, IM*	*J1200*
Hyzine	*25 mg*	*IM*	*J3410*
Hyzine-50	*up to 25 mg*	*IM*	*J3410*
I			
Ibandronate sodium	1 mg		**J1740**
Ibutilide fumarate	1 mg	IV	**J1742**
Idamycin	*5 mg*	*IV*	*J9211*
Idarubicin HCl	5 mg	IV	**J9211**
Idursulfase	1 mg		**J1743**
Ifex	*1 g*	*IV*	*J9208*
Ifex/Mesnex			*J9999*
Ifosfamide	1 g	IV	**J9208**
IL-2	*per single use vial*		*J9015*
Iletin	*per 5 units*		*J1815*
	Per 50 units		*J1817*

◀▶ New   ←→ Revised   ✔ Reinstated   ✖ Deleted

DRUG NAME	DOSAGE	METHOD OF ADMINISTRATION	HCPCS CODE
Ilotycin, see Erythromycin gluceptate			
Imferon	*50 mg*		*J1750, J1752*
Imiglucerase	per unit	IV	**J1785**
Imitrex	*6 mg*	*SC*	*J3030*
Immune globulin			
Flebogamma	500 mg	IV	**J1572**
Gammagard Liquid	500 mg	IV	**J1569**
Gamunex	500 mg	IV	**J1561**
HepaGam B	0.5 ml	IM	**J1571**
	0.5 ml	IV	**J1573** ◀
Human	*1 cc*		*J1460*
NOS	500 mg	IV	**J1566**
Octagam	500 mg	IV	**J1568**
Privigen	500 mg	IV	**J1459** ◀
Rhophylac	100 IU	IM	**J2791**
Subcutaneous	100 mg		**J1562**
Immunosuppressive drug, not otherwise classified			**J7599**
Implanon			*J7307*
Imuran	*50 mg*	*ORAL*	*J7500*
	100 mg		*J7501*
Inamrinone Lactate			*J3490*
Inapsine	*up to 5 mg*	*IM, IV*	*J1790*
Increlex	*1 mg*		*J2170*
Inderal	*up to 1 mg*	*IV*	*J1800*
Infed	*50 mg*		*J1750*
Infergen	*1 mcg*	*SC*	*J9212*
Infliximab, injection	10 mg	IM, IV	**J1745**
Infumorph	*up to 10 mg*		*J2270*
	100 mg		*J2271*
	Per 10 mg		*J2275*
Innohep	*1,000 iu*	*SC*	*J1655*
Innolet	*per 50 units*		*J1817*
Innovar	*up to 2 ml ampule*	*IM, IV*	*J1810*
Insulin	5 units	SC	**J1815**
Insulin lispro	50 units	SC	**J1817**
Intal	*per 10 mg*	*INH*	*J7631, J7632*
Integrilin	*5 mg*	*IM, IV*	*J1327*
Intera-BMWD	*per square centimeter*		*Q4104*
Integra			
Bilayer Matrix Wound Dressing (BMWD)	*per square centimeter*		*Q4104*
Dermal Regeneration Template (DRT)	*per square centimeter*		*Q4105*

◀▶ New   ←→ Revised   ✔ Reinstated   ✖ Deleted

TABLE OF DRUGS

DRUG NAME	DOSAGE	METHOD OF ADMINISTRATION	HCPCS CODE
Integra—cont'd			
Flowable Wound Matrix	*1 cc*		*Q4114*
Matrix	*per square centimeter*		*Q4108*
Interferon alphacon-1, recombinant	1 mcg	SC	**J9212**
Interferon alfa-2a, recombinant	3 million units	SC, IM	**J9213**
Interferon alfa-2b, recombinant	1 million units	SC, IM	**J9214**
Interferon alfa-n3 (human leukocyte derived)	250,000 IU	IM	**J9215**
Interferon beta-1a	33 mcg	IM	**J1825**
	11 mcg	IM	**Q3025**
	11 mcg	SC	**Q3026**
Interferon beta-1b	0.25 mg	SC	**J1830**
Interferon gamma-1b	3 million units	SC	**J9216**
Interleukin	*per single use vial*		*J9015*
Intrauterine copper contraceptive		OTH	J7300
Intron-A	*1 million units*		*J9214*
Invanz	*500 mg*		*J1335*
Invirase	*200 mg*	*ORAL*	*S0140*
Iplex	*1 m*		*J2170*
Ipratropium bromide, unit dose form	per mg	INH	**J7644, J7645**
Iressa	*250 mg*	*ORAL*	*J8565*
Irinotecan	20 mg	IV	**J9206**
Iron dextran	*50 mg*	*IV, IM*	**J1750,** ~~J1751, J1752~~
Iron sucrose	1 mg	IV	**J1756**
Irrigation solution for Tx of bladder calculi	per 50 ml	OTH	**Q2004**
Isocal	*1 unit*		*B4150*
Isocal HCN	*1 unit*		*B4152*
Isocaine HCl	*per 10 ml*	*VAR*	*J0670*
Isoetharine HCl			
concentrated form	per mg	INH	**J7647, J7648**
unit dose form	per mg	INH	**J7649, J7650**
Isoproterenol HCl			
concentrated form	per mg	INH	**J7657, J7658**
unit dose form	per mg	INH	**J7659, J7660**
Isotein HN	*1 unit*		*B4153*
Isovue-200	*per ml*		*Q9966*
Isovue-250	*per ml*		*Q9966*
Isovue-300	*per ml*		*Q9967*
Isovue-370	*per ml*		*Q9967*
Isovue-M-200	*per ml*		*Q9966*
Isovue-M-300	*per ml*		*Q9967*

◄ ► New   ← → Revised   ✔ Reinstated   ✖ Deleted

DRUG NAME	DOSAGE	METHOD OF ADMINISTRATION	HCPCS CODE
Isuprel			
concentrated form	*per mg*	*INH*	**J7657, J7658**
unit dose form	*per mg*	*INH*	**J7659, J7660**
Itraconazole	50 mg	IV	**J1835**
Iveegam EN	*500 m*		*J1566*
Ixabepilone	1 mg		**J9207** ◄
Ixempra	*1 mg*		*J9207*
J			
Jenamicin	*up to 80 mg*	*IM, IV*	*J1580*
K			
Kabikinase	*per 250,000 IU*	*IV*	*J2995*
Kaleinate	*per 10 ml*	*IV*	*J0610*
Kanamycin sulfate	up to 75 mg	IM, IV	**J1850**
	up to 500 mg	IM, IV	**J1840**
Kantrex	*up to 75 mg*	*IM, IV*	*J1850*
	up to 500 mg	*IM, IV*	*J1840*
Kay-Pred 25	*up to 1 ml*		*J2650*
Keflin	*up to 1 g*	*IM, IV*	*J1890*
Kefurox, see Cufuroxime sodium			
	per 750 mg		*J0697*
Kefzol	*500 mg*	*IV, IM*	*J0690*
Kenaject-40	*per 10 mg*	*IM*	*J3301*
	1 mg		*J3300*
Kenalog-10	*per 10 mg*	*IM*	*J3301*
	1 mg		*J3300*
Kenalog-40	*per 10 mg*	*IM*	*J3301*
	1 mg		*J3300*
Kepivance	*50 mcg*		*J2425*
Keppra	*10 mg*		*J1953*
Kestrone 5	*per 1 mg*	*IM*	*J1435*
Ketorolac tromethamine	per 15 mg	IM, IV	**J1885**
Key-Pred 25	*up to 1 ml*	*IM*	*J2650*
Key-Pred 50	*up to 1 ml*	*IM*	*J2650*
Key-Pred-SP, see Prednisolone sodium phosphate			
K-Flex	*up to 60 mg*	*IV, IM*	*J2360*
Kineret			*J3490*
Kinevac	*5 mcg*		*J2805*
Kinlytic	*5,000 IU*		*J3364*
	250,000 IU		*J3365*
Klebcil	*up to 75 mg*	*IM, IV*	*J1850*
	up to 500 mg	*IM, IV*	*J1840*

◄► New   ←→ Revised   ✔ Reinstated   ✖ Deleted

DRUG NAME	DOSAGE	METHOD OF ADMINISTRATION	HCPCS CODE
Koate-HP (anti-hemophilic factor)			
human	*per IU*	*IV*	*J7190*
porcine	*per IU*	*IV*	*J7191*
recombinant	*per IU*	*IV*	*J7192*
Kogenate			
human	per IU	IV	**J7190**
porcine	per IU	IV	**J7191**
recombinant	per IU	IV	**J7192**
Konakion	*per 1 mg*	*IM, SC, IV*	*J3430*
Konyne-80	*per IU*	*IV*	*J7194, J7195*
Kytril	*1 mg*	*ORAL*	*Q0166*
	1 mg	*IV*	*S0091*
	100 mcg	*IV*	*J1626*
L			
LA-12	*up to 1,000 mcg*		*J3420*
L.A.E. 20	*up to 10 mg*	*IM*	*J1380*
	up to 20 mg	*IM*	*J1390*
	up to 40 mg	*IM*	*J0970*
Laetrile, Amygdalin, vitamin B-17			**J3570**
Lanoxin	*up to 0.5 mg*	*IM, IV*	*J1160*
Lanreotide	1 mg		**J1930**
Lantus	*per 5 units*		*J1815*
	per 50 units		*J1817*
Largon, see Propiomazine HCl			
Laronidase	0.1 mg		**J1931**
Lasix	*up to 20 mg*	*IM, IV*	*J1940*
L-Caine	*10 mg*	*IV*	*J2001*
L-Carnitine	*per 1 gm*		*J1955*
Lepirudin	50 mg		**J1945**
Leucovorin calcium	per 50 mg	IM, IV	**J0640**
Leukeran			*J8999*
Leukine	*50 mcg*	*IV*	*J2820*
Leuprolide acetate (for depot suspension)	per 3.75 mg	IM	**J1950**
	7.5 mg	IM	**J9217**
Leuprolide acetate	per 1 mg	IM	**J9218**
Leuprolide acetate implant	65 mg		**J9219**
Leustatin	*per mg*	*IV*	*J9065*
Levalbuterol HCl			
concentrated form	0.5 mg	INH	~~J7602,~~ **J7607, J7612**
unit dose form	0.5 mg	INH	~~J7603,~~ **J7614, J7615**

◀▶ New   ←→ Revised   ✔ Reinstated   ✖ Deleted

DRUG NAME	DOSAGE	METHOD OF ADMINISTRATION	HCPCS CODE
Levaquin I.U.	250 mg	IV	J1956
Levemir	per 5 units		J1815
Levetiracetam	10 mg		J1953 ◄
Levocarnitine	per 1 gm	IV	J1955
Levo-Dromoran	up to 2 mg	SC, IV	J1960
Levofloxacin	250 mg	IV	J1956
Levoleucovorin calcium	0.5 mg		J0641 ◄
Levonorgestrel implant			J7306
Levonorgestrel-releasing intrauterine contraceptive system	52 mg	OTH	J7302
Levorphanol tartrate	up to 2 mg	SC, IV	J1960
Levsin	up to 0.25 mg	SC, IM, IV	J1980
Levulan Kerastick	unit dose (354 mg)	OTH	J7308
Lexiscan	0.1 mg		J2785
Librium	up to 100 mg	IM, IV	J1990
Lidocaine HCl	10 mg	IV	J2001
Lidoject-1	10 mg	IV	J2001
Lidoject-2	10 mg	IV	J2001
Lincocin	up to 300 mg	IV	J2010
Lincomycin HCl	up to 300 mg	IV	J2010
Linezolid	200 mg	IV	J2020
Liquaemin Sodium	1,000 units	IV, SC	J1644
Liquid Pred	5 mg		J7506
Lioresal	10 mg	IT	J0475
			J0476
Lispro-PFC	per 50 units		J1817
LMD (10%)	500 ml	IV	J7100
Lok-Pak	per 10 mg		J1642
Lonalac Powder	1 unit		B4150
Loniten	10 mg	ORAL	S0139
Lovenox	10 mg	SC	J1650
Lorazepam	2 mg	IM, IV	J2060
L-phenylalanine mustard	50 mg		J9245
Lucentis	0.1 mg		J2778
Lufyllin	up to 500 mg	IM	J1180
Luminal	up to 120 mg		J2560
Luminal Sodium	up to 120 mg	IM, IV	J2560
Lunelle	5 mg/25 mg	IM	J1056
Lupon Depot	7.5 mg		J9216
Lupon Depot-Ped	7.5 mg		J9216
Lupron	per 1 mg	IM	J9218
	per 3.75 mg	IM	J1950
	7.5 mg	IM	J9217

◄ ▶ New   ← → Revised   ✔ Reinstated   ✖ Deleted

DRUG NAME	DOSAGE	METHOD OF ADMINISTRATION	HCPCS CODE
Lupron-3	3.75 mg	SC	J1950
Lupron-4	3.75 mg	SC	J1950
Lupron depot	3.75 mg	IM	J1950
	7.5 mg	IM	J9217
Lupron implant	65 mg	OTH	J9219
Lutrepulse	per 100 mcg		J1620
Lymphocyte immune globulin			
anti-thymocyte globulin, equine	250 mg	IV	J7504
anti-thymocyte globulin, rabbit	25 mg	IV	J7511
Lyophilized	100 mg	IV	J9093
	200 mg	IV	J9094
	500 mg	IV	J9095
	1 g	IV	J9096
	2 g	IV	J9097
M			
Macugen	0.3 mg		J2503
Magnacal	1 unit		B4152
Magnavist	up to 25 millicurie		A9539
	Up to 75 millicurie		A9567
Magnesium sulfate	500 mg		J3475
Magnes Sulf	per 500 mg		J3475
Magnevist	per ml		A9579
Malulane			J8999
Mannitol	25% in 50 ml	IV	J2150
other			J7799
Marcaine			J3490
Marinol	2.5 mg	ORAL	Q0167
	5 mg	ORAL	Q0168
Marmine	up to 50 mg	IM, IV	J1240
Maxipime	500 mg	IV	J0692
MCT Oil	1 unit		B4155
MD-76R	per ml		Q9963
MD Gastroview	per ml		Q9963
MDP-Bracco	up to 30 millicuries		A9503
Mecasermin	1 mg		J2170
Mechlorethamine HCl (nitrogen mustard), HN2	10 mg	IV	J9230
Medidex	1 mg		J1100
Medracone	80 mg		J1040
Medralone 40	20 mg	IM	J1020
	40 mg	IM	J1030
	80 mg	IM	J1040

◀▶ New   ←→ Revised   ✔ Reinstated   ✖ Deleted

DRUG NAME	DOSAGE	METHOD OF ADMINISTRATION	HCPCS CODE
Medralone 80	20 mg	IM	J1020
	40 mg	IM	J1030
	80 mg	IM	J1040
Medrol	per 4 mg	ORAL	J7509
Medroxyprogesterone acetate	50 mg	IM	J1051
	150 mg	IM	J1055
Medroxyprogesterone acetate/estradiol cypionate	5 mg/25 mg	IM	J1056
Mefoxin	1 g	IV, IM	J0694
Megace			J8999
Megestrol Acetate			J8999
Melphalan HCl	50 mg	IV	J9245
Melphalan, oral	2 mg	ORAL	J8600
Menadione	per 1 mg		J3430
Menoject LA	up to 1 ml	IM	J1060
Mepergan Injection	up to 50 mg	IM, IV	J2180
Meperidine HCl	per 100 mg	IM, IV, SC	J2175
Meperidine and promethazine HCl	up to 50 mg	IM, IV	J2180
Meritate	per 150 mg		J3520
Mepivacaine HCL	per 10 ml	VAR	J0670
Meprozine	up to 50 mg		J2180
Mercaptopurine			J8999
Meritene	1 unit		B4150
Meropenem	100 mg		J2185
Merrem	100 m		J2185
Mesna	200 mg	IV	J9209
Mesnex	200 mg	IV	J9209
Metaprel			
concentrated form	per 10 mg	INH	J7667, J7668
unit dose form	per 10 mg	INH	J7669, J7670
Metaproterenol sulfate			
concentrated form	per 10 mg	INH	J7667, J7668
unit dose form	per 10 mg	INH	J7669, J7670
Metaraminol bitartrate	per 10 mg	IV, IM, SC	J0380
Metastron	per millicurie		A9600
Methacholine chloride	1 mg		J7674
Methadone HCl	up to 10 mg	IM, SC	J1230
Methergine, see Methylergonovine maleate			
Methocarbamol	up to 10 ml	IV, IM	J2800
Method M Monoclonal Purified	per IU		J7192
Methotrexate, oral	2.5 mg	ORAL	J8610
Methotrexate sodium	5 mg	IV, IM, IT, IA	J9250
	50 mg	IV, IM, IT, IA	J9260

◀▶ New   ←→ Revised   ✔ Reinstated   ✖ Deleted

DRUG NAME	DOSAGE	METHOD OF ADMINISTRATION	HCPCS CODE
Methotrexate LPF	5 mg	IV, IM, IT, IA	J9250
	50 mg	IV, IM, IT, IA	J9260
Methylcotolone	80 mg		J1040
Methyldopate HCl	up to 250 mg	IV	J0210
Methylene blue	1 ml		A9535
Methylpred 40	40 mg		J1030
Methylpred DP	per 4 mg		J7509
Methylprednisolone, oral	per 4 mg	ORAL	J7509
Methylprednisolone acetate	20 mg	IM	J1020
	40 mg	IM	J1030
	80 mg	IM	J1040
Methylprednisolone sodium succinate	up to 40 mg	IM, IV	J2920
	up to 125 mg	IM, IV	J2930
Meticorten	5 mg		J7506
Metoclopramide HCl	up to 10 mg	IV	J2765
Metrodin	75 IU		J3355
Metronidazole			J3490
Miacalcin	up to 400 units	SC, IM	J0630
MIBG	Per 0.5 millicurie		A9508
Micafungin sodium	1 mg		J2248
MicRhoGAM	50 mcg		J2788
Microlipids	1 unit		B4155
Midazolam HCl	per 1 mg	IM, IV	J2250
Mifoprex	200 mg	ORAL	S0190
Milrinone lactate	5 mg	IV	J2260
Mirena	52 mg	OTH	J7302
Mithracin	2,500 mcg	IV	J9270
Mithramycin	2.5 mg		J9270
Mitomycin	5 mg	IV	J9280
	20 mg	IV	J9290
	40 mg	IV	J9291
Mitoxana	1 gm		J9208
Mitoxantrone HCl	per 5 mg	IV	J9293
Moducal	1 unit		B4155
Monarc	per IU		J7190
Monocid, see Cefonicic sodium			
Monoclate-P			
human	per IU	IV	J7190
porcine	per IU	IV	J7191
recombinant	per IU	IV	J7192
Monoclonal antibodies, parenteral	5 mg	IV	J7505

◀▶ New   ←→ Revised   ✔ Reinstated   ✖ Deleted

DRUG NAME	DOSAGE	METHOD OF ADMINISTRATION	HCPCS CODE
Monoject LA	up to 1 ml		J1060
Monoject Prefill	per 10 units		J1642
Monoject Prefill Advanced	10 ml		A4216
Mononine	per IU	IV	J7193
Morphine sulfate	up to 10 mg	IM, IV, SC	J2270
	100 mg	IM, IV, SC	J2271
preservative-free	per 10 mg	SC, IM, IV	J2275
Moxifloxacin	100 mg		J2280
MPI-DMSA Kidney Reagent	up to 10 millicurie		A9551
MPI-DTPA Kit-Chelate	up to 25 millicurie		A9539
	Up to 75 millicurie		A9567
MPI Indium DTPA IN-111	up to 25 millicurie		A9539
	Up to 75 millicurie		A9567
M-Prednisol-40	20 mg	IM	J1020
	40 mg	IM	J1030
	80 mg	IM	J1040
M-Prednisol-80	20 mg	IM	J1020
	40 mg	IM	J1030
	80 mg	IM	J1040
Mucomyst			
injection	100 mg		J0132
unit dose form	per gram	INH	J7604, J7608
Mucosil	per gram		J7608
Mucosol			
injection	100 mg		J0132
unit dose	per gram	INH	J7604, J7608
Muromonab-CD3	5 mg	IV	J7505
Muse		OTH	J0275
	1.25 mcg	OTH	J0270
Mustargen	10 mg	IV	J9230
Mutamycin	5 mg	IV	J9280
	20 mg	IV	J9290
	40 mg	IV	J9291
Mycamine	1 mg		J2248
Mycophenolic acid	180 mg		J7518
Mycophenolate Mofetil	250 mg	ORAL	J7517
Myfortic	180 mg		J7518
Myleran	1 mg		J0594
	2 mg	ORAL	J8510
Mylocel	500 mg	ORAL	S0176
Mylotarg	5 mg	IV	J9300

◄ ► New   ← → Revised   ✓ Reinstated   ✖ Deleted

DRUG NAME	DOSAGE	METHOD OF ADMINISTRATION	HCPCS CODE
Myobloc	per 100 units	IM	J0587
Myochrysine	up to 50 mg	IM	J1600
Myolin	up to 60 mg	IV, IM	J2360
Myoview	up to 40 millicuries		A9502
Myozyme	10 mg		J0220
N			
N-Acetyl-L-Cysteine			J7699
Nabi-HB			J3490
Nabilone	1 mg	ORAL	**J8650**
Nafcillin Sodium			J3490
Naglazyme	1 mg		J1458
Nalbuphine HCl	per 10 mg	IM, IV, SC	**J2300**
Nallpen	2 gm		S0032
Naloxone HCl	per 1 mg	IM, IV, SC	**J2310**
Naltrexone, depot form	1 mg		**J2315**
Nandrobolic L.A	up to 50 mg	IM	J2320
	up to 100 mg	IM	J2321
	up to 200 mg	IM	J2322
Nandrolone decanoate	up to 50 mg	IM	**J2320**
	up to 100 mg	IM	**J2321**
	up to 200 mg	IM	**J2322**
Narcan	1 mg	IM, IV, SC	J2310
Naropin	1 mg		J2795
Nasahist B	per 10 mg	IM, SC, IV	J0945
Nasalcrom	per 10 mg		J7631
Nasal vaccine inhalation		INH	**J3530**
Natalizumab	1 mg		**J2323**
Natrecor	0.1 mg		J2325
Natural Estrogenic Substance	per 25 mg		J1410
Navane, see Thiothixene			
Navelbine	per 10 mg	IV	J9390
ND Stat	per 10 mg	IM, SC, IV	J0945
Nebcin	up to 80 mg	IM, IV	J3260
	per 300 mg		J7682
NebuPent	per 300 mg	INH	J2545, J7676
	300 mg	IM, IV	S0080
inhalation solution			J7699
Nelarabine	50 mg	IV	**J9261**
Nembutal Sodium Solution	per 50 mg	IM, IV, OTH	J2515
Neocyten	up to 60 mg	IV, IM	J2360
Neo-Durabolic	up to 50 mg	IM	J2320

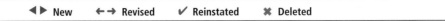

◀ ▶ New   ← → Revised   ✔ Reinstated   ✖ Deleted

TABLE OF DRUGS

DRUG NAME	DOSAGE	METHOD OF ADMINISTRATION	HCPCS CODE
Neoral	*100 mg*		**J7502**
	25 mg		**J7515**
	250 mg		**J7516**
Neoquess	*up to 20 mg*	*IM*	**J0500**
Neosar			
	100 mg	*IV*	**J9070**
	200 mg	*IV*	**J9080**
	500 mg	*IV*	**J9090**
	1 g	*IV*	**J9091**
	2 g	*IV*	**J9092**
	100 mg		**J9093**
	200 mg		**J9094**
	500 mg		**J9095**
	1 gm		**J9096**
	2 gm		**J9097**
Neostigmine methylsulfate	up to 0.5 mg	*IM, IV, SC*	**J2710**
Neo-Synephrine	*up to 1 ml*	*SC, IM, IV*	**J2370**
NephrAmine	*premix*		**B5000**
Nervidox-6 S	*up to 1,000 mcg*		**J3420**
Nervidox S	*up to 1,000 mcg*		**J3420**
Nervocaine 1%	*10 mg*	*IV*	**J2001**
Nervocaine 2%	*10 mg*	*IV*	**J2001**
Nesacaine	*per 30 ml*	*VAR*	**J2400**
Nesacaine-MPF	*per 30 ml*	*VAR*	**J2400**
Nesiritide	**0.1 mg**		**J2325**
Neulasta	*6 mg*		**J2505**
Neumega	*5 mg*	*SC*	**J2355**
Neupogen	*300 mcg*	*SC, IV*	**J1440**
	480 mcg	*SC, IV*	**J1441**
Neuro B-12	*up to 1,000 mcg*		**J3420**
Neuro B-12 Forte S	*up to 1,000 mcg*		**J3420**
Neurolite	*up to 25 millicurie*		**A9557**
Neutrexin	*per 25 mg*	*IV*	**J3305**
Nipent	*per 10 mg*	*IV*	**J9268**
Nolvadex			**J8999**
Nordiflex	*1 mg*		**J2941**
Norditropin	*1 mg*		**J2941**
Nordryl	*up to 50 mg*	*IV, IM*	**J1200**
	50 mg	*ORAL*	**Q0163**
Norflex	*up to 60 mg*	*IV, IM*	**J2360**
Norplant II			**J7306**

◀ ▶ New   ← → Revised   ✔ Reinstated   ✖ Deleted

DRUG NAME	DOSAGE	METHOD OF ADMINISTRATION	HCPCS CODE
Norplant System			*J3590*
Norzine			
injection	*up to 10 mg*	*IM*	*J3280*
oral	*10 mg*	*ORAL*	*Q0174*
Not otherwise classified drugs			**J3490**
other than inhalation solution administered thru DME			**J7799**
inhalation solution administered thru DME			**J7699**
anti-neoplastic			**J9999**
chemotherapeutic		ORAL	**J8999**
immunosuppressive			**J7599**
nonchemotherapeutic		ORAL	**J8499**
Novantrone	*per 5 mg*	*IV*	*J9293*
Novarel	*per 1,000 USP Units*		*J0725*
Novolin	*per 5 units*		*J1815*
	per 50 units		*J1817*
Novolog	*per 5 units*		*J1815*
	per 50 units		*J1817*
Novo Nordsik	*per 5 mg*		*J1815*
Nov-onxol	*30 mg*		*J9265*
Novo Seven	*1 mcg*	*IV*	*J7189*
NPH	*5 units*	*SC*	*J1815*
Nubain	*per 10 mg*	*IM, IV, SC*	*J2300*
Nulicaine	*10 mg*	*IV*	*J2001*
Numorphan	*up to 1 mg*	*IV, SC, IM*	*J2410*
Numorphan H.P.	*up to 1 mg*	*IV, SC, IM*	*J2410*
Nutri-source	*1 unit*		*B4155*
Nutri-twelve	*up to 1,000 mcg*		*J3420*
Nutropin	*1 mg*		*J2941*
NuvaRing	*each*		*J7303*
O			
Oasis Burn Matrix	*per square centimeter*		*Q4103*
Oasis Wound Matrix	*per square centimeter*		*Q4102*
Octagam	500 mg		**J1568**
Octreotide Acetate, injection	1 mg	IM	**J2353**
	25 mcg	IV, SQ	**J2354**
Oculinum	*per unit*	*IM*	*J0585*
O-Flex	*up to 60 mg*	*IV, IM*	*J2360*
Omalizumab	5 mg		**J2357**
Omnipaque 140	*per ml*		*Q9965*
Omnipaque 180	*per ml*		*Q9965*
Omnipaque 300	*per ml*		*Q9967*

◄► New   ←→ Revised   ✔ Reinstated   ✖ Deleted

DRUG NAME	DOSAGE	METHOD OF ADMINISTRATION	HCPCS CODE
Omnipaque 350	per ml		Q9967
Omnipen-N			
sodium	up to 500 mg	IM, IV	J0290
sodium/sulbactam sodium	per 1.5 gm	IM, IV	J0295
Omniscan	per ml		A9579
Oncaspar	per single dose vial	IM, IV	J9266
Oncovin	1 mg	IV	J9370
	2 mg	IV	J9375
	5 mg	IV	J9380
Ondansetron HCl	1 mg	IV	J2405
Ondansetron HCl	8 mg	ORAL	Q0179
Ontak	300 mcg		J9160
Onxol	30 mg		J9265
Opana	up to 1 mg		J2410
Oprelvekin	5 mg	SC	J2355
Optimark	per ml		A9579
Optiray 160	per ml		Q9965
Optiray 300	per ml		Q9967
Optiray 320	per ml		Q9967
Optiray 350	per ml		Q9967
Optison	per ml		Q9956
Oraminic II	per 10 mg	IM, SC, IV	J0945
Orapred ODT	per 5 mg		J7510
Orasong	5 mg		J7506
Ormazine	10 mg	ORAL	Q0171
	25 mg	ORAL	Q0172
	up to 50 mg	IM, IV	J3230
Orphenadrine citrate	up to 60 mg	IV, IM	J2360
Orphenate	up to 60 mg	IV, IM	J2360
Orencia	10 mg		J0129
Orthoclone OKT3	5 mg		J7505
Ortho Evra	each		J7304
Orthovisc			J7324
Or-Tyl	up to 20 mg	IM	J0500
Osmitrol	25% in 50 ml		J2150
Osmitrol, other			J7799
Osmolite	1 unit		B4150
Ostreoscan	up to 6 millicuries		A9572
Ovidrel			J3490
Oxacillin sodium	up to 250 mg	IM, IV	J2700
Oxaliplatin	0.5 mg		J9263

◄ ► New   ← → Revised   ✔ Reinstated   ✖ Deleted

TABLE OF DRUGS

DRUG NAME	DOSAGE	METHOD OF ADMINISTRATION	HCPCS CODE
Oxilan 300	*per ml*		*Q9967*
Oxilan 350	*per ml*		*Q9967*
Oxymorphone HCl	up to 1 mg	IV, SC, IM	**J2410**
Oxytetracycline HCl	up to 50 mg	IM	**J2460**
Oxytocin	up to 10 units	IV, IM	**J2590**
P			
Pacis	*per installation*		*J9031*
Paclitaxel	30 mg	IV	**J9265**
Paclitaxel protein-bound particles	1 mg		**J9264**
Palifermin	50 mcg		**J2425**
Palonosetron HCl	25 mcg		**J2469**
Pamidronate disodium	per 30 mg	IV	**J2430**
Panglobulin NF	*500 mg*		*J1566*
Panhematin	*1 mg*		*J1640*
Panitumumab	10 mg		**J9303**
Panmycin	*up to 250 mg*	*IM, IV*	*J0120*
Papaverine HCl	up to 60 mg	IV, IM	**J2440**
Paragard T 380 A		OTH	*J7300*
Paraplatin	*50 mg*	*IV*	*J9045*
Paricalcitol, injection	1 mcg	IV, IM	**J2501**
Pavagen TD	*up to 60 mg*		*J2440*
Pediapred	*5 mg*		*J7510*
Pegademase bovine	25 iu		**J2504**
Pegaptinib	0.3 mg		**J2503**
Pegaspargase	per single dose vial	IM, IV	**J9266**
Pegasys			*J3490*
Pegfilgrastim	6 mg		**J2505**
Peg-Intron			*J3490*
Pemetrexed	10 mg		**J9305**
Penicillin G benzathine	up to 600,000 units	IM	**J0560**
	up to 1,200,000 units	IM	**J0570**
	up to 2,400,000 units	IM	**J0580**
Penicillin G benzathine and penicillin G procaine			
	up to 600,000 units	IM	**J0530**
	up to 1,200,000 units	IM	**J0540**
	up to 2,400,000 units	IM	**J0550**
Penicillin G potassium	up to 600,000 units	IM, IV	**J2540**
Penicillin G procaine, aqueous	up to 600,000 units	IM, IV	**J2510**
Pentacarinat	*per 300 mg*		*J2545*
	300 mg		*S0080*
Pentam	*per 300 mg*		*J2545*

◀ ▶ New   ← → Revised   ✔ Reinstated   ✖ Deleted

DRUG NAME	DOSAGE	METHOD OF ADMINISTRATION	HCPCS CODE
Pentam 300	*300 mg*		*S0080*
Pentam, inhalation solution			*J7699*
Pentamidine isethionate	per 300 mg	INH	J2545, J7676
Pentaspan	*100 ml*		*J2513*
Pentastarch, 10%	100 ml		J2513
Pentate Calcium Trisodium	*per 25 millicuries*		*A9539*
	Up to 75 millicuries		*A9567*
Pentate Zinc Trisodium	*per 25 millicuries*		*A9539*
	Up to 75 millicuries		*A9567*
Pentazocine HCl	30 mg	IM, SC, IV	J3070
Pentobarbital sodium	per 50 mg	IM, IV, OTH	J2515
Pentostatin	per 10 mg	IV	J9268
Peforomist	*20 mcg*		*J7606*
Pepcid			*J3490*
Pergonal	*75 IU*		*S0122*
Permapen	*up to 600,000*	*IM*	*J0560*
	up to 1,200,000 units	*IM*	*J0570*
	up to 2,400,000 units	*IM*	*J0580*
Perphenazine			
injection	up to 5 mg	IM, IV	J3310
tablets	4 mg	ORAL	Q0175
	8 mg	ORAL	Q0176
Persantine IV	*per 10 mg*	*IV*	*J1245*
Pfizerpen	*up to 600,000 units*	*IM, IV*	*J2540*
Pfizerpen A.S.	*up to 600,000 units*	*IM, IV*	*J2510*
Phenadoz			*J8498*
Phenazine 25	*up to 50 mg*	*IM, IV*	*J2550*
	12.5 mg	*ORAL*	*Q0169*
	25 mg	*ORAL*	*Q0170*
Phenazine 50	*up to 50 mg*	*IM, IV*	*J2550*
	12.5 mg	*ORAL*	*Q0169*
	25 mg	*ORAL*	*Q0170*
Phenergan	*12.5 mg*	*ORAL*	*Q0169*
	25 mg	*ORAL*	*Q0170*
	up to 50 mg	*IM, IV*	*J2550, J8498*
Phenobarbital sodium	up to 120 mg	IM, IV	J2560
Phentolamine mesylate	up to 5 mg	IM, IV	J2760
Phenylephrine HCl	up to 1 ml	SC, IM, IV	J2370
Phenylephrine HCL, other			*J7799*
Phenytoin sodium	per 50 mg	IM, IV	J1165
Phosphocol (P32)	*per millicurie*		*A9564*

◄► New   ←→ Revised   ✔ Reinstated   ✖ Deleted

TABLE OF DRUGS

DRUG NAME	DOSAGE	METHOD OF ADMINISTRATION	HCPCS CODE
Phosphotec	*up to 25 millicuries*		*A9538*
Photofrin	*75 mg*	*IV*	*J9600*
Phytonadione (Vitamin K)	per 1 mg	IM, SC, IV	**J3430**
Piperacillin/Tazobactam Sodium, injection	1.125 g	IV	**J2543**
Pipracil	*500 mg*		*S0081*
Pitocin	*up to 10 units*	*IV, IM*	*J2590*
Plantinol AQ	*10 mg*	*IV*	*J9060*
	50 mg	*IV*	*J9062*
Plas+SD	*each unit*	*IV*	*P9023*
Plasma			
cryoprecipitate reduced	each unit		**P9044**
pooled multiple donor, frozen	each unit	IV	**P9023**
Platinol	50 mg	IV	**J9062**
Plenaxis	*10 mg*		*J0128*
Plicamycin	2,500 mcg	IV	**J9270**
Pneumorax II			*S0195*
Polocaine	*per 10 ml*	*VAR*	*J0670*
Polycillin-N			
sodium	*up to 500 mg*	*IM, IV*	*J0290*
sodium/sulbactam sodium	*per 1.5 gm*	*IM, IV*	*J0295*
Polycose Liquid or Powder	*1 unit*		*B4155*
Polygam S/D	*500 mg*		*J1566*
Porex	*up to 50 mg*		*J2550*
Porfimer Sodium	75 mg	IV	**J9600**
Portagen Powder	*1 unit*		*B4150*
Potassium chloride	per 2 mEq	IV	**J3480**
Potassium Chloride Solution	*up to 1,000 cc*		*J7120*
Pralidoxime chloride	up to 1 g	IV, IM, SC	**J2730**
Precision HN	*1 unit*		*B4153*
Precision Isotonic	*1 unit*		*B4153*
Predacort 50	*up to 1 ml*		*J2650*
Predalone-50	*up to 1 ml*	*IM*	*J2650*
Predcor-25	*up to 1 ml*	*IM*	*J2650*
Predcor-50	*up to 1 ml*	*IM*	*J2650*
Predicort-50	*up to 1 ml*	*IM*	*J2650*
Pred-Ject-50	*up to 1 ml*		*J2650*
Prelone	*5 mg*		*J7510*
Prednicen-M	*5 mg*		*J7506*
Prednicot	*5 mg*		*J7506*
Prednisone	*per 5 mg*	*ORAL*	**J7506**
Prednisolone, oral	*5 mg*	*ORAL*	**J7510**

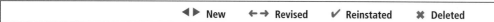

◀▶ New ←→ Revised ✔ Reinstated ✘ Deleted

DRUG NAME	DOSAGE	METHOD OF ADMINISTRATION	HCPCS CODE
Prednisolone acetate	up to 1 ml	IM	**J2650**
Prednoral	*5 mg*		*J7510*
Predoject-50	*up to 1 ml*	*IM*	*J2650*
Predone	*5 mg*		*J7506*
Pregnyl	*per 1,000 USP units*	*IM*	*J0725*
Premarin	*per 25 mg*		*J1410*
Premarin Aqueous	*per 25 mg*		*J1410*
Premarin Intravenous	*per 25 mg*	*IV, IM*	*J1410*
Prescription, chemotherapeutic, not otherwise specified		ORAL	**J8999**
Prescription, nonchemotherapeutic, not otherwise specified		ORAL	**J8499**
Prialt	*1 mcg*		*J2278*
Pri-Andriol LA	*up to 200 mg*		*J2322*
Pridoxine HCL			*J3490*
Primacor	*5 mg*	*IV*	*J2260*
Primatrix	*per square centimeter*		*Q4110*
Primaxin			
IM	*per 250 mg*	*IV, IM*	*J0743*
IV	*per 250 mg*	*IV, IM*	*J0743*
Primetheasone	*1 mg*		*J1100*
Pri-Methylate	*80 mg*		*J1040*
Priscoline HCl	*up to 25 mg*	*IV*	*J2670*
Privigen	500 mg		**J1459** ◄
Pro-Depo, see Hydroxyprogesterone Caproate			
Procainamide HCl	up to 1 g	IM, IV	**J2690**
Prochlorperazine	up to 10 mg	IM, IV	**J0780**
			J8498
Prochlorperazine HCL			*J8498*
Prochlorperazine maleate	5 mg	ORAL	**Q0164**
	10 mg	ORAL	**Q0165**
			S0183
Procrit			*J0885*
			J0886
			Q4081
Profasi HP	*per 1,000 USP units*	*IM*	*J0725*
Profilnine Heat-Treated			
non-recombinant	*per IU*	*IV*	*J7193*
recombinant	*per IU*	*IV*	*J7195*
complex	*per IU*	*IV*	*J7194*
Profilnine-SD	*per IU*		*J7193, J7194, J7195*
Progest	*per 50 mg*		*J2675*

◄ ▶ New   ← → Revised   ✓ Reinstated   ✗ Deleted

DRUG NAME	DOSAGE	METHOD OF ADMINISTRATION	HCPCS CODE
Progestaject	*per 50 mg*		*J2675*
Progesterone	per 50 mg		**J2675**
Prograf			
oral	*per 1 mg*	*ORAL*	*J7507*
parenteral	*5 mg*		*J7525*
Prohance	*per ml*		*A9579*
Prokine	*50 mcg*	*IV*	*J2820*
Prolastin	*10 mg*	*IV*	*J0256*
Proleukin	*per single use vial*	*IM, IV*	*J9015*
Prolixin Decanoate, see Fluphenazine decanoate			
	25 mg	*IM, SC*	*J2680*
Promazine HCl	up to 25 mg	IM	**J2950**
Prometh-50	*up to 50 mg*		*J2550*
Promethazine			*J8498*
Promethazine HCl			
injection	up to 50 mg	IM, IV	**J2550**
oral	12.5 mg	ORAL	**Q0169**
oral	25 mg	ORAL	**Q0170**
Promethegan			*J8498*
Promix	*1 unit*		*B4155*
Pronestyl	*up to 1 g*	*IM, IV*	*J2690*
Propac	*1 unit*		*B4155*
Propecia	*5 mg*	*ORAL*	*S0138*
Proplex T			
non-recombinant	per IU	IV	**J7193**
recombinant	per IU	IV	**J7195**
complex	per IU	IV	**J7194**
Proplex SX-T			
non-recombinant	per IU	IV	**J7193**
recombinant	per IU	IV	**J7195**
complex	per IU	IV	**J7194**
Propofol			*J3490*
Propranolol HCl	up to 1 mg	IV	**J1800**
Prorex-25			
	up to 50 mg	*IM, IV*	*J2550*
	12.5 mg	*ORAL*	*Q0169*
	25 mg	*ORAL*	*Q0170*
Prorex-50			
	up to 50 mg	*IM, IV*	*J2550*
	12.5 mg	*ORAL*	*Q0169*
	25 mg	*ORAL*	*Q0170*

 New   ←→ Revised   ✔ Reinstated   ✖ Deleted

DRUG NAME	DOSAGE	METHOD OF ADMINISTRATION	HCPCS CODE
Proscar	*5 mg*	*ORAL*	*S0138*
Prostaglandin	*per 1.25 millicurie*		*J0270*
Prostaphlin	*up to 1 g*	*IM, IV*	*J2690*
	up to 250 mg		*J2700*
Prostascint	*up to 10 millicurie*		*A9507*
Prostigmin	*up to 0.5 mg*	*IM, IV, SC*	*J2710*
Prostin	*per 1.25 millicurie*		*J0270*
Protamine sulfate	per 10 mg	IV	J2720
Protein C Concentrate	10 IU		J2724
Protirelin	per 250 mcg	IV	J2725
Prothazine	*up to 50 mg*	*IM, IV*	*J2550*
	12.5 mg	*ORAL*	*Q0169*
	25 mg	*ORAL*	*Q0170*
Protonix IV	*40 mg*		*S0164*
Protopam Chloride	*up to 1 g*	*IV, IM, SC*	*J2730*
Protropin	*1 mg*		*J2940*
Proventil			
concentrated form	*1 mg*	*INH*	*J7610, J7611*
unit dose form	*1 mg*	*INH*	*J7609, J7613*
Provocholine	*per 1 mg*		*J7674*
Prozine-50	*up to 25 mg*	*IM*	*J2950*
Pulmicort	*0.25 mg*	*INH*	*J7633*
	up to 0.5 mg		*J7626*
Pulmicort Flexhaler	*per 0.25 mg*		*J7633*
	up to 0.5 mg		*J7626*
Pulmicort Respules	*0.5 mg*	*INH*	*J7627, J7626*
	per 0.25 mg		*J7633*
	up to 0.5 mg		*J7626*
noncompounded, concentrated	*0.25 mg*	*INH*	*J7626*
Pulmozyme	*per mg*		*J7639*
Purinethol	*50 mg*		*S0108*
Pyridoxine HCl	100 mg		J3415
Q			
Quadramet	*per 50 millicurie*		*A9605*
Quelicin	*up to 20 mg*	*IV, IM*	*J0330*
Quelicin Chloride	*20 mg*	*IM, IV*	*J0330*
Quinupristin/dalfopristin	500 mg (150/350)	IV	J2770
Qvar	*per mg*		*J7622*
R			
Ranibizumab	0.1 mg		J2778
Ranitidine HCL, injection	25 mg	IV, IM	J2780

◀ ▶ New   ← → Revised   ✔ Reinstated   ✖ Deleted

DRUG NAME	DOSAGE	METHOD OF ADMINISTRATION	HCPCS CODE
Rapamune	1 mg	ORAL	J7520
Raptiva			J3490
Rasburicase	0.5 mg		**J2783**
Rebetron Kit	1 million units		J9214
Rebif	33 mcg		J1825
	11 mcg		Q3026
Reclast	1 mg		**J3488**
Recombinate (anti-hemophilic factor)			
human	per IU	IV	J7190
porcine	per IU	IV	J7191
recombinant	per IU	IV	J7192
Recombivax			J3490
Redisol	up to 1,000 mcg	IM, SC	J3420
Regadenoson	0.1 mg		**J2785** ◀
Refacto	per IU		J7192
Refludan	50 m		J1945
Regitine	up to 5 mg	IM, IV	J2760
Reglan	up to 10 mg	IV	J2765
Regranex Gel	0.5 gm		S0157
Regular	5 units	SC	J1815
Relefact TRH	per 250 mcg	IV	J2725
Relion	per 5 units		J1815
	per 50 units		J1817
Remicade	10 mg	IM, IV	J1745
Remodulin	1 mg		J3285
Renacidin	500 ml		Q2004
RenAmin	premix		B5000
Reno-30	per ml		Q9958
Reno-60	per ml		Q9961
Reno-Dip	per ml		Q9958
Renocal-76	per ml		Q9963
Renografin-60	per ml		Q9961
Reno-M60	per ml		Q9961
Renu	1 unit		B4150
ReoPro	10 mg	IV	J0130
Rep-Pred 40	20 mg	IM	J1020
	40 mg	IM	J1030
	80 mg	IM	J1040
Rep-Pred 80	20 mg	IM	J1020
	40 mg	IM	J1030
	80 mg	IM	J1040

◀▶ New   ←→ Revised   ✔ Reinstated   ✖ Deleted

DRUG NAME	DOSAGE	METHOD OF ADMINISTRATION	HCPCS CODE
Repronex	*75 IU*		*S0122*
Resectisol			*J7799*
RespiGam	*50 mg*	*IV*	*J1565*
Respiratory Syncytial Virus Immuneglobulin	50 mg	IV	**J1565**
Restall	*up to 25 mg*		*J3410*
Retavase	*18.1 mg*	*IV*	*J2993*
Reteplase	18.1 mg	IV	**J2993**
Retisert			*J7311*
Retrovir	*10 mg*	*IV*	*J3485*
ReVia	*1 mg*		*J2315*
Rheomacrodex	*500 ml*	*IV*	*J7100*
Rhesonativ	*1 dose package/ 300 mcg*	*IM*	*J2790*
	50 mg		*J2788*
Rheumatrex	*5 mg*		*J9250*
	50 mg		*J9260*
Rheumatrex Dose Pack	*2.5 mg*	*ORAL*	*J8610*
Rho(D)			
immune globulin			**J2791**
immune globulin, human	1 dose package/ 300 mcg	IM	**J2790**
	50 mg		**J2788**
immune globulin, human, solvent detergent	100	IU, IV	**J2792**
RhoGAM	*1 dose package, 300 mcg*	*IM*	*J2790*
	50 mg		*J2788*
Rhophylac	100 IU		**J2791**
Rifadin			*J3490*
Rimso-50	*50 ml*		*J1212*
Ringers lactate infusion	up to 1,000 cc	IV	**J7120**
Risperdal Costa	*0.5 mg*		*J2794*
Risperidone	0.5 mg		**J2794**
Rituxan	*100 mg*	*IV*	*J9310*
Rituximab	100 mg	IV	**J9310**
Robaxin	*up to 10 ml*	*IV, IM*	*J2800*
Robinul	*per mg*		*J7643*
Rocephin	*per 250 mg*	*IV, IM*	*J0696*
Roferon-A	*3 million units*	*SC, IM*	*J9213*
Ropivacaine Hydrochloride	1 mg		**J2795**
Rubex	*10 mg*	*IV*	*J9000*
Rubidomycin	*10 mg*		*J9150*
Rubramin PC	*up to 1,000 mcg*	*IM, SC*	*J3420*

◀▶ New   ←→ Revised   ✔ Reinstated   ✘ Deleted

DRUG NAME	DOSAGE	METHOD OF ADMINISTRATION	HCPCS CODE
S			
Sadol NS	*25 mg*		*S0012*
Saizen	*1 mg*		*J2941*
Saline solution	*10 ml*		*A4216*
5% dextrose	500 ml	IV	**J7042**
infusion	250 cc	IV	**J7050**
	1,000 cc	IV	**J7030**
sterile	500 ml = 1 unit	IV, OTH	**J7040**
Salyrgan-Theophylline	*per 40 mg*		*J2810*
Sandimmune	25 mg	ORAL	J7515
	100 mg	ORAL	J7502
	250 mg	OTH	J7516
Sandoglobulin, see Immune globin intravenous (human)			
Sangcya	*100 mg*		*J7502*
	25 mg		*J7515*
	250 mg		*J7516*
Sandostatin	*25 mcg*		*J2354*
Sandostatin Lar Depot	1 mg	IM	J2353
Sano-Drol	*40 mg*		*J1030, J1040*
Sargramostim (GM-CSF)	50 mcg	IV	**J2820**
Scandonest	*per 10 ml*		*J0670*
SecreFlo	*1 mcg*		*J2850*
Selestoject	per 4 mg	IM, IV	J0704
Sensi-Touch Lumbar Puncture Tray	*10 mg*		*J2001*
Sensorcaine			*J3490*
Septra IV	10 ml		S0039
Septra Infusion			*J3490*
Sermorelin acetate	1 mcg		**Q0515**
Serostim	*1 mg*		*J2941*
Simulect	*20 mg*		*J0480*
Sincalide	5 mcg		**J2805**
Sinografin	*per ml*		*Q9963*
Sinusol-B	per 10 mg	IM, SC, IV	J0945
Sirolimus	1 mg	ORAL	**J7520**
Smz-TMP			*J3490*
~~Sodium chloride, 0.9%~~	~~per 2 ml~~		~~J2912~~ ✖
Sodium Chloride	1,000 cc		J7030
	10 ml		A4216
	500 ml = 1 unit		J7040
	500 ml		A4217
	250 cc		J7050
inhalation solution			J7699, J7799

◄▶ New   ←→ Revised   ✔ Reinstated   ✖ Deleted

DRUG NAME	DOSAGE	METHOD OF ADMINISTRATION	HCPCS CODE
Sodium Chloride/Respiratory Therapy	*10 ml*		*A4216*
Sodium ferricgluconate in sucrose	12.5 mg		**J2916**
Sodium Hyaluronate			
Euflexxa			**J7323**
Hyalgan			**J7321**
Orthovisc			**J7324**
Supartz			**J7321**
Solganal	*up to 50 mg*	*IM*	*J2910*
Soliris	*10 mg*		*J1300*
Soltamox			*J8999*
Solu-Cortef	*up to 50 mg*	*IV, IM, SC*	*J1710*
	100 mg		*J1720*
Solu-Medrol	*up to 40 mg*	*IM, IV*	*J2920*
	up to 125 mg	*IM, IV*	*J2930*
Solurex	*1 mg*	*IM, IV, OTH*	*J1100*
Solurex LA	*1 mg*	*IM*	*J1094*
Somatrem	1 mg		**J2940**
Somatropin	1 mg		**J2941**
Somatulin Depot	*1 mg*		*J1930*
Sparine	*up to 25 mg*	*IM*	*J2950*
Spasmoject	*up to 20 mg*	*IM*	*J0500*
Spectinomycin HCl	up to 2 g	IM	**J3320**
Sporanox	*50 mg*	*IV*	*J1835*
Stadol	*1 mg*		*J0595*
	25 mg		*S0012*
Staphcillin, see Methicillin sodium			
Stilphostrol	*250 mg*	*IV*	*J9165*
Streptase	*250,000 iu*	*IV*	*J2995*
Streptokinase	per 250,000	IU, IV	**J2995**
Streptomycin Sulfate	*up to 1 g*	*IM*	*J3000*
Streptomycin	up to 1 g	IM	**J3000**
Streptozocin	1 gm	IV	**J9320**
Sterapred	*5 mg*		*J7506*
Strontium-89 chloride	per millicurie		**A9600**
Sublimaze	*0.1 mg*	*IM, IV*	*J3010*
Succinylcholine chloride	up to 20 mg	IV, IM	**J0330**
Sucostrin	*up to 20 mg*		*J0330*
Sufenta			*J3490*
Sufentanil Citrate			*J3490*
Sulfa Magg	*per 500 mg*		*J3475*
Sulfatrim	*10 ml*		*S0039*

◀▶ New   ←→ Revised   ✔ Reinstated   ✖ Deleted

DRUG NAME	DOSAGE	METHOD OF ADMINISTRATION	HCPCS CODE
Sumacal	1 unit		B4155
Sumatriptan succinate	6 mg	SC	J3030
Sumycin	up to 250 mg	IM, IV	J0120
Supartz			J7321
Supperlin LA	50 mg		J9225
Surostrin	up to 20 mg	IV, IM	J0330
Sus-Phrine	up to 1 ml ampule	SC, IM	J0170
Sustacal	1 unit		B4150
Sustacal HC	1 unit		B4152
Sustagen Powder	1 unit		B4150
Synagis	per 50 mg		C9003
Synercid	500 mg (150/350)	IV	J2770
Synkavite	per 1 mg	IM, SC, IV	J3430
Syntocinon	up to 10 units	IV, IM	J2590
Synvisc			J7322
Syrex	10 ml		A4216
Sytobex	1,000 mcg	IM, SC	J3420
T			
Tac-3	per 10 mg		J3301
Tach-40	per 10 mg		J3301
Tacrolimus			
oral	per 1 mg	ORAL	J7507
parenteral	5 mg		J7525
Tagamet	300 mg		S0023
Talwin	30 mg	IM, SC, IV	J3070
Tamiflu	per 75 mg		G9035
Tamoxifen Citrate			J8999
Tarabin CFS	100 mg		J9100
Taractan, see Chlorprothixene			
Taxol	30 mg	IV	J9265
Taxotere	20 mg	IV	J9170
Tazicef	per 500 mg		J0713
Tazidime, see Ceftazidime Technetium TC Sestambi	per dose		A9500
			J0713
Technalite	per millicurie		A9512
TechneScan HDP	Up to 30 millicuries		A9561
TechneScan MAG-3	up to 15 millicuries		A9562
TechneScan PYP	up to 25 millicuries		A9538
Technetium Tc-99m MPI-MDP	up to 30 millicuries		A9503
TEEV	up to 1 cc	IM	J0900
Temodar	5 mg	ORAL	J8700

 New   Revised   Reinstated   ✖ Deleted

DRUG NAME	DOSAGE	METHOD OF ADMINISTRATION	HCPCS CODE	
Temozolmide	5 mg	ORAL	**J8700**	
Temsirolimus	1 mg		**J9330**	◄
Tenecteplase	1 ~~50~~ mg		~~J3100,~~ **J3101**	←
Teniposide	50 mg		**Q2017**	
Tequin	*10 mg*	*IV*	*J1590*	
Terbutaline sulfate	up to 1 mg	SC, IV	**J3105**	
concentrated form	per 1 mg	INH	**J7680**	
unit dose form	per 1 mg	INH	**J7681**	
Teriparatide	10 mcg		**J3110**	
Terramycin IM	*up to 50 mg*	*IM*	*J2460*	
Testa-C	*up to 100 mg*	*IM*	*J1070*	
	1 cc, 200 mg	*IM*	*J1080*	
Testadiate	*up to 1 cc*	*IM*	*J0900*	
Testadiate-Depo	*up to 100 mg*	*IM*	*J1070*	
	1 cc, 200 mg	*IM*	*J1080*	
Testaject-LA	*up to 100 mg*	*IM*	*J1070*	
	1 cc, 200 mg	*IM*	*J1080*	
Testaqua	*up to 50 mg*	*IM*	*J3140*	
Test-Estro Cypionates	*up to 1 ml*	*IM*	*J1060*	
Test-Estro-C	*up to 1 ml*	*IM*	*J1060*	
Testex	*up to 100 mg*	*IM*	*J3150*	
Testoject-50	*up to 50 mg*	*IM*	*J3140*	
Testoject-LA	*up to 100 mg*	*IM*	*J1070*	
	1 cc, 200 mg	*IM*	*J1080*	
Testone				
LA 200	*up to 100 mg*	*IM*	*J3120*	
	up to 200 mg	*IM*	*J3130*	
LA 100	*up to 100 mg*	*IM*	*J3120*	
	up to 200 mg	*IM*	*J3130*	
Testosterone	*up to 50 mg*		*J3140*	
Testosterone Aqueous	*up to 50 mg*	*IM*	*J3140*	
Testosterone enanthate and estradiol valerate	up to 1 cc	IM	**J0900**	
Testosterone enanthate	up to 100 mg	IM	**J3120**	
	up to 200 mg	IM	**J3130**	
Testosterone cypionate	up to 100 mg	IM	**J1070**	
	1 cc, 200 mg	IM	**J1080**	
Testosterone cypionate and estradiol cypionate	up to 1 ml	IM	**J1060**	
Testosterone propionate	up to 100 mg	IM	**J3150**	
Testosterone suspension	up to 50 mg	IM	**J3140**	
Testradiol 90/4	*up to 1 cc*	*IM*	*J0900*	

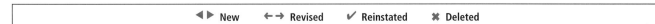

◄▶ New   ←→ Revised   ✔ Reinstated   ✖ Deleted

DRUG NAME	DOSAGE	METHOD OF ADMINISTRATION	HCPCS CODE
Testrin PA	up to 100 mg	IM	J3120
	up to 200 mg	IM	J3130
Testro AQ	up to 50 mg		J3140
Testro-L.A. 200	up to 200 mg		J3130
Tetanus immune globulin, human	up to 250 units	IM	J1670
Tetra-Con	up to 250 mg	IM, IV	J0120
Tetracycline	up to 250 mg	IM, IV	J0120
Tev-Tropin	1 mg		J2941
Thallous Chloride TI–201	per MCI		A9505
Theelin Aqueous	per 1 mg	IM	J1435
Theophylline	per 40 mg	IV	J2810
TheraCys	per vial	IV	J9031
Thiamine HCl	100 mg		J3411
Thiethylperazine maleate			
injection	up to 10 mg	IM	J3280
oral	10 mg	ORAL	Q0174
Thioplex	15 mg		J9340
Thiotepa	15 mg	IV	J9340
Thorazine	10 mg	ORAL	Q0171
	25 mg	ORAL	Q0172
	up to 50 mg		J3230, J8498
Thrombate III	per IU		J7197
Thymoglobulin, see Immune globin, anti-thymocyte			
	25 mg		J7511
Thypinone	per 250 mcg	IV	J2725
Thyprel TRH	per 250 mcg		J2725
Thyrel TRH	per 250 mcg		J2725
Thyrogen	0.9 mg	IM, SC	J3240
Thyrotropin Alfa, injection	0.9 mg	IM, SC	J3240
Tia-Doce S	up to 1,000 mcg		J3420
Tice BCG	per vial	IV	J9031
injection	up to 200 mg	IM	J3250
Ticon			
injection	up to 200 mg	IM	J3250
oral	250 mg	ORAL	Q0173
Tigan			
injection	up to 200 mg	IM	J3250
oral	250 mg	ORAL	Q0173
Tigecycline	1 mg		J3243

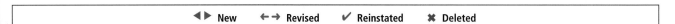

◀▶ New   ←→ Revised   ✔ Reinstated   ✖ Deleted

DRUG NAME	DOSAGE	METHOD OF ADMINISTRATION	HCPCS CODE	
Tiject-20	up to 200 mg	IM	J3250	
	250 mg	ORAL	Q0173	
Timentin			J3490	
Tinzaparin	1000 IU	SC	J1655	
Tirofiban Hydrochloride, injection	0.25 mg	IM, IV	J3246	
TissueMend	per square centimeter		Q4109	
TNKase	1 mg		~~J3100,~~ J3101	←
Tobi	300 mg	INH	J7682, J7685	
Tobramycin, inhalation solution	300 mg	INH	J7682, J7685	
Tobramycin sulfate	up to 80 mg	IM, IV	J3260	
Tofranil, see Imipramine HCl				
Tolazoline HCl	up to 25 mg	IV	J2670	
Toposar	10 mg		J9181	
Topotecan	0.25 mg	ORAL	J8705	◄
	4 mg	IV	J9350	
Toradol	per 15 mg	IM, IV	J1885	
Torecan	10 mg	ORAL	Q0174	
	up to 10 mg	IM	J3280	
Torisel	1 mg		J9330	
Tornalate				
concentrated form	per mg	INH	J7628	
unit dose	per mg	INH	J7629	
Torsemide	10 mg/ml	IV	J3265	
Tosylate			J3490	
Totacillin-N				
sodium	up to 500 mg	IM, IV	J0290	
sodium/sulbactam sodium	per 1.5 gm	IM, IV	J0295	
Tramacal	1 unit		B4154	
Tramonide 40	per 10 mg		J3301	
Trastuzumab	10 mg	IV	J9355	
Treanda	1 mg		J9033	
Trasylol	10,000 KIU		J0365	
Traumin-acid	1 unit		B4154	
Travasorb	1 unit		B4150	
Travasorb Hepatic	1 unit		B4154	
Travasorb HN	1 unit		B4153	
Travasorb MCT	1 unit		B4154	
Travasorb Renal	1 unit		B4154	
Travenol	500 ml		A4217	
Trelstar Depot	3.75 mg		J3315	
Trelstar LA	3.75 mg		J3315	

◄▶ New   ←→ Revised   ✔ Reinstated   ✖ Deleted

DRUG NAME	DOSAGE	METHOD OF ADMINISTRATION	HCPCS CODE
Treprostinil	1 mg		**J3285**
Trexall	*2.5 mg*	*ORAL*	*J8610*
	5 mg		*J9250*
	50 mg		*J9260*
Triethylenethosphoramide	*15 mg*		*J9340*
Tri-Kort	*1 mg*		*J3300*
	per 10 mg	*IM*	*J3301*
Triam-A	*1 mg*		*J3300*
	per 10 mg	*IM*	*J3301*
Triamcinolone			
concentrated form	per 1 mg	INH	**J7683**
unit dose	per 1 mg	INH	**J7684**
Triamcinolone acetonide	1 ~~10~~ mg	~~IM~~	**J3300**, ~~J3301~~
	per 10 mg	IM	**J3301**
Triamcinolone diacetate	per 5 mg	IM	**J3302**
Triamcinolone hexacetonide	per 5 mg	VAR	**J3303**
Triam ForteTristoject	*per 5 mg*		*J3302*
Triesence	*1 mg*		*J3300*
	per 10 mg	*IM*	*J3301*
Triflupromazine HCl	up to 20 mg	IM, IV	**J3400**
Tri-Kort	*per 10 mg*		*J3301*
Trilafon	*4 mg*	*ORAL*	*Q0175*
	8 mg	*ORAL*	*Q0176*
	up to 5 mg	*IM, IV*	*J3310*
Trilog	*1 mg*		*J3300*
	per 10 mg	*IM*	*J3301*
Trilone	*per 5 mg*		*J3302*
Trimethobenzamide HCl			
injection	up to 200 mg	IM	**J3250**
oral	250 mg	ORAL	**Q0173**
Trimetrexate glucuronate	per 25 mg	IV	**J3305**
Triptorelin Pamoate	3.75 mg		**J3315**
Trisenox	*1 mg*	*IV*	*J9017*
Trobicin	up to 2 g	IM	*J3320*
Trovan	*100 mg*	*IV*	*J0200*
Truxadryl	*50 mg*		*Q0163*
Twinject	*1 ml*		*J0170*
Twinrix			*J3490*
Tygacil	*1 mg*		*J3243*
Tysabri	*1 mg*		*J2323*
Tysabri	*1 mg*		*J2323*

◀▶ New   ←→ Revised   ✔ Reinstated   ✖ Deleted

DRUG NAME	DOSAGE	METHOD OF ADMINISTRATION	HCPCS CODE
U			
Ultra Filtered	*50 mcg*		*J2788*
Ultra Filtered Plus	*50 mcg*		*J2788*
Ultra-TechneKow	*per millicurie*		*A9512*
Ultravist 150	*per ml*		*Q9965*
Ultravist 240	*per ml*		*Q9966*
Ultravist 300	*per ml*		*Q9966*
Ultravist 370	*per ml*		*Q9967*
Ultrazine-10	*up to 10 mg*	*IM, IV*	*J0780*
Unasyn	*per 1.5 gm*	*IM, IV*	*J0295*
Unclassified drugs (see also **Not elsewhere classified**)			**J3490**
Unipen	*3 gm*		*S0032*
Unspecified oral antiemetic			**Q0181**
Urea	up to 40 g	IV	J3350
Ureaphil	*up to 40 g*	*IV*	*J3350*
Urecholine	*up to 5 mg*	*SC*	*J0520*
Urofollitropin	75 iu		**J3355**
Urokinase	5,000 IU vial	IV	J3364
	250,000 IU vial	IV	J3365
V			
V-Gan 25	*up to 50 mg*	*IM, IV*	*J2550*
	12.5 mg	*ORAL*	*Q0169*
	25 mg	*ORAL*	*Q0170*
V-Gan 50	*up to 50 mg*	*IM, IV*	*J2550*
	12.5 mg	*ORAL*	*Q0169*
	25 mg	*ORAL*	*Q0170*
Valergen			
	10 mg	*IM*	*J1380*
	20 mg	*IM*	*J1390*
	up to 40 mg	*IM*	*J0970*
Valergen 10	*10 mg*	*IM*	*J1380*
	20 mg	*IM*	*J1390*
	up to 40 mg	*IM*	*J0970*
Valergen 20	*10 mg*	*IM*	*J1380*
	20 mg	*IM*	*J1390*
	up to 40 mg	*IM*	*J0970*
Valergen 40	*up to 10 mg*	*IM*	*J1380*
	up to 20 mg	*IM*	*J1390*
	up to 40 mg	*IM*	*J0970*
Valertest No. 1	*up to 1 cc*	*IM*	*J0900*
			J1060

◄► New   ←→ Revised   ✔ Reinstated   ✖ Deleted

DRUG NAME	DOSAGE	METHOD OF ADMINISTRATION	HCPCS CODE
Valertest No. 2	up to 1 cc	IM	J0900
Valium	up to 5 mg	IM, IV	J3360
Valrubicin, intravesical	200 mg	OTH	**J9357**
Valstar	200 mg	OTH	J9357
Vanatrip	20 mg		J1320
Vanceril	per mg		J7622
Vancenase	per mg		J7622
Vancocin	500 mg	IV, IM	J3370
Vancoled	500 mg	IV, IM	J3370
Vancomycin HCl	500 mg	IV, IM	**J3370**
Vasceze	per 10 mg		J1642
Vasoxyl, see Methoxamine HCl			
Vazol	per 10 mg		J0945
Vectibix	10 mg		J9303
Velban	1 mg	IV	J9360
Velcade	0.1 mg		J9041
Velosulin BR (RDNA)	per 5 units		J1815
	per 50 units		J1817
Velsar	1 mg	IV	J9360
Venofer	1 mg	IV	J1756
Ventavis	20 mcg		Q4080
Ventolin	0.5 mg	INH	J7620
concentrated form	1 mg	INH	J7610, J7611
unit dose form	1 mg	INH	J7609, J7613
VePesid			
	10 mg	IV	J9181
	50 mg	ORAL	J8560
Versed	per 1 mg	IM, IV	J2250
Verteporfin	0.1 mg	IV	**J3396**
Vesolin BR	per 50 units		J1817
Vesprin	up to 20 mg	IM, IV	J3400
VFEND IV	10 mg		J3465
VGan	up to 50 mg		J2550
Viadur	65 mg		J9219
Vidaza	1 mg		J9025
Videx	25 mg		S0137
Viagra	25 mg		S0090
Vinblastine sulfate	1 mg	IV	**J9360**
Vincasar PFS	1 mg	IV	J9370
	2 mg	IV	J9375
	5 mg	IV	J9380

◄► New   ←→ Revised   ✔ Reinstated   ✖ Deleted

DRUG NAME	DOSAGE	METHOD OF ADMINISTRATION	HCPCS CODE
Vincristine sulfate	1 mg	IV	**J9370**
	2 mg	IV	**J9375**
	5 mg	IV	**J9380**
Vinorelbine tartrate	per 10 mg	IV	**J9390**
Virilon	200 mg		J1080
Vispaque 320	per ml		Q9967
Vistacot	up to 25 mg		J3410
Vistaject-25	up to 25 mg	IM	J3410
Vistaril	up to 25 mg	IM	J3410
	25 mg	ORAL	Q0177
	50 mg	ORAL	Q0178
Vistide	375 mg	IV	J0740
Visudyne	0.1 mg	IV	J3396
Vital (Vital HN)	1 unit		B4153
Vitamin B1	100 mg		J3411
Vitamin B6	100 mg		J2415
Vitamin K, phytonadione, menadione, menadiol sodium diphosphate	per 1 mg	IM, SC, IV	**J3430**
Vitamin B-12 cyanocobalamin	up to 1,000 mcg	IM, SC	**J3420**
Vitrase	up to 150 units		J3470
	per 1 USP unit		J3471
	per 1,000 USP units		J3472
Vitrasert	4.5 mg		J7310
Vitravene	1.65 mg		J1452
Vivitrol	1 mg		J2315
Vivonex HN	1 unit		B4153
Vivonex t.e.n.	1 unit		B4153
Von Willebrand Factor Complex, human	per IU VWF:RCo	IV	**J7187**
Voriconazole	10 mg		**J3465**
Vumon	50 mg		Q2017
W			
Water for Inhalation	10 ml		A4216
Water for Injection	10 ml		A4216
	500 ml		A4217
Water for irrigation	500 ml		A4217
Wehamine	up to 50 mg	IM, IV	J1240
Wehdryl	up to 50 mg	IM, IV	J1200
	50 mg	ORAL	Q0163
Wellbutrin SR Tablets	150 mg/ bottle of 60 tablets		S0106
Wellcovorin	per 50 mg	IM, IV	J0640
Win Rho SD	100 IU	IV	J2792

◀▶ New   ←→ Revised   ✔ Reinstated   ✖ Deleted

DRUG NAME	DOSAGE	METHOD OF ADMINISTRATION	HCPCS CODE
Wyamine Sulfate, see Mephentermine sulfate			
Wycillin	up to 600,000 units	IM, IV	J2510
Wydase	up to 150 units	SC, IV	J3470
X			
Xeloda	150 mg	ORAL	J8520
	500 mg	ORAL	J8521
Xolair	5 mg		J2357
Xopenex	0.5 mg	INH	J7620
concentrated form	1 mg	INH	J7610, J7611
unit dose form	1 mg	INH	J7609, J7613
Xylocaine HCl	10 mg	IV	J2001
Z			
Zanosar	1 gm	IV	J9320
Zantac	25 mg	IV, IM	J2780
Zemaira	10 mg	IV	J0256
Zemplar	1 mcg	IM, IV	J2501
Zenapax	25 mg	IV	J7513
Zetran	up to 5 mg	IM, IV	J3360
Zevalin	up to 5 millicurie		A9542
Ziconotide	1 mcg		**J2278**
Zidovudine	10 mg	IV	**J3485**
Zinacef	per 750 mg	IM, IV	J0697
Zinecard	500 mg		J1180
Ziprasidone Mesylate	10 mg		**J3486**
Zithromax	1 g	ORAL	Q0144
I.V.	500 mg	IV	J0456
Zmax	1 gm		Q0144
Zofran	1 mg	IV	J2405
	4 mg	ORAL	S0181
	8 mg	ORAL	Q0179
Zoladex	per 3.6 mg	SC	J9202
Zoledronic Acid	1 mg		**J3487**
Zolicef	500 mg	IV, IM	J0690
Zometa	1 mg		**J3487**
Zorbtive	1 mg		J2941
Zosyn	1.125 g	IV	J2543
Zovirax	5 mg		J0133, J8499
Zyprexa	2.5 mg		S0166
Zyvox	200 mg	IV	J2020

◄► New   ←→ Revised   ✔ Reinstated   ✖ Deleted

HCPCS 2009: LEVEL II NATIONAL CODES

2009 HCPCS quarterly updates available on the companion website at: http://evolve.elsevier.com/Buck/HCPCS/

DISCLAIMER

Every effort has been made to make this text complete and accurate, but no guarantee, warranty, or representation is made for its accuracy or completeness. This text is based on the Centers for Medicare and Medicaid Services Healthcare Common Procedure Coding System (HCPCS).

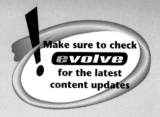

INTRODUCTION

2009 HCPCS quarterly updates available on the companion website at: http:/evolve.elsevier.com/Buck/HCPCS/.

The Centers for Medicare and Medicaid Services (CMS) (formerly Health Care Financing Administration [HCFA]) Healthcare Common Procedure Coding System (HCPCS) is a collection of codes and descriptors that represent procedures, supplies, products, and services that may be provided to Medicare beneficiaries and to individuals enrolled in private health insurance programs. The codes are divided as follows:

Level I: Codes and descriptors copyrighted by the American Medical Association's (AMA's) Current Procedural Terminology, ed. 4 (CPT-4). These are 5 position numeric codes representing physician and nonphysician services.

Level II: 5 position alpha-numeric codes representing primarily items and nonphysician services that are not represented in the Level I codes. Codes and descriptors copyrighted by the American Dental Association's current dental terminology, seventh edition (CDT 7/8), are 5 position alpha-numeric codes comprising the D series. **This book does not contain codes D0100 through D9999.** They can be purchased from the ADA. All other Level II codes and descriptors are approved and maintained jointly by the alpha-numeric editorial panel.

Level III: The CMS eliminated Level III local codes. See Program Memorandum AB-02-113.

Headings are provided as a means of grouping similar or closely related items. The placement of a code under a heading does not indicate additional means of classification, nor does it relate to any health insurance coverage categories.

HCPCS also contains modifiers, which are two-position codes and descriptors used to indicate that a service or procedure that has been performed has been altered by some specific circumstance but not changed in its definition or code. Modifiers are grouped by the levels. Level I modifiers and descriptors are copyrighted by the AMA. Level II modifiers are HCPCS modifiers. Modifiers in the D series are copyrighted by the ADA. **This book does not contain D series modifiers.**

HCPCS is designed to promote uniform reporting and statistical data collection of medical procedures, supplies, products, and services.

HCPCS Disclaimer

Inclusion or exclusion of a procedure, supply, product, or service does not imply any health insurance coverage or reimbursement policy.

HCPCS makes as much use as possible of generic descriptions, but the inclusion of brand names to describe devices or drugs is intended only for indexing purposes; it is not meant to convey endorsement of any particular product or drug.

Updating HCPCS

The primary updates are made annually. Quarterly updates are also issued by CMS.

Legend

◄▶ New
←→ Revised
✔ Reinstated
✖ Deleted
⊙ Special coverage instructions
◆ Not covered or valid by Medicare
✳ Carrier discretion
▶ ASC paid separately when provided integral to a surgical procedure on ASC list

The revised symbol is placed in front of items with data, payment, or miscellaneous changes. The ASC (Ambulatory Surgery Centers) symbol appears after the code.

◄▶ New	←→ Revised	✔ Reinstated	✖ Deleted
⊙ Special coverage instructions	◆ Not covered or valid by Medicare	✳ Carrier discretion	▶ ASC payment group

INTRODUCTION

LEVEL II NATIONAL MODIFIERS

✳ **A1**   Dressing for one wound

✳ **A2**   Dressing for two wounds

✳ **A3**   Dressing for three wounds

✳ **A4**   Dressing for four wounds

✳ **A5**   Dressing for five wounds

✳ **A6**   Dressing for six wounds

✳ **A7**   Dressing for seven wounds

✳ **A8**   Dressing for eight wounds

✳ **A9**   Dressing for nine or more wounds

✿ **AA**   Anesthesia services performed personally by anesthesiologist

IOM: 100-04, 12, 90.4

✿ **AD**   Medical supervision by a physician: more than four concurrent anesthesia procedures

IOM: 100-04, 12, 90.4

✳ **AE**   Registered dietician

✳ **AF**   Specialty physician

✳ **AG**   Primary physician

✿ **AH**   Clinical psychologist

IOM: 100-04, 12, 170

✿ **AJ**   Clinical social worker

IOM: 100-04, 12, 170

✳ **AK**   Nonparticipating physician

✿ **AM**   Physician, team member service

Cross Reference QM

✳ **AP**   Determination of refractive state was not performed in the course of diagnostic ophthalmological examination

✳ **AQ**   Physician providing a service in an unlisted health professional shortage area (HPSA)

✳ **AR**   Physician provider services in a physician scarcity area

✳ **AS**   Physician assistant, nurse practitioner, or clinical nurse specialist services for assistant at surgery

✳ **AT**   Acute treatment (this modifier should be used when reporting service 98940, 98941, 98942)

✳ **AU**   Item furnished in conjunction with a urological, ostomy, or tracheostomy supply

✳ **AV**   Item furnished in conjunction with a prosthetic device, prosthetic or orthotic

✳ **AW**   Item furnished in conjunction with a surgical dressing

✳ **AX**   Item furnished in conjunction with dialysis services

✳ **BA**   Item furnished in conjunction with parenteral enteral nutrition (PEN) services

✳ **BL**   Special acquisition of blood and blood products

✳ **BO**   Orally administered nutrition, not by feeding tube

✳ **BP**   The beneficiary has been informed of the purchase and rental options and has elected to purchase the item

✳ **BR**   The beneficiary has been informed of the purchase and rental options and has elected to rent the item

✳ **BU**   The beneficiary has been informed of the purchase and rental options and after 30 days has not informed the supplier of his/her decision

✳ **CA**   Procedure payable only in the inpatient setting when performed emergently on an outpatient who expires prior to admission

✳ **CB**   Service ordered by a renal dialysis facility (RDF) physician as part of the ESRD beneficiary's dialysis benefit, is not part of the composite rate, and is separately reimbursable

✳ **CC**   Procedure code change (Use 'CC' when the procedure code submitted was changed either for administrative reasons or because an incorrect code was filed)

✿ **CD**   AMCC test has been ordered by an ESRD facility or MCP physician that is part of the composite rate and is not separately billable

✿ **CE**   AMCC test has been ordered by an ESRD facility or MCP physician that is a composite rate test but is beyond the normal frequency covered under the rate and is separately reimbursable based on medical necessity

✿ **CF**   AMCC test has been ordered by an ESRD facility or MCP physician that is not part of the composite rate and is separately billable

▶ ✳ **CG**   Policy criteria applied

✳ **CR**   Catastrophe/Disaster related

✳ **E1**   Upper left, eyelid

✳ **E2**   Lower left, eyelid

✳ **E3**   Upper right, eyelid

◀▶ **New**   ←→ **Revised**   ✔ **Reinstated**   ✖ **Deleted**

✿ **Special coverage instructions**   ◆ **Not covered or valid by Medicare**   ✳ **Carrier discretion**   ▶ **ASC payment group**

✳ **E4** Lower right, eyelid

⊛ **EA** Erythropoetic stimulating agent (ESA) administered to treat anemia due to anti-cancer chemotherapy

⊛ **EB** Erythropoetic stimulating agent (ESA) administered to treat anemia due to anti-cancer radiotherapy

⊛ **EC** Erythropoetic stimulating agent (ESA) administered to treat anemia not due to anti-cancer radiotherapy or anti-cancer chemotherapy

⊛ **ED** Hematocrit level has exceeded 39% (or hemoglobin level has exceeded 13.0 g/dl) for 3 or more consecutive billing cycles immediately prior to and including the current cycle

⊛ **EE** Hematocrit level has not exceeded 39% (or hemoglobin level has not exceeded 13.0 g/dl) for 3 or more consecutive billing cycles immediately prior to and including the current cycle

⊛ **EJ** Subsequent claims for a defined course of therapy, e.g., EPO, sodium hyaluronate, infliximab

⊛ **EM** Emergency reserve supply (for ESRD benefit only)

✳ **EP** Service provided as part of Medicaid early periodic screening diagnosis and treatment (EPSDT) program

✳ **ET** Emergency services

✳ **EY** No physician or other licensed health care provider order for this item or service

✳ **F1** Left hand, second digit

✳ **F2** Left hand, third digit

✳ **F3** Left hand, fourth digit

✳ **F4** Left hand, fifth digit

✳ **F5** Right hand, thumb

✳ **F6** Right hand, second digit

✳ **F7** Right hand, third digit

✳ **F8** Right hand, fourth digit

✳ **F9** Right hand, fifth digit

✳ **FA** Left hand, thumb

◆ **FB** Item provided without cost to provider, supplier or practitioner, or full credit received for replaced device (examples, but not limited to, covered under warranty, replaced due to defect, free samples)

⊛ **FC** Partial credit received for replaced device

✳ **FP** Service provided as part of family planning program

✳ **G1** Most recent URR reading of less than 60

✳ **G2** Most recent URR reading of 60 to 64.9

✳ **G3** Most recent URR reading of 65 to 69.9

✳ **G4** Most recent URR reading of 70 to 74.9

✳ **G5** Most recent URR reading of 75 or greater

✳ **G6** ESRD patient for whom less than six dialysis sessions have been provided in a month

⊛ **G7** Pregnancy resulted from rape or incest or pregnancy certified by physician as life threatening

IOM: 100-02, 15, 20.1; 100-03, 3, 170.3

✳ **G8** Monitored anesthesia care (MAC) for deep complex, complicated, or markedly invasive surgical procedure

✳ **G9** Monitored anesthesia care for patient who has history of severe cardiopulmonary condition

✳ **GA** Waiver of liability statement on file

✳ **GB** Claim being resubmitted for payment because it is no longer covered under a global payment demonstration

⊛ **GC** This service has been performed in part by a resident under the direction of a teaching physician.

IOM: 100-04, 12, 90.4

✳ **GD** Units of service exceeds medically unlikely edit value and represents reasonable and necessary services

⊛ **GE** This service has been performed by a resident without the presence of a teaching physician under the primary care exception

✳ **GF** Non-physician (e.g. nurse practitioner (NP), certified registered nurse anesthetist (CRNA), certified registered nurse (CRN), clinical nurse specialist (CNS), physician assistant (PA)) services in a critical access hospital

✳ **GG** Performance and payment of a screening mammogram and diagnostic mammogram on the same patient, same day

✳ **GH** Diagnostic mammogram converted from screening mammogram on same day

✳ **GJ** "Opt out" physician or practitioner emergency or urgent service

---

◀ ▶ New   ← → Revised   ✓ Reinstated   ✺ Deleted

⊛ Special coverage instructions   ◆ Not covered or valid by Medicare   ✳ Carrier discretion   ▶ ASC payment group

* **GK** Reasonable and necessary item/service associated with a GA or GZ modifier

* **GL** Medically unnecessary upgrade provided instead of non-upgraded item, no charge, no Advance Beneficiary Notice (ABN)

* **GM** Multiple patients on one ambulance trip

* **GN** Services delivered under an outpatient speech language pathology plan of care

* **GO** Services delivered under an outpatient occupational therapy plan of care

* **GP** Services delivered under an outpatient physical therapy plan of care

* **GQ** Via asynchronous telecommunications system

* **GR** This service was performed in whole or in part by a resident in a department of Veterans Affairs medical center or clinic, supervised in accordance with VA policy

☺ **GS** Dosage of EPO or darbepoetin alfa has been reduced and maintained in response to hematocrit or hemoglobin level

☺ **GT** Via interactive audio and video telecommunication systems

☺ **GV** Attending physician not employed or paid under arrangement by the patient's hospice provider

☺ **GW** Service not related to the hospice patient's terminal condition

◆ **GY** Item or service statutorily excluded, does not meet the definition of any Medicare benefit or, for non-Medicare insurers, is not a contract benefit

◆ **GZ** Item or service expected to be denied as not reasonable or necessary

◆ **H9** Court-ordered

◆ **HA** Child/adolescent program

◆ **HB** Adult program, nongeriatric

◆ **HC** Adult program, geriatric

◆ **HD** Pregnant/parenting women's program

◆ **HE** Mental health program

◆ **HF** Substance abuse program

◆ **HG** Opioid addiction treatment program

◆ **HH** Integrated mental health/substance abuse program

◆ **HI** Integrated mental health and mental retardation/developmental disabilities program

◆ **HJ** Employee assistance program

◆ **HK** Specialized mental health programs for high-risk populations

◆ **HL** Intern

◆ **HM** Less than bachelor degree level

◆ **HN** Bachelors degree level

◆ **HO** Masters degree level

◆ **HP** Doctoral level

◆ **HQ** Group setting

◆ **HR** Family/couple with client present

◆ **HS** Family/couple without client present

◆ **HT** Multi-disciplinary team

◆ **HU** Funded by child welfare agency

◆ **HV** Funded state addictions agency

◆ **HW** Funded by state mental health agency

◆ **HX** Funded by county/local agency

◆ **HY** Funded by juvenile justice agency

◆ **HZ** Funded by criminal justice agency

* **J1** Competitive acquisition program no-pay submission for a prescription number

* **J2** Competitive acquisition program, restocking of emergency drugs after emergency administration

* **J3** Competitive acquisition program (CAP), drug not available through CAP as written, reimbursed under average sales price methodology

* **JA** Administered intravenously

* **JB** Administered subcutaneously

▶ * **JC** Skin substitute used as a graft

▶ * **JD** Skin substitute not used as a graft

* **JW** Drug amount discarded/not administered to any patient

* **K0** Lower extremity prosthesis functional Level 0 - does not have the ability or potential to ambulate or transfer safely with or without assistance and a prosthesis does not enhance their quality of life or mobility

* **K1** Lower extremity prosthesis functional Level 1 - has the ability or potential to use a prosthesis for transfers or ambulation on level surfaces at fixed cadence. Typical of the limited and unlimited household ambulator.

◀▶ New ←→ Revised ✔ Reinstated ✖ Deleted
☺ Special coverage instructions ◆ Not covered or valid by Medicare * Carrier discretion ▶ ASC payment group

* **K2**   Lower extremity prosthesis functional Level 2 - has the ability or potential for ambulation with the ability to traverse low level environmental barriers such as curbs, stairs or uneven surfaces. Typical of the limited community ambulator.

* **K3**   Lower extremity prosthesis functional Level 3 - has the ability or potential for ambulation with variable cadence. Typical of the community ambulator who has the ability to traverse most environmental barriers and may have vocational, therapeutic, or exercise activity that demands prosthetic utilization beyond simple locomotion.

* **K4**   Lower extremity prosthesis functional Level 4 - has the ability or potential for prosthetic ambulation that exceeds the basic ambulation skills, exhibiting high impact, stress, or energy levels, typical of the prosthetic demands of the child, active adult, or athlete.

* **KA**   Add on option/accessory for wheelchair

* **KB**   Beneficiary requested upgrade for ABN, more than 4 modifiers identified on claim

* **KC**   Replacement of special power wheelchair interface

* **KD**   Drug or biological infused through DME

▶ * **KE**   Bid under round one of the DMEPOS competitive bidding program for use with non-competitive bid base equipment

* **KF**   Item designated by FDA as Class III device

* **KG**   DMEPOS item subject to DMEPOS competitive bidding program number 1

* **KH**   DMEPOS item, initial claim, purchase or first month rental

* **KI**   DMEPOS item, second or third month rental

* **KJ**   DMEPOS item, parenteral enteral nutrition (PEN) pump or capped rental, months four to fifteen

* **KK**   DMEPOS item subject to DMEPOS competitive bidding program number 2

→ * **KL**   DMEPOS item delivered via mail

* **KM**   Replacement of facial prosthesis including new impression/moulage

* **KN**   Replacement of facial prosthesis using previous master model

* **KO**   Single drug unit dose formulation

* **KP**   First drug of a multiple drug unit dose formulation

* **KQ**   Second or subsequent drug of a multiple drug unit dose formulation

* **KR**   Rental item, billing for partial month

◎ **KS**   Glucose monitor supply for diabetic beneficiary not treated with insulin

→ * **KT**   Beneficiary resides in a competitive bidding area and travels outside that competitive bidding area and receives a competitive bid item

* **KU**   DMEPOS item subject to DMEPOS competitive bidding program number 3

* **KV**   DMEPOS item subject to DMEPOS competitive bidding program that is furnished as part of a professional service

* **KW**   DMEPOS item subject to DMEPOS competitive bidding program number 4

* **KX**   Requirements specified in the medical policy have been met

* **KY**   DMEPOS item subject to DMEPOS competitive bidding program number 5

* **KZ**   New coverage not implemented by managed care

* **LC**   Left circumflex coronary artery

* **LD**   Left anterior descending coronary artery

* **LL**   Lease/rental (use the 'LL' modifier when DME equipment rental is to be applied against the purchase price)

* **LR**   Laboratory round trip

◎ **LS**   FDA-monitored intraocular lens implant

* **LT**   Left side (used to identify procedures performed on the left side of the body)

* **M2**   Medicare secondary payer (MSP)

* **MS**   Six month maintenance and servicing fee for reasonable and necessary parts and labor which are not covered under any manufacturer or supplier warranty

* **NR**   New when rented (use the NR modifier when DME which was new at the time of rental is subsequently purchased)

* **NU**   New equipment

* **P1**   A normal healthy patient

* **P2**   A patient with mild systemic disease

* **P3**   A patient with severe systemic disease

* **P4**   A patient with severe systemic disease that is a constant threat to life

---

◀▶ New   ←→ Revised   ✔ Reinstated   ✖ Deleted

◎ Special coverage instructions   ◆ Not covered or valid by Medicare   * Carrier discretion   ▶ ASC payment group

* **P5**   A moribund patient who is not expected to survive without the operation

* **P6**   A declared brain-dead patient whose organs are being removed for donor purposes

* **PL**   Progressive addition lenses

☼ **Q0**   Investigational clinical service provided in a clinical research study that is in an approved clinical research study

☼ **Q1**   Routine clinical service provided in a clinical research study that is in an approved clinical research study

* **Q2**   HCFA/ORD demonstration project procedure/service

* **Q3**   Live kidney donor surgery and related services

* **Q4**   Service for ordering/referring physician qualifies as a service exemption

☼ **Q5**   Service furnished by a substitute physician under a reciprocal billing arrangement

IOM: 100-04, 1, 30.2.10

☼ **Q6**   Service furnished by a locum tenens physician

IOM: 100-04, 1, 30.2.11

* **Q7**   One Class A finding

* **Q8**   Two Class B findings

* **Q9**   One Class B and two Class C findings

* **QC**   Single channel monitoring

* **QD**   Recording and storage in solid state memory by a digital recorder

* **QE**   Prescribed amount of oxygen is less than 1 liter per minute (LPM)

* **QF**   Prescribed amount of oxygen exceeds 4 liters per minute (LPM) and portable oxygen is prescribed

* **QG**   Prescribed amount of oxygen is greater than 4 liters per minute (LPM)

* **QH**   Oxygen conserving device is being used with an oxygen delivery system

☼ **QJ**   Services/items provided to a prisoner or patient in state or local custody, however the state or local government, as applicable, meets the requirements in 42 CFR 411.4 (B)

☼ **QK**   Medical direction of two, three, or four concurrent anesthesia procedures involving qualified individuals

IOM: 100-04, 12, 90

* **QL**   Patient pronounced dead after ambulance called

* **QM**   Ambulance service provided under arrangement by a provider of services

* **QN**   Ambulance service furnished directly by a provider of services

☼ **QP**   Documentation is on file showing that the laboratory test(s) was ordered individually or ordered as a CPT-recognized panel other than automated profile codes 80002-80019, G0058, G0059, and G0060.

☼ **QS**   Monitored anesthesia care service

IOM: 100-04, 12, 30.6

* **QT**   Recording and storage on tape by an analog tape recorder

* **QW**   CLIA-waived test

* **QX**   CRNA service: with medical direction by a physician

☼ **QY**   Medical direction of one certified registered nurse anesthetist (CRNA) by an anesthesiologist

IOM: 100-04, 12, 90

* **QZ**   CRNA service: without medical direction by a physician

▶ * **RA**   Replacement of a DME item

▶ * **RB**   Replacement of a part of DME furnished as part of a repair

* **RC**   Right coronary artery

* **RD**   Drug provided to beneficiary, but not administered "incident-to"

▶ * **RE**   Furnished in full compliance with FDA-mandated risk evaluation and mitigation strategy (REMS)

~~**RP**   Replacement and repair RP may be used to indicate replacement of DME, orthotic and prosthetic devices which have been in use for sometime. The claim shows the code for the part, followed by the 'RP' modifier and the charge for the part.~~ ✖

* **RR**   Rental (use the 'RR' modifier when DME is to be rented)

* **RT**   Right side (used to identify procedures performed on the right side of the body)

◆ **SA**   Nurse practitioner rendering service in collaboration with a physician

◆ **SB**   Nurse midwife

◆ **SC** Medically necessary service or supply

◆ **SD** Services provided by registered nurse with specialized, highly technical home infusion training

◆ **SE** State and/or federally funded programs/services

✳ **SF** Second opinion ordered by a professional review organization (PRO) per Section 9401, P.L. 99-272 (100% reimbursement - no Medicare deductible or coinsurance)

✳ **SG** Ambulatory surgical center (ASC) facility service

◆ **SH** Second concurrently administered infusion therapy

◆ **SJ** Third or more concurrently administered infusion therapy

◆ **SK** Member of high risk population (use only with codes for immunization)

◆ **SL** State supplied vaccine

◆ **SM** Second surgical opinion

◆ **SN** Third surgical opinion

◆ **SQ** Item ordered by home health

◆ **SS** Home infusion services provided in the infusion suite of the IV therapy provider

◆ **ST** Related to trauma or injury

◆ **SU** Procedure performed in physician's office (to denote use of facility and equipment)

◆ **SV** Pharmaceuticals delivered to patient's home but not utilized

✳ **SW** Services provided by a certified diabetic educator

◆ **SY** Persons who are in close contact with member of high-risk population (use only with codes for immunization)

✳ **T1** Left foot, second digit

✳ **T2** Left foot, third digit

✳ **T3** Left foot, fourth digit

✳ **T4** Left foot, fifth digit

✳ **T5** Right foot, great toe

✳ **T6** Right foot, second digit

✳ **T7** Right foot, third digit

✳ **T8** Right foot, fourth digit

✳ **T9** Right foot, fifth digit

✳ **TA** Left foot, great toe

✳ **TC** Technical component. Under certain circumstances, a charge may be made for the technical component alone. Under those circumstances the technical component charge is identified by adding modifier 'TC' to the usual procedure number. Technical component charges are institutional charges and not billed separately by physicians. However, portable x-ray suppliers only bill for technical component and should utilize modifier TC. The charge data from portable x-ray suppliers will then be used to build customary and prevailing profiles.

◆ **TD** RN

◆ **TE** LPN/LVN

◆ **TF** Intermediate level of care

◆ **TG** Complex/high tech level of care

◆ **TH** Obstetrical treatment/services, prenatal or postpartum

◆ **TJ** Program group, child and/or adolescent

◆ **TK** Extra patient or passenger, non-ambulance

◆ **TL** Early intervention/individualized family service plan (IFSP)

◆ **TM** Individualized education program (IEP)

◆ **TN** Rural/outside providers' customary service area

◆ **TP** Medical transport, unloaded vehicle

◆ **TQ** Basic life support transport by a volunteer ambulance provider

◆ **TR** School-based individual education program (IEP) services provided outside the public school district responsible for the student

✳ **TS** Follow-up service

◆ **TT** Individualized service provided to more than one patient in same setting

◆ **TU** Special payment rate, overtime

◆ **TV** Special payment rates, holidays/weekends

◆ **TW** Back-up equipment

◆ **U1** Medicaid Level of Care 1, as defined by each State

◆ **U2** Medicaid Level of Care 2, as defined by each State

◆ **U3** Medicaid Level of Care 3, as defined by each State

◆ **U4** Medicaid Level of Care 4, as defined by each State

LEVEL II NATIONAL MODIFIERS

◀▶ New ← → Revised ✔ Reinstated ✖ Deleted
⊚ Special coverage instructions ◆ Not covered or valid by Medicare ✳ Carrier discretion ▶ ASC payment group

◆ **U5**   Medicaid Level of Care 5, as defined by each State

◆ **U6**   Medicaid Level of Care 6, as defined by each State

◆ **U7**   Medicaid Level of Care 7, as defined by each State

◆ **U8**   Medicaid Level of Care 8, as defined by each State

◆ **U9**   Medicaid Level of Care 9, as defined by each State

◆ **UA**   Medicaid Level of Care 10, as defined by each State

◆ **UB**   Medicaid Level of Care 11, as defined by each State

◆ **UC**   Medicaid Level of Care 12, as defined by each State

◆ **UD**   Medicaid Level of Care 13, as defined by each State

✳ **UE**   Used durable medical equipment

◆ **UF**   Services provided in the morning

◆ **UG**   Services provided in the afternoon

◆ **UH**   Services provided in the evening

◆ **UJ**   Services provided at night

◆ **UK**   Services provided on behalf of the client to someone other than the client (collateral relationship)

✳ **UN**   Two patients served

✳ **UP**   Three patients served

✳ **UQ**   Four patients served

✳ **UR**   Five patients served

✳ **US**   Six or more patients served

✳ **VP**   Aphakic patient

Ambulance Modifiers

Modifiers that are used on claims for ambulance services are created by combining two alpha characters. Each alpha character, with the exception of X, represents an origin (source) code or a destination code. The pair of alpha codes creates one modifier. The first position alpha-code = origin; the second position alpha-code = destination. On form CMS-1491, used to report ambulance services, Item 12 should contain the origin code and Item 13 should contain the destination code. Origin and destination codes and their descriptions are as follows:

D	Diagnostic or therapeutic site other than P or H when these are used as origin codes
E	Residential, domiciliary, custodial facility (other than an 1819 facility)
G	Hospital-based dialysis facility (hospital or hospital related)
H	Hospital
I	Site of transfer (e.g., airport or helicopter pad) between modes of ambulance transport
J	Non–hospital-based dialysis facility
N	Skilled nursing facility (SNF) (1819 facility)
P	Physician's office (includes HMO non-hospital facility, clinic, etc.)
R	Residence
S	Scene of accident or acute event
X	Destination code only. Intermediate stop at physician's office en route to the hospital (includes non-hospital facility, clinic, etc.)

TRANSPORT SERVICES INCLUDING AMBULANCE (A0000-A0999)

◆ **A0021**   Ambulance service, outside state per mile, transport (Medicaid only)
Cross Reference A0030

◆ **A0080**   Non-emergency transportation, per mile - vehicle provided by volunteer (individual or organization), with no vested interest

◆ **A0090**   Non-emergency transportation, per mile - vehicle provided by individual (family member, self, neighbor) with vested interest

◆ **A0100**   Non-emergency transportation; taxi

◆ **A0110**   Non-emergency transportation and bus, intra or inter state carrier

◆ **A0120**   Non-emergency transportation: mini-bus, mountain area transports, or other transportation systems

◆ **A0130**   Non-emergency transportation: wheel chair van

◆ **A0140**   Non-emergency transportation and air travel (private or commercial), intra or inter state

◆ **A0160**   Non-emergency transportation: per mile - caseworker or social worker

◆ **A0170**   Transportation: ancillary: parking fees, tolls, other

◆ **A0180**   Non-emergency transportation: ancillary: lodging - recipient

◆ **A0190**   Non-emergency transportation: ancillary: meals - recipient

◆ **A0200**   Non-emergency transportation: ancillary: lodging - escort

◆ **A0210**   Non-emergency transportation: ancillary: meals - escort

◆ **A0225**   Ambulance service, neonatal transport, base rate, emergency transport, one way

◆ **A0380**   BLS mileage (per mile)
Cross Reference A0425

✳ **A0382**   BLS routine disposable supplies

✳ **A0384**   BLS specialized service disposable supplies; defibrillation (used by ALS ambulances and BLS ambulances in jurisdictions where defibrillation is permitted in BLS ambulances)

◆ **A0390**   ALS mileage (per mile)
Cross Reference A0425

✳ **A0392**   ALS specialized service disposable supplies; defibrillation (to be used only in jurisdictions where defibrillation cannot be performed in BLS ambulances)

✳ **A0394**   ALS specialized service disposable supplies; IV drug therapy

✳ **A0396**   ALS specialized service disposable supplies; esophageal intubation

✳ **A0398**   ALS routine disposable supplies

✳ **A0420**   Ambulance waiting time (ALS or BLS), one half (½) hour increments

Waiting Time Table			
UNITS	TIME	UNITS	TIME
1	½ to 1 hr.	6	3 to 3½ hrs.
2	1 to 1½ hrs.	7	3½ to 4 hrs.
3	1½ to 2 hrs.	8	4 to 4½ hrs.
4	2 to 2½ hrs.	9	4½ to 5 hrs.
5	2½ to 3 hrs.	10	5 to 5½ hrs.

◀▶ New   ←→ Revised   ✔ Reinstated   ✖ Deleted
☺ Special coverage instructions   ◆ Not covered or valid by Medicare   ✳ Carrier discretion   ▶ ASC payment group

✳ **A0422** Ambulance (ALS or BLS) oxygen and oxygen supplies, life sustaining situation

✳ **A0424** Extra ambulance attendant, ground (ALS or BLS) or air (fixed or rotary winged); (requires medical review)

✳ **A0425** Ground mileage, per statute mile

✳ **A0426** Ambulance service, advanced life support, non-emergency transport, Level 1 (ALS1)

✳ **A0427** Ambulance service, advanced life support, emergency transport, Level 1 (ALS1-Emergency)

✳ **A0428** Ambulance service, basic life support, non-emergency transport (BLS)

✳ **A0429** Ambulance service, basic life support, emergency transport (BLS-Emergency)

✳ **A0430** Ambulance service, conventional air services, transport, one way (fixed wing)

✳ **A0431** Ambulance service, conventional air services, transport, one way (rotary wing)

✳ **A0432** Paramedic intercept (PI), rural area, transport furnished by a volunteer ambulance company, which is prohibited by state law from billing third party payers

✳ **A0433** Advanced life support, Level 2 (ALS2)

✳ **A0434** Specialty care transport (SCT)

✳ **A0435** Fixed wing air mileage, per statute mile

✳ **A0436** Rotary wing air mileage, per statute mile

◆ **A0888** Noncovered ambulance mileage, per mile (e.g., for miles traveled beyond closest appropriate facility) MCM 2125

◆ **A0998** Ambulance response and treatment, no transport
IOM: 100-02, 10, 20

⊘ **A0999** Unlisted ambulance service
IOM: 100-02, 10, 20

MEDICAL AND SURGICAL SUPPLIES (A4000-A9999)

✳ **A4206** Syringe with needle, sterile 1cc or less, each

✳ **A4207** Syringe with needle, sterile 2cc, each

✳ **A4208** Syringe with needle, sterile 3cc, each

✳ **A4209** Syringe with needle, sterile 5cc or greater, each

◆ **A4210** Needle-free injection device, each
IOM: 100-03, 4, 280.1

⊘ **A4211** Supplies for self-administered injections
IOM: 100-02, 15, 50

✳ **A4212** Non-coring needle or stylet with or without catheter

✳ **A4213** Syringe, sterile, 20 cc or greater, each

✳ **A4215** Needle, sterile, any size, each

⊘ **A4216** Sterile water, saline and/or dextrose diluent/flush, 10 ml

Other: Sodium Chloride, Water for Injection, BD Posiflush, Monoject Prefill advanced, HSA Sterile Diluent, Sodium Chloride/Respiratory therapy, Water for Inhalation, Saline Solution, Broncho Saline, Syrex, Normal Saline IV Flush Syringe

IOM: 100-02, 15, 50

⊘ **A4217** Sterile water/saline, 500 ml

Other: Water for Injection, Sodium Chloride, Water for Irrigation, Travenol, Curity Sterile Water, Curity Sterile Saline

IOM: 100-02, 15, 50

⊘ **A4218** Sterile saline or water, metered dose dispenser, 10 ml

⊘ **A4220** Refill kit for implantable infusion pump
IOM: 100-03, 4, 280.14

✳ **A4221** Supplies for maintenance of drug infusion catheter, per week (list drug separately)

✳ **A4222** Infusion supplies for external drug infusion pump, per cassette or bag (list drug separately)

✳ **A4223** Infusion supplies not used with external infusion pump, per cassette or bag (list drugs separately)
IOM: 100-03, 4, 280.14

⊘ **A4230** Infusion set for external insulin pump, non-needle cannula type

(Requires prior authorization and copy of invoice)

IOM: 100-03, 4, 280.14

⊘ **A4231** Infusion set for external insulin pump, needle type

(Requires prior authorization and copy of invoice)

IOM: 100-03, 4, 280.14

◆ **A4232** Syringe with needle for external insulin pump, sterile, 3cc
IOM: 100-03, 4, 280.14

✳ **A4233** Replacement battery, alkaline (other than J cell), for use with medically necessary home blood glucose monitor owned by patient, each

---

◀ ▶ **New**   ← → **Revised**   ✔ **Reinstated**   ✖ **Deleted**

⊘ **Special coverage instructions**   ◆ **Not covered or valid by Medicare**   ✳ **Carrier discretion**   ▌ **ASC payment group**

MEDICAL AND SURGICAL SUPPLIES

＊ **A4234** Replacement battery, alkaline, J cell, for use with medically necessary home blood glucose monitor owned by patient, each

＊ **A4235** Replacement battery, lithium, for use with medically necessary home blood glucose monitor owned by patient, each

＊ **A4236** Replacement battery, silver oxide, for use with medically necessary home blood glucose monitor owned by patient, each

＊ **A4244** Alcohol or peroxide, per pint

＊ **A4245** Alcohol wipes, per box

＊ **A4246** Betadine or pHisoHex solution, per pint

＊ **A4247** Betadine or iodine swabs/wipes, per box

＊ **A4248** Chlorhexidine containing antiseptic, 1 ml

◆ **A4250** Urine test or reagent strips or tablets (100 tablets or strips)

IOM: 100-02, 15, 110

◆ **A4252** Blood ketone test or reagent strip, each Medicare Statute 1861(n)

❂ **A4253** Blood glucose test or reagent strips for home blood glucose monitor, per 50 strips

IOM: 100-03, 1, 40.2

❂ **A4254** Glucose monitor owned by patient, each

IOM: 100-03, 1, 40.2

❂ **A4255** Platforms for home blood glucose monitor, 50 per box

IOM: 100-03, 1, 40.2

❂ **A4256** Normal, low and high calibrator solution/chips

IOM: 100-03, 1, 40.2

＊ **A4257** Replacement lens shield cartridge for use with laser skin piercing device, each

❂ **A4258** Spring-powered device for lancet, each

IOM: 100-03, 1, 40.2

❂ **A4259** Lancets, per box of 100

IOM: 100-03, 1, 40.2

◆ **A4261** Cervical cap for contraceptive use Medicare Statute 1862a1

❂ **A4262** Temporary, absorbable lacrimal duct implant, each

❂ **A4263** Permanent, long term, non-dissolvable lacrimal duct implant, each

IOM: 100-04, 12, 30.4

❂ **A4265** Paraffin, per pound

IOM: 100-03, 4, 280.1

◆ **A4266** Diaphragm for contraceptive use

◆ **A4267** Contraceptive supply, condom, male, each

(Provider must bill at least 10 units at a time)

◆ **A4268** Contraceptive supply, condom, female, each

(Provider must bill at least 10 units at a time)

◆ **A4269** Contraceptive supply, spermicide (e.g., foam, gel), each

＊ **A4270** Disposable endoscope sheath, each

＊ **A4280** Adhesive skin support attachment for use with external breast prosthesis, each

＊ **A4281** Tubing for breast pump, replacement

＊ **A4282** Adapter for breast pump, replacement

＊ **A4283** Cap for breast pump bottle, replacement

＊ **A4284** Breast shield and splash protector for use with breast pump, replacement

＊ **A4285** Polycarbonate bottle for use with breast pump, replacement

＊ **A4286** Locking ring for breast pump, replacement

＊ **A4290** Sacral nerve stimulation test lead, each

Vascular Catheters

❂ **A4300** Implantable access catheter, (e.g., venous, arterial, epidural subarachnoid, or peritoneal, etc.) external access

IOM: 100-02, 15, 120

＊ **A4301** Implantable access total; catheter, port/reservoir (e.g., venous, arterial, epidural, subarachnoid, peritoneal, etc.)

＊ **A4305** Disposable drug delivery system, flow rate of 50 ml or greater per hour

＊ **A4306** Disposable drug delivery system, flow rate of less than 50 ml per hour

Incontinence Appliances and Care Supplies

❂ **A4310** Insertion tray without drainage bag and without catheter (accessories only)

IOM: 100-02, 15, 20

❂ **A4311** Insertion tray without drainage bag with indwelling catheter, Foley type, two-way latex with coating (Teflon, silicone, silicone elastomer, or hydrophilic, etc.)

IOM: 100-02, 15, 20

◀▶ New   ←→ Revised   ✔ Reinstated   ✖ Deleted

❂ Special coverage instructions   ◆ Not covered or valid by Medicare   ＊ Carrier discretion   ▶ ASC payment group

⚙ **A4312**   Insertion tray without drainage bag with indwelling catheter, Foley type, two-way, all silicone
IOM: 100-02, 15, 20

⚙ **A4313**   Insertion tray without drainage bag with indwelling catheter, Foley type, three-way, for continuous irrigation
IOM: 100-02, 15, 20

⚙ **A4314**   Insertion tray with drainage bag with indwelling catheter, Foley type, two-way latex with coating (Teflon, silicone, silicone elastomer or hydrophilic, etc.)
IOM: 100-02, 15, 20

⚙ **A4315**   Insertion tray with drainage bag with indwelling catheter, Foley type, two-way, all silicone
IOM: 100-02, 15, 20

⚙ **A4316**   Insertion tray with drainage bag with indwelling catheter, Foley type, three-way, for continuous irrigation
IOM: 100-02, 15, 20

⚙ **A4320**   Irrigation tray with bulb or piston syringe, any purpose
IOM: 100-02, 15, 20

⚙ **A4321**   Therapeutic agent for urinary catheter irrigation

⚙ **A4322**   Irrigation syringe, bulb, or piston, each
IOM: 100-02, 15, 20

⚙ **A4326**   Male external catheter with integral collection chamber, any type, each
IOM: 100-02, 15, 20

⚙ **A4327**   Female external urinary collection device; meatal cup, each
IOM: 100-02, 15, 20

⚙ **A4328**   Female external urinary collection device; pouch, each
IOM: 100-02, 15, 20

⚙ **A4330**   Perianal fecal collection pouch with adhesive, each
IOM: 100-02, 15, 20

⚙ **A4331**   Extension drainage tubing, any type, any length, with connector/adaptor, for use with urinary leg bag or urostomy pouch, each
IOM: 100-02, 15, 20

⚙ **A4332**   Lubricant, individual sterile packet, each
IOM: 100-02, 15, 20

⚙ **A4333**   Urinary catheter anchoring device, adhesive skin attachment, each
IOM: 100-02, 15, 20

⚙ **A4334**   Urinary catheter anchoring device, leg strap, each
IOM: 100-02, 15, 20

⚙ **A4335**   Incontinence supply; miscellaneous
IOM: 100-02, 15, 20

⚙ **A4338**   Indwelling catheter; Foley type, two-way latex with coating (Teflon, silicone, silicone elastomer, or hydrophilic, etc.), each
IOM: 100-02, 15, 20

⚙ **A4340**   Indwelling catheter; specialty type (e.g., coude, mushroom, wing, etc.), each
IOM: 100-02, 15, 20

⚙ **A4344**   Indwelling catheter, Foley type, two-way, all silicone, each
IOM: 100-02, 15, 20

⚙ **A4346**   Indwelling catheter; Foley type, three way for continuous irrigation, each
IOM: 100-02, 15, 20

⚙ **A4349**   Male external catheter, with or without adhesive, disposable, each
IOM: 100-02, 15, 20

⚙ **A4351**   Intermittent urinary catheter; straight tip, with or without coating (Teflon, silicone, silicone elastomer, or hydrophilic, etc.), each
IOM: 100-02, 15, 20

⚙ **A4352**   Intermittent urinary catheter; coude (curved) tip, with or without coating (Teflon, silicone, silicone elastomeric, or hydrophilic, etc.), each
IOM: 100-02, 15, 20

⚙ **A4353**   Intermittent urinary catheter, with insertion supplies
IOM: 100-02, 15, 20

⚙ **A4354**   Insertion tray with drainage bag but without catheter
IOM: 100-02, 15, 20

⚙ **A4355**   Irrigation tubing set for continuous bladder irrigation through a three-way indwelling Foley catheter, each
IOM: 100-02, 15, 20

External Urinary Supplies

⚙ **A4356**   External urethral clamp or compression device (not to be used for catheter clamp), each
IOM: 100-02, 15, 20

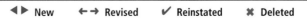

◄ ► New   ← → Revised   ✔ Reinstated   ✖ Deleted
⚙ Special coverage instructions   ◆ Not covered or valid by Medicare   ✳ Carrier discretion   ▶ ASC payment group

⊕ **A4357** Bedside drainage bag, day or night, with or without anti-reflux device, with or without tube, each

IOM: 100-02, 15, 20

⊕ **A4358** Urinary drainage bag, leg or abdomen, vinyl, with or without tube, with straps, each

IOM: 100-02, 15, 20

Ostomy Supplies

⊕ **A4361** Ostomy faceplate, each

IOM: 100-02, 15, 20

⊕ **A4362** Skin barrier; solid, 4 × 4 or equivalent; each

IOM: 100-02, 15, 20

⊕ **A4363** Ostomy clamp, any type, replacement only, each

⊕ **A4364** Adhesive, liquid or equal, any type, per oz

IOM: 100-02, 15, 20

⊕ **A4365** Adhesive remover wipes, any type, per 50

IOM: 100-02, 15, 20

✳ **A4366** Ostomy vent, any type, each

⊕ **A4367** Ostomy belt, each

IOM: 100-02, 15, 20

✳ **A4368** Ostomy filter, any type, each

⊕ **A4369** Ostomy skin barrier, liquid (spray, brush, etc), per oz

IOM: 100-02, 15, 20

⊕ **A4371** Ostomy skin barrier, powder, per oz

IOM: 100-02, 15, 20

⊕ **A4372** Ostomy skin barrier, solid 4 × 4 or equivalent, standard wear, with built-in convexity, each

IOM: 100-02, 15, 20

⊕ **A4373** Ostomy skin barrier, with flange (solid, flexible, or accordian), with built-in convexity, any size, each

IOM: 100-02, 15, 20

⊕ **A4375** Ostomy pouch, drainable, with faceplate attached, plastic, each

IOM: 100-02, 15, 20

⊕ **A4376** Ostomy pouch, drainable, with faceplate attached, rubber, each

IOM: 100-02, 15, 20

⊕ **A4377** Ostomy pouch, drainable, for use on faceplate, plastic, each

IOM: 100-02, 15, 20

⊕ **A4378** Ostomy pouch, drainable, for use on faceplate, rubber, each

IOM: 100-02, 15, 20

⊕ **A4379** Ostomy pouch, urinary, with faceplate attached, plastic, each

IOM: 100-02, 15, 20

⊕ **A4380** Ostomy pouch, urinary, with faceplate attached, rubber, each

IOM: 100-02, 15, 20

⊕ **A4381** Ostomy pouch, urinary, for use on faceplate, plastic, each

IOM: 100-02, 15, 20

⊕ **A4382** Ostomy pouch, urinary, for use on faceplate, heavy plastic, each

IOM: 100-02, 15, 20

⊕ **A4383** Ostomy pouch, urinary, for use on faceplate, rubber, each

IOM: 100-02, 15, 20

⊕ **A4384** Ostomy faceplate equivalent, silicone ring, each

IOM: 100-02, 15, 20

⊕ **A4385** Ostomy skin barrier, solid 4 × 4 or equivalent, extended wear, without built-in convexity, each

IOM: 100-02, 15, 20

⊕ **A4387** Ostomy pouch closed, with barrier attached, with built-in convexity (1 piece), each

IOM: 100-02, 15, 20

⊕ **A4388** Ostomy pouch, drainable, with extended wear barrier attached (1 piece), each

IOM: 100-02, 15, 20

⊕ **A4389** Ostomy pouch, drainable, with barrier attached, with built-in convexity (1 piece), each

IOM: 100-02, 15, 20

⊕ **A4390** Ostomy pouch, drainable, with extended wear barrier attached, with built-in convexity (1 piece), each

IOM: 100-02, 15, 20

⊕ **A4391** Ostomy pouch, urinary, with extended wear barrier attached (1 piece), each

IOM: 100-02, 15, 20

⊕ **A4392** Ostomy pouch, urinary, with standard wear barrier attached, with built-in convexity (1 piece), each

IOM: 100-02, 15, 20

◀▶ New   ←→ Revised   ✔ Reinstated   ✘ Deleted

⊕ Special coverage instructions   ◆ Not covered or valid by Medicare   ✳ Carrier discretion   ▶ ASC payment group

⊕ **A4393** Ostomy pouch, urinary, with extended wear barrier attached, with built-in convexity (1 piece), each
IOM: 100-02, 15, 20

⊕ **A4394** Ostomy deodorant, with or without lubricant, for use in ostomy pouch, per fluid ounce
IOM: 100-02, 15, 20

⊕ **A4395** Ostomy deodorant for use in ostomy pouch, solid, per tablet
IOM: 100-02, 15, 20

⊕ **A4396** Ostomy belt with peristomal hernia support
IOM: 100-02, 15, 20

⊕ **A4397** Irrigation supply; sleeve, each
IOM: 100-02, 15, 20

⊕ **A4398** Ostomy irrigation supply; bag, each
IOM: 100-02, 15, 20

⊕ **A4399** Ostomy irrigation supply; cone/catheter, including brush
IOM: 100-02, 15, 20

⊕ **A4400** Ostomy irrigation set
IOM: 100-02, 15, 20

⊕ **A4402** Lubricant, per ounce
IOM: 100-02, 15, 20

⊕ **A4404** Ostomy ring, each
IOM: 100-02, 15, 20

⊕ **A4405** Ostomy skin barrier, non-pectin based, paste, per ounce
IOM: 100-02, 15, 20

⊕ **A4406** Ostomy skin barrier, pectin-based, paste, per ounce
IOM: 100-02, 15, 20

⊕ **A4407** Ostomy skin barrier, with flange (solid, flexible, or accordion), extended wear, with built-in convexity, 4 × 4 inches or smaller, each
IOM: 100-02, 15, 20

⊕ **A4408** Ostomy skin barrier, with flange (solid, flexible, or accordion), extended wear, with built-in convexity, larger than 4 × 4 inches, each
IOM: 100-02, 15, 20

⊕ **A4409** Ostomy skin barrier, with flange (solid, flexible, or accordion), extended wear, without built-in convexity, 4 × 4 inches or smaller, each
IOM: 100-02, 15, 20

⊕ **A4410** Ostomy skin barrier, with flange (solid, flexible, or accordion), extended wear, without built-in convexity, larger than 4 × 4 inches, each
IOM: 100-02, 15, 20

⊕ **A4411** Ostomy skin barrier, solid 4 × 4 or equivalent, extended wear, with built-in convexity, each

⊕ **A4412** Ostomy pouch, drainable, high output, for use on a barrier with flange (2 piece system), without filter, each
IOM: 100-02, 15, 20

⊕ **A4413** Ostomy pouch, drainable, high output, for use on a barrier with flange (2 piece system), with filter, each
IOM: 100-02, 15, 20

⊕ **A4414** Ostomy skin barrier, with flange (solid, flexible, or accordion), without built-in convexity, 4 × 4 inches or smaller, each
IOM: 100-02, 15, 20

⊕ **A4415** Ostomy skin barrier, with flange (solid, flexible, or accordion), without built-in convexity, larger than 4 × 4 inches, each
IOM: 100-02, 15, 20

✳ **A4416** Ostomy pouch, closed, with barrier attached, with filter (1 piece), each

✳ **A4417** Ostomy pouch, closed, with barrier attached, with built-in convexity, with filter (1 piece), each

✳ **A4418** Ostomy pouch, closed; without barrier attached, with filter (1 piece), each

✳ **A4419** Ostomy pouch, closed; for use on barrier with non-locking flange, with filter (2 piece), each

✳ **A4420** Ostomy pouch, closed; for use on barrier with locking flange (2 piece), each

✳ **A4421** Ostomy supply; miscellaneous

⊕ **A4422** Ostomy absorbent material (sheet/pad/crystal packet) for use in ostomy pouch to thicken liquid stomal output, each
IOM: 100-02, 15, 20

✳ **A4423** Ostomy pouch, closed; for use on barrier with locking flange, with filter (2 piece), each

✳ **A4424** Ostomy pouch, drainable, with barrier attached, with filter (1 piece), each

✳ **A4425** Ostomy pouch, drainable; for use on barrier with non-locking flange, with filter (2 piece system), each

✳ **A4426** Ostomy pouch, drainable; for use on barrier with locking flange (2 piece system), each

---

◄ ► **New**   ← → **Revised**   ✔ **Reinstated**   ✖ **Deleted**

⊕ **Special coverage instructions**   ◆ **Not covered or valid by Medicare**   ✳ **Carrier discretion**   ▸ **ASC payment group**

✳ **A4427** Ostomy pouch, drainable; for use on barrier with locking flange, with filter (2 piece system), each

✳ **A4428** Ostomy pouch, urinary, with extended wear barrier attached, with faucet-type tap with valve (1 piece), each

✳ **A4429** Ostomy pouch, urinary, with barrier attached, with built-in convexity, with faucet-type tap with valve (1 piece), each

✳ **A4430** Ostomy pouch, urinary, with extended wear barrier attached, with built-in convexity, with faucet-type tap with valve (1 piece), each

✳ **A4431** Ostomy pouch, urinary; with barrier attached, with faucet-type tap with valve (1 piece), each

✳ **A4432** Ostomy pouch, urinary; for use on barrier with non-locking flange, with faucet-type tap with valve (2 piece), each

✳ **A4433** Ostomy pouch, urinary; for use on barrier with locking flange (2 piece), each

✳ **A4434** Ostomy pouch, urinary; for use on barrier with locking flange, with faucet-type tap with valve (2 piece), each

Miscellaneous Supplies

☉ **A4450** Tape, non-waterproof, per 18 square inches
IOM: 100-02, 15, 20

☉ **A4452** Tape, waterproof, per 18 square inches
IOM: 100-02, 15, 20

☉ **A4455** Adhesive remover or solvent (for tape, cement or other adhesive), per ounce
IOM: 100-02, 15, 20

✳ **A4458** Enema bag with tubing, reusable

✳ **A4461** Surgical dressing holder, non-reusable, each

✳ **A4463** Surgical dressing holder, reusable, each

✳ **A4465** Non-elastic binder for extremity

☉ **A4470** Gravlee jet washer
IOM: 100-02, 16, 90; 100-03, 4, 230.5

☉ **A4480** VABRA aspirator
IOM: 100-02, 16, 90; 100-03, 4, 230.6

☉ **A4481** Tracheostoma filter, any type, any size, each
IOM: 100-02, 15, 20

☉ **A4483** Moisture exchanger, disposable, for use with invasive mechanical ventilation
IOM: 100-02, 15, 20

◆ **A4490** Surgical stockings above knee length, each
IOM: 100-02, 15, 100; 100-02, 15, 110; 100-03, 4, 280.1

◆ **A4495** Surgical stockings thigh length, each
IOM: 100-02, 15, 100; 100-02, 15, 110; 100-03, 4, 280.1

◆ **A4500** Surgical stockings below knee length, each
IOM: 100-02, 15, 100; 100-02, 15, 110; 100-03, 4, 280.1

◆ **A4510** Surgical stockings full length, each
IOM: 100-02, 15, 100; 100-02, 15, 110; 100-03, 4, 280.1

◆ **A4520** Incontinence garment, any type, (e.g. brief, diaper), each
IOM: 100-03, 4, 280.1

☉ **A4550** Surgical trays
IOM: 100-04, 12, 30.4

◆ **A4554** Disposable underpads, all sizes
IOM: 100-02, 15, 120; 100-03, 4, 280.1

✳ **A4556** Electrodes, (e.g., apnea monitor), per pair

✳ **A4557** Lead wires, (e.g., apnea monitor), per pair

✳ **A4558** Conductive gel or paste, for use with electrical device (e.g., TENS, NMES), per oz

✳ **A4559** Coupling gel or paste, for use with ultrasound device, per oz

✳ **A4561** Pessary, rubber, any type

✳ **A4562** Pessary, non rubber, any type

✳ **A4565** Slings

◆ **A4570** Splint
IOM: 100-02, 6, 10; 100-02, 15, 100; 100-04, 4, 240

◆ **A4575** Topical hyperbaric oxygen chamber, disposable
IOM: 100-03, 1, 20.29

◆ **A4580** Cast supplies (e.g. plaster)
IOM: 100-02, 6, 10; 100-02, 15, 100; 100-04, 4, 240

◆ **A4590** Special casting material (e.g. fiberglass)
IOM: 100-02, 6, 10; 100-02, 15, 100; 100-04, 4, 240

◀▶ New   ←→ Revised   ✔ Reinstated   ✖ Deleted
☉ Special coverage instructions   ◆ Not covered or valid by Medicare   ✳ Carrier discretion   ▶ ASC payment group

⊙ **A4595** Electrical stimulator supplies, 2 lead, per month, (e.g. TENS, NMES)

IOM: 100-03, 2, 160.13

✳ **A4600** Sleeve for intermittent limb compression device, replacement only, each

✳ **A4601** Lithium ion battery for non-prosthetic use, replacement

Supplies for Respiratory and Oxygen Equipment

✳ **A4604** Tubing with integrated heating element for use with positive airway pressure device

✳ **A4605** Tracheal suction catheter, closed system, each

✳ **A4606** Oxygen probe for use with oximeter device, replacement

→ ✳ **A4608** Transtracheal oxygen catheter, each

✳ **A4611** Battery, heavy duty; replacement for patient owned ventilator

✳ **A4612** Battery cables; replacement for patient-owned ventilator

✳ **A4613** Battery charger; replacement for patient-owned ventilator

✳ **A4614** Peak expiratory flow rate meter, hand held

→ ⊙ **A4615** Cannula, nasal

IOM: 100-03, 2, 160.6; 100-04, 20, 100.2

→ ⊙ **A4616** Tubing (oxygen), per foot

IOM: 100-03, 2, 160.6; 100-04, 20, 100.2

→ ⊙ **A4617** Mouth piece

IOM: 100-03, 2, 160.6; 100-04, 20, 100.2

⊙ **A4618** Breathing circuits

IOM: 100-03, 2, 160.6; 100-04, 20, 100.2

⊙ **A4619** Face tent

IOM: 100-03, 2, 160.6; 100-04, 20, 100.2

→ ⊙ **A4620** Variable concentration mask

IOM: 100-03, 2, 160.6; 100-04, 20, 100.2

⊙ **A4623** Tracheostomy, inner cannula

IOM: 100-02, 15, 120; 100-03, 1, 20.9

✳ **A4624** Tracheal suction catheter, any type, other than closed system, each

⊙ **A4625** Tracheostomy care kit for new tracheostomy

IOM: 100-02, 15, 120

⊙ **A4626** Tracheostomy cleaning brush, each

IOM: 100-02, 15, 120

◆ **A4627** Spacer, bag, or reservoir, with or without mask, for use with metered dose inhaler

IOM: 100-02, 15, 110

✳ **A4628** Oropharyngeal suction catheter, each

⊙ **A4629** Tracheostomy care kit for established tracheostomy

IOM: 100-02, 15, 120

Supplies for Other Durable Medical Equipment

⊙ **A4630** Replacement batteries, medically necessary, transcutaneous electrical stimulator, owned by patient

IOM: 100-03, 3, 160.7

✳ **A4633** Replacement bulb/lamp for ultraviolet light therapy system, each

✳ **A4634** Replacement bulb for therapeutic light box, tabletop model

⊙ **A4635** Underarm pad, crutch, replacement, each

IOM: 100-03, 4, 280.1

⊙ **A4636** Replacement, handgrip, cane, crutch, or walker, each

IOM: 100-03, 4, 280.1

⊙ **A4637** Replacement, tip, cane, crutch, walker, each

IOM: 100-03, 4, 280.1

✳ **A4638** Replacement battery for patient-owned ear pulse generator, each

✳ **A4639** Replacement pad for infrared heating pad system, each

⊙ **A4640** Replacement pad for use with medically necessary alternating pressure pad owned by patient

IOM: 100-03, 4, 280.1; 100-08, 5, 5.2.3

Supplies for Radiological Procedures

✳ **A4641** Radiopharmaceutical, diagnostic, not otherwise classified

✳ **A4642** Indium In-111 satumomab pendetide, diagnostic, per study dose, up to 6 millicuries

◆ **A4643** Imaging, e.g., gadoteridol injection

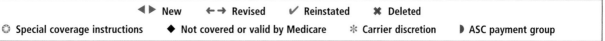

◀ ▶ **New**   ←→ **Revised**   ✔ **Reinstated**   ✖ **Deleted**

⊙ **Special coverage instructions**   ◆ **Not covered or valid by Medicare**   ✳ **Carrier discretion**   ▶ **ASC payment group**

Miscellaneous Supplies

* **A4648** Tissue marker, implantable, any type, each

* **A4649** Surgical supply; miscellaneous

* **A4650** Implantable radiation dosimeter, each

⊛ **A4651** Calibrated microcapillary tube, each
IOM: 100-04, 3, 40.3

⊛ **A4652** Microcapillary tube sealant
IOM: 100-04, 3, 40.3

Supplies for Dialysis

* **A4653** Peritoneal dialysis catheter anchoring device, belt, each

⊛ **A4657** Syringe, with or without needle, each
IOM: 100-04, 3, 40.3

⊛ **A4660** Sphygmomanometer/blood pressure apparatus with cuff and stethoscope
IOM: 100-04, 3, 40.3

⊛ **A4663** Blood pressure cuff only
IOM: 100-04, 3, 40.3

◆ **A4670** Automatic blood pressure monitor
IOM: 100-04, 3, 40.3

⊛ **A4671** Disposable cycler set used with cycler dialysis machine, each
IOM: 100-04, 3, 40.3

⊛ **A4672** Drainage extension line, sterile, for dialysis, each
IOM: 100-04, 3, 40.3

⊛ **A4673** Extension line with easy lock connectors, used with dialysis
IOM: 100-04, 3, 40.3

⊛ **A4674** Chemicals/antiseptics solution used to clean/sterilize dialysis equipment, per 8 oz
IOM: 100-04, 3, 40.3

⊛ **A4680** Activated carbon filters for hemodialysis, each
IOM: 100-04, 3, 40.3

⊛ **A4690** Dialyzers (artificial kidneys), all types, all sizes, for hemodialysis, each
IOM: 100-04, 3, 40.3

⊛ **A4706** Bicarbonate concentrate, solution, for hemodialysis, per gallon
IOM: 100-04, 3, 40.3

⊛ **A4707** Bicarbonate concentrate, powder, for hemodialysis, per packet
IOM: 100-04, 3, 40.3

⊛ **A4708** Acetate concentrate solution, for hemodialysis, per gallon
IOM: 100-04, 3, 40.3

⊛ **A4709** Acid concentrate, solution, for hemodialysis, per gallon
IOM: 100-04, 3, 40.3

⊛ **A4714** Treated water (deionized, distilled, or reverse osmosis) for peritoneal dialysis, per gallon
IOM: 100-03, 4, 230.7; 100-04, 3, 40.3

⊛ **A4719** "Y set" tubing for peritoneal dialysis
IOM: 100-04, 3, 40.3

⊛ **A4720** Dialysate solution, any concentration of dextrose, fluid volume greater than 249cc, but less than or equal to 999cc, for peritoneal dialysis
IOM: 100-04, 3, 40.3

⊛ **A4721** Dialysate solution, any concentration of dextrose, fluid volume greater than 999cc but less than or equal to 1999cc, for peritoneal dialysis
IOM: 100-04, 3, 40.3

⊛ **A4722** Dialysate solution, any concentration of dextrose, fluid volume greater than 1999cc but less than or equal to 2999cc, for peritoneal dialysis
IOM: 100-04, 3, 40.3

⊛ **A4723** Dialysate solution, any concentration of dextrose, fluid volume greater than 2999cc but less than or equal to 3999cc, for peritoneal dialysis
IOM: 100-04, 3, 40.3

⊛ **A4724** Dialysate solution, any concentration of dextrose, fluid volume greater than 3999cc but less than or equal to 4999cc for peritoneal dialysis
IOM: 100-04, 3, 40.3

⊛ **A4725** Dialysate solution, any concentration of dextrose, fluid volume greater than 4999cc but less than or equal to 5999cc, for peritoneal dialysis
IOM: 100-04, 3, 40.3

⊛ **A4726** Dialysate solution, any concentration of dextrose, fluid volume greater than 5999cc, for peritoneal dialysis
IOM: 100-04, 3, 40.3

* **A4728** Dialysate solution, non-dextrose containing, 500 ml

◀▶ New   ←→ Revised   ✔ Reinstated   ✖ Deleted

⊛ Special coverage instructions   ◆ Not covered or valid by Medicare   * Carrier discretion   ▶ ASC payment group

⊕ **A4730** Fistula cannulation set for hemodialysis, each

IOM: 100-04, 3, 40.3

⊕ **A4736** Topical anesthetic, for dialysis, per gram

IOM: 100-04, 3, 40.3

⊕ **A4737** Injectable anesthetic, for dialysis, per 10 ml

IOM: 100-04, 3, 40.3

⊕ **A4740** Shunt accessory, for hemodialysis, any type, each

IOM: 100-04, 3, 40.3

⊕ **A4750** Blood tubing, arterial or venous, for hemodialysis, each

IOM: 100-04, 3, 40.3

⊕ **A4755** Blood tubing, arterial and venous combined, for hemodialysis, each

IOM: 100-04, 3, 40.3

⊕ **A4760** Dialysate solution test kit, for peritoneal dialysis, any type, each

IOM: 100-04, 3, 40.3

⊕ **A4765** Dialysate concentrate, powder, additive for peritoneal dialysis, per packet

IOM: 100-04, 3, 40.3

⊕ **A4766** Dialysate concentrate, solution, additive for peritoneal dialysis, per 10 ml

IOM: 100-04, 3, 40.3

⊕ **A4770** Blood collection tube, vacuum, for dialysis, per 50

IOM: 100-04, 3, 40.3

⊕ **A4771** Serum clotting time tube, for dialysis, per 50

IOM: 100-04, 3, 40.3

⊕ **A4772** Blood glucose test strips, for dialysis, per 50

IOM: 100-04, 3, 40.3

⊕ **A4773** Occult blood test strips, for dialysis, per 50

IOM: 100-04, 3, 40.3

⊕ **A4774** Ammonia test strips, for dialysis, per 50

IOM: 100-04, 3, 40.3

⊕ **A4802** Protamine sulfate, for hemodialysis, per 50 mg

IOM: 100-04, 3, 40.3

⊕ **A4860** Disposable catheter tips for peritoneal dialysis, per 10

IOM: 100-04, 3, 40.3

⊕ **A4870** Plumbing and/or electrical work for home hemodialysis equipment

IOM: 100-04, 3, 40.3

⊕ **A4890** Contracts, repair and maintenance, for hemodialysis equipment

IOM: 100-02, 15, 110.2

⊕ **A4911** Drain bag/bottle, for dialysis, each

⊕ **A4913** Miscellaneous dialysis supplies, not otherwise specified

⊕ **A4918** Venous pressure clamp, for hemodialysis, each

⊕ **A4927** Gloves, non-sterile, per 100

⊕ **A4928** Surgical mask, per 20

⊕ **A4929** Tourniquet for dialysis, each

⊕ **A4930** Gloves, sterile, per pair

✳ **A4931** Oral thermometer, reusable, any type, each

✳ **A4932** Rectal thermometer, reusable, any type, each

Additional Ostomy Supplies

⊕ **A5051** Ostomy pouch, closed; with barrier attached (1 piece), each

IOM: 100-02, 15, 120

⊕ **A5052** Ostomy pouch, closed; without barrier attached (1 piece), each

IOM: 100-02, 15, 120

⊕ **A5053** Ostomy pouch, closed; for use on faceplate, each

IOM: 100-02, 15, 120

⊕ **A5054** Ostomy pouch, closed; for use on barrier with flange (2 piece), each

IOM: 100-02, 15, 120

⊕ **A5055** Stoma cap

IOM: 100-02, 15, 120

✳ **A5061** Ostomy pouch, drainable; with barrier attached, (1 piece), each

IOM: 100-02, 15, 120

⊕ **A5062** Ostomy pouch, drainable; without barrier attached (1 piece), each

IOM: 100-02, 15, 120

⊕ **A5063** Ostomy pouch, drainable; for use on barrier with flange (2 piece system), each

IOM: 100-02, 15, 120

⊕ **A5071** Ostomy pouch, urinary; with barrier attached (1 piece), each

IOM: 100-02, 15, 120

⊕ **A5072** Ostomy pouch, urinary; without barrier attached (1 piece), each

IOM: 100-02, 15, 120

MEDICAL AND SURGICAL SUPPLIES

A4730 – A5072

◀▶ New   ←→ Revised   ✔ Reinstated   ✖ Deleted

⊕ Special coverage instructions   ◆ Not covered or valid by Medicare   ✳ Carrier discretion   ▶ ASC payment group

⊚ **A5073** Ostomy pouch, urinary; for use on barrier with flange (2 piece), each
IOM: 100-02, 15, 120

⊚ **A5081** Continent device; plug for continent stoma
IOM: 100-02, 15, 120

⊚ **A5082** Continent device; catheter for continent stoma
IOM: 100-02, 15, 120

✳ **A5083** Continent device, stoma absorptive cover for continent stoma

⊚ **A5093** Ostomy accessory; convex insert
IOM: 100-02, 15, 120

Additional Incontinence Appliances/Supplies

⊚ **A5102** Bedside drainage bottle with or without tubing, rigid or expandable, each
IOM: 100-02, 15, 120

⊚ **A5105** Urinary suspensory, with leg bag, with or without tube, each
IOM: 100-02, 15, 120

⊚ **A5112** Urinary leg bag; latex
IOM: 100-02, 15, 120

⊚ **A5113** Leg strap; latex, replacement only, per set
IOM: 100-02, 15, 120

⊚ **A5114** Leg strap; foam or fabric, replacement only, per set
IOM: 100-02, 15, 120

Supplies for Either Incontinence or Ostomy Appliances

⊚ **A5120** Skin barrier, wipes or swabs, each
IOM: 100-02, 15, 120

⊚ **A5121** Skin barrier; solid, 6 × 6 or equivalent, each
IOM: 100-02, 15, 120

⊚ **A5122** Skin barrier; solid, 8 × 8 or equivalent, each
IOM: 100-02, 15, 120

⊚ **A5126** Adhesive or non-adhesive; disk or foam pad
IOM: 100-02, 15, 120

⊚ **A5131** Appliance cleaner, incontinence and ostomy appliances, per 16 oz
IOM: 100-02, 15, 120

⊚ **A5200** Percutaneous catheter/tube anchoring device, adhesive skin attachment
IOM: 100-02, 15, 120

Diabetic Shoes, Fitting, and Modifications

⊚ **A5500** For diabetics only, fitting (including follow-up), custom preparation and supply of off-the-shelf depth-inlay shoe manufactured to accommodate multi-density insert(s), per shoe
IOM: 100-02, 15, 140

⊚ **A5501** For diabetics only, fitting (including follow-up), custom preparation and supply of shoe molded from cast(s) of patient's foot (custom-molded shoe), per shoe
IOM: 100-02, 15, 140

⊚ **A5503** For diabetics only, modification (including fitting) of off-the-shelf depth-inlay shoe or custom-molded shoe with roller or rigid rocker bottom, per shoe
IOM: 100-02, 15, 140

⊚ **A5504** For diabetics only, modification (including fitting) of off-the-shelf depth-inlay shoe or custom-molded shoe with wedge(s), per shoe
IOM: 100-02, 15, 140

⊚ **A5505** For diabetics only, modification (including fitting) of off-the-shelf depth-inlay shoe or custom-molded shoe with metatarsal bar, per shoe
IOM: 100-02, 15, 140

⊚ **A5506** For diabetics only, modification (including fitting) of off-the-shelf depth-inlay shoe or custom-molded shoe with off-set heel(s), per shoe
IOM: 100-02, 15, 140

⊚ **A5507** For diabetics only, not otherwise specified modification (including fitting) of off-the-shelf depth-inlay shoe or custom-molded shoe, per shoe
IOM: 100-02, 15, 140

⊚ **A5508** For diabetics only, deluxe feature of off-the-shelf depth-inlay shoe or custom-molded shoe, per shoe

⊚ **A5510** For diabetics only, direct formed, compression molded to patient's foot without external heat source, multiple-density insert(s) prefabricated, per shoe
IOM: 100-02, 15, 140

◀▶ New   ←→ Revised   ✔ Reinstated   ✖ Deleted
⊚ Special coverage instructions   ◆ Not covered or valid by Medicare   ✳ Carrier discretion   ▶ ASC payment group

✳ **A5512** For diabetics only, multiple density insert, direct formed, molded to foot after external heat source of 230 degrees Fahrenheit or higher, total contact with patient's foot, including arch, base layer minimum of 1/4 inch material of shore a 35 durometer or 3/16 inch material of shore a 40 durometer (or higher), prefabricated, each

✳ **A5513** For diabetics only, multiple density insert, custom molded from model of patient's foot, total contact with patient's foot, including arch, base layer minimum of 3/16 inch material of shore a 35 durometer (or higher), includes arch filler and other shaping material, custom fabricated, each

Dressings

◆ **A6000** Non-contact wound warming wound cover for use with the non-contact wound warming device and warming card

IOM: 100-02, 16, 20

→ ✿ **A6010** Collagen based wound filler, dry form, sterile, per gram of collagen

IOM: 100-02, 15, 100

→ ✿ **A6011** Collagen based wound filler, gel/paste, sterile, per gram of collagen

IOM: 100-02, 15, 100

→ ✿ **A6021** Collagen dressing, sterile, pad size 16 sq. in. or less, each

IOM: 100-02, 15, 100

→ ✿ **A6022** Collagen dressing, sterile, pad size more than 16 sq. in. but less than or equal to 48 sq. in., each

IOM: 100-02, 15, 100

→ ✿ **A6023** Collagen dressing, sterile, pad size more than 48 sq. in., each

IOM: 100-02, 15, 100

→ ✿ **A6024** Collagen dressing wound filler, sterile, per 6 inches

IOM: 100-02, 15, 100

✳ **A6025** Gel sheet for dermal or epidermal application, (e.g., silicone, hydrogel, other), each

✿ **A6154** Wound pouch, each

IOM: 100-02, 15, 100

→ ✿ **A6196** Alginate or other fiber gelling dressing, wound cover, sterile, pad size 16 sq. in. or less, each dressing

IOM: 100-02, 15, 100

→ ✿ **A6197** Alginate or other fiber gelling dressing, wound cover, sterile, pad size more than 16 sq. in., but less than or equal to 48 sq. in., each dressing

IOM: 100-02, 15, 100

→ ✿ **A6198** Alginate or other fiber gelling dressing, wound cover, sterile, pad size more than 48 sq. in., each dressing

IOM: 100-02, 15, 100

→ ✿ **A6199** Alginate or other fiber gelling dressing, wound filler, sterile, per 6 inches

IOM: 100-02, 15, 100

→ ✳ **A6200** Composite dressing, pad size 16 sq. in. or less, without adhesive border, each dressing

IOM: 100-02, 15, 100

→ ✳ **A6201** Composite dressing, pad size more than 16 sq. in. but less than or equal to 48 sq. in., without adhesive border, each dressing

IOM: 100-02, 15, 100

→ ✳ **A6202** Composite dressing, sterile, pad size more than 48 sq. in., without adhesive border, each dressing

IOM: 100-02, 15, 100

→ ✿ **A6203** Composite dressing, sterile, pad size 16 sq. in. or less, with any size adhesive border, each dressing

IOM: 100-02, 15, 100

→ ✿ **A6204** Composite dressing, sterile, pad size more than 16 sq. in. but less than or equal to 48 sq. in., with any size adhesive border, each dressing

IOM: 100-02, 15, 100

→ ✿ **A6205** Composite dressing, sterile, pad size more than 48 sq. in., with any size adhesive border, each dressing

IOM: 100-02, 15, 100

→ ✿ **A6206** Contact layer, sterile, 16 sq. in. or less, each dressing

IOM: 100-02, 15, 100

→ ✿ **A6207** Contact layer, sterile, more than 16 sq. in. but less than or equal to 48 sq. in., each dressing

IOM: 100-02, 15, 100

→ ✿ **A6208** Contact layer, sterile, more than 48 sq. in., each dressing

IOM: 100-02, 15, 100

→ ✿ **A6209** Foam dressing, wound cover, sterile, pad size 16 sq. in. or less, without adhesive border, each dressing

IOM: 100-02, 15, 100

◄▶ New   ←→ Revised   ✔ Reinstated   ✖ Deleted
✿ Special coverage instructions   ◆ Not covered or valid by Medicare   ✳ Carrier discretion   ▶ ASC payment group

→ ⊕ **A6210** Foam dressing, wound cover, sterile, pad size more than 16 sq. in. but less than or equal to 48 sq. in., without adhesive border, each dressing

IOM: 100-02, 15, 100

→ ⊕ **A6211** Foam dressing, wound cover, sterile, pad size more than 48 sq. in., without adhesive border, each dressing

IOM: 100-02, 15, 100

→ ⊕ **A6212** Foam dressing, wound cover, sterile, pad size 16 sq. in. or less, with any size adhesive border, each dressing

IOM: 100-02, 15, 100

→ ⊕ **A6213** Foam dressing, wound cover, sterile, pad size more than 16 sq. in. but less than or equal to 48 sq. in., with any size adhesive border, each dressing

IOM: 100-02, 15, 100

→ ⊕ **A6214** Foam dressing, wound cover, sterile, pad size more than 48 sq. in., with any size adhesive border, each dressing

IOM: 100-02, 15, 100

→ ⊕ **A6215** Foam dressing, wound filler, sterile, per gram

IOM: 100-02, 15, 100

⊕ **A6216** Gauze, non-impregnated, non-sterile, pad size 16 sq. in. or less, without adhesive border, each dressing

IOM: 100-02, 15, 100

⊕ **A6217** Gauze, non-impregnated, non-sterile, pad size more than 16 sq. in. but less than or equal to 48 sq. in., without adhesive border, each dressing

IOM: 100-02, 15, 100

⊕ **A6218** Gauze, non-impregnated, non-sterile, pad size more than 48 sq. in., without adhesive border, each dressing

IOM: 100-02, 15, 100

→ ⊕ **A6219** Gauze, non-impregnated, sterile, pad size 16 sq. in. or less, with any size adhesive border, each dressing

IOM: 100-02, 15, 100

→ ⊕ **A6220** Gauze, non-impregnated, sterile, pad size more than 16 sq. in. but less than or equal to 48 sq. in., with any size adhesive border, each dressing

IOM: 100-02, 15, 100

→ ⊕ **A6221** Gauze, non-impregnated, sterile, pad size more than 48 sq. in., with any size adhesive border, each dressing

IOM: 100-02, 15, 100

→ ⊕ **A6222** Gauze, impregnated with other than water, normal saline, or hydrogel, sterile, pad size 16 sq. in. or less, without adhesive border, each dressing

IOM: 100-02, 15, 100

→ ⊕ **A6223** Gauze, impregnated with other than water, normal saline, or hydrogel, sterile, pad size more than 16 sq. in. but less than or equal to 48 sq. in., without adhesive border, each dressing

IOM: 100-02, 15, 100

→ ⊕ **A6224** Gauze, impregnated with other than water, normal saline, or hydrogel, sterile, pad size more than 48 square inches, without adhesive border, each dressing

IOM: 100-02, 15, 100

→ ⊕ **A6228** Gauze, impregnated, water or normal saline, sterile, pad size 16 sq. in. or less, without adhesive border, each dressing

IOM: 100-02, 15, 100

→ ⊕ **A6229** Gauze, impregnated, water or normal saline, sterile, pad size more than 16 sq. in. but less than or equal to 48 sq. in., without adhesive border, each dressing

IOM: 100-02, 15, 100

→ ⊕ **A6230** Gauze, impregnated, water or normal saline, sterile, pad size more than 48 sq. in., without adhesive border, each dressing

IOM: 100-02, 15, 100

→ ⊕ **A6231** Gauze, impregnated, hydrogel, for direct wound contact, sterile, pad size 16 sq. in. or less, each dressing

IOM: 100-02, 15, 100

→ ⊕ **A6232** Gauze, impregnated, hydrogel, for direct wound contact, sterile, pad size greater than 16 sq. in., but less than or equal to 48 sq. in., each dressing

IOM: 100-02, 15, 100

→ ⊕ **A6233** Gauze, impregnated, hydrogel, for direct wound contact, sterile, pad size more than 48 sq. in., each dressing

IOM: 100-02, 15, 100

→ ⊕ **A6234** Hydrocolloid dressing, wound cover, sterile, pad size 16 sq. in. or less, without adhesive border, each dressing

IOM: 100-02, 15, 100

→ ⊕ **A6235** Hydrocolloid dressing, wound cover, sterile, pad size more than 16 sq. in. but less than or equal to 48 sq. in., without adhesive border, each dressing

IOM: 100-02, 15, 100

◀ ▶ New   ←→ Revised   ✔ Reinstated   ✖ Deleted

⊕ Special coverage instructions   ◆ Not covered or valid by Medicare   ✳ Carrier discretion   ▶ ASC payment group

→ ❂ **A6236** Hydrocolloid dressing, wound cover, sterile, pad size more than 48 sq. in., without adhesive border, each dressing

IOM: 100-02, 15, 100

→ ❂ **A6237** Hydrocolloid dressing, wound cover, sterile, pad size 16 sq. in. or less, with any size adhesive border, each dressing

IOM: 100-02, 15, 100

→ ❂ **A6238** Hydrocolloid dressing, wound cover, sterile, pad size more than 16 sq. in. but less than or equal to 48 sq. in., with any size adhesive border, each dressing

IOM: 100-02, 15, 100

→ ❂ **A6239** Hydrocolloid dressing, wound cover, sterile, pad size more than 48 sq. in., with any size adhesive border, each dressing

IOM: 100-02, 15, 100

→ ❂ **A6240** Hydrocolloid dressing, wound filler, paste, sterile, per ounce

IOM: 100-02, 15, 100

→ ❂ **A6241** Hydrocolloid dressing, wound filler, dry form, sterile, per gram

IOM: 100-02, 15, 100

→ ❂ **A6242** Hydrogel dressing, wound cover, sterile, pad size 16 sq. in. or less, without adhesive border, each dressing

IOM: 100-02, 15, 100

→ ❂ **A6243** Hydrogel dressing, wound cover, sterile, pad size more than 16 sq. in. but less than or equal to 48 sq. in., without adhesive border, each dressing

IOM: 100-02, 15, 100

→ ❂ **A6244** Hydrogel dressing, wound cover, sterile, pad size more than 48 sq. in., without adhesive border, each dressing

IOM: 100-02, 15, 100

→ ❂ **A6245** Hydrogel dressing, wound cover, sterile, pad size 16 sq. in. or less, with any size adhesive border, each dressing

IOM: 100-02, 15, 100

→ ❂ **A6246** Hydrogel dressing, wound cover, sterile, pad size more than 16 sq. in. but less than or equal to 48 sq. in., with any size adhesive border, each dressing

IOM: 100-02, 15, 100

→ ❂ **A6247** Hydrogel dressing, wound cover, sterile, pad size more than 48 sq. in., with any size adhesive border, each dressing

IOM: 100-02, 15, 100

→ ❂ **A6248** Hydrogel dressing, wound filler, gel, sterile, per fluid ounce

IOM: 100-02, 15, 100

❂ **A6250** Skin sealants, protectants, moisturizers, ointments, any type, any size

IOM: 100-02, 15, 100

→ ❂ **A6251** Specialty absorptive dressing, wound cover, sterile, pad size 16 sq. in. or less, without adhesive border, each dressing

IOM: 100-02, 15, 100

→ ❂ **A6252** Specialty absorptive dressing, wound cover, sterile, pad size more than 16 sq. in. but less than or equal to 48 sq. in., without adhesive border, each dressing

IOM: 100-02, 15, 100

→ ❂ **A6253** Specialty absorptive dressing, wound cover, sterile, pad size more than 48 sq. in., without adhesive border, each dressing

IOM: 100-02, 15, 100

→ ❂ **A6254** Specialty absorptive dressing, wound cover, sterile, pad size 16 sq. in. or less, with any size adhesive border, each dressing

IOM: 100-02, 15, 100

→ ❂ **A6255** Specialty absorptive dressing, wound cover, sterile, pad size more than 16 sq. in. but less than or equal to 48 sq. in., with any size adhesive border, each dressing

IOM: 100-02, 15, 100

→ ❂ **A6256** Specialty absorptive dressing, wound cover, sterile, pad size more than 48 sq. in., with any size adhesive border, each dressing

IOM: 100-02, 15, 100

→ ❂ **A6257** Transparent film, sterile, 16 sq. in. or less, each dressing

IOM: 100-02, 15, 100

→ ❂ **A6258** Transparent film, sterile, more than 16 sq. in. but less than or equal to 48 sq. in., each dressing

IOM: 100-02, 15, 100

→ ❂ **A6259** Transparent film, sterile, more than 48 sq. in., each dressing

IOM: 100-02, 15, 100

→ ❂ **A6260** Wound cleansers, sterile, any type, any size

IOM: 100-02, 15, 100

→ ❂ **A6261** Wound filler, gel/paste, sterile, per fluid ounce, not otherwise specified

IOM: 100-02, 15, 100

◀▶ New   ←→ Revised   ✔ Reinstated   ✖ Deleted

❂ Special coverage instructions   ◆ Not covered or valid by Medicare   ✳ Carrier discretion   ▷ ASC payment group

→ ⊙ **A6262** Wound filler, dry form, sterile, per gram, not otherwise specified
IOM: 100-02, 15, 100

→ ⊙ **A6266** Gauze, impregnated, other than water, normal saline, or zinc paste, sterile, any width, per linear yard
IOM: 100-02, 15, 100

⊙ **A6402** Gauze, non-impregnated, sterile, pad size 16 sq. in. or less, without adhesive border, each dressing
IOM: 100-02, 15, 100

⊙ **A6403** Gauze, non-impregnated, sterile, pad size more than 16 sq. in., less than or equal to 48 sq. in., without adhesive border, each dressing
IOM: 100-02, 15, 100

⊙ **A6404** Gauze, non-impregnated, sterile, pad size more than 48 sq. in., without adhesive border, each dressing
IOM: 100-02, 15, 100

→ ✳ **A6407** Packing strips, non-impregnated, sterile, up to 2 inches in width, per linear yard
IOM: 100-02, 15, 100

⊙ **A6410** Eye pad, sterile, each
IOM: 100-02, 15, 100

⊙ **A6411** Eye pad, non-sterile, each
IOM: 100-02, 15, 100

✳ **A6412** Eye patch, occlusive, each

◆ **A6413** Adhesive bandage, first-aid type, any size, each
Medicare Statute 1861(s)(5)

✳ **A6441** Padding bandage, non-elastic, non-woven/non-knitted, width greater than or equal to three inches and less than five inches, per yard

✳ **A6442** Conforming bandage, non-elastic, knitted/woven, non-sterile, width less than three inches, per yard

✳ **A6443** Conforming bandage, non-elastic, knitted/woven, non-sterile, width greater than or equal to three inches and less than five inches, per yard

✳ **A6444** Conforming bandage, non-elastic, knitted/woven, non-sterile, width greater than or equal to five inches, per yard

✳ **A6445** Conforming bandage, non-elastic, knitted/woven, sterile, width less than three inches, per yard

✳ **A6446** Conforming bandage, non-elastic, knitted/woven, sterile, width greater than or equal to three inches and less than five inches, per yard

✳ **A6447** Conforming bandage, non-elastic, knitted/woven, sterile, width greater than or equal to five inches, per yard

✳ **A6448** Light compression bandage, elastic, knitted/woven, width less than three inches, per yard

✳ **A6449** Light compression bandage, elastic, knitted/woven, width greater than or equal to three inches and less than five inches, per yard

✳ **A6450** Light compression bandage, elastic, knitted/woven, width greater than or equal to five inches, per yard

✳ **A6451** Moderate compression bandage, elastic, knitted/woven, load resistance of 1.25 to 1.34 foot pounds at 50% maximum stretch, width greater than or equal to three inches and less than five inches, per yard

✳ **A6452** High compression bandage, elastic, knitted/woven, load resistance greater than or equal to 1.35 foot pounds at 50% maximum stretch, width greater than or equal to three inches and less than five inches, per yard

✳ **A6453** Self-adherent bandage, elastic, non-knitted/non-woven, width less than three inches, per yard

✳ **A6454** Self-adherent bandage, elastic, non-knitted/non-woven, width greater than or equal to three inches and less than five inches, per yard

✳ **A6455** Self-adherent bandage, elastic, non-knitted/non-woven, width greater than or equal to five inches, per yard

✳ **A6456** Zinc paste impregnated bandage, non-elastic, knitted/woven, width greater than or equal to three inches and less than five inches, per yard

✳ **A6457** Tubular dressing with or without elastic, any width, per linear yard

⊙ **A6501** Compression burn garment, bodysuit (head to foot), custom fabricated
IOM: 100-02, 15, 100

⊙ **A6502** Compression burn garment, chin strap, custom fabricated
IOM: 100-02, 15, 100

⊙ **A6503** Compression burn garment, facial hood, custom fabricated
IOM: 100-02, 15, 100

◀▶ New   ←→ Revised   ✔ Reinstated   ✖ Deleted

⊙ Special coverage instructions   ◆ Not covered or valid by Medicare   ✳ Carrier discretion   ▶ ASC payment group

⊛ **A6504**   Compression burn garment, glove to wrist, custom fabricated

IOM: 100-02, 15, 100

⊛ **A6505**   Compression burn garment, glove to elbow, custom fabricated

IOM: 100-02, 15, 100

⊛ **A6506**   Compression burn garment, glove to axilla, custom fabricated

IOM: 100-02, 15, 100

⊛ **A6507**   Compression burn garment, foot to knee length, custom fabricated

IOM: 100-02, 15, 100

⊛ **A6508**   Compression burn garment, foot to thigh length, custom fabricated

IOM: 100-02, 15, 100

⊛ **A6509**   Compression burn garment, upper trunk to waist including arm openings (vest), custom fabricated

IOM: 100-02, 15, 100

⊛ **A6510**   Compression burn garment, trunk, including arms down to leg openings (leotard), custom fabricated

IOM: 100-02, 15, 100

⊛ **A6511**   Compression burn garment, lower trunk including leg openings (panty), custom fabricated

IOM: 100-02, 15, 100

⊛ **A6512**   Compression burn garment, not otherwise classified

IOM: 100-02, 15, 100

✳ **A6513**   Compression burn mask, face and/or neck, plastic or equal, custom fabricated

GRADIENT COMPRESSION STOCKINGS (A6530-A6549)

◆ **A6530**   Gradient compression stocking, below knee, 18–30 mmHg, each

IOM: 100-03, 4, 280.1

⊛ **A6531**   Gradient compression stocking, below knee, 30–40 mmHg, each

IOM: 100-02, 15, 100

⊛ **A6532**   Gradient compression stocking, below knee, 40–50 mmHg, each

IOM: 100-02, 15, 100

◆ **A6533**   Gradient compression stocking, thigh length, 18–30 mmHg, each

IOM: 100-02, 15, 130; 100-03, 4, 280.1

◆ **A6534**   Gradient compression stocking, thigh length, 30–40 mmHg, each

IOM: 100-02, 15, 130; 100-03, 4, 280.1

◆ **A6535**   Gradient compression stocking, thigh length, 40–50 mmHg, each

IOM: 100-02, 15, 130; 100-03, 4, 280.1

◆ **A6536**   Gradient compression stocking, full length/chap style, 18–30 mmHg, each

IOM: 100-02, 15, 130; 100-03, 4, 280.1

◆ **A6537**   Gradient compression stocking, full length/chap style, 30–40 mmHg, each

IOM: 100-02, 15, 130; 100-03, 4, 280.1

◆ **A6538**   Gradient compression stocking, full length/chap style, 40–50 mmHg, each

IOM: 100-02, 15, 130; 100-03, 4, 280.1

◆ **A6539**   Gradient compression stocking, waist length, 18–30 mmHg, each

IOM: 100-02, 15, 130; 100-03, 4, 280.1

◆ **A6540**   Gradient compression stocking, waist length, 30–40 mmHg, each

IOM: 100-02, 15, 130; 100-03, 4, 280.1

◆ **A6541**   Gradient compression stocking, waist length, 40–50 mmHg, each

IOM: 100-02, 15, 130; 100-03, 4, 280.1

◆ **A6542**   Gradient compression stocking, custom made

IOM: 100-02, 15, 130; 100-03, 4, 280.1

◆ **A6543**   Gradient compression stocking, lymphedema

IOM: 100-02, 15, 130; 100-03, 4, 280.1

◆ **A6544**   Gradient compression stocking, garter belt

IOM: 100-02, 15, 130; 100-03, 4, 280.1

▶ ⊛ **A6545**   Gradient compression wrap, non-elastic, below knee, 30-50 mm hg, each

IOM: 10-02, 15, 100

◆ **A6549**   Gradient compression stocking, not otherwise specified

IOM: 100-02, 15, 130; 100-03, 4, 280.1

✳ **A6550**   Wound care set, for negative pressure wound therapy electrical pump, includes all supplies and accessories

---

◀ ▶ New   ← → Revised   ✔ Reinstated   ✖ Deleted

⊛ Special coverage instructions   ◆ Not covered or valid by Medicare   ✳ Carrier discretion   ▶ ASC payment group

RESPIRATORY DURABLE MEDICAL EQUIPMENT, INEXPENSIVE AND ROUTINELY PURCHASED (A7000-A7509)

✳ **A7000** Canister, disposable, used with suction pump, each

✳ **A7001** Canister, non-disposable, used with suction pump, each

✳ **A7002** Tubing, used with suction pump, each

✳ **A7003** Administration set, with small volume nonfiltered pneumatic nebulizer, disposable

✳ **A7004** Small volume nonfiltered pneumatic nebulizer, disposable

✳ **A7005** Administration set, with small volume nonfiltered pneumatic nebulizer, non-disposable

✳ **A7006** Administration set, with small volume filtered pneumatic nebulizer

✳ **A7007** Large volume nebulizer, disposable, unfilled, used with aerosol compressor

✳ **A7008** Large volume nebulizer, disposable, prefilled, used with aerosol compressor

✳ **A7009** Reservoir bottle, nondisposable, used with large volume ultrasonic nebulizer

✳ **A7010** Corrugated tubing, disposable, used with large volume nebulizer, 100 feet

✳ **A7011** Corrugated tubing, non-disposable, used with large volume nebulizer, 10 feet

✳ **A7012** Water collection device, used with large volume nebulizer

✳ **A7013** Filter, disposable, used with aerosol compressor

✳ **A7014** Filter, non-disposable, used with aerosol compressor or ultrasonic generator

✳ **A7015** Aerosol mask, used with DME nebulizer

✳ **A7016** Dome and mouthpiece, used with small volume ultrasonic nebulizer

☺ **A7017** Nebulizer, durable, glass or autoclavable plastic, bottle type, not used with oxygen

IOM: 100-03, 4, 280.1

✳ **A7018** Water, distilled, used with large volume nebulizer, 1000 ml

✳ **A7025** High frequency chest wall oscillation system vest, replacement for use with patient owned equipment, each

✳ **A7026** High frequency chest wall oscillation system hose, replacement for use with patient owned equipment, each

✳ **A7027** Combination oral/nasal mask, used with continuous positive airway pressure device, each

✳ **A7028** Oral cushion for combination oral/nasal mask, replacement only, each

✳ **A7029** Nasal pillows for combination oral/nasal mask, replacement only, pair

✳ **A7030** Full face mask used with positive airway pressure device, each

✳ **A7031** Face mask interface, replacement for full face mask, each

✳ **A7032** Cushion for use on nasal mask interface, replacement only, each

✳ **A7033** Pillow for use on nasal cannula type interface, replacement only, pair

✳ **A7034** Nasal interface (mask or cannula type) used with positive airway pressure device, with or without head strap

✳ **A7035** Headgear used with positive airway pressure device

✳ **A7036** Chinstrap used with positive airway pressure device

✳ **A7037** Tubing used with positive airway pressure device

✳ **A7038** Filter, disposable, used with positive airway pressure device

✳ **A7039** Filter, non disposable, used with positive airway pressure device

✳ **A7040** One way chest drain valve

✳ **A7041** Water seal drainage container and tubing for use with implanted chest tube

✳ **A7042** Implanted pleural catheter, each

✳ **A7043** Vacuum drainage bottle and tubing for use with implanted catheter

✳ **A7044** Oral interface used with positive airway pressure device, each

☺ **A7045** Exhalation port with or without swivel used with accessories for positive airway devices, replacement only

IOM: 100-03, 4, 230.17

☺ **A7046** Water chamber for humidifier, used with positive airway pressure device, replacement, each

IOM: 100-03, 4, 230.17

☺ **A7501** Tracheostoma valve, including diaphragm, each

IOM: 100-02, 15, 120

◄▶ New   ←→ Revised   ✔ Reinstated   ✖ Deleted

☺ Special coverage instructions   ◆ Not covered or valid by Medicare   ✳ Carrier discretion   ▶ ASC payment group

⊙ **A7502** Replacement diaphragm/faceplate for tracheostoma valve, each

IOM: 100-02, 15, 120

⊙ **A7503** Filter holder or filter cap, reusable, for use in a tracheostoma heat and moisture exchange system, each

IOM: 100-02, 15, 120

⊙ **A7504** Filter for use in a tracheostoma heat and moisture exchange system, each

IOM: 100-02, 15, 120

⊙ **A7505** Housing, reusable without adhesive, for use in a heat and moisture exchange system and/or with a tracheostoma valve, each

IOM: 100-02, 15, 120

⊙ **A7506** Adhesive disc for use in a heat and moisture exchange system and/or with tracheostoma valve, any type, each

IOM: 100-02, 15, 120

⊙ **A7507** Filter holder and integrated filter without adhesive, for use in a tracheostoma heat and moisture exchange system, each

IOM: 100-02, 15, 120

⊙ **A7508** Housing and integrated adhesive, for use in a tracheostoma heat and moisture exchange system and/or with a tracheostoma valve, each

IOM: 100-02, 15, 120

⊙ **A7509** Filter holder and integrated filter housing, and adhesive, for use as a tracheostoma heat and moisture exchange system, each

IOM: 100-02, 15, 120

✳ **A7520** Tracheostomy/laryngectomy tube, non-cuffed, polyvinylchloride (PVC), silicone or equal, each

✳ **A7521** Tracheostomy/laryngectomy tube, cuffed, polyvinylchloride (PVC), silicone or equal, each

✳ **A7522** Tracheostomy/laryngectomy tube, stainless steel or equal (sterilizable and reusable), each

✳ **A7523** Tracheostomy shower protector, each

✳ **A7524** Tracheostoma stent/stud/button, each

✳ **A7525** Tracheostomy mask, each

✳ **A7526** Tracheostomy tube collar/holder, each

✳ **A7527** Tracheostomy/laryngectomy tube plug/stop, each

HELMETS (A8000-A8004)

✳ **A8000** Helmet, protective, soft, prefabricated, includes all components and accessories

✳ **A8001** Helmet, protective, hard, prefabricated, includes all components and accessories

✳ **A8002** Helmet, protective, soft, custom fabricated, includes all components and accessories

✳ **A8003** Helmet, protective, hard, custom fabricated, includes all components and accessories

✳ **A8004** Soft interface for helmet, replacement only

ADMINISTRATIVE, MISCELLANEOUS, AND INVESTIGATIONAL (A9000-A9999)

NOTE: The following codes do not imply that codes in other sections are necessarily covered.

⊙ **A9150** Non-prescription drugs

IOM: 100-02, 15, 50

◆ **A9152** Single vitamin/mineral/trace element, oral, per dose, not otherwise specified

◆ **A9153** Multiple vitamins, with or without minerals and trace elements, oral, per dose, not otherwise specified

✳ **A9155** Artificial saliva, 30 ml

◆ **A9180** Pediculosis (lice infestation) treatment, topical, for administration by patient/caretaker

◆ **A9270** Non-covered item or service

IOM: 100-02, 16, 20

◆ **A9274** External ambulatory insulin delivery system, disposable, each, includes all supplies and accessories

◆ **A9275** Home glucose disposable monitor, includes test strips

◆ **A9276** Sensor; invasive (e.g. subcutaneous), disposable, for use with interstitial continuous glucose monitoring system, one unit = 1 day supply
Medicare Statute 1861(n)

◆ **A9277** Transmitter; external, for use with interstitial continuous glucose monitoring system
Medicare Statute 1861(n)

◀▶ New   ←→ Revised   ✔ Reinstated   ✖ Deleted

⊙ Special coverage instructions   ◆ Not covered or valid by Medicare   ✳ Carrier discretion   ▶ ASC payment group

◆ **A9278** Receiver (monitor); external, for use with interstitial continuous glucose monitoring system
Medicare Statute 1861(n)

◆ **A9279** Monitoring feature/device, stand-alone or integrated, any type, includes all accessories, components and electronics, not otherwise classified

◆ **A9280** Alert or alarm device, not otherwise classified
Medicare Statute 1861

◆ **A9281** Reaching/grabbing device, any type, any length, each
Medicare Statute 1862 SSA

◆ **A9282** Wig, any type, each
Medicare Statute 1862 SSA

◆ **A9283** Foot pressure off loading/supportive device, any type, each
Medicare Statute 1862a(i)13

▶ ✪ **A9284** Spirometer, non-electronic, includes all accessories

◆ **A9300** Exercise equipment
IOM: 100-02, 15, 110.1; 100-03, 4, 280.1

Supplies for Radiology Procedures (Radiopharmaceuticals)

∗ **A9500** Technetium Tc-99m sestamibi, diagnostic, per study dose, up to 40 millicuries
Other: Cardiolite; TC Sestamibi

∗ **A9501** Technetium Tc-99m teboroxime, diagnostic, per study dose

→ ∗ **A9502** Technetium Tc-99m tetrofosmin, diagnostic, per study dose
Other: Myoview

∗ **A9503** Technetium Tc-99m medronate, diagnostic, per study dose, up to 30 millicuries
Other: CIS-MDP, Draximage MDP-10, Draximage MDP-25, MDP-Bracco, Technetium Tc-99m MPI-MDP

∗ **A9504** Technetium Tc-99m apcitide, diagnostic, per study dose, up to 20 millicuries
Other: Acutect

∗ **A9505** Thallium Tl-201 thallous chloride, diagnostic, per millicurie
Other: Thallous chloride USP, Thallous Chloride TL-201

∗ **A9507** Indium In-111 capromab pendetide, diagnostic, per study dose, up to 10 millicuries
Other: Prostascint

∗ **A9508** Iodine I-131 iobenguane sulfate, diagnostic, per 0.5 millicurie
Other: MIBG

∗ **A9509** Iodine I-123 sodium iodide, diagnostic, per millicurie

∗ **A9510** Technetium Tc-99m disofenin, diagnostic, per study dose, up to 15 millicuries
Other: Hepatolite

∗ **A9512** Technetium Tc-99m pertechnetate, diagnostic, per millicurie
Other: Technalite, Ultra-TechneKow

∗ **A9516** Iodine I-123 sodium iodide, diagnostic, per 100 microcuries, up to 999 microcuries

∗ **A9517** Iodine I-131 sodium iodide capsule(s), therapeutic, per millicurie

∗ **A9521** Technetium Tc-99m exametazime, diagnostic, per study dose, up to 25 millicuries
Other: Ceretec

∗ **A9524** Iodine I-131 iodinated serum albumin, diagnostic, per 5 microcuries

∗ **A9526** Nitrogen N-13 ammonia, diagnostic, per study dose, up to 40 millicuries

∗ **A9527▶** Iodine I-125, sodium iodide solution, therapeutic, per millicurie

∗ **A9528** Iodine I-131 sodium iodide capsule(s), diagnostic, per millicurie

∗ **A9529** Iodine I-131 sodium iodide solution, diagnostic, per millicurie

∗ **A9530** Iodine I-131 sodium iodide solution, therapeutic, per millicurie

∗ **A9531** Iodine I-131 sodium iodide, diagnostic, per microcurie (up to 100 microcuries)

∗ **A9532** Iodine I-125 serum albumin, diagnostic, per 5 microcuries

∗ **A9535** Injection, methylene blue, 1 ml
Other: Methylene blue

∗ **A9536** Technetium Tc-99m depreotide, diagnostic, per study dose, up to 35 millicuries

∗ **A9537** Technetium Tc-99m mebrofenin, diagnostic, per study dose, up to 15 millicuries

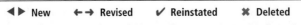

◀ ▶ New   ← → Revised   ✔ Reinstated   ✖ Deleted
✪ Special coverage instructions   ◆ Not covered or valid by Medicare   ∗ Carrier discretion   ▶ ASC payment group

* **A9538** Technetium Tc-99m pyrophosphate, diagnostic, per study dose, up to 25 millicuries

 Other: CIS-PYRO, Phosphotec, TechneScan PYP

* **A9539** Technetium Tc-99m pentetate, diagnostic, per study dose, up to 25 millicuries

 Other: AN-DTPA, DTPA, Magnavist, MPI-DTPA Kit-Chelate, MPI Indium DTPA IN-111, Pentate Calcium Trisodium, Pentate Zinc Trisodium

* **A9540** Technetium Tc-99m macroaggregated albumin, diagnostic, per study dose, up to 10 millicuries

* **A9541** Technetium Tc-99m sulfur colloid, diagnostic, per study dose, up to 20 millicuries

* **A9542** Indium In-111 ibritumomab tiuxetan, diagnostic, per study dose, up to 5 millicuries

 Other: Zevalin

* **A9543** Yttrium Y-90 ibritumomab tiuxetan, therapeutic, per treatment dose, up to 40 millicuries

* **A9544** Iodine I-131 tositumomab, diagnostic, per study dose

* **A9545** Iodine I-131 tositumomab, therapeutic, per treatment dose

 Other: Bexxar

* **A9546** Cobalt Co-57/58, cyanocobalamin, diagnostic, per study dose, up to 1 microcurie

* **A9547** Indium In-111 oxyquinoline, diagnostic, per 0.5 millicurie

* **A9548** Indium In-111 pentetate, diagnostic, per 0.5 millicurie

* **A9550** Technetium Tc-99m sodium gluceptate, diagnostic, per study dose, up to 25 millicuries

* **A9551** Technetium Tc-99m succimer, diagnostic, per study dose, up to 10 millicuries

 Other: MPI-DMSA Kidney Reagent

* **A9552** Fluorodeoxyglucose F-18 FDG, diagnostic, per study dose, up to 45 millicuries

* **A9553** Chromium Cr-51 sodium chromate, diagnostic, per study dose, up to 250 microcuries

 Other: Chromitope Sodium

* **A9554** Iodine I-125 sodium Iothalamate, diagnostic, per study dose, up to 10 microcuries

 Other: Golkil-125

* **A9555** Rubidium Rb-82, diagnostic, per study dose, up to 60 millicuries

 Other: Cardiogen 82

* **A9556** Gallium Ga-67 citrate, diagnostic, per millicurie

 Other: Ganite

* **A9557** Technetium Tc-99m bicisate, diagnostic, per study dose, up to 25 millicuries

 Other: Neurolite

* **A9558** Xenon Xe-133 gas, diagnostic, per 10 millicuries

* **A9559** Cobalt Co-57 cyanocobalamin, oral, diagnostic, per study dose, up to 1 microcurie

* **A9560** Technetium Tc-99m labeled red blood cells, diagnostic, per study dose, up to 30 millicuries

* **A9561** Technetium Tc-99m oxidronate, diagnostic, per study dose, up to 30 millicuries

 Other: TechneScan HDP

* **A9562** Technetium Tc-99m mertiatide, diagnostic, per study dose, up to 15 millicuries

 Other: TechneScan MAG-3

* **A9563** Sodium phosphate P-32, therapeutic, per millicurie

* **A9564** Chromic phosphate P-32 suspension, therapeutic, per millicurie

 Other: Phosphocol (P32)

* **A9566** Technetium Tc-99m fanolesomab, diagnostic, per study dose, up to 25 millicuries

* **A9567** Technetium Tc-99m pentetate, diagnostic, aerosol, per study dose, up to 75 millicuries

 Other: AN-DTPA, DTPA, Magnavist, MPI-DTPA Kit-Chelate, MPI Indium DTPA IN-111, Pentate Calcium Trisodium, Pentate Zinc Trisodium

* **A9568** Technetium TC-99m arcitumomab, diagnostic, per study dose, up to 45 millicuries

 Other: CEAScan

* **A9569** Technetium Tc-99m exametazime labeled autologous white blood cells, diagnostic, per study dose

 Other: Ceretec

◄► New   ←→ Revised   ✔ Reinstated   ✖ Deleted
☼ Special coverage instructions   ◆ Not covered or valid by Medicare   ✳ Carrier discretion   ▶ ASC payment group

* **A9570** Indium In-111 labeled autologous white blood cells, diagnostic, per study dose

* **A9571** Indium In-111 labeled autologous platelets, diagnostic, per study dose

* **A9572** Indium In-111 pentetreotide, diagnostic, per study dose, up to 6 millicuries

Other: Ostreoscan

* **A9576** Injection, gadoteridol, (ProHance Multipack), per ml

* **A9577** Injection, gadobenate dimeglumine (MultiHance), per ml

* **A9578** Injection, gadobenate dimeglumine (MultiHance Multipack), per ml

* **A9579** Injection, gadolinium-based magnetic resonance contrast agent, not otherwise specified (NOS), per ml

NDC: Omniscan; Optimark, Prohance, Magnevist

Other: NovaPlus® Omniscan

▶ * **A9580** Sodium fluoride F-18, diagnostic, per study dose, up to 30 millicuries

* **A9600** Strontium Sr-89 chloride, therapeutic, per millicurie

Other: Metastron; Strontium-89 Chloride

* **A9605** Samarium Sm-153 lexidronamm, therapeutic, per 50 millicuries

Other: Quadramet

⊘ **A9698** Non-radioactive contrast imaging material, not otherwise classified, per study

IOM: 100-04, 12, 70; 100-04, 13, 20

* **A9699** Radiopharmaceutical, therapeutic, not otherwise classified

⊘ **A9700** Supply of injectable contrast material for use in echocardiography, per study

IOM: 100-04, 12, 30.4

Miscellaneous Service Component

* **A9900** Miscellaneous DME supply, accessory, and/or service component of another HCPCS code

* **A9901** DME delivery, set up, and/or dispensing service component of another HCPCS code

* **A9999** Miscellaneous DME supply or accessory, not otherwise specified

◀▶ New   ←→ Revised   ✔ Reinstated   ✖ Deleted

⊘ Special coverage instructions   ◆ Not covered or valid by Medicare   * Carrier discretion   ▶ ASC payment group

ENTERAL AND PARENTERAL THERAPY (B4000-B9999)

Enteral Formulae and Enteral Medical Supplies

⚙ **B4034** Enteral feeding supply kit; syringe fed, per day

IOM: 100-02, 15, 120; 100-03, 3, 180.2; 100-04, 20, 100.2.2

⚙ **B4035** Enteral feeding supply kit; pump fed, per day

IOM: 100-02, 15, 120; 100-03, 3, 180.2; 100-04, 20, 100.2.2

⚙ **B4036** Enteral feeding supply kit; gravity fed, per day

IOM: 100-02, 15, 120; 100-03, 3, 180.2; 100-04, 20, 100.2.2

⚙ **B4081** Nasogastric tubing with stylet

IOM: 100-02, 15, 120; 100-03, 3, 180.2; 100-04, 20, 100.2.2

⚙ **B4082** Nasogastric tubing without stylet

IOM: 100-02, 15, 120; 100-03, 3, 180.2; 100-04, 20, 100.2.2

⚙ **B4083** Stomach tube - Levine type

IOM: 100-02, 15, 120; 100-03, 3, 180.2; 100-04, 20, 100.2.2

✳ **B4087** Gastrostomy/jejunostomy tube, standard, any material, any type, each

✳ **B4088** Gastrostomy/jejunostomy tube, low-profile, any material, any type, each

◆ **B4100** Food thickener, administered orally, per ounce

IOM: 100-03, 4, 208.1

⚙ **B4102** Enteral formula, for adults, used to replace fluids and electrolytes (e.g. clear liquids), 500 ml = 1 unit

IOM: 100-03, 3, 180.2

⚙ **B4103** Enteral formula, for pediatrics, used to replace fluids and electrolytes (e.g. clear liquids), 500 ml = 1 unit

IOM: 100-03, 3, 180.2

⚙ **B4104** Additive for enteral formula (e.g. fiber)

IOM: 100-03, 3, 180.2

⚙ **B4149** Enteral formula, manufactured blenderized natural foods with intact nutrients, includes proteins, fats, carbohydrates, vitamins and minerals, may include fiber, administered through an enteral feeding tube, 100 calories = 1 unit

IOM: 100-02, 15, 120; 100-03, 3, 180.2; 100-04, 20, 100.2.2

⚙ **B4150** Enteral formulae, nutritionally complete with intact nutrients, includes proteins, fats, carbohydrates, vitamins, and minerals, may include fiber, administered through an enteral feeding tube, 100 calories = 1 unit

Other: Enrich, Ensure, Ensure HN, Ensure Powder, Isocal, Lonalac Powder, Meritene, Meritene Powder, Osmolite, Osmolite HN, Portagen Powder, Sustacal, Renu, Sustagen Powder, Travasorb

IOM: 100-02, 15, 120; 100-03, 3, 180.2; 100-04, 20, 100.2.2

⚙ **B4152** Enteral formula, nutritionally complete, calorically dense (equal to or greater than 1.5 kcal/ml) with intact nutrients, includes proteins, fats, carbohydrates, vitamins and minerals, may include fiber, administered through an enteral feeding tube, 100 calories = 1 unit

Other: Magnacal, Isocal HCN, Sustacal HC, Ensure HN, Ensure Plus, Ensure Plus HN

IOM: 100-02, 15, 120; 100-03, 3, 180.2; 100-04, 20, 100.2.2

⚙ **B4153** Enteral formula, nutritionally complete, hydrolyzed proteins (amino acids and peptide chain), includes fats, carbohydrates, vitamins and minerals, may include fiber, administered through an enteral feeding tube, 100 calories = 1 unit

Other: Criticare HN, Vivonex t.e.n. (Total Enteral Nutrition), Vivonex HN, Vital (Vital HN), Travasorb HN, Isotein HN, Precision HN, Precision Isotonic

IOM: 100-02, 15, 120; 100-03, 3, 180.2; 100-04, 20, 100.2.2

⚙ **B4154** Enteral formula, nutritionally complete, for special metabolic needs, excludes inherited disease of metabolism, includes altered composition of proteins, fats, carbohydrates, vitamins and/or minerals, may include fiber, administered through an enteral feeding tube, 100 calories = 1 unit

Other: Hepatic-aid, Travasorb Hepatic, Travasorb MCT, Travasorb Renal, Traum-aid, Tramacal, Aminaid, Traumin-acid

IOM: 100-02, 15, 120; 100-03, 3, 180.2; 100-04, 20, 100.2.2

◀▶ New   ←→ Revised   ✔ Reinstated   ✘ Deleted

⚙ Special coverage instructions   ◆ Not covered or valid by Medicare   ✳ Carrier discretion   ▶ ASC payment group

⊛ **B4155** Enteral formula, nutritionally incomplete/modular nutrients, includes specific nutrients, carbohydrates (e.g. glucose polymers), proteins/amino acids (e.g. glutamine, arginine), fat (e.g. medium chain triglycerides) or combination, administered through an enteral feeding tube, 100 calories = 1 unit

Other: Casec, Propac, Gerval Protein, Promix, Casec, Moducal, Controlyte, Polycose Liquid or Powder, Sumacal, Microlipids, MCT Oil, Nutri-source

IOM: 100-02, 15, 120; 100-03, 3, 180.2; 100-04, 20, 100.2.2

⊛ **B4157** Enteral formula, nutritionally complete, for special metabolic needs for inherited disease of metabolism, includes proteins, fats, carbohydrates, vitamins and minerals, may include fiber, administered through an enteral feeding tube, 100 calories = 1 unit

IOM: 100-03, 3, 180.2

⊛ **B4158** Enteral formula, for pediatrics, nutritionally complete with intact nutrients, includes proteins, fats, carbohydrates, vitamins and minerals, may include fiber and/or iron, administered through an enteral feeding tube, 100 calories = 1 unit

IOM: 100-03, 3, 180.2

⊛ **B4159** Enteral formula, for pediatrics, nutritionally complete soy based with intact nutrients, includes proteins, fats, carbohydrates, vitamins and minerals, may include fiber and/or iron, administered through an enteral feeding tube, 100 calories = 1 unit

IOM: 100-03, 3, 180.2

⊛ **B4160** Enteral formula, for pediatrics, nutritionally complete calorically dense (equal to or greater than 0.7 kcal/ml) with intact nutrients, includes proteins, fats, carbohydrates, vitamins and minerals, may include fiber, administered through an enteral feeding tube, 100 calories = 1 unit

IOM: 100-03, 3, 180.2

⊛ **B4161** Enteral formula, for pediatrics, hydrolyzed/amino acids and peptide chain proteins, includes fats, carbohydrates, vitamins and minerals, may include fiber, administered through an enteral feeding tube, 100 calories = 1 unit

IOM: 100-03, 3, 180.2

⊛ **B4162** Enteral formula, for pediatrics, special metabolic needs for inherited disease of metabolism, includes proteins, fats, carbohydrates, vitamins and minerals, may include fiber, administered through an enteral feeding tube, 100 calories = 1 unit

IOM: 100-03, 3, 180.2

Parenteral Nutritional Solutions and Supplies

⊛ **B4164** Parenteral nutrition solution: carbohydrates (dextrose), 50% or less (500 ml = 1 unit) - homemix

IOM: 100-02, 15, 120; 100-03, 3, 180.2; 100-04, 20, 100.2.2

⊛ **B4168** Parenteral nutrition solution; amino acid, 3.5%, (500 ml = 1 unit) - homemix

IOM: 100-02, 15, 120; 100-03, 3, 180.2; 100-04, 20, 100.2.2

⊛ **B4172** Parenteral nutrition solution; amino acid, 5.5% through 7%, (500 ml = 1 unit) - homemix

IOM: 100-02, 15, 120; 100-03, 3, 180.2; 100-04, 20, 100.2.2

⊛ **B4176** Parenteral nutrition solution; amino acid, 7% through 8.5%, (500 ml = 1 unit) - homemix

IOM: 100-02, 15, 120; 100-03, 3, 180.2; 100-04, 20, 100.2.2

⊛ **B4178** Parenteral nutrition solution: amino acid, greater than 8.5%, (500 ml = 1 unit) - homemix

IOM: 100-02, 15, 120; 100-03, 3, 180.2; 100-04, 20, 100.2.2

⊛ **B4180** Parenteral nutrition solution; carbohydrates (dextrose), greater than 50% (500 ml = 1 unit)—home mix

IOM: 100-02, 15, 120; 100-03, 3, 180.2; 100-04, 20, 100.2.2

⊛ **B4185** Parenteral nutrition solution, per 10 grams lipids

⊛ **B4189** Parenteral nutrition solution; compounded amino acid and carbohydrates with electrolytes, trace elements, and vitamins, including preparation, any strength, 10 to 51 grams of protein - premix

IOM: 100-02, 15, 120; 100-03, 3, 180.2; 100-04, 20, 100.2.2

◀▶ New ←→ Revised ✔ Reinstated ✖ Deleted
⊛ Special coverage instructions ◆ Not covered or valid by Medicare ✳ Carrier discretion ▶ ASC payment group

⊕ **B4193** Parenteral nutrition solution; compounded amino acid and carbohydrates with electrolytes, trace elements, and vitamins, including preparation, any strength, 52 to 73 grams of protein - premix

IOM: 100-02, 15, 120; 100-03, 3, 180.2; 100-04, 20, 100.2.2

⊕ **B4197** Parenteral nutrition solution; compounded amino acid and carbohydrates with electrolytes, trace elements and vitamins, including preparation, any strength, 74 to 100 grams of protein - premix

IOM: 100-02, 15, 120; 100-03, 3, 180.2; 100-04, 20, 100.2.2

⊕ **B4199** Parenteral nutrition solution; compounded amino acid and carbohydrates with electrolytes, trace elements and vitamins, including preparation, any strength, over 100 grams of protein - premix

IOM: 100-02, 15, 120; 100-03, 3, 180.2; 100-04, 20, 100.2.2

⊕ **B4216** Parenteral nutrition; additives (vitamins, trace elements, heparin, electrolytes) homemix per day

IOM: 100-02, 15, 120; 100-03, 3, 180.2; 100-04, 20, 100.2.2

⊕ **B4220** Parenteral nutrition supply kit; premix, per day

IOM: 100-02, 15, 120; 100-03, 3, 180.2; 100-04, 20, 100.2.2

⊕ **B4222** Parenteral nutrition supply kit; home mix, per day

IOM: 100-02, 15, 120; 100-03, 3, 180.2; 100-04, 20, 100.2.2

⊕ **B4224** Parenteral nutrition administration kit, per day

IOM: 100-02, 15, 120; 100-03, 3, 180.2; 100-04, 20, 100.2.2

⊕ **B5000** Parenteral nutrition solution: compounded amino acid and carbohydrates with electrolytes, trace elements, and vitamins, including preparation, any strength, renal - Amirosyn-RF, NephrAmine, RenAmine - premix

Other: Amirosyn-RF, NephrAmine, RenAmin

IOM: 100-02, 15, 120; 100-03, 3, 180.2; 100-04, 20, 100.2.2

⊕ **B5100** Parenteral nutrition solution: compounded amino acid and carbohydrates with electrolytes, trace elements, and vitamins, including preparation, any strength, hepatic - FreAmine HBC, HepatAmine - premix

Other: FerAmine HBC, HepatAmine

IOM: 100-02, 15, 120; 100-03, 3, 180.2; 100-04, 20, 100.2.2

⊕ **B5200** Parenteral nutrition solution; compounded amino acid and carbohydrates with electrolytes, trace elements, and vitamins, including preparation, any strength, stress - branch chain amino acids - premix

IOM: 100-02, 15, 120; 100-03, 3, 180.2; 100-04, 20, 100.2.2

Enteral and Parenteral Pumps

⊕ **B9000** Enteral nutrition infusion pump - without alarm

IOM: 100-02, 15, 120; 100-03, 3, 180.2; 100-04, 20, 100.2.2

⊕ **B9002** Enteral nutrition infusion pump - with alarm

IOM: 100-02, 15, 120; 100-03, 3, 180.2; 100-04, 20, 100.2.2

⊕ **B9004** Parenteral nutrition infusion pump, portable

IOM: 100-02, 15, 120; 100-03, 3, 180.2; 100-04, 20, 100.2.2

⊕ **B9006** Parenteral nutrition infusion pump, stationary

IOM: 100-02, 15, 120; 100-03, 3, 180.2; 100-04, 20, 100.2.2

⊕ **B9998** NOC for enteral supplies

IOM: 100-02, 15, 120; 100-03, 3, 180.2; 100-04, 20, 100.2.2

⊕ **B9999** NOC for parenteral supplies

(Determine if an alternative HCPCS Level II or a CPT code better describes the service being reported. This code should be used only if a more specific code is unavailable.)

IOM: 100-02, 15, 120; 100-03, 3, 180.2; 100-04, 20, 100.2.2

◄▶ New ←→ Revised ✔ Reinstated ✖ Deleted
⊕ Special coverage instructions ◆ Not covered or valid by Medicare ✱ Carrier discretion ▶ ASC payment group

CMS HOSPITAL OUTPATIENT PAYMENT SYSTEM (C1000-C9999)

NOTE: C codes are used ONLY as a part of Hospital Outpatient Prospective Payment System (OPPS) and are not to be used to report other services. C codes are updated quarterly by the Centers for Medicare and Medicaid Services.

⊗ **C1300** Hyperbaric oxygen under pressure, full body chamber, per 30-minute interval
Medicare Statute 1833(t)

⊗ **C1713** Anchor/Screw for opposing bone-to-bone or soft tissue-to-bone (implantable)
Medicare Statute 1833(t)

⊗ **C1714** Catheter, transluminal atherectomy, directional
Medicare Statute 1833(t)

⊗ **C1715** Brachytherapy needle
Medicare Statute 1833(t)

⊗ **C1716▶** Brachytherapy source, non-stranded, gold-198, per source
Medicare Statute 1833(t)

⊗ **C1717▶** Brachytherapy source, non-stranded, high dose rate iridium 192, per source
Medicare Statute 1833(t)

⊗ **C1719▶** Brachytherapy source, non-stranded, non-high dose rate iridium-192, per source
Medicare Statute 1833(t)

⊗ **C1721** Cardioverter-defibrillator, dual chamber (implantable)
Medicare Statute 1833(t)

⊗ **C1722** Cardioverter-defibrillator, single chamber (implantable)
Medicare Statute 1833(t)

⊗ **C1724** Catheter, transluminal atherectomy, rotational
Medicare Statute 1833(t)

⊗ **C1725** Catheter, transluminal angioplasty, non-laser (may include guidance, infusion/perfusion capability)
Medicare Statute 1833(t)

⊗ **C1726** Catheter, balloon dilatation, non-vascular
Medicare Statute 1833(t)

⊗ **C1727** Catheter, balloon tissue dissector, non-vascular (insertable)
Medicare Statute 1833(t)

⊗ **C1728** Catheter, brachytherapy seed administration
Medicare Statute 1833(t)

⊗ **C1729** Catheter, drainage
Medicare Statute 1833(t)

⊗ **C1730** Catheter, electrophysiology, diagnostic, other than 3D mapping (19 or fewer electrodes)
Medicare Statute 1833(t)

⊗ **C1731** Catheter, electrophysiology, diagnostic, other than 3D mapping (20 or more electrodes)
Medicare Statute 1833(t)

⊗ **C1732** Catheter, electrophysiology, diagnostic/ablation, 3D or vector mapping
Medicare Statute 1833(t)

⊗ **C1733** Catheter, electrophysiology, diagnostic/ablation, other than 3D or vector mapping, other than cool-tip
Medicare Statute 1833(t)

⊗ **C1750** Catheter, hemodialysis/peritoneal, long-term
Medicare Statute 1833(t)

⊗ **C1751** Catheter, infusion, inserted peripherally, centrally, or midline (other than hemodialysis)
Medicare Statute 1833(t)

⊗ **C1752** Catheter, hemodialysis/peritoneal, short-term
Medicare Statute 1833(t)

⊗ **C1753** Catheter, intravascular ultrasound
Medicare Statute 1833(t)

⊗ **C1754** Catheter, intradiscal
Medicare Statute 1833(t)

⊗ **C1755** Catheter, instraspinal
Medicare Statute 1833(t)

⊗ **C1756** Catheter, pacing, transesophageal
Medicare Statute 1833(t)

⊗ **C1757** Catheter, thrombectomy/embolectomy
Medicare Statute 1833(t)

⊗ **C1758** Catheter, ureteral
Medicare Statute 1833(t)

⊗ **C1759** Catheter, intracardiac echocardiography
Medicare Statute 1833(t)

⊗ **C1760** Closure device, vascular (implantable/insertable)
Medicare Statute 1833(t)

⊗ **C1762** Connective tissue, human (includes fascia lata)
Medicare Statute 1833(t)

⊗ **C1763** Connective tissue, non-human (includes synthetic)
Medicare Statute 1833(t)

⊗ **C1764** Event recorder, cardiac (implantable)
Medicare Statute 1833(t)

⊗ **C1765** Adhesion barrier
Medicare Statute 1833 (t)

◀ ▶ New   ← → Revised   ✔ Reinstated   ✘ Deleted
⊗ Special coverage instructions   ◆ Not covered or valid by Medicare   ✳ Carrier discretion   ▶ ASC payment group

⊛ **C1766** Introducer/sheath, guiding, intracardiac electrophysiological, steerable, other than peel-away
Medicare Statute 1833(t)

⊛ **C1767** Generator, neurostimulator (implantable), nonrechargeable
Medicare Statute 1833(t)

⊛ **C1768** Graft, vascular
Medicare Statute 1833(t)

⊛ **C1769** Guide wire
Medicare Statute 1833(t)

⊛ **C1770** Imaging coil, magnetic reasonance (insertable)
Medicare Statute 1833(t)

⊛ **C1771** Repair device, urinary, incontinence, with sling graft
Medicare Statute 1833(t)

⊛ **C1772** Infusion pump, programmable (implantable)
Medicare Statute 1833(t)

⊛ **C1773** Retrieval device, insertable (used to retrieve fractured medical devices)
Medicare Statute 1833(t)

⊛ **C1776** Joint device (implantable)
Medicare Statute 1833(t)

⊛ **C1777** Lead, cardioverter-defibrillator, endocardial single coil (implantable)
Medicare Statute 1833(t)

⊛ **C1778** Lead, neurostimulator (implantable)
Medicare Statute 1833(t)

⊛ **C1779** Lead, pacemaker, trasvenous VDD single pass
Medicare Statute 1833(t)

⊛ **C1780** Lens, intraocular (new technology)
Medicare Statute 1833(t)

⊛ **C1781** Mesh (implantable)
Medicare Statute 1833(t)

⊛ **C1782** Morcellator
Medicare Statute 1833(t)

⊛ **C1783** Ocular implant, aqueous drainage assist device
Medicare Statute 1833(t)

⊛ **C1784** Ocular device, intraoperative, detached retina
Medicare Statute 1833(t)

⊛ **C1785** Pacemaker, dual chamber, rate-responsive (implantable)
Medicare Statute 1833(t)

⊛ **C1786** Pacemaker, single chamber, rate-responsive (implantable)
Medicare Statute 1833(t)

⊛ **C1787** Patient programmer, neurostimulator
Medicare Statute 1833(t)

⊛ **C1788** Port, indwelling (implantable)
Medicare Statute 1833(t)

⊛ **C1789** Prosthesis, breast (implantable)
Medicare Statute 1833(t)

⊛ **C1813** Prosthesis, penile, inflatable
Medicare Statute 1833(t)

⊛ **C1814** Retinal tamponade device, silicone oil
Medicare Statute 1833(t)

⊛ **C1815** Prosthesis, urinary sphincter (implantable)
Medicare Statute 1833(t)

⊛ **C1816** Receiver and/or transmitter, neurostimulator (implantable)
Medicare Statute 1833(t)

⊛ **C1817** Septal defect implant system, intracardiac
Medicare Statute 1833(t)

⊛ **C1818** Integrated keratoprosthesic
Medicare Statute 1833(t)

⊛ **C1819** Surgical tissue localization and excision device (implantable)
Medicare Statute 1833(t)

⊛ **C1820** Generator, neurostimulator (implantable), with rechargeable battery and charging system
Medicare Statute 1833(t)

⊛ **C1821** Interspinous process distraction device (implantable)
Medicare Statute 1833(t)

⊛ **C1874** Stent, coated/covered, with delivery system
Medicare Statute 1833(t)

⊛ **C1875** Stent, coated/covered, without delivery system
Medicare Statute 1833(t)

⊛ **C1876** Stent, non-coated/non-covered, with delivery system
Medicare Statute 1833(t)

⊛ **C1877** Stent, non-coated/non-covered, without delivery system
Medicare Statute 1833(t)

⊛ **C1878** Material for vocal cord medialization, synthetic (implantable)
Medicare Statute 1833(t)

⊛ **C1879** Tissue marker (implantable)
Medicare Statute 1833(t)

⊛ **C1880** Vena cava filter
Medicare Statute 1833(t)

⊛ **C1881** Dialysis access system (implantable)
Medicare Statute 1833(t)

⊛ **C1882** Cardioverter-defibrillator, other than single or dual chamber (implantable)
Medicare Statute 1833(t)

⊛ **C1883** Adaptor/Extension, pacing lead or neurostimulator lead (implantable)
Medicare Statute 1833(t)

◀▶ New ←→ Revised ✔ Reinstated ✖ Deleted
⊛ Special coverage instructions ◆ Not covered or valid by Medicare ✳ Carrier discretion ▶ ASC payment group

⊛ **C1884** Embolization protective system
Medicare Statute 1833(t)

⊛ **C1885** Catheter, transluminal angioplasty, laser
Medicare Statute 1833(t)

⊛ **C1887** Catheter, guiding (may include infusion/perfusion capability)
Medicare Statute 1833(t)

⊛ **C1888** Catheter, ablation, non-cardiac, endovascular (implantable)
Medicare Statute 1833(t)

⊛ **C1891** Infusion pump, non-programmable, permanent (implantable)
Medicare Statute 1833(t)

⊛ **C1892** Introducer/sheath, guiding, intracardiac electrophysiological, fixed-curve, peel-away
Medicare Statute 1833(t)

⊛ **C1893** Introducer/sheath, guiding, intracardiac electrophysiological, fixed-curve, other than peel-away
Medicare Statute 1833(t)

⊛ **C1894** Introducer/sheath, other than guiding, other than intracardiac electrophysiological, non-laser
Medicare Statute 1833(t)

⊛ **C1895** Lead, cardioverter-defibrillator, endocardial dual coil (implantable)
Medicare Statute 1833(t)

⊛ **C1896** Lead, cardioverter-defibrillator, other than endocardial single or dual coil (implantable)
Medicare Statute 1833(t)

⊛ **C1897** Lead, neurostimulator test kit (implantable)
Medicare Statute 1833(t)

⊛ **C1898** Lead, pacemaker, other than transvenous VDD single pass
Medicare Statute 1833(t)

⊛ **C1899** Lead, pacemaker/cardioverter-defibrillator combination (implantable)
Medicare Statute 1833(t)

⊛ **C1900** Lead, left ventricular coronary venous system
Medicare Statute 1833(t)

⊛ **C2614** Probe, percutaneous lumbar discectomy
Medicare Statute 1833(t)

⊛ **C2615** Sealant, pulmonary, liquid
Medicare Statute 1833(t)

⊛ **C2616▶** Brachytherapy source, non-stranded, yttrium-90, per source
Medicare Statute 1833(T)

⊛ **C2617** Stent, non-coronary, temporary, without delivery system
Medicare Statute 1833(t)

⊛ **C2618** Probe, cryoablation
Medicare Statute 1833(t)

⊛ **C2619** Pacemaker, dual chamber, non rate-responsive (implantable)
Medicare Statute 1833(t)

⊛ **C2620** Pacemaker, single chamber, non rate-responsive (implantable)
Medicare Statute 1833(t)

⊛ **C2621** Pacemaker, other than single or dual chamber (implantable)
Medicare Statute 1833(t)

⊛ **C2622** Prosthesis, penile, non-inflatable
Medicare Statute 1833(t)

⊛ **C2625** Stent, non-coronary, temporary, with delivery system
Medicare Statute 1833(t)

⊛ **C2626** Infusion pump, non-programmable, temporary (implantable)
Medicare Statute 1833(t)

⊛ **C2627** Catheter, suprapubic/cystoscopic
Medicare Statute 1833(t)

⊛ **C2628** Catheter, occlusion
Medicare Statute 1833(t)

⊛ **C2629** Introducer/Sheath, other than guiding, intracardiac electrophysiological, laser
Medicare Statute 1833(t)

⊛ **C2630** Catheter, electrophysiology, diagnostic/ablation, other than 3D or vector mapping, cool-tip
Medicare Statute 1833(t)

⊛ **C2631** Repair device, urinary, incontinence, without sling graft
Medicare Statute 1833(t)

⊛ **C2634▶** Brachytherapy source, non-stranded, high activity, iodine-125, greater than 1.01 mci (NIST), per source
Medicare Statute 1833(t)

⊛ **C2635▶** Brachytherapy source, non-stranded, high activity, paladium-103, greater than 2.2 mci (NIST), per source
Medicare Statute 1833(t)

⊛ **C2636▶** Brachytherapy linear source, non-stranded, paladium-103, per 1 mm

⊛ **C2637** Brachytherapy source, non-stranded, Ytterbium-169, per source
Medicare Statute 1833(t)

⊛ **C2638▶** Brachytherapy source, stranded, iodine-125, per source
Medicare Statute 1833(t)(2)

⊛ **C2639▶** Brachytherapy source, non-stranded, iodine-125, per source
Medicare Statute 1833(t)(2)

⊛ **C2640▶** Brachytherapy source, stranded, palladium-103, per source
Medicare Statute 1833(t)(2)

◀ ▶ **New**   ←→ **Revised**   ✔ **Reinstated**   ✖ **Deleted**
⊛ **Special coverage instructions**   ◆ **Not covered or valid by Medicare**   ✳ **Carrier discretion**   ▶ **ASC payment group**

⊗ **C2641**▶ Brachytherapy source, non-stranded, palladium-103, per source
Medicare Statute 1833(t)(2)

⊗ **C2642**▶ Brachytherapy source, stranded, cesium-131, per source
Medicare Statute 1833(t)(2)

⊗ **C2643**▶ Brachytherapy source, non-stranded, cesium-131, per source
Medicare Statute 1833(t)(2)

⊗ **C2698**▶ Brachytherapy source, stranded, not otherwise specified, per source
Medicare Statute 1833(t)(2)

⊗ **C2699**▶ Brachytherapy source, non-stranded, not otherwise specified, per source
Medicare Statute 1833(t)(2)

⊗ **C8900**▶ Magnetic resonance angiography with contrast, abdomen
Medicare Statute 1833(t)(2)

⊗ **C8901**▶ Magnetic resonance angiography without contrast, abdomen
Medicare Statute 1833(t)(2)

⊗ **C8902**▶ Magnetic resonance angiography without contrast followed by with contrast, abdomen
Medicare Statute 1833(t)(2)

⊗ **C8903**▶ Magnetic resonance imaging with contrast, breast; unilateral
Medicare Statute 1833(t)(2)

⊗ **C8904**▶ Magnetic resonance imaging without contrast, breast; unilateral
Medicare Statute 1833(t)(2)

⊗ **C8905**▶ Magnetic resonance imaging without contrast followed by with contrast, breast; unilateral
Medicare Statute 1833(t)(2)

⊗ **C8906**▶ Magnetic resonance imaging with contrast, breast; bilateral
Medicare Statute 1833(t)(2)

⊗ **C8907**▶ Magnetic resonance imaging without contrast, breast; bilateral
Medicare Statute 1833(t)(2)

⊗ **C8908**▶ Magnetic resonance imaging without contrast followed by with contrast, breast; bilateral
Medicare Statute 1833(t)(2)

⊗ **C8909**▶ Magnetic resonance angiography with contrast, chest (excluding myocardium)
Medicare Statute 1833(t)(2)

⊗ **C8910**▶ Magnetic resonance angiography without contrast, chest (excluding myocardium)
Medicare Statute 1833(t)(2)

⊗ **C8911**▶ Magnetic resonance angiography without contrast followed by with contrast, chest (excluding myocardium)
Medicare Statute 1833(t)(2)

⊗ **C8912**▶ Magnetic resonance angiography with contrast, lower extremity
Medicare Statute 1833(t)(2)

⊗ **C8913**▶ Magnetic resonance angiography without contrast, lower extremity
Medicare Statute 1833(t)(2)

⊗ **C8914**▶ Magnetic resonance angiography without contrast followed by with contrast, lower extremity
Medicare Statute 1833(t)(2)

⊗ **C8918**▶ Magnetic resonance angiography with contrast, pelvis
Medicare Statute 1833(t)(2)

⊗ **C8919**▶ Magnetic resonance angiography without contrast, pelvis
Medicare Statute 1833(t)(2)

⊗ **C8920**▶ Magnetic resonance angiography without contrast followed by with contrast, pelvis
Medicare Statute 1833(t)(2)

→ ⊗ **C8921** Transthoracic echocardiography with contrast, or without contrast followed by with contrast, for congenital cardiac anomalies; complete
Medicare Statute 1833(t)(2)

→ ⊗ **C8922** Transthoracic echocardiography with contrast, or without contrast followed by with contrast, for congenital cardiac anomalies; follow-up or limited study
Medicare Statute 1833(t)(2)

→ ⊗ **C8923** Transthoracic echocardiography with contrast, or without contrast followed by with contrast, real-time with image documentation (2D) with or without M-mode recording; complete
Medicare Statute 1833(t)(2)

→ ⊗ **C8924** Transthoracic echocardiography with contrast, or without contrast followed by with contrast, real-time with image documentation (2D) with or without M-mode recording; follow-up or limited study
Medicare Statute 1833(t)(2)

→ ⊗ **C8925** Transesophageal echocardiography (TEE) with contrast, or without contrast followed by with contrast, real time with image documentation (2D) (with or without M-mode recording); including probe placement, image acquisition, interpretation and report
Medicare Statute 1833(t)(2)

→ ⊗ **C8926** Transesophageal echocardiography (TEE) with contrast, or without contrast followed by with contrast, for congenital cardiac anomalies; including probe placement, image acquisition, interpretation and report
Medicare Statute 1833(t)(2)

→ ☼ **C8927** Transesophageal echocardiography (TEE) with contrast, or without contrast followed by with contrast, for monitoring purposes, including probe placement, real time 2-dimensional image acquisition and interpretation leading to ongoing (continuous) assessment of (dynamically changing) cardiac pumping function and to therapeutic measures on an immediate time basis
Medicare Statute 1833(t)(2)

→ ☼ **C8928** Transthoracic echocardiography with contrast, or without contrast followed by with contrast, real-time with image documentation (2D), with or without M-mode recording, during rest and cardiovascular stress test using treadmill, bicycle exercise and/or pharmacologically induced stress, with interpretation and report
Medicare Statute 1833(t)(2)

▶ ☼ **C8929** Transthoracic echocardiography with contrast, or without contrast followed by with contrast, real-time with image documentation (2D), includes M-mode recording, when performed, complete, with spectral Doppler echocardiography, and with color flow Doppler echocardiography
Medicare Statute 1833(t)(2)

▶ ☼ **C8930** Transthoracic echocardiography, with contrast, or without contrast followed by with contrast, real-time with image documentation (2D), includes M-mode recording, when performed, during rest and cardiovascular stress test using treadmill, bicycle exercise and/or pharmacologically induced stress, with interpretation and report; including performance of continuous electrocardiographic monitoring, with physician supervision
Medicare Statute 1833(t)(2)

☼ **C8957** Intravenous infusion for therapy/ diagnosis; initiation of prolonged infusion (more than 8 hours), requiring use of portable or implantable pump
Medicare Statute 1833(t)

~~C9003~~ ~~Palivizumab RSV IGM, per 50 mg~~ ✖
Cross Reference CPT 90378

☼ **C9113** Injection, pantoprazole sodium, per vial
Medicare Statute 1833(t)

☼ **C9121▶** Injection, argatroban, per 5 mg
Medicare Statute 1833(t)

~~C9237~~ ~~Injection, lanreotide acetate, 1 mg~~ ✖
Cross Reference J1930

~~C9238~~ ~~Injection, levetiracetam, 10 mg~~ ✖
Cross Reference J1953

~~C9239~~ ~~Injection, temsirolimus, 1 mg~~ ✖
Cross Reference J9330

~~C9240~~ ~~Injection, ixabepilone, 1 mg~~ ✖
Cross Reference J9207

~~C9241~~ ~~Injection, doripenem, 10 mg~~ ✖
Cross Reference J1267

~~C9242~~ ~~Injection, fosaprepitant, 1 mg~~ ✖
Cross Reference J1453

~~C9243~~ ~~Injection, bendamustine hcl, 1 mg~~ ✖
Cross Reference J9033

~~C9244~~ ~~Injection, regadenoson, 0.4 mg~~ ✖
Cross Reference J2785

▶ ☼ **C9245▶** Injection, romiplostim, 10 mcg
Medicare Statute 1833(t)

▶ ☼ **C9246▶** Injection, gadoxetate disodium, per ml
Medicare Statute 1833(t)

▶ ☼ **C9247** Iobenguane, I-123, diagnostic, per study dose, up to 10 millicuries
Medicare Statute 1833(t)

▶ ☼ **C9248▶** Injection, clevidipien butyrate, 1 mg
Medicare Statute 1833(t)

☼ **C9352** Microporous collagen implantable tube (NeuraGen Nerve Guide), per centimeter length
621MMA

☼ **C9353** Microporous collagen implantable slit tube (NeuraWrap Nerve Protector), per centimeter length
621MMA

☼ **C9354▶** Acellular pericardial tissue matrix of non-human origin (Veritas), per square centimeter
621 MMA

☼ **C9355▶** Collagen nerve cuff (NeuroMatrix), per 0.5 centimeter length
621 MMA

▶ ☼ **C9356▶** Tendon, porous matrix of cross-linked collagen and glycosaminoglycan matrix (TenoGlide Tendon Protector Sheet), per square centimeter
621 MMA

~~C9357~~ ~~Dermal substitute, granulated cross-linked collagen and glycosaminoglycan matrix (flowable wound matrix), 1 cc~~ ✖
Cross Reference Q4114

▶ ☼ **C9358▶** Dermal substitute, native, non-denatured collagen (SurgiMend Collagen Matrix), per 0.5 square centimeters
621 MMA

◀▶ New   ←→ Revised   ✔ Reinstated   ✖ Deleted

☼ Special coverage instructions   ◆ Not covered or valid by Medicare   ✳ Carrier discretion   ▶ ASC payment group

▶ ✪ **C9359** Porous purified collagen matrix bone void filler (Integra Mozaik Osteoconductive Scaffold Putty, Integra OS Osteoconductive Scaffold Putty), per 0.5 cc
Medicare Statute 1833(t)

✪ **C9399** Unclassified drugs or biologicals
621MMA

✪ **C9716** Creations of thermal anal lesions by radiofrequency energy
Medicare Statute 1833(t)

~~**C9723** Dynamic infrared blood perfusion imaging (DIRI)~~ ✖

✪ **C9724** Endoscopic full-thickness plication in the gastric cardia using endoscopic plication system (EPS); includes endoscopy
Medicare Statute 1833(t)

✪ **C9725** Placement of endorectal intracavitary applicator for high intensity brachytherapy
Medicare Statute 1833(t)

✪ **C9726** Placement and removal (if performed) of applicator into breast for radiation therapy
Medicare Statute 1833(t)

✪ **C9727** Insertion of implants into the soft palate; minimum of three implants
Medicare Statute 1833(t)

✪ **C9728** Placement of interstitial device(s) for radiation therapy/surgery guidance (e.g., fiducial markers, dosimeter), other than prostate (any approach), single or multiple
Medicare Statute 1833(t)

▶ ✪ **C9898** Radiolabeled product provided during a hospital inpatient stay

▶ ✪ **C9899** Implanted prosthetic device, payable only for inpatients who do not have inpatient coverage
Medicare Statute 1833(t)

◀▶ New   ←→ Revised   ✔ Reinstated   ✖ Deleted
✪ Special coverage instructions   ◆ Not covered or valid by Medicare   ✲ Carrier discretion   ▶ ASC payment group

DURABLE MEDICAL EQUIPMENT (E0100–E9999)

Canes

⊚ **E0100** Cane, includes canes of all materials, adjustable or fixed, with tip

IOM: 100-02, 15, 110.1; 100-03, 4, 280.1; 100-03, 4, 280.2

⊚ **E0105** Cane, quad or three prong, includes canes of all materials, adjustable or fixed, with tips

IOM: 100-02, 15, 110.1; 100-03, 4, 280.1; 100-03, 4, 280.2

Crutches

⊚ **E0110** Crutches, forearm, includes crutches of various materials, adjustable or fixed, pair, complete with tips and handgrips

IOM: 100-02, 15, 110.1; 100-03, 4, 280.1

⊚ **E0111** Crutch forearm, includes crutches of various materials, adjustable or fixed, each, with tips and handgrips

IOM: 100-02, 15, 110.1; 100-03, 4, 280.1

⊚ **E0112** Crutches, underarm, wood, adjustable or fixed, pair, with pads, tips, and handgrips

IOM: 100-02, 15, 110.1; 100-03, 4, 280.1

⊚ **E0113** Crutch underarm, wood, adjustable or fixed, each, with pad, tip, and handgrip

IOM: 100-02, 15, 110.1; 100-03, 4, 280.1

⊚ **E0114** Crutches, underarm, other than wood, adjustable or fixed, pair, with pads, tips and handgrips

IOM: 100-02, 15, 110.1; 100-03, 4, 280.1

⊚ **E0116** Crutch, underarm, other than wood, adjustable or fixed, with pad, tip, handgrip, with or without shock absorber, each

IOM: 100-02, 15, 110.1; 100-03, 4, 280.1

⊚ **E0117** Crutch, underarm, articulating, spring assisted, each

IOM: 100-02, 15, 110.1

✳ **E0118** Crutch substitute, lower leg platform, with or without wheels, each

Walkers

⊚ **E0130** Walker, rigid (pickup), adjustable or fixed height

IOM: 100-02, 15, 110.1; 100-03, 4, 280.1

⊚ **E0135** Walker, folding (pickup), adjustable or fixed height

IOM: 100-02, 15, 110.1; 100-03, 4, 280.1

⊚ **E0140** Walker, with trunk support, adjustable or fixed height, any type

IOM: 100-02, 15, 110.1; 100-03, 4, 280.1

⊚ **E0141** Walker, rigid, wheeled, adjustable or fixed height

IOM: 100-02, 15, 110.1; 100-03, 4, 280.1

⊚ **E0143** Walker, folding, wheeled, adjustable or fixed height

IOM: 100-02, 15, 110.1; 100-03, 4, 280.1

⊚ **E0144** Walker, enclosed, four sided framed, rigid or folding, wheeled, with posterior seat

IOM: 100-02, 15, 110.1; 100-03, 4, 280.1

⊚ **E0147** Walker, heavy duty, multiple braking system, variable wheel resistance

IOM: 100-02, 15, 110.1; 100-03, 4, 280.1

✳ **E0148** Walker, heavy duty, without wheels, rigid or folding, any type, each

✳ **E0149** Walker, heavy duty, wheeled, rigid or folding, any type

✳ **E0153** Platform attachment, forearm crutch, each

✳ **E0154** Platform attachment, walker, each

✳ **E0155** Wheel attachment, rigid pick-up walker, per pair

Attachments

✳ **E0156** Seat attachment, walker

✳ **E0157** Crutch attachment, walker, each

✳ **E0158** Leg extensions for walker, per set of four (4)

✳ **E0159** Brake attachment for wheeled walker, replacement, each

Commodes

⊚ **E0160** Sitz type bath or equipment, portable, used with or without commode

IOM: 100-03, 4, 280.1

◀▶ New   ←→ Revised   ✔ Reinstated   ✖ Deleted

⊚ Special coverage instructions   ◆ Not covered or valid by Medicare   ✳ Carrier discretion   ▶ ASC payment group

© **E0161** Sitz type bath or equipment, portable, used with or without commode, with faucet attachment/ s

IOM: 100-03, 4, 280.1

© **E0162** Sitz bath chair

IOM: 100-03, 4, 280.1

© **E0163** Commode chair, mobile or stationary, with fixed arms

IOM: 100-02, 15, 110.1; 100-03, 4, 280.1

© **E0165** Commode chair, mobile or stationary, with detachable arms

IOM: 100-02, 15, 110.1; 100-03, 4, 280.1

© **E0167** Pail or pan for use with commode chair, replacement only

IOM: 100-03, 4, 280.1

✳ **E0168** Commode chair, extra wide and/or heavy duty, stationary or mobile, with or without arms, any type, each

✳ **E0170** Commode chair with integrated seat lift mechanism, electric, any type

✳ **E0171** Commode chair with integrated seat lift mechanism, non-electric, any type

◆ **E0172** Seat lift mechanism placed over or on top of toilet, any type

Medicare Statute 1861 SSA

✳ **E0175** Foot rest, for use with commode chair, each

Decubitus Care Equipment

© **E0181** Powered pressure reducing mattress overlay/pad, alternating, with pump, includes heavy duty

IOM: 100-03, 4, 280.1; 100-08, 5, 5.2.3

© **E0182** Pump for alternating pressure pad, for replacement only

IOM: 100-03, 4, 280.1; 100-08, 5, 5.2.3

© **E0184** Dry pressure mattress

IOM: 100-03, 4, 280.1; 100-08, 5, 5.2.3

© **E0185** Gel or gel-like pressure pad for mattress, standard mattress length and width

IOM: 100-03, 4, 280.1; 100-08, 5, 5.2.3

© **E0186** Air pressure mattress

IOM: 100-03, 4, 280.1

© **E0187** Water pressure mattress

IOM: 100-03, 4, 280.1

© **E0188** Synthetic sheepskin pad

IOM: 100-03, 4, 280.1; 100-08, 5, 5.2.3

© **E0189** Lambswool sheepskin pad, any size

IOM: 100-03, 4, 280.1; 100-08, 5, 5.2.3

© **E0190** Positioning cushion/pillow/wedge, any shape or size, includes all components and accessories

IOM: 100-02, 15, 110.1

✳ **E0191** Heel or elbow protector, each

✳ **E0193** Powered air flotation bed (low air loss therapy)

© **E0194** Air fluidized bed

IOM: 100-03, 4, 280.1

© **E0196** Gel pressure mattress

IOM: 100-03, 4, 280.1

© **E0197** Air pressure pad for mattress, standard mattress length and width

IOM: 100-03, 4, 280.1

© **E0198** Water pressure pad for mattress, standard mattress length and width

IOM: 100-03, 4, 280.1

© **E0199** Dry pressure pad for mattress, standard mattress length and width

IOM: 100-03, 4, 280.1

Heat/Cold Application

© **E0200** Heat lamp, without stand (table model), includes bulb, or infrared element

IOM: 100-02, 15, 110.1; 100-03, 4, 280.1

✳ **E0202** Phototherapy (bilirubin) light with photometer

◆ **E0203** Therapeutic lightbox, minimum 10,000 lux, table top model

IOM: 100-03, 4, 280.1

© **E0205** Heat lamp, with stand, includes bulb, or infrared element

IOM: 100-02, 15, 110.1; 100-03, 4, 280.1

© **E0210** Electric heat pad, standard

IOM: 100-03, 4, 280.1

© **E0215** Electric heat pad, moist

IOM: 100-03, 4, 280.1

© **E0217** Water circulating heat pad with pump

IOM: 100-03, 4, 280.1

© **E0218** Water circulating cold pad with pump

IOM: 100-03, 4, 280.1

✳ **E0220** Hot water bottle

✳ **E0221** Infrared heating pad system

◀▶ New   ←→ Revised   ✔ Reinstated   ✖ Deleted

© Special coverage instructions   ◆ Not covered or valid by Medicare   ✳ Carrier discretion   ▶ ASC payment group

⊛ **E0225** Hydrocollator unit, includes pads
IOM: 100-02, 15, 230; 100-03, 4, 280.1

✳ **E0230** Ice cap or collar

◆ **E0231** Non-contact wound warming device (temperature control unit, AC adapter and power cord) for use with warming card and wound cover
IOM: 100-02, 16, 20

◆ **E0232** Warming card for use with the non-contact wound warming device and non contact wound warming wound cover
IOM: 100-02, 16, 20

⊛ **E0235** Paraffin bath unit, portable (see medical supply code A4265 for paraffin)
IOM: 100-02, 15, 230; 100-03, 4, 280.1

⊛ **E0236** Pump for water circulating pad
IOM: 100-03, 4, 280.1

⊛ **E0238** Non-electric heat pad, moist
IOM: 100-03, 4, 280.1

⊛ **E0239** Hydrocollator unit, portable
IOM: 100-02, 15, 230; 100-03, 4, 280.1

Bath and Toilet Aids

◆ **E0240** Bath/shower chair, with or without wheels, any size
IOM: 100-03, 4, 280.1

◆ **E0241** Bath tub wall rail, each
IOM: 100-02, 15, 110.1; 100-03, 4, 280.1

◆ **E0242** Bath tub rail, floor base
IOM: 100-02, 15, 110.1; 100-03, 4, 280.1

◆ **E0243** Toilet rail, each
IOM: 100-02, 15, 110.1; 100-03, 4, 280.1

◆ **E0244** Raised toilet seat
IOM: 100-03, 4, 280.1

◆ **E0245** Tub stool or bench
IOM: 100-03, 4, 280.1

✳ **E0246** Transfer tub rail attachment

⊛ **E0247** Transfer bench for tub or toilet with or without commode opening
IOM: 100-03, 4, 280.1

⊛ **E0248** Transfer bench, heavy duty, for tub or toilet with or without commode opening
IOM: 100-03, 4, 280.1

⊛ **E0249** Pad for water circulating heat unit
IOM: 100-03, 4, 280.1

Hospital Beds and Accessories

⊛ **E0250** Hospital bed, fixed height, with any type side rails, with mattress
IOM: 100-02, 15, 110.1; 100-03, 4, 280.7

⊛ **E0251** Hospital bed, fixed height, with any type side rails, without mattress
IOM:100-02, 15, 110.1; 100-03, 4, 280.7

⊛ **E0255** Hospital bed, variable height, hi-lo, with any type side rails, with mattress
IOM: 100-02, 15, 110.1; 100-03, 4, 280.7

⊛ **E0256** Hospital bed, variable height, hi-lo, with any type side rails, without mattress
IOM: 100-02, 15, 110.1; 100-03, 4, 280.7

⊛ **E0260** Hospital bed, semi-electric (head and foot adjustment), with any type side rails, with mattress
IOM: 100-02, 15, 110.1; 100-03, 4, 280.7

⊛ **E0261** Hospital bed, semi-electric (head and foot adjustment), with any type side rails, without mattress
IOM: 100-02, 15, 110.1; 100-03, 4, 280.7

⊛ **E0265** Hospital bed, total electric (head, foot and height adjustments), with any type side rails, with mattress
IOM: 100-02, 15, 110.1; 100-03, 4, 280.7

⊛ **E0266** Hospital bed, total electric (head, foot and height adjustments), with any type side rails, without mattress
IOM: 100-02, 15, 110.1; 100-03, 4, 280.7

◆ **E0270** Hospital bed, institutional type includes: oscillating, circulating and Stryker frame, with mattress
IOM: 100-03, 4, 280.1

⊛ **E0271** Mattress, innerspring
IOM: 100-03, 4, 280.1; 100-03, 4, 280.7

⊛ **E0272** Mattress, foam rubber
IOM: 100-03, 4, 280.1; 100-03, 4, 280.7

◆ **E0273** Bed board
IOM: 100-03, 4, 280.1

◆ **E0274** Over-bed table
IOM: 100-03, 4, 280.1

⊛ **E0275** Bed pan, standard, metal or plastic
IOM: 100-03, 4, 280.1

⊛ **E0276** Bed pan, fracture, metal or plastic
IOM: 100-03, 4, 280.1

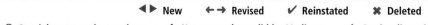

◀▶ New   ←→ Revised   ✔ Reinstated   ✖ Deleted
⊛ Special coverage instructions   ◆ Not covered or valid by Medicare   ✳ Carrier discretion   ▶ ASC payment group

⊛ **E0277** Powered pressure-reducing air mattress
IOM: 100-03, 4, 280.1

✳ **E0280** Bed cradle, any type

⊛ **E0290** Hospital bed, fixed height, without side rails, with mattress
IOM: 100-02, 15, 110.1; 100-03, 4, 280.7

⊛ **E0291** Hospital bed, fixed height, without side rails, without mattress
IOM: 100-02, 15, 110.1; 100-03, 4, 280.7

⊛ **E0292** Hospital bed, variable height, hi-lo, without side rails, with mattress
IOM: 100-02, 15, 110.1; 100-03, 4, 280.7

⊛ **E0293** Hospital bed, variable height, hi-lo, without side rails, without mattress
IOM: 100-02, 15, 110.1; 100-03, 4, 280.7

⊛ **E0294** Hospital bed, semi-electric (head and foot adjustment), without side rails, with mattress
IOM: 100-02, 15, 110.1; 100-03, 4, 280.7

⊛ **E0295** Hospital bed, semi-electric (head and foot adjustment), without side rails, without mattress
IOM: 100-02, 15, 110.1; 100-03, 4, 280.7

⊛ **E0296** Hospital bed, total electric (head, foot and height adjustments). Without side rails, with mattress
IOM: 100-02, 15, 110.1; 100-03, 4, 280.7

⊛ **E0297** Hospital bed, total electric (head, foot and height adjustments), without side rails, without mattress
IOM: 100-02, 15, 110.1; 100-03, 4, 280.7

✳ **E0300** Pediatric crib, hospital grade, fully enclosed

⊛ **E0301** Hospital bed, heavy duty, extra wide, with weight capacity greater than 350 pounds, but less than or equal to 600 pounds, with any type side rails, without mattress
IOM: 100-03, 4, 280.7

⊛ **E0302** Hospital bed, extra heavy duty, extra wide, with weight capacity greater than 600 pounds, with any type side rails, without mattress
IOM: 100-03, 4, 280.7

⊛ **E0303** Hospital bed, heavy duty, extra wide, with weight capacity greater than 350 pounds, but less than or equal to 600 pounds, with any type side rails, with mattress
IOM: 100-03, 4, 280.7

⊛ **E0304** Hospital bed, extra heavy duty, extra wide, with weight capacity greater than 600 pounds, with any type side rails, with mattress
IOM: 100-03, 4, 280.7

⊛ **E0305** Bed side rails, half length
IOM: 100-03, 4, 280.7

⊛ **E0310** Bed side rails, full length
IOM: 100-03, 4, 280.7

◆ **E0315** Bed accessory: board, table, or support device, any type
IOM: 100-03, 4, 280.1

✳ **E0316** Safety enclosure frame/canopy for use with hospital bed, any type

⊛ **E0325** Urinal; male, jug-type, any material
IOM: 100-03, 4, 280.1

⊛ **E0326** Urinal; female, jug-type, any material
IOM: 100-03, 4, 280.1

✳ **E0328** Hospital bed, pediatric, manual, 360 degree side enclosures, top of headboard, footboard and side rails up to 24 inches above the spring, includes mattress

✳ **E0329** Hospital bed, pediatric, electric or semi-electric, 360 degree side enclosures, top of headboard, footboard and side rails up to 24 inches above the spring, includes mattress

✳ **E0350** Control unit for electronic bowel irrigation/evacuation system

✳ **E0352** Disposable pack (water reservoir bag, speculum, valving mechanism and collection bag/box) for use with the electronic bowel irrigation/evacuation system

✳ **E0370** Air pressure elevator for heel

✳ **E0371** Non powered advanced pressure reducing overlay for mattress, standard mattress length and width

✳ **E0372** Powered air overlay for mattress, standard mattress length and width

✳ **E0373** Non powered advanced pressure reducing mattress

Oxygen and Related Respiratory Equipment

⊛ **E0424** Stationary compressed gaseous oxygen system, rental; includes container, contents, regulator, flowmeter, humidifier, nebulizer, cannula or mask, and tubing
IOM: 100-03, 4, 280.1; 100-04, 20, 30.6

◄► New ←→ Revised ✔ Reinstated ✖ Deleted
⊛ Special coverage instructions ◆ Not covered or valid by Medicare ✳ Carrier discretion ▶ ASC payment group

DURABLE MEDICAL EQUIPMENT

⊛ **E0425** Stationary compressed gas system, purchase; includes regulator, flowmeter, humidifier, nebulizer, cannula or mask, and tubing

IOM: 100-03, 4, 280.1; 100-04, 20, 30.6

⊛ **E0430** Portable gaseous oxygen system, purchase; includes regulator, flowmeter, humidifier, cannula or mask, and tubing

IOM: 100-03, 4, 280.1; 100-04, 20, 30.6

⊛ **E0431** Portable gaseous oxygen system, rental; includes portable container, regulator, flowmeter, humidifier, cannula or mask, and tubing

IOM: 100-03, 4, 280.1; 100-04, 20, 30.6

⊛ **E0434** Portable liquid oxygen system, rental; includes portable container, supply reservoir, humidifier, flowmeter, refill adaptor, contents gauge, cannula or mask, and tubing

IOM: 100-03, 4, 280.1; 100-04, 20, 30.6

⊛ **E0435** Portable liquid oxygen system, purchase; includes portable container, supply reservoir, flowmeter, humidifier, contents gauge, cannula or mask, tubing and refill adaptor

IOM: 100-03, 4, 280.1; 100-04, 20, 30.6

⊛ **E0439** Stationary liquid oxygen system, rental; includes container, contents, regulator, flowmeter, humidifier, nebulizer, cannula or mask, & tubing

IOM: 100-03, 4, 280.1; 100-04, 20, 30.6

⊛ **E0440** Stationary liquid oxygen system, purchase; includes use of reservoir, contents indicator, regulator, flowmeter, humidifier, nebulizer, cannula or mask, and tubing

IOM: 100-03, 4, 280.1; 100-04, 20, 30.6

⊛ **E0441** Oxygen contents, gaseous (for use with owned gaseous stationary systems or when both a stationary and portable gaseous system are owned), 1 month's supply = 1 unit

IOM: 100-03, 4, 280.1; 100-04, 20, 30.6

⊛ **E0442** Oxygen contents, liquid (for use with owned liquid stationary systems or when both a stationary and portable liquid system are owned), 1 month's supply = 1 unit

IOM: 100-03, 4, 280.1; 100-04, 20, 30.6

⊛ **E0443** Portable oxygen contents, gaseous (for use only with portable gaseous systems when no stationary gas or liquid system is used), 1 month's supply = 1 unit

IOM: 100-03, 4, 280.1; 100-04, 20, 30.6

⊛ **E0444** Portable oxygen contents, liquid (for use only with portable liquid systems when no stationary gas or liquid system is used), 1 month's supply = 1 unit

IOM: 100-03, 4, 280.1; 100-04, 20, 30.6

✷ **E0445** Oximeter device for measuring blood oxygen levels non-invasively

⊛ **E0450** Volume control ventilator, without pressure support mode, may include pressure control mode, used with invasive interface (e.g., tracheostomy tube)

IOM: 100-03, 4, 280.1

⊛ **E0455** Oxygen tent, excluding croup or pediatric tents

IOM: 100-03, 4, 280.1; 100-04, 20, 30.6

✷ **E0457** Chest shell (cuirass)

✷ **E0459** Chest wrap

⊛ **E0460** Negative pressure ventilator; portable or stationary

IOM: 100-03, 4, 240.2

⊛ **E0461** Volume control ventilator, without pressure support mode, may include pressure control mode, used with non-invasive interface (e.g. mask)

IOM: 100-03, 4, 240.2

✷ **E0462** Rocking bed with or without side rails

✷ **E0463** Pressure support ventilator with volume control mode, may include pressure control mode, used with invasive interface (e.g., tracheostomy tube)

✷ **E0464** Pressure support ventilator with volume control mode, may include pressure control mode, used with non-invasive interface (e.g., mask)

⊛ **E0470** Respiratory assist device, bi-level pressure capability, without backup rate feature, used with noninvasive interface, e.g., nasal or facial mask (intermittent assist device with continuous positive airway pressure device)

IOM: 100-03, 4, 240.2

⊛ **E0471** Respiratory assist device, bi-level pressure capability, with back-up rate feature, used with noninvasive interface, e.g., nasal or facial mask (intermittent assist device with continuous positive airway pressure device)

IOM: 100-03, 4, 240.2

◀▶ New ←→ Revised ✔ Reinstated ✖ Deleted
⊛ Special coverage instructions ◆ Not covered or valid by Medicare ✷ Carrier discretion ▶ ASC payment group

132

⚙ **E0472** Respiratory assist device, bi-level pressure capability, with backup rate feature, used with invasive interface, e.g., tracheostomy tube (intermittent assist device with continuous positive airway pressure device)

IOM: 100-03, 4, 240.2

⚙ **E0480** Percussor, electric or pneumatic, home model

IOM: 100-03, 4, 240.2

◆ **E0481** Intrapulmonary percussive ventilation system and related accessories

IOM: 100-03, 4, 240.2

✳ **E0482** Cough stimulating device, alternating positive and negative airway pressure

✳ **E0483** High frequency chest wall oscillation air-pulse generator system, (includes hoses and vest), each

✳ **E0484** Oscillatory positive expiratory pressure device, non-electric, any type, each

✳ **E0485** Oral device/appliance used to reduce upper airway collapsibility, adjustable or non-adjustable, prefabricated, includes fitting and adjustment

✳ **E0486** Oral device/appliance used to reduce upper airway collapsibility, adjustable or non-adjustable, custom fabricated, includes fitting and adjustment

▶ ⚙ **E0487** Spirometer, electronic, includes all accessories

IPPB Machines

⚙ **E0500** IPPB machine, all types, with built-in nebulization; manual or automatic valves; internal or external power source

IOM: 100-03, 4, 240.2

Humidifiers/Nebulizers/Compressors for Use with Oxygen IPPB Equipment

⚙ **E0550** Humidifier, durable for extensive supplemental humidification during IPPB treatments or oxygen delivery

IOM: 100-03, 4, 240.2

⚙ **E0555** Humidifier, durable, glass or autoclavable plastic bottle type, for use with regulator or flowmeter

IOM: 100-03, 4, 280.1; 100-04, 20, 30.6

⚙ **E0560** Humidifier, durable for supplemental humidification during IPPB treatment or oxygen delivery

IOM: 100-03, 4, 280.1

✳ **E0561** Humidifier, non-heated, used with positive airway pressure device

✳ **E0562** Humidifier, heated, used with positive airway pressure device

✳ **E0565** Compressor, air power source for equipment which is not self-contained or cylinder driven

⚙ **E0570** Nebulizer, with compressor

IOM: 100-03, 4, 240.2; 100-03, 4, 280.1

⚙ **E0571** Aerosol compressor, battery powered, for use with small volume nebulizer

IOM: 100-03, 4, 240.2

✳ **E0572** Aerosol compressor, adjustable pressure, light duty for intermittent use

✳ **E0574** Ultrasonic/electronic aerosol generator with small volume nebulizer

⚙ **E0575** Nebulizer, ultrasonic, large volume

IOM: 100-03, 4, 240.2

⚙ **E0580** Nebulizer, durable, glass or autoclavable plastic, bottle type, for use with regulator or flowmeter

IOM: 100-03, 4, 240.2; 100-03, 4, 280.1

⚙ **E0585** Nebulizer, with compressor and heater

IOM: 100-03, 4, 240.2; 100-03, 4, 280.1

Suction Pump/Room Vaporizers

⚙ **E0600** Respiratory suction pump, home model, portable or stationary, electric

IOM: 100-03, 4, 240.2

⚙ **E0601** Continuous airway pressure (CPAP) device

IOM: 100-03, 4, 240.4

✳ **E0602** Breast pump, manual, any type

✳ **E0603** Breast pump, electric (AC and/or DC), any type

✳ **E0604** Breast pump, hospital grade, electric (AC and/or DC), any type

⚙ **E0605** Vaporizer, room type

IOM: 100-03, 4, 240.2

⚙ **E0606** Postural drainage board

IOM: 100-03, 4, 240.2

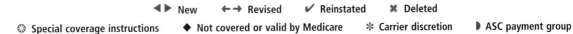

◀ ▶ New   ← → Revised   ✔ Reinstated   ✖ Deleted
⚙ Special coverage instructions   ◆ Not covered or valid by Medicare   ✳ Carrier discretion   ▶ ASC payment group

Monitoring Equipment

⊚ **E0607** Home blood glucose monitor

IOM: 100-03, 4, 230.16

Pacemaker Monitor

⊚ **E0610** Pacemaker monitor, self-contained, (checks battery depletion, includes audible and visible check systems)

IOM: 100-03, 1, 20.8

⊚ **E0615** Pacemaker monitor, self-contained, checks battery depletion and other pacemaker components, includes digital/visible check systems

IOM: 100-03, 1, 20.8

∗ **E0616** Implantable cardiac event recorder with memory, activator and programmer

∗ **E0617** External defibrillator with integrated electrocardiogram analysis

∗ **E0618** Apnea monitor, without recording feature

∗ **E0619** Apnea monitor, with recording feature

∗ **E0620** Skin piercing device for collection of capillary blood, laser, each

Patient Lifts

⊚ **E0621** Sling or seat, patient lift, canvas or nylon

IOM: 100-03, 4, 240.2

◆ **E0625** Patient lift, bathroom or toilet, not otherwise classified

IOM: 100-03, 4, 240.2

⊚ **E0627** Seat lift mechanism incorporated into a combination lift-chair mechanism

IOM: 100-03, 4, 280.4; 100-04, 4, 20

Cross Reference Q0080

⊚ **E0628** Separate seat lift mechanism for use with patient owned furniture - electric

IOM: 100-03, 4, 280.4; 100-04, 4, 20

Cross Reference Q0078

⊚ **E0629** Separate seat lift mechanism for use with patient owned furniture - non-electric

IOM: 100-04, 4, 20

Cross Reference Q0079

⊚ **E0630** Patient lift, hydraulic or mechanical, includes any seat, sling, strap(s) or pad(s)

IOM: 100-03, 4, 240.2

⊚ **E0635** Patient lift, electric, with seat or sling

IOM: 100-03, 4, 240.2

∗ **E0636** Multipositional patient support system, with integrated lift, patient accessible controls

⊚ **E0637** Combination sit to stand system, any size including pediatric, with seatlift feature, with or without wheels

IOM: 100-03, 4, 240.2

◆ **E0638** Standing frame system, one position (e.g. upright, supine or prone stander), any size including pediatric, with or without wheels

IOM: 100-03, 4, 240.2

∗ **E0639** Patient lift, moveable from room to room with disassembly and reassembly, includes all components/accessories

∗ **E0640** Patient lift, fixed system, includes all components/accessories

◆ **E0641** Standing frame system, multi-position (e.g. three-way stander), any size including pediatric, with or without wheels

IOM: 100-03, 4, 240.2

◆ **E0642** Standing frame system, mobile (dynamic stander), any size including pediatric

IOM: 100-03, 4, 240.2

Pneumatic Compressor and Appliances

⊚ **E0650** Pneumatic compressor, non-segmental home model

IOM: 100-03, 4, 280.6

⊚ **E0651** Pneumatic compressor, segmental home model without calibrated gradient pressure

IOM: 100-03, 4, 280.6

⊚ **E0652** Pneumatic compressor, segmental home model with calibrated gradient pressure

IOM: 100-03, 4, 280.6

⊚ **E0655** Non-segmental pneumatic appliance for use with pneumatic compressor, half arm

IOM: 100-03, 4, 280.6

◀▶ New   ←→ Revised   ✔ Reinstated   ✖ Deleted

⊚ Special coverage instructions   ◆ Not covered or valid by Medicare   ∗ Carrier discretion   ▶ ASC payment group

▶ ✪ **E0656** Segmental pneumatic appliance for use with pneumatic compressor, trunk

▶ ✪ **E0657** Segmental pneumatic appliance for use with pneumatic compressor, chest

✪ **E0660** Non-segmental pneumatic appliance for use with pneumatic compressor, full leg

IOM: 100-03, 4, 280.6

✪ **E0665** Non-segmental pneumatic appliance for use with pneumatic compressor, full arm

IOM: 100-03, 4, 280.6

✪ **E0666** Non-segmental pneumatic appliance for use with pneumatic compressor, half leg

IOM: 100-03, 4, 280.6

✪ **E0667** Segmental pneumatic appliance for use with pneumatic compressor, full leg

IOM: 100-03, 4, 280.6

✪ **E0668** Segmental pneumatic appliance for use with pneumatic compressor, full arm

IOM: 100-03, 4, 280.6

✪ **E0669** Segmental pneumatic appliance for use with pneumatic compressor, half leg

IOM: 100-03, 4, 280.6

✪ **E0671** Segmental gradient pressure pneumatic appliance, full leg

IOM: 100-03, 4, 280.6

✪ **E0672** Segmental gradient pressure pneumatic appliance, full arm

IOM: 100-03, 4, 280.6

✪ **E0673** Segmental gradient pressure pneumatic appliance, half leg

IOM: 100-03, 4, 280.6

✳ **E0675** Pneumatic compression device, high pressure, rapid inflation/deflation cycle, for arterial insufficiency (unilateral or bilateral system)

✳ **E0676** Intermittent limb compression device (includes all accessories), not otherwise specified

Ultraviolet Cabinet

✳ **E0691** Ultraviolet light therapy system panel, includes bulbs/lamps, timer and eye protection; treatment area 2 square feet or less

✳ **E0692** Ultraviolet light therapy system panel, includes bulbs/lamps, timer and eye protection, 4 foot panel

✳ **E0693** Ultraviolet light therapy system panel, includes bulbs/lamps, timer and eye protection, 6 foot panel

✳ **E0694** Ultraviolet multidirectional light therapy system in 6 foot cabinet, includes bulbs/lamps, timer and eye protection

Safety Equipment

✳ **E0700** Safety equipment (e.g., belt, harness or vest)

✪ **E0705** Transfer device, any type, each

Restraints

✳ **E0710** Restraints, any type (body, chest, wrist or ankle)

Transcutaneous and/or Neuromuscular Electrical Nerve Stimulators (TENS)

✪ **E0720** Transcutaneous electrical nerve stimulation (TENS) device, two lead, localized stimulation

IOM: 100-03, 2, 160.2; 100-03, 4, 280.1

✪ **E0730** Transcutaneous electrical nerve stimulation (TENS) device, four or more leads, for multiple nerve stimulation

IOM: 100-03, 2, 160.2; 100-03, 4, 280.1

✪ **E0731** Form fitting conductive garment for delivery of TENS or NMES (with conductive fibers separated from the patient's skin by layers of fabric)

IOM: 100-03, 2, 160.13

✪ **E0740** Incontinence treatment system, pelvic floor stimulator, monitor, sensor and/or trainer

IOM: 100-03, 4, 230.8

✳ **E0744** Neuromuscular stimulator for scoliosis

✪ **E0745** Neuromuscular stimulator, electronic shock unit

IOM: 100-03, 2, 160.12

✪ **E0746** Electromyography (EMG), biofeedback device

IOM: 100-03, 1, 30.1

✪ **E0747** Osteogenesis stimulator, electrical, non-invasive, other than spinal applications

---

◀ ▶ **New**   ← → **Revised**   ✔ **Reinstated**   ✖ **Deleted**

✪ **Special coverage instructions**   ◆ **Not covered or valid by Medicare**   ✳ **Carrier discretion**   ▌ **ASC payment group**

⊛ **E0748** Osteogensis stimulator, electrical, non-invasive, spinal applications

⊛ **E0749** Osteogenesis stimulator, electrical, surgically implanted

✳ **E0755** Electronic salivary reflex stimulator (intra-oral/non-invasive)

✳ **E0760** Osteogenesis stimulator, low intensity ultrasound, non-invasive

⊛ **E0761** Non-thermal pulsed high frequency radiowaves, high peak power electromagnetic energy treatment device

✳ **E0762** Transcutaneous electrical joint stimulation device system, includes all accessories

⊛ **E0764** Functional neuromuscular stimulator, transcutaneous stimulation of muscles of ambulation with computer control, used for walking by spinal cord injured, entire system, after completion of training program

IOM: 100-03, 2, 160.12

✳ **E0765** FDA approved nerve stimulator, with replaceable batteries, for treatment of nausea and vomiting

⊛ **E0769** Electrical stimulation or electromagnetic wound treatment device, not otherwise classified

IOM: 100-04, 32, 11.1

▶ ⊛ **E0770** Functional electrical stimulator, transcutaneous stimulation of nerve and/or muscle groups, any type, complete system, not otherwise specified

Infusion Supplies

✳ **E0776** IV pole

✳ **E0779** Ambulatory infusion pump, mechanical, reusable, for infusion 8 hours or greater

(Requires prior authorization and copy of invoice)

✳ **E0780** Ambulatory infusion pump, mechanical, reusable, for infusion less than 8 hours

(Requires prior authorization and copy of invoice)

⊛ **E0781** Ambulatory infusion pump, single or multiple channels, electric or battery operated with administrative equipment, worn by patient

IOM: 100-03, 1, 50.3

⊛ **E0782** Infusion pump, implantable, non-programmable (includes all components, e.g., pump, cathether, connectors, etc.)

IOM: 100-03, 1, 50.3

⊛ **E0783** Infusion pump system, implantable, programmable (includes all components, e.g., pump, catheter, connectors, etc.)

IOM: 100-03, 1, 50.3

⊛ **E0784** External ambulatory infusion pump, insulin

IOM: 100-03, 1, 50.3

⊛ **E0785** Implantable intraspinal (epidural/intrathecal) catheter used with implantable infusion pump, replacement

IOM: 100-03, 1, 50.3

⊛ **E0786** Implantable programmable infusion pump, replacement (excludes implantable intraspinal catheter)

IOM: 100-03, 1, 50.3

⊛ **E0791** Parenteral infusion pump, stationary, single or multi-channel

IOM: 100-02, 15, 120; 100-03, 3, 180.2; 100-04, 20, 100.2.2

Traction Equipment: All Types and Cervical

⊛ **E0830** Ambulatory traction device, all types, each

IOM: 100-03, 4, 280.1

⊛ **E0840** Traction frame, attached to headboard, cervical traction

IOM: 100-03, 4, 280.1

✳ **E0849** Traction equipment, cervical, free-standing stand/frame, pneumatic, applying traction force to other than mandible

⊛ **E0850** Traction stand, free standing, cervical traction

IOM: 100-03, 4, 280.1

✳ **E0855** Cervical traction equipment not requiring additional stand or frame

✳ **E0856** Cervical traction device, cervical collar with inflatable air bladder

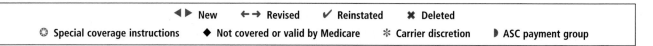

Traction: Overdoor

⚙ **E0860** Traction equipment, overdoor, cervical
IOM: 100-03, 4, 280.1

Traction: Extremity

⚙ **E0870** Traction frame, attached to footboard, extremity traction, (e.g., Buck's)
IOM: 100-03, 4, 280.1

⚙ **E0880** Traction stand, free standing, extremity traction, (e.g., Buck's)
IOM: 100-03, 4, 280.1

Traction: Pelvic

⚙ **E0890** Traction frame, attached to footboard, pelvic traction
IOM: 100-03, 4, 280.1

⚙ **E0900** Traction stand, free standing, pelvic traction, (e.g., Buck's)
IOM: 100-03, 4, 280.1

Trapeze Equipment, Fracture Frame, and Other Orthopedic Devices

⚙ **E0910** Trapeze bars, A/K/A patient helper, attached to bed, with grab bar
IOM: 100-03, 4, 280.1

⚙ **E0911** Trapeze bar, heavy duty, for patient weight capacity greater than 250 pounds, attached to bed, with grab bar
IOM: 100-03, 4, 280.1

⚙ **E0912** Trapeze bar, heavy duty, for patient weight capacity greater than 250 pounds, free standing, complete with grab bar
IOM: 100-03, 4, 280.1

⚙ **E0920** Fracture frame, attached to bed, includes weights
IOM: 100-03, 4, 280.1

⚙ **E0930** Fracture frame, free standing, includes weights
IOM: 100-03, 4, 280.1

⚙ **E0935** Continuous passive motion exercise device for use on knee only
IOM: 100-03, 4, 280.1

◆ **E0936** Continuous passive motion exercise device for use other than knee

⚙ **E0940** Trapeze bar, free standing, complete with grab bar
IOM: 100-03, 4, 280.1

⚙ **E0941** Gravity assisted traction device, any type
IOM: 100-03, 4, 280.1

✳ **E0942** Cervical head harness/halter

✳ **E0944** Pelvic belt/harness/boot

✳ **E0945** Extremity belt/harness

⚙ **E0946** Fracture, frame, dual with cross bars, attached to bed, (e.g. Balken, 4 poster)
IOM: 100-03, 4, 280.1

⚙ **E0947** Fracture frame, attachments for complex pelvic traction
IOM: 100-03, 4, 280.1

⚙ **E0948** Fracture frame, attachments for complex cervical traction
IOM: 100-03, 4, 280.1

Wheelchairs Accessories

⚙ **E0950** Wheelchair accessory, tray, each
IOM: 100-03, 4, 280.1

✳ **E0951** Heel loop/holder, any type, with or without ankle strap, each

⚙ **E0952** Toe loop/holder, any type, each
IOM: 100-03, 4, 280.1

✳ **E0955** Wheelchair accessory, headrest, cushioned, any type, including fixed mounting hardware, each

✳ **E0956** Wheelchair accessory, lateral trunk or hip support, any type, including fixed mounting hardware, each

✳ **E0957** Wheelchair accessory, medial thigh support, any type, including fixed mounting hardware, each

⚙ **E0958** Manual wheelchair accessory, one-arm drive attachment, each
IOM: 100-03, 4, 280.1

✳ **E0959** Manual wheelchair accessory, adapter for amputee, each
IOM: 100-03, 4, 280.1

✳ **E0960** Wheelchair accessory, shoulder harness/straps or chest strap, including any type mounting hardware

✳ **E0961** Manual wheelchair accessory, wheel lock brake extension (handle), each
IOM: 100-03, 4, 280.1

◄► New   ←→ Revised   ✔ Reinstated   ✘ Deleted
⚙ Special coverage instructions   ◆ Not covered or valid by Medicare   ✳ Carrier discretion   ▶ ASC payment group

* **E0966** Manual wheelchair accessory, headrest extension, each

  IOM: 100-03, 4, 280.1

⊘ **E0967** Manual wheelchair accessory, hand rim with projections, any type, each

  IOM: 100-03, 4, 280.1

⊘ **E0968** Commode seat, wheelchair

  IOM: 100-03, 4, 280.1

⊘ **E0969** Narrowing device, wheelchair

  IOM: 100-03, 4, 280.1

◆ **E0970** No.2 footplates, except for elevating leg rest

  IOM: 100-03, 4, 280.1

  Cross Reference CPT K0037, K0042

* **E0971** Manual wheelchair accessory, anti-tipping device, each

  IOM: 100-03, 4, 280.1

  Cross Reference CPT K0021

⊘ **E0973** Wheelchair accessory, adjustable height, detachable armrest, complete assembly, each

  IOM: 100-03, 4, 280.1

⊘ **E0974** Manual wheelchair accessory, anti-rollback device, each

  IOM: 100-03, 4, 280.1

* **E0978** Wheelchair accessory, positioning belt/safety belt/pelvic strap, each

* **E0980** Safety vest, wheelchair

* **E0981** Wheelchair accessory, seat upholstery, replacement only, each

* **E0982** Wheelchair accessory, back upholstery, replacement only, each

* **E0983** Manual wheelchair accessory, power add-on to convert manual wheelchair to motorized wheelchair, joystick control

* **E0984** Manual wheelchair accessory, power add-on to convert manual wheelchair to motorized wheelchair, tiller control

* **E0985** Wheelchair accessory, seat lift mechanism

* **E0986** Manual wheelchair accessory, push activated power assist, each

* **E0990** Wheelchair accessory, elevating leg rest, complete assembly, each

  IOM: 100-03, 4, 280.1

* **E0992** Manual wheelchair accessory, solid seat insert

⊘ **E0994** Arm rest, each

  IOM: 100-03, 4, 280.1

* **E0995** Wheelchair accessory, calf rest/pad, each

  IOM: 100-03, 4, 280.1

* **E1002** Wheelchair accessory, power seating system, tilt only

* **E1003** Wheelchair accessory, power seating system, recline only, without shear reduction

* **E1004** Wheelchair accessory, power seating system, recline only, with mechanical shear reduction

* **E1005** Wheelchair accessory, power seating system, recline only, with power shear reduction

* **E1006** Wheelchair accessory, power seating system, combination tilt and recline, without shear reduction

* **E1007** Wheelchair accessory, power seating system, combination tilt and recline, with mechanical shear reduction

* **E1008** Wheelchair accessory, power seating system, combination tilt and recline, with power shear reduction

* **E1009** Wheelchair accessory, addition to power seating system, mechanically linked leg elevation system, including pushrod and leg rest, each

* **E1010** Wheelchair accessory, addition to power seating system, power leg elevation system, including leg rest, pair

⊘ **E1011** Modification to pediatric size wheelchair, width adjustment package (not to be dispensed with initial chair)

  IOM: 100-03, 4, 280.1

⊘ **E1014** Reclining back, addition to pediatric size wheelchair

  IOM: 100-03, 4, 280.1

⊘ **E1015** Shock absorber for manual wheelchair, each

  IOM: 100-03, 4, 280.1

⊘ **E1016** Shock absorber for power wheelchair, each

  IOM: 100-03, 4, 280.1

⊘ **E1017** Heavy duty shock absorber for heavy duty or extra heavy duty manual wheelchair, each

  IOM: 100-03, 4, 280.1

◀▶ New   ←→ Revised   ✔ Reinstated   ✖ Deleted

⊘ Special coverage instructions   ◆ Not covered or valid by Medicare   ✻ Carrier discretion   ▶ ASC payment group

⊗ **E1018**   Heavy duty shock absorber for heavy duty or extra heavy duty power wheelchair, each

IOM: 100-03, 4, 280.1

⊗ **E1020**   Residual limb support system for wheelchair

IOM: 100-03, 3, 280.3

✳ **E1028**   Wheelchair accessory, manual swingaway, retractable or removable mounting hardware for joystick, other control interface or positioning accessory

✳ **E1029**   Wheelchair accessory, ventilator tray, fixed

✳ **E1030**   Wheelchair accessory, ventilator tray, gimbaled

Rollabout Chair and Transfer System

⊗ **E1031**   Rollabout chair, any and all types with castors 5" or greater

IOM: 100-03, 4, 280.1

⊗ **E1035**   Multi-positional patient transfer system, with integrated seat, operated by care giver

IOM: 100-02, 15, 110

⊗ **E1037**   Transport chair, pediatric size

IOM: 100-03, 4, 280.1

⊗ **E1038**   Transport chair, adult size, patient weight capacity up to and including 300 pounds

IOM: 100-03, 4, 280.1

✳ **E1039**   Transport chair, adult size, heavy duty, patient weight capacity greater than 300 pounds

Wheelchair: Fully Reclining

⊗ **E1050**   Fully-reclining wheelchair, fixed full length arms, swing away detachable elevating leg rests

IOM: 100-03, 4, 280.1

⊗ **E1060**   Fully-reclining wheelchair, detachable arms, desk or full length, swing away detachable elevating legrests

IOM: 100-03, 4, 280.1

⊗ **E1070**   Fully-reclining wheelchair, detachable arms (desk or full length) swing away detachable footrests

IOM: 100-03, 4, 280.1

⊗ **E1083**   Hemi-wheelchair, fixed full length arms, swing away detachable elevating leg rest

IOM: 100-03, 4, 280.1

⊗ **E1084**   Hemi-wheelchair, detachable arms desk or full length arms, swing away detachable elevating leg rests

IOM: 100-03, 4, 280.1

◆ **E1085**   Hemi-wheelchair, fixed full length arms, swing away detachable foot rests

IOM: 100-03, 4, 280.1

Cross Reference CPT K0002

◆ **E1086**   Hemi-wheelchair, detachable arms desk or full length, swing away detachable footrests

IOM: 100-03, 4, 280.1

Cross Reference CPT K0002

⊗ **E1087**   High strength lightweight wheelchair, fixed full length arms, swing away detachable elevating leg rests

IOM: 100-03, 4, 280.1

⊗ **E1088**   High strength lightweight wheelchair, detachable arms desk or full length, swing away detachable elevating leg rests

IOM: 100-03, 4, 280.1

◆ **E1089**   High strength lightweight wheelchair, fixed length arms, swing away detachable footrest

IOM: 100-03, 4, 280.1

Cross Reference CPT K0004

◆ **E1090**   High strength lightweight wheelchair, detachable arms desk or full length, swing away detachable foot rests

IOM: 100-03, 4, 280.1

Cross Reference CPT K0004

⊗ **E1092**   Wide heavy duty wheelchair, detachable arms (desk or full length) swing away detachable elevating leg rests

IOM: 100-03, 4, 280.1

⊗ **E1093**   Wide heavy duty wheelchair, detachable arms (desk or full length arms), swing away detachable foot rests

IOM: 100-03, 4, 280.1

Wheelchair: Semi-reclining

⊗ **E1100**   Semi-reclining wheelchair, fixed full length arms, swing away detachable elevating leg rests

IOM: 100-03, 4, 280.1

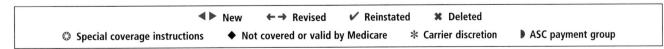

◀▶ **New**   ←→ **Revised**   ✔ **Reinstated**   ✖ **Deleted**

⊗ **Special coverage instructions**   ◆ **Not covered or valid by Medicare**   ✳ **Carrier discretion**   ▶ **ASC payment group**

⊘ **E1110** Semi-reclining wheelchair, detachable arms (desk or full length), elevating leg rest

IOM: 100-03, 4, 280.1

Wheelchair: Standard

◆ **E1130** Standard wheelchair, fixed full length arms, fixed or swing away detachable footrests

IOM: 100-03, 4, 280.1

Cross Reference CPT K0001

◆ **E1140** Wheelchair, detachable arms, desk or full length, swing away detachable footrests

IOM: 100-03, 4, 280.1

Cross Reference CPT K0001

⊘ **E1150** Wheelchair, detachable arms, desk or full length, swing away detachable elevating legrests

IOM: 100-03, 4, 280.1

⊘ **E1160** Wheelchair, fixed full length arms, swing away detachable elevating legrests

IOM: 100-03, 4, 280.1

✳ **E1161** Manual adult size wheelchair, includes tilt in space

Wheelchair: Amputee

⊘ **E1170** Amputee wheelchair, fixed full length arms, swing away detachable elevating legrests

IOM: 100-03, 4, 280.1

⊘ **E1171** Amputee wheelchair, fixed full length arms, without footrests or legrest

IOM: 100-03, 4, 280.1

⊘ **E1172** Amputee wheelchair, detachable arms (desk or full length) without footrests or legrest

IOM: 100-03, 4, 280.1

⊘ **E1180** Amputee wheelchair, detachable arms (desk or full length) swing away detachable footrests

IOM: 100-03, 4, 280.1

⊘ **E1190** Amputee wheelchair, detachable arms (desk or full length), swing away detachable elevating legrests

IOM: 100-03, 4, 280.1

⊘ **E1195** Heavy duty wheelchair, fixed full length arms, swing away detachable elevating legrests

IOM: 100-03, 4, 280.1

⊘ **E1200** Amputee wheelchair, fixed full length arms, swing away detachable footrest

IOM: 100-03, 4, 280.1

Wheelchair: Special Size

⊘ **E1220** Wheelchair; specially sized or constructed, (indicate brand name, model number, if any) and justification

IOM: 100-03, 4, 280.3

⊘ **E1221** Wheelchair with fixed arm, footrests

IOM: 100-03, 4, 280.3

⊘ **E1222** Wheelchair with fixed arm, elevating legrests

IOM: 100-03, 4, 280.3

⊘ **E1223** Wheelchair with detachable arms, footrests

IOM: 100-03, 4, 280.3

⊘ **E1224** Wheelchair with detachable arms, elevating legrests

IOM: 100-03, 4, 280.3

⊘ **E1225** Wheelchair accessory, manual semi-reclining back, (recline greater than 15 degrees, but less than 80 degrees), each

IOM: 100-03, 4, 280.3

⊘ **E1226** Wheelchair accessory, manual fully reclining back, (recline greater than 80 degrees), each

IOM: 100-03, 4, 280.1

⊘ **E1227** Special height arms for wheelchair

IOM: 100-03, 4, 280.3

⊘ **E1228** Special back height for wheelchair

IOM: 100-03, 4, 280.3

✳ **E1229** Wheelchair, pediatric size, not otherwise specified

⊘ **E1230** Power operated vehicle (three or four wheel non-highway), specify brand name and model number

IOM: 100-08, 5, 5.2.3

→ ⊘ **E1231** Wheelchair, pediatric size, tilt-in-space, rigid, adjustable, with seating system

IOM: 100-03, 4, 280.1

→ ⊘ **E1232** Wheelchair, pediatric size, tilt-in-space, folding, adjustable, with seating system

IOM: 100-03, 4, 280.1

◀▶ New	←→ Revised	✔ Reinstated	✖ Deleted
⊘ Special coverage instructions	◆ Not covered or valid by Medicare	✳ Carrier discretion	▸ ASC payment group

→ ⊕ **E1233** Wheelchair, pediatric size, tilt-in-space, rigid, adjustable, without seating system

IOM: 100-03, 4, 280.1

→ ⊕ **E1234** Wheelchair, pediatric size, tilt-in-space, folding, adjustable, without seating system

IOM: 100-03, 4, 280.1

→ ⊕ **E1235** Wheelchair, pediatric size, rigid, adjustable, with seating system

IOM: 100-03, 4, 280.1

→ ⊕ **E1236** Wheelchair, pediatric size, folding, adjustable, with seating system

IOM: 100-03, 4, 280.1

→ ⊕ **E1237** Wheelchair, pediatric size, rigid, adjustable, without seating system

IOM: 100-03, 4, 280.1

→ ⊕ **E1238** Wheelchair, pediatric size, folding, adjustable, without seating system

IOM: 100-03, 4, 280.1

✳ **E1239** Power wheelchair, pediatric size, not otherwise specified

Wheelchair: Lightweight

⊕ **E1240** Lightweight wheelchair, detachable arms, (desk or full length) swing away detachable, elevating leg rests

IOM: 100-03, 4, 280.1

◆ **E1250** Lightweight wheelchair, fixed full length arms, swing away detachable footrest

IOM: 100-03, 4, 280.1

Cross Reference CPT K0003

◆ **E1260** Lightweight wheelchair, detachable arms (desk or full length) swing away detachable footrest

IOM: 100-03, 4, 280.1

Cross Reference CPT K0003

⊕ **E1270** Lightweight wheelchair, fixed full length arms, swing away detachable elevating legrests

IOM: 100-03, 4, 280.1

Wheelchair: Heavy Duty

⊕ **E1280** Heavy duty wheelchair, detachable arms (desk or full length), elevating legrests

IOM: 100-03, 4, 280.1

◆ **E1285** Heavy duty wheelchair, fixed full length arms, swing away detachable footrest

IOM: 100-03, 4, 280.1

Cross Reference CPT K0006

◆ **E1290** Heavy duty wheelchair, detachable arms (desk or full length) swing away detachable footrest

IOM: 100-03, 4, 280.1

Cross Reference CPT K0006

⊕ **E1295** Heavy duty wheelchair, fixed full length arms, elevating legrest

IOM: 100-03, 4, 280.1

⊕ **E1296** Special wheelchair seat height from floor

IOM: 100-03, 4, 280.3

⊕ **E1297** Special wheelchair seat depth, by upholstery

IOM: 100-03, 4, 280.3

⊕ **E1298** Special wheelchair seat depth and/or width, by construction

IOM: 100-03, 4, 280.3

Whirlpool Equipment

◆ **E1300** Whirlpool, portable (overtub type)

IOM: 100-03, 4, 280.1

⊕ **E1310** Whirlpool, non-portable (built-in type)

IOM: 100-03, 4, 280.1

Repairs and Replacement Parts

⊕ **E1340** Repair or nonroutine service for durable medical equipment requiring the skill of a technician, labor component, per 15 minutes

IOM: 100-02, 15, 110.2

Additional Oxygen Related Equipment

→ ⊕ **E1353** Regulator

IOM: 100-03, 4, 240.2

▶ ✳ **E1354** Oxygen accessory, wheeled cart for portable cylinder or portable concentrator, any type, replacement only, each

→ ⊕ **E1355** Stand/rack

IOM: 100-03, 4, 240.2

▶ ✳ **E1356** Oxygen accessory, battery pack/cartridge for portable concentrator, any type, replacement only, each

◀ ▶ New   ←→ Revised   ✔ Reinstated   ✖ Deleted

⊕ Special coverage instructions   ◆ Not covered or valid by Medicare   ✳ Carrier discretion   ▶ ASC payment group

DURABLE MEDICAL EQUIPMENT

E1233 – E1356

▶ ✳ **E1357** Oxygen accessory, battery charger for portable concentrator, any type, replacement only, each

▶ ◆ **E1358** Oxygen accessory, DC power adapter for portable concentrator, any type, replacement only, each

⊗ **E1372** Immersion external heater for nebulizer

IOM: 100-03, 4, 240.2

⊗ **E1390** Oxygen concentrator, single delivery port, capable of delivering 85 percent or greater oxygen concentration at the prescribed flow rate

IOM: 100-03, 4, 240.2

⊗ **E1391** Oxygen concentrator, dual delivery port, capable of delivering 85 percent or greater oxygen concentration at the prescribed flow rate, each

IOM: 100-03, 4, 240.2

⊗ **E1392** Portable oxygen concentrator, rental

IOM: 100-03, 4, 240.2

✳ **E1399** Durable medical equipment, miscellaneous

⊗ **E1405** Oxygen and water vapor enriching system with heated delivery

IOM: 100-03, 4, 240.2

⊗ **E1406** Oxygen and water vapor enriching system without heated delivery

IOM: 100-03, 4, 240.2

Artificial Kidney Machines and Accessories

⊗ **E1500** Centrifuge, for dialysis

⊗ **E1510** Kidney, dialysate delivery syst. kidney machine, pump recirculating, air removal syst. flowrate meter, power off, heater and temperature control with alarm, I.V. poles, pressure gauge, concentrate container

⊗ **E1520** Heparin infusion pump for hemodialysis

⊗ **E1530** Air bubble detector for hemodialysis, each, replacement

⊗ **E1540** Pressure alarm for hemodialysis, each, replacement

⊗ **E1550** Bath conductivity meter for hemodialysis, each

⊗ **E1560** Blood leak detector for hemodialysis, each, replacement

⊗ **E1570** Adjustable chair, for ESRD patients

⊗ **E1575** Transducer protectors/fluid barriers for hemodialysis, any size, per 10

⊗ **E1580** Unipuncture control system for hemodialysis

⊗ **E1590** Hemodialysis machine

⊗ **E1592** Automatic intermittent peritoneal dialysis system

⊗ **E1594** Cycler dialysis machine for peritoneal dialysis

⊗ **E1600** Delivery and/or installation charges for hemodialysis equipment

⊗ **E1610** Reverse osmosis water purification system, for hemodialysis

IOM: 100-03, 4, 230.7

⊗ **E1615** Deionizer water purification system, for hemodialysis

IOM: 100-03, 4, 230.7

⊗ **E1620** Blood pump for hemodialysis replacement

⊗ **E1625** Water softening system, for hemodialysis

IOM: 100-03, 4, 230.7

✳ **E1630** Reciprocating peritoneal dialysis system

⊗ **E1632** Wearable artificial kidney, each

⊗ **E1634** Peritoneal dialysis clamps, each

IOM: 100-04, 8, 60.4.2; 100-04, 8, 90.1; 100-04, 18, 80; 100-04, 18, 90

⊗ **E1635** Compact (portable) travel hemodialyzer system

⊗ **E1636** Sorbent cartridges, for hemodialysis, per 10

⊗ **E1637** Hemostats, each

⊗ **E1639** Scale, each

⊗ **E1699** Dialysis equipment, not otherwise specified

Jaw Motion Rehabilitation System and Accessories

✳ **E1700** Jaw motion rehabilitation system

✳ **E1701** Replacement cushions for jaw motion rehabilitation system, pkg. of 6

✳ **E1702** Replacement measuring scales for jaw motion rehabilitation system, pkg. of 200

◀▶ New   ←→ Revised   ✔ Reinstated   ✖ Deleted

⊗ Special coverage instructions   ◆ Not covered or valid by Medicare   ✳ Carrier discretion   ▶ ASC payment group

Other Orthopedic Devices

✳ **E1800** Dynamic adjustable elbow extension/ flexion device, includes soft interface material

✳ **E1801** Static progressive stretch elbow device, extension and/or flexion, with or without range of motion adjustment, includes all components and accessories

✳ **E1802** Dynamic adjustable forearm pronation/ supination device, includes soft interface material

✳ **E1805** Dynamic adjustable wrist extension/ flexion device, includes soft interface material

✳ **E1806** Static progressive stretch wrist device, flexion and/or extension, with or without range of motion adjustment, includes all components and accessories

✳ **E1810** Dynamic adjustable knee extension/ flexion device, includes soft interface material

✳ **E1811** Static progressive stretch knee device, extension and/or flexion, with or without range of motion adjustment, includes all components and accessories

✳ **E1812** Dynamic knee, extension/flexion device with active resistance control

✳ **E1815** Dynamic adjustable ankle extension/ flexion device, includes soft interface material

✳ **E1816** Static progressive stretch ankle device, flexion and/or extension, with or without range of motion adjustment, includes all components and accessories

✳ **E1818** Static progressive stretch forearm pronation/supination device with or without range of motion adjustment, includes all components and accessories

✳ **E1820** Replacement soft interface material, dynamic adjustable extension/flexion device

✳ **E1821** Replacement soft interface material/ cuffs for bi-directional static progressive stretch device

✳ **E1825** Dynamic adjustable finger extension/ flexion device, includes soft interface material

✳ **E1830** Dynamic adjustable toe extension/ flexion device, includes soft interface material

✳ **E1840** Dynamic adjustable shoulder flexion/ abduction/rotation device, includes soft interface material

✳ **E1841** Static progressive stretch shoulder device, with or without range of motion adjustment, includes all components and accessories

✳ **E1902** Communication board, non-electronic augmentative or alternative communication device

✳ **E2000** Gastric suction pump, home model, portable or stationary, electric

☺ **E2100** Blood glucose monitor with integrated voice synthesizer

IOM: 100-03, 4, 230.16

☺ **E2101** Blood glucose monitor with integrated lancing/blood sample

IOM: 100-03, 4, 230.16

✳ **E2120** Pulse generator system for tympanic treatment of inner ear endolymphatic fluid

Wheelchair Assessories

✳ **E2201** Manual wheelchair accessory, nonstandard seat frame, width greater than or equal to 20 inches and less than 24 inches

✳ **E2202** Manual wheelchair accessory, nonstandard seat frame width, 24-27 inches

✳ **E2203** Manual wheelchair accessory, nonstandard seat frame depth, 20 to less than 22 inches

✳ **E2204** Manual wheelchair accessory, nonstandard seat frame depth, 22 to 25 inches

✳ **E2205** Manual wheelchair accessory, handrim without projections (includes ergonomic or contoured), any type, replacement only, each

✳ **E2206** Manual wheelchair accessory, wheel lock assembly, complete, each

✳ **E2207** Wheelchair accessory, crutch and cane holder, each

✳ **E2208** Wheelchair accessory, cylinder tank carrier, each

✳ **E2209** Accessory arm trough, with or without hand support, each

---

◄► New   ←→ Revised   ✔ Reinstated   ✖ Deleted

☺ Special coverage instructions   ◆ Not covered or valid by Medicare   ✳ Carrier discretion   ▶ ASC payment group

* **E2210** Wheelchair accessory, bearings, any type, replacement only, each

* **E2211** Manual wheelchair accessory, pneumatic propulsion tire, any size, each

* **E2212** Manual wheelchair accessory, tube for pneumatic propulsion tire, any size, each

* **E2213** Manual wheelchair accessory, insert for pneumatic propulsion tire (removable), any type, any size, each

* **E2214** Manual wheelchair accessory, pneumatic caster tire, any size, each

* **E2215** Manual wheelchair accessory, tube for pneumatic caster tire, any size, each

* **E2216** Manual wheelchair accessory, foam filled propulsion tire, any size, each

* **E2217** Manual wheelchair accessory, foam filled caster tire, any size, each

* **E2218** Manual wheelchair accessory, foam propulsion tire, any size, each

* **E2219** Manual wheelchair accessory, foam caster tire, any size, each

* **E2220** Manual wheelchair accessory, solid (rubber/plastic) propulsion tire, any size, each

* **E2221** Manual wheelchair accessory, solid (rubber/plastic) caster tire (removable), any size, each

* **E2222** Manual wheelchair accessory, solid (rubber/plastic) caster tire with integrated wheel, any size, each

* **E2223** Manual wheelchair accessory, valve, any type, replacement only, each

* **E2224** Manual wheelchair accessory, propulsion wheel excludes tire, any size, each

* **E2225** Manual wheelchair accessory, caster wheel excludes tire, any size, replacement only, each

* **E2226** Manual wheelchair accessory, caster fork, any size, replacement only, each

* **E2227** Manual wheelchair accessory, gear reduction drive wheel, each

* **E2228** Manual wheelchair accessory, wheel braking system and lock, complete, each

▶ ◆ **E2230** Manual wheelchair accessory, manual standing system

▶ * **E2231** Manual wheelchair accessory, solid seat support base (replaces sling seat), includes any type mounting hardware

* **E2291** Back, planar, for pediatric size wheelchair including fixed attaching hardware

* **E2292** Seat, planar, for pediatric size wheelchair including fixed attaching hardware

* **E2293** Back, contoured, for pediatric size wheelchair including fixed attaching hardware

* **E2294** Seat, contoured, for pediatric size wheelchair including fixed attaching hardware

▶ * **E2295** Manual wheelchair accessory, for pediatric size wheelchair, dynamic seating frame, allows coordinated movement of multiple positioning features

* **E2300** Power wheelchair accessory, power seat elevation system

→ * **E2301** Power wheelchair accessory, power standing system

* **E2310** Power wheelchair accessory, electronic connection between wheelchair controller and one power seating system motor, including all related electronics, indicator feature, mechanical function selection switch, and fixed mounting hardware

* **E2311** Power wheelchair accessory, electronic connection between wheelchair controller and two or more power seating system motors, including all related electronics, indicator feature, mechanical function selection switch, and fixed mounting hardware

* **E2312** Power wheelchair accessory, hand or chin control interface, mini-proportional remote joystick, proportional, including fixed mounting hardware

* **E2313** Power wheelchair accessory, harness for upgrade to expandable controller, including all fasteners, connectors and mounting hardware, each

* **E2321** Power wheelchair accessory, hand control interface, remote joystick, nonproportional, including all related electronics, mechanical stop switch, and fixed mounting hardware

* **E2322** Power wheelchair accessory, hand control interface, multiple mechanical switches, nonproportional, including all related electronics, mechanical stop switch, and fixed mounting hardware

---

◀ ▶ **New**   ← → **Revised**   ✔ **Reinstated**   ✖ **Deleted**

☺ **Special coverage instructions**   ◆ **Not covered or valid by Medicare**   * **Carrier discretion**   ▶ **ASC payment group**

* **E2323** Power wheelchair accessory, specialty joystick handle for hand control interface, prefabricated

* **E2324** Power wheelchair accessory, chin cup for chin control interface

* **E2325** Power wheelchair accessory, sip and puff interface, nonproportional, including all related electronics, mechanical stop switch, and manual swingaway mounting hardware

* **E2326** Power wheelchair accessory, breath tube kit for sip and puff interface

* **E2327** Power wheelchair accessory, head control interface, mechanical, proportional, including all related electronics, mechanical direction change switch, and fixed mounting hardware

* **E2328** Power wheelchair accessory, head control or extremity control interface, electronic, proportional, including all related electronics and fixed mounting hardware

* **E2329** Power wheelchair accessory, head control interface, contact switch mechanism, nonproportional, including all related electronics, mechanical stop switch, mechanical direction change switch, head array, and fixed mounting hardware

* **E2330** Power wheelchair accessory, head control interface, proximity switch mechanism, nonproportional, including all related electronics, mechanical stop switch, mechanical direction change switch, head array, and fixed mounting hardware

* **E2331** Power wheelchair accessory, attendant control, proportional, including all related electronics and fixed mounting hardware

* **E2340** Power wheelchair accessory, nonstandard seat frame width, 20-23 inches

* **E2341** Power wheelchair accessory, nonstandard seat frame width, 24-27 inches

* **E2342** Power wheelchair accessory, nonstandard seat frame depth, 20 or 21 inches

* **E2343** Power wheelchair accessory, nonstandard seat frame depth, 22-25 inches

* **E2351** Power wheelchair accessory, electronic interface to operate speech generating device using power wheelchair control interface

* **E2360** Power wheelchair accessory, 22 NF non-sealed lead acid battery, each

* **E2361** Power wheelchair accessory, 22NF sealed lead acid battery, each, (e.g. gel cell, absorbed glassmat)

* **E2362** Power wheelchair accessory, group 24 non-sealed lead acid battery, each

* **E2363** Power wheelchair accessory, group 24 sealed lead acid battery, each (e.g. gel cell, absorbed glassmat)

* **E2364** Power wheelchair accessory, U-1 non-sealed lead acid battery, each

* **E2365** Power wheelchair accessory, U-1 sealed lead acid battery, each (e.g. gel cell, absorbed glassmat)

* **E2366** Power wheelchair accessory, battery charger, single mode, for use with only one battery type, sealed or non-sealed, each

* **E2367** Power wheelchair accessory, battery charger, dual mode, for use with either battery type, sealed or non-sealed, each

* **E2368** Power wheelchair component, motor, replacement only

* **E2369** Power wheelchair component, gear box, replacement only

* **E2370** Power wheelchair component, motor and gear box combination, replacement only

* **E2371** Power wheelchair accessory, group 27 sealed lead acid battery, (e.g. gel cell, absorbed glass mat), each

* **E2372** Power wheelchair accessory, group 27 non-sealed lead acid battery, each

* **E2373** Power wheelchair accessory, hand or chin control interface, compact remote joystick, proportional, including fixed mounting hardware

☼ **E2374** Power wheelchair accessory, hand or chin control interface, standard remote joystick (not including controller), proportional, including all related electronics and fixed mounting hardware, replacement only

☼ **E2375** Power wheelchair accessory, non-expandable controller, including all related electronics and mounting hardware, replacement only

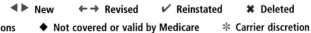

◄ ▶ **New**   ← → **Revised**   ✔ **Reinstated**   ✖ **Deleted**
☼ **Special coverage instructions**   ◆ **Not covered or valid by Medicare**   * **Carrier discretion**   ▶ **ASC payment group**

☺ **E2376** Power wheelchair accessory, expandable controller, including all related electronics and mounting hardware, replacement only

☺ **E2377** Power wheelchair accessory, expandable controller, including all related electronics and mounting hardware, upgrade provided at initial issue

☺ **E2381** Power wheelchair accessory, pneumatic drive wheel tire, any size, replacement only, each

☺ **E2382** Power wheelchair accessory, tube for pneumatic drive wheel tire, any size, replacement only, each

☺ **E2383** Power wheelchair accessory, insert for pneumatic drive wheel tire (removable), any type, any size, replacement only, each

☺ **E2384** Power wheelchair accessory, pneumatic caster tire, any size, replacement only, each

☺ **E2385** Power wheelchair accessory, tube for pneumatic caster tire, any size, replacement only, each

☺ **E2386** Power wheelchair accessory, foam filled drive wheel tire, any size, replacement only, each

☺ **E2387** Power wheelchair accessory, foam filled caster tire, any size, replacement only, each

☺ **E2388** Power wheelchair accessory, foam drive wheel tire, any size, replacement only, each

☺ **E2389** Power wheelchair accessory, foam caster tire, any size, replacement only, each

☺ **E2390** Power wheelchair accessory, solid (rubber/plastic) drive wheel tire, any size, replacement only, each

☺ **E2391** Power wheelchair accessory, solid (rubber/plastic) caster tire (removable), any size, replacement only, each

☺ **E2392** Power wheelchair accessory, solid (rubber/plastic) caster tire with integrated wheel, any size, replacement only, each

☺ **E2393** Power wheelchair accessory, valve for pneumatic tire tube, any type, replacement only, each

☺ **E2394** Power wheelchair accessory, drive wheel excludes tire, any size, replacement only, each

☺ **E2395** Power wheelchair accessory, caster wheel excludes tire, any size, replacement only, each

☺ **E2396** Power wheelchair accessory, caster fork, any size, replacement only, each

✳ **E2397** Power wheelchair accessory, lithium-based battery, each

✳ **E2399** Power wheelchair accessory, not otherwise classified interface, including all related electronics and any type mounting hardware

Negative Pressure

✳ **E2402** Negative pressure wound therapy electrical pump, stationary or portable

Speech Device

☺ **E2500** Speech generating device, digitized speech, using pre-recorded messages, less than or equal to 8 minutes recording time

IOM: 100-03, 1, 50.1

☺ **E2502** Speech generating device, digitized speech, using pre-recorded messages, greater than 8 minutes but less than or equal to 20 minutes recording time

IOM: 100-03, 1, 50.1

☺ **E2504** Speech generating device, digitized speech, using pre-recorded messages, greater than 20 minutes but less than or equal to 40 minutes recording time

IOM: 100-03, 1, 50.1

☺ **E2506** Speech generating device, digitized speech, using pre-recorded messages, greater than 40 minutes recording time

IOM: 100-03, 1, 50.1

☺ **E2508** Speech generating device, synthesized speech, requiring message formulation by spelling and access by physical contact with the device

IOM: 100-03, 1, 50.1

☺ **E2510** Speech generating device, synthesized speech, permitting multiple methods of message formulation and multiple methods of device access

IOM: 100-03, 1, 50.1

☺ **E2511** Speech generating software program, for personal computer or personal digital assistant

IOM: 100-03, 1, 50.1

☺ **E2512** Accessory for speech generating device, mounting system

IOM: 100-03, 1, 50.1

◀▶ **New** ←→ **Revised** ✔ **Reinstated** ✖ **Deleted**
☺ **Special coverage instructions** ◆ **Not covered or valid by Medicare** ✳ **Carrier discretion** ▶ **ASC payment group**

⚙ **E2599**   Accessory for speech generating device, not otherwise classified

IOM: 100-03, 1, 50.1

Wheelchair, Miscellaneous

✱ **E2601**   General use wheelchair seat cushion, width less than 22 inches, any depth

✱ **E2602**   General use wheelchair seat cushion, width 22 inches or greater, any depth

✱ **E2603**   Skin protection wheelchair seat cushion, width less than 22 inches, any depth

✱ **E2604**   Skin protection wheelchair seat cushion, width 22 inches or greater, any depth

✱ **E2605**   Positioning wheelchair seat cushion, width less than 22 inches, any depth

✱ **E2606**   Positioning wheelchair seat cushion, width 22 inches or greater, any depth

✱ **E2607**   Skin protection and positioning wheelchair seat cushion, width less than 22 inches, any depth

✱ **E2608**   Skin protection and positioning wheelchair seat cushion, width 22 inches or greater, any depth

✱ **E2609**   Custom fabricated wheelchair seat cushion, any size

✱ **E2610**   Wheelchair seat cushion, powered

✱ **E2611**   General use wheelchair back cushion, width less than 22 inches, any height, including any type mounting hardware

✱ **E2612**   General use wheelchair back cushion, width 22 inches or greater, any height, including any type mounting hardware

✱ **E2613**   Positioning wheelchair back cushion, posterior, width less than 22 inches, any height, including any type mounting hardware

✱ **E2614**   Positioning wheelchair back cushion, posterior, width 22 inches or greater, any height, including any type mounting hardware

✱ **E2615**   Positioning wheelchair back cushion, posterior-lateral, width less than 22 inches, any height, including any type mounting hardware

✱ **E2616**   Positioning wheelchair back cushion, posterior-lateral, width 22 inches or greater, any height, including any type mounting hardware

✱ **E2617**   Custom fabricated wheelchair back cushion, any size, including any type mounting hardware

✱ **E2619**   Replacement cover for wheelchair seat cushion or back cushion, each

✱ **E2620**   Positioning wheelchair back cushion, planar back with lateral supports, width less than 22 inches, any height, including any type mounting hardware

✱ **E2621**   Positioning wheelchair back cushion, planar back with lateral supports, width 22 inches or greater, any height, including any type mounting hardware

Gait Trainer

◆ **E8000**   Gait trainer, pediatric size, posterior support, includes all accessories and components

◆ **E8001**   Gait trainer, pediatric size, upright support, includes all accessories and components

◆ **E8002**   Gait trainer, pediatric size, anterior support, includes all accessories and components

◀▶ New   ←→ Revised   ✔ Reinstated   ✖ Deleted

⚙ Special coverage instructions   ◆ Not covered or valid by Medicare   ✱ Carrier discretion   ▌ ASC payment group

TEMPORARY PROCEDURES/PROFESSIONAL SERVICES (G0000-G9999)

NOTE: This section contains national codes assigned by CMS on a temporary basis to identify procedures/professional services.

* **G0008** Administration of influenza virus vaccine

* **G0009** Administration of pneumococcal vaccine

* **G0010** Administration of hepatitis B vaccine

* **G0027** Semen analysis; presence and/or motility of sperm excluding Huhner

  Laboratory Certification: Hematology

⊙ **G0101** Cervical or vaginal cancer screening; pelvic and clinical breast examination

⊙ **G0102** Prostate cancer screening; digital rectal examination

  IOM: 100-02, 6, 10; 100-04, 4, 240

⊙ **G0103** Prostate cancer screening; prostate specific antigen test (PSA)

  IOM: 100-02, 6, 10; 100-04, 4, 240

⊙ **G0104** Colorectal cancer screening; flexible sigmoidoscopy

⊙ **G0105** Colorectal cancer screening; colonoscopy on individual at high risk

⊙ **G0106** Colorectal cancer screening; alternative to G0104, screening sigmoidoscopy, barium enema

* **G0108** Diabetes outpatient self-management training services, individual, per 30 minutes

* **G0109** Diabetes outpatient self-management training services, group session (2 or more) per 30 minutes

* **G0117** Glaucoma screening for high risk patients furnished by an optometrist or ophthalmologist

* **G0118** Glaucoma screening for high risk patient furnished under the direct supervision of an optometrist or ophthalmologist

⊙ **G0120** Colorectal cancer screening; alternative to G0105, screening colonoscopy, barium enema.

⊙ **G0121** Colorectal cancer screening; colonoscopy on individual not meeting criteria for high risk

◆ **G0122** Colorectal cancer screening; barium enema

⊙ **G0123** Screening cytopathology, cervical or vaginal (any reporting system), collected in preservative fluid, automated thin layer preparation, screening by cytotechnologist under physician supervision

  IOM: 100-03, 3, 190.2;

  Laboratory Certification: Cytology

⊙ **G0124** Screening cytopathology, cervical or vaginal (any reporting system), collected in preservative fluid, automated thin layer preparation, requiring interpretation by physician

  IOM: 100-03, 3, 190.2;

  Laboratory Certification: Cytology

⊙ **G0127** Trimming of dystrophic nails, any number

  (Limit 1 unit of service)

  IOM: 100-02, 15, 290

⊙ **G0128** Direct (face-to-face with patient) skilled nursing services of a registered nurse provided in a comprehensive outpatient rehabilitation facility, each 10 minutes beyond the first 5 minutes

  Medicare Statute 1833(a)

→ * **G0129** Occupational therapy services requiring the skills of a qualified occupational therapist, furnished as a component of a partial hospitalization treatment program, per session (45 minutes or more)

⊙ **G0130▶** Single energy x-ray absorptiometry (SEXA) bone density study, one or more sites; appendicular skeleton (peripheral) (eg, radius, wrist, heel)

  IOM: 100-03, 2, 150.3

* **G0141** Screening cytopathology smears, cervical or vaginal, performed by automated system, with manual rescreening, requiring interpretation by physician
  Laboratory Certification: cytology

* **G0143** Screening cytopathology, cervical or vaginal (any reporting system), collected in preservative fluid, automated thin layer preparation, with manual screening and rescreening by cytotechnologist under physician supervision
  Laboratory Certification: Cytology

◀▶ New   ←→ Revised   ✔ Reinstated   ✖ Deleted

⊙ Special coverage instructions   ◆ Not covered or valid by Medicare   * Carrier discretion   ▶ ASC payment group

148

✳ **G0144** Screening cytopathology, cervical or vaginal (any reporting system), collected in preservative fluid, automated thin layer preparation, with screening by automated system, under physician supervision
Laboratory Certification: Cytology

✳ **G0145** Screening cytopathology, cervical or vaginal (any reporting system), collected in preservative fluid, automated thin layer preparation, with screening by automated system and manual rescreening under physician supervision
Laboratory Certification: Cytology

✳ **G0147** Screening cytopathology smears, cervical or vaginal; performed by automated system under physician supervision; Laboratory Certification: Cytology

✳ **G0148** Screening cytopathology smears, cervical or vaginal; performed by automated system with manual rescreening; Laboratory Certification: Cytology

✳ **G0151** Services of physical therapist in home health setting, each 15 minutes

✳ **G0152** Services of occupational therapist in home health setting, each 15 minutes

✳ **G0153** Services of speech and language pathologist in home health setting, each 15 minutes

✳ **G0154** Services of skilled nurse in home health setting, each 15 minutes

✳ **G0155** Services of clinical social worker in home health setting, each 15 minutes

✳ **G0156** Services of home health aide in home health setting, each 15 minutes

☼ **G0166** External counterpulsation, per treatment session
IOM: 100-03, 1, 20.20

✳ **G0168** Wound closure utilizing tissue adhesive(s) only

☼ **G0173▶** Linear accelerator based stereotactic radiosurgery, complete course of therapy in one session

✳ **G0175** Scheduled interdisciplinary team conference (minimum of three exclusive of patient care nursing staff) with patient present

☼ **G0176** Activity therapy, such as music, dance, art or play therapies not for recreation, related to the care and treatment of patient's disabling mental health problems, per session (45 minutes or more)

☼ **G0177** Training and educational services related to the care and treatment of patient's disabling mental health problems per session (45 minutes or more)

✳ **G0179** Physician re-certification for Medicare-covered home health services under a home health plan of care (patient not present), including contacts with home health agency and review of reports of patient status required by physicians to affirm the initial implementation of the plan of care that meets patient's needs, per re-certification period

✳ **G0180** Physician certification for Medicare-covered home health services under a home health plan of care (patient not present), including contacts with home health agency and review of reports of patient status required by physicians to affirm the initial implementation of the plan of care that meets patient's needs, per certification period

✳ **G0181** Physician supervision of a patient receiving Medicare-covered services provided by a participating home health agency (patient not present) requiring complex and multidisciplinary care modalities involving regular physician development and/or revision of care plans, review of subsequent reports of patient status, review of laboratory and other studies, communication (including telephone calls) with other health care professionals involved in the patient's care, integration of new information into the medical treatment plan and/or adjustment of medical therapy, within a calendar month, 30 minutes or more

✳ **G0182** Physician supervision of a patient under a Medicare-approved hospice (patient not present) requiring complex and multidisciplinary care modalities involving regular physician development and/or revision of care plans, review of subsequent reports of patient status, review of laboratory and other studies, communication (including telephone calls) with other health care professionals involved in the patient's care, integration of new information into the medical treatment plan and/or adjustment of medical therapy, within a calendar month, 30 minutes or more

◄▶ New   ←→ Revised   ✔ Reinstated   ✖ Deleted
☼ Special coverage instructions   ◆ Not covered or valid by Medicare   ✳ Carrier discretion   ▶ ASC payment group

* **G0186** Destruction of localized lesion of choroid (for example, choroidal neovascularization); photocoagulation, feeder vessel technique (one or more sessions)

* **G0202** Screening mammography, producing direct digital image, bilateral, all views

* **G0204** Diagnostic mammography, producing direct digital image, bilateral, all views

* **G0206** Diagnostic mammography, producing direct digital image, unilateral, all views

◆ **G0219** PET imaging whole body; melanoma for non-covered indications

IOM: 100-03, 4, 220.6

◆ **G0235** PET imaging, any site, not otherwise specified

IOM: 100-03, 4, 220.6

* **G0237** Therapeutic procedures to increase strength or endurance of respiratory muscles, face to face, one on one, each 15 minutes (includes monitoring)

* **G0238** Therapeutic procedures to improve respiratory function, other than described by G0237, one on one, face to face, per 15 minutes (includes monitoring)

* **G0239** Therapeutic procedures to improve respiratory function or increase strength or endurance of respiratory muscles, two or more individuals (includes monitoring)

☺ **G0245** Initial physician evaluation and management of a diabetic patient with diabetic sensory neuropathy resulting in a loss of protective sensation (LOPS) which must include (1) the diagnosis of LOPS, (2) a patient history, (3) a physical examination that consist of at least the following elements: (A) visual inspection of the forefoot, hindfoot and toe web spaces, (B) evaluation of a protective sensation, (C) evaluation of foot structure and biomechanics, (D) evaluation of vascular status and skin integrity, and (E) evaluation and recommendation of footwear, and (4) patient education

IOM: 100-03, 1, 70.2.1

☺ **G0246** Follow-up physician evaluation and management of a diabetic patient with diabetic sensory neuropathy resulting in a loss of protective sensation (LOPS) to include at least the following: (1) a patient history, (2) a physical examination that includes: (A) visual inspection of the forefoot, hindfoot and toe web spaces, (B) evaluation of protective sensation, (C) evaluation of foot structure and biomechanics, (D) evaluation of vascular status and skin integrity, and (E) evaluation and recommendation of footwear, and (3) patient education

IOM: 100-03, 1, 70.2.1

☺ **G0247** Routine foot care by a physician of a diabetic patient with diabetic sensory neuropathy resulting in a loss of protective sensation (LOPS) to include, the local care of superficial wounds (i.e. superficial to muscle and fascia) and at least the following if present: (1) local care of superficial wounds, (2) debridement of corns and calluses, and (3) trimming and debridement of nails

IOM: 100-03, 1, 70.2.1

→ ☺ **G0248** Demonstration, prior to initial use, of home INR monitoring for patient with either mechanical heart valve(s), chronic atrial fibrillation, or venous thromboembolism who meets Medicare coverage criteria, under the direction of a physician; includes: face-to-face demonstration of use and care of the INR monitor, obtaining at least one blood sample, provision of instructions for reporting home INR test results, and documentation of patient ability to perform testing prior to its use

IOM: 100-03, 4, 210.1

→ ☺ **G0249** Provision of test materials and equipment for home INR monitoring of patient with either mechanical heart valve(s), chronic atrial fibrillation, or venous thromboembolism who meets Medicare coverage criteria; includes provision of materials for use in the home and reporting of test results to physician; not occurring more frequently than once a week

IOM: 100-03, 4, 210.1

◀ ▶ New   ← → Revised   ✔ Reinstated   ✖ Deleted

☺ Special coverage instructions   ◆ Not covered or valid by Medicare   * Carrier discretion   ▶ ASC payment group

→ ⊙ **G0250** Physician review, interpretation, and patient management of home INR testing for a patient with either mechanical heart valve(s), chronic atrial fibrillation, or venous thromboembolism who meets Medicare coverage criteria; includes face-to-face verification by the physician at least once a year (e.g. during an evaluation and management service) that the patient uses the device in the context of the management of the anticoagulation therapy following initiation of the home INR monitoring; not occurring more frequently than once a week

IOM: 100-03, 4, 210.1

⊙ **G0251▶** Linear accelerator based stereotactic radiosurgery, delivery including collimator changes and custom plugging, fractionated treatment, all lesions, per session, maximum five sessions per course of treatment

◆ **G0252** PET imaging, full and partial-ring PET scanners only, for initial diagnosis of breast cancer and/or surgical planning for breast cancer (e.g. initial staging of axillary lymph nodes)

IOM: 100-03, 4, 220.6

◆ **G0255** Current perception threshold/sensory nerve conduction test, (SNCT) per limb, any nerve

IOM: 100-03, 2, 160.23

⊙ **G0257** Unscheduled or emergency dialysis treatment for an ESRD patient in a hospital outpatient department that is not certified as an ESRD facility

⊙ **G0259** Injection procedure for sacroiliac joint; arthrography

⊙ **G0260** Injection procedure for sacroiliac joint; provision of anesthetic, steroid and/or other therapeutic agent, with or without arthrography

✳ **G0268** Removal of impacted cerumen (one or both ears) by physician on same date of service as audiologic function testing

⊙ **G0269** Placement of occlusive device into either a venous or arterial access site, post surgical or interventional procedure (e.g. angioseal plug, vascular plug)

✳ **G0270** Medical nutrition therapy; reassessment and subsequent intervention(s) following second referral in same year for change in diagnosis, medical condition or treatment regimen (including additional hours needed for renal disease), individual, face to face with the patient, each 15 minutes

✳ **G0271** Medical nutrition therapy, reassessment and subsequent intervention(s) following second referral in same year for change in diagnosis, medical condition, or treatment regimen (including additional hours needed for renal disease), group (2 or more individuals), each 30 minutes

→ ✳ **G0275** Renal angiography, non-selective, one or both kidneys, performed at the same time as cardiac catheterization and/or coronary angiography, includes positioning or placement of any catheter in the abdominal aorta at or near the origins (OSTIA) of the renal arteries, injection of dye, flush aortogram, production of permanent images, and radiologic supervision and interpretation (list separately in addition to primary procedure)

→ ✳ **G0278** Iliac and/or femoral artery angiography, non-selective, bilateral or ipsilateral to catheter insertion, performed at the same time as cardiac catheterization and/or coronary angiography, includes positioning or placement of the catheter in the distal aorta or ipsilateral femoral or iliac artery, injection of dye, production of permanent images, and radiologic supervision and interpretation (list separately in addition to primary procedure)

✳ **G0281** Electrical stimulation, (unattended), to one or more areas, for chronic stage III and stage IV pressure ulcers, arterial ulcers, diabetic ulcers, and venous stasis ulcers not demonstrating measurable signs of healing after 30 days of conventional care, as part of a therapy plan of care

◆ **G0282** Electrical stimulation, (unattended), to one or more areas, for wound care other than described in G0281

IOM: 100-03, 4, 270.1

◀▶ New   ←→ Revised   ✔ Reinstated   ✖ Deleted
⊙ Special coverage instructions   ◆ Not covered or valid by Medicare   ✳ Carrier discretion   ▶ ASC payment group

* **G0283** Electrical stimulation (unattended), to one or more areas for indication(s) other than wound care, as part of a therapy plan of care

* **G0288** Reconstruction, computed tomographic angiography of aorta for surgical planning for vascular surgery

* **G0289** Arthroscopy, knee, surgical, for removal of loose body, foreign body, debridement/shaving of articular cartilage (chondroplasty) at the time of other surgical knee arthroscopy in a different compartment of the same knee

⊙ **G0290** Transcatheter placement of a drug eluting intracoronary stent(s), percutaneous, with or without other therapeutic intervention, any method; single vessel

⊙ **G0291** Transcatheter placement of a drug eluting intracoronary stent(s), percutaneous, with or without other therapeutic intervention, any method; each additional vessel

⊙ **G0293** Noncovered surgical procedure(s) using conscious sedation, regional, general or spinal anesthesia in a Medicare qualifying clinical trial, per day

⊙ **G0294** Noncovered procedure(s) using either no anesthesia or local anesthesia only, in a Medicare qualifying clinical trial, per day

◆ **G0295** Electromagnetic therapy, to one or more areas, for wound care other than described in G0329 or for other uses

IOM: 100-03, 4, 270.1

G0297 Insertion of single chamber pacing cardioverter defibrillator pulse generator ✖

G0300 Insertion or repositioning of electrode lead(s) for dual chamber pacing cardioverter defibrillator and insertion of pulse generator ✖

* **G0302** Pre-operative pulmonary surgery services for preparation for LVRS, complete course of services, to include a minimum of 16 days of services

* **G0303** Pre-operative pulmonary surgery services for preparation for LVRS, 10 to 15 days of services

* **G0304** Pre-operative pulmonary surgery services for preparation for LVRS, 1 to 9 days of services

* **G0305** Post-discharge pulmonary surgery services after LVRS, minimum of 6 days of services

* **G0306** Complete CBC, automated (HgB, HCT, RBC, WBC, without platelet count) and automated WBC differential count

Laboratory Certification: Hematology

* **G0307** Complete CBC, automated (HgB, HCT, RBC, WBC; without platelet count)

Laboratory Certification: Hematology

G0308 End-stage renal disease (ESRD) related services during the course of treatment, for patients under 2 years of age to include monitoring for the adequacy of nutrition, assessment of growth and development, and counseling of parents; with 4 or more face-to-face physician visits per month ✖

G0309 End-stage renal disease (ESRD) related services during the course of treatment, for patients under 2 years of age to include monitoring for the adequacy of nutrition, assessment of growth and development, and counseling of parents; with 2 or 3 face-to-face physician visits per month ✖

G0310 End-stage renal disease (ESRD) related services during the course of treatment, for patients under 2 years of age to include monitoring for the adequacy of nutrition, assessment of growth and development, and counseling of parents; with 1 face-to-face physician visit per month ✖

G0311 End-stage renal disease (ESRD) related services during the course of treatment, for patients between 2 and 11 years of age to include monitoring for the adequacy of nutrition, assessment of growth and development, and counseling of parents; with 4 or more face-to-face physician visits per month ✖

G0312 End-stage renal disease (ESRD) related services during the course of treatment, for patients between 2 and 11 years of age to include monitoring for the adequacy of nutrition, assessment of growth and development, and counseling of parents; with 2 or 3 face-to-face physician visits per month ✖

G0313 End-stage renal disease (ESRD) related services during the course of treatment, for patients between 2 and 11 years of age to include monitoring for the adequacy of nutrition, assessment of growth and development, and counseling of parents; with 1 face-to-face physician visits per month ✖

◀ ▶ New   ← → Revised   ✔ Reinstated   ✖ Deleted

⊙ Special coverage instructions   ◆ Not covered or valid by Medicare   * Carrier discretion   ▶ ASC payment group

G0314 ~~End-stage renal disease (ESRD) related services during the course of treatment, for patients between 12 and 19 years of age to include monitoring for the adequacy of nutrition, assessment of growth and development, and counseling of parents; with 4 or more face-to-face physician visits per month~~ ✖

G0315 ~~End-stage renal disease (ESRD) related services during the course of treatment, for patients between 12 and 19 years of age to include monitoring for the adequacy of nutrition, assessment of growth and development, and counseling of parents; with 2 or 3 face-to-face physician visits per month~~ ✖

G0316 ~~End-stage renal disease (ESRD) related services during the course of treatment, for patients between 12 and 19 years of age to include monitoring for the adequacy of nutrition, assessment of growth and development, and counseling of parents; with 1 face-to-face physician visit per month~~ ✖

G0317 ~~End-stage renal disease (ESRD) related services during the course of treatment, for patients 20 years of age and over; with 4 or more face-to-face physician visits per month~~ ✖

G0318 ~~End-stage renal disease (ESRD) related services during the course of treatment, for patients 20 years of age and over; with 2 or 3 face-to-face physician visits per month~~ ✖

G0319 ~~End-stage renal disease (ESRD) related services during the course of treatment, for patients 20 years of age and over; with 1 face-to-face physician visit per month~~ ✖

G0320 ~~End-stage renal disease (ESRD) related services for home dialysis patients per full month; for patients under two years of age to include monitoring for adequacy of nutrition, assessment of growth and development, and counseling of parents~~ ✖

G0321 ~~End-stage renal disease (ESRD) related services for home dialysis patients per full month; for patients two to eleven years of age to include monitoring for adequacy of nutrition, assessment of growth and development, and counseling of parents~~ ✖

G0322 ~~End-stage renal disease (ESRD) related services for home dialysis patients per full month; for patients twelve to nineteen years of age to include monitoring for adequacy of nutrition, assessment of growth and development, and counseling of parents~~ ✖

G0323 ~~End-stage renal disease (ESRD) related services for home dialysis patients per full month; for patients twenty years of age and older~~ ✖

G0324 ~~End-stage renal disease (ESRD) related services for home dialysis (less than full month), per day; for patients under two years of age~~ ✖

G0325 ~~End-stage renal disease (ESRD) related services for home dialysis (less than full month), per day; for patients between two and eleven years of age~~ ✖

G0326 ~~End-stage renal disease (ESRD) related services for home dialysis (less than full month), per day; for patients between twelve and nineteen years of age~~ ✖

G0327 ~~End-stage renal disease (ESRD) related services for home dialysis (less than full month), per day; for patients twenty years of age and over~~ ✖

✪ G0328 Colorectal cancer screening; fecal occult blood test, immunoassay, 1-3 simultaneous

Laboratory Certification: Routine Chemistry, Hematology

✳ G0329 Electromagnetic therapy, to one or more areas for chronic stage III and stage IV pressure ulcers, arterial ulcers, and diabetic ulcers and venous stasis ulcers not demonstrating measurable signs of healing after 30 days of conventional care as part of a therapy plan of care

G0332 ~~Services for intravenous infusion of immunoglobulin prior to administration (this service is to be billed in conjunction with administration of immunoglobulin)~~ ✖

✪ G0333 Pharmacy dispensing fee for inhalation drug(s); initial 30-day supply as a beneficiary

✳ G0337 Hospice evaluation and counseling services, pre-election

✳ G0339▶ Image-guided robotic linear accelerator-based stereotactic radiosurgery, complete course of therapy in one session or first session of fractionated treatment

---

◀▶ New   ←→ Revised   ✔ Reinstated   ✖ Deleted

✪ Special coverage instructions   ◆ Not covered or valid by Medicare   ✳ Carrier discretion   ▶ ASC payment group

* **G0340** Image-guided robotic linear accelerator-based stereotactic radiosurgery, delivery including collimator changes and custom plugging, fractionated treatment, all lesions, per session, second through fifth sessions, maximum five sessions per course of treatment

☺ **G0341** Percutaneous islet cell transplant, includes portal vein catheterization and infusion

IOM: 100-03, 4, 260.3; 100-04, 32, 70

☺ **G0342** Laparoscopy for islet cell transplant, includes portal vein catheterization and infusion

IOM: 100-03, 4, 260.3

☺ **G0343** Laparotomy for islet cell transplant, includes portal vein catheterization and infusion

IOM: 100-03, 4, 260.3

~~G0344~~ ~~Initial preventive physical examination; face-to-face visit, services limited to new beneficiary during the first six months of Medicare enrollment~~ ✖

* **G0364** Bone marrow aspiration performed with bone marrow biopsy through the same incision on the same date of service

* **G0365** Vessel mapping of vessels for hemodialysis access (services for preoperative vessel mapping prior to creation of hemodialysis access using an autogenous hemodialysis conduit, including arterial inflow and venous outflow)

~~G0366~~ ~~Electrocardiogram, routine ECG with 12 leads, performed as a component of the initial preventive examination with interpretation and report~~ ✖

~~G0367~~ ~~Tracing only, without interpretation and report; performed as a component of the initial preventive examination~~ ✖

~~G0368~~ ~~Interpretation and report only, performed as a component of the initial preventive examination~~ ✖

☺ **G0372** Physician service required to establish and document the need for a power mobility device

~~G0377~~ ~~Administration of vaccine for Part D drug~~ ✖

☺ **G0378** Hospital observation service, per hour

☺ **G0379** Direct admission of patient for hospital observation care

* **G0380** Level 1 hospital emergency department visit provided in a type B emergency department; (the ED must meet at least one of the following requirements: (1) it is licensed by the state in which it is located under applicable state law as an emergency room or emergency department; (2) it is held out to the public (by name, posted signs, advertising, or other means) as a place that provides care for emergency medical conditions on an urgent basis without requiring a previously scheduled appointment; or (3) during the calendar year immediately preceding the calendar year in which a determination under 42 CFR § 489.24 is being made, based on a representative sample of patient visits that occurred during that calendar year, it provides at least one-third of all of its outpatient visits for the treatment of emergency medical conditions on an urgent basis without requiring a previously scheduled appointment)

* **G0381** Level 2 hospital emergency department visit provided in a type B emergency department; (the ED must meet at least one of the following requirements: (1) it is licensed by the state in which it is located under applicable state law as an emergency room or emergency department; (2) it is held out to the public (by name, posted signs, advertising, or other means) as a place that provides care for emergency medical conditions on an urgent basis without requiring a previously scheduled appointment; or (3) during the calendar year immediately preceding the calendar year in which a determination under 42 CFR § 489.24 is being made, based on a representative sample of patient visits that occurred during that calendar year, it provides at least one-third of all of its outpatient visits for the treatment of emergency medical conditions on an urgent basis without requiring a previously scheduled appointment)

◀▶ New   ←→ Revised   ✔ Reinstated   ✖ Deleted

☺ Special coverage instructions   ◆ Not covered or valid by Medicare   * Carrier discretion   ▶ ASC payment group

✳ **G0382** Level 3 hospital emergency department visit provided in a type B emergency department; (the ED must meet at least one of the following requirements: (1) it is licensed by the state in which it is located under applicable state law as an emergency room or emergency department; (2) it is held out to the public (by name, posted signs, advertising, or other means) as a place that provides care for emergency medical conditions on an urgent basis without requiring a previously scheduled appointment; or (3) during the calendar year immediately preceding the calendar year in which a determination under 42 CFR § 489.24 is being made, based on a representative sample of patient visits that occurred during that calendar year, it provides at least one-third of all of its outpatient visits for the treatment of emergency medical conditions on an urgent basis without requiring a previously scheduled appointment)

✳ **G0383** Level 4 hospital emergency department visit provided in a type B emergency department; (the ED must meet at least one of the following requirements: (1) it is licensed by the state in which it is located under applicable state law as an emergency room or emergency department; (2) it is held out to the public (by name, posted signs, advertising, or other means) as a place that provides care for emergency medical conditions on an urgent basis without requiring a previously scheduled appointment; or (3) during the calendar year immediately preceding the calendar year in which a determination under 42 CFR § 489.24 is being made, based on a representative sample of patient visits that occurred during that calendar year, it provides at least one-third of all of its outpatient visits for the treatment of emergency medical conditions on an urgent basis without requiring a previously scheduled appointment)

✳ **G0384** Level 5 hospital emergency department visit provided in a type B emergency department; (the ED must meet at least one of the following requirements: (1) it is licensed by the state in which it is located under applicable state law as an emergency room or emergency department; (2) it is held out to the public (by name, posted signs, advertising, or other means) as a place that provides care for emergency medical conditions on an urgent basis without requiring a previously scheduled appointment; or (3) during the calendar year immediately preceding the calendar year in which a determination under 42 CFR § 489.24 is being made, based on a representative sample of patient visits that occurred during that calendar year, it provides at least one-third of all of its outpatient visits for the treatment of emergency medical conditions on an urgent basis without requiring a previously scheduled appointment)

☺ **G0389** Ultrasound B-scan and/or real time with image documentation; for abdominal aortic aneurysm (AAA) screening

☺ **G0390** Trauma response team associated with hospital critical care service

✳ **G0392** Transluminal balloon angioplasty, percutaneous; for maintenance of hemodialysis access, arteriovenous fistula or graft; arterial

✳ **G0393** Transluminal balloon angioplasty, percutaneous; for maintenance of hemodialysis access, arteriovenous fistula or graft; venous

✳ **G0394** Blood occult test (e.g., guaiac), feces, for single determination for colorectal neoplasm (i.e., patient was provided three cards or single triple card for consecutive collection)

✳ **G0396** Alcohol and/or substance (other than tobacco) abuse structured assessment (e.g., AUDIT, DAST), and brief intervention 15 to 30 minutes

Bill instead of 99408 and 99409

✳ **G0397** Alcohol and/or substance (other than tobacco) abuse structured assessment (e.g., AUDIT, DAST), and intervention, greater than 30 minutes

Bill instead of 99408 and 99409

◀▶ New   ←→ Revised   ✔ Reinstated   ✖ Deleted

☺ Special coverage instructions   ◆ Not covered or valid by Medicare   ✳ Carrier discretion   ▶ ASC payment group

▶ ✳ **G0398**   Home sleep study test (HST) with type II portable monitor, unattended; minimum of 7 channels: EEG, EOG, EMG, ECG/heart rate, airflow, respiratory effort and oxygen saturation

▶ ✳ **G0399**   Home sleep test (HST) with type III portable monitor, unattended; minimum of 4 channels: 2 respiratory movement/airflow, 1 ECG/heart rate and 1 oxygen saturation

▶ ✳ **G0400**   Home sleep test (HST) with type IV portable monitor, unattended; minimum of 3 channels

▶ ✳ **G0402**   Initial preventive physical examination; face-to-face visit, services limited to new beneficiary during the first 12 months of Medicare enrollment

▶ ✳ **G0403**   Electrocardiogram, routine ECG with 12 leads; performed as a screening for the initial preventive physical examination with interpretation and report

▶ ✳ **G0404**   Electrocardiogram, routine ECG with 12 leads; tracing only, without interpretation and report, performed as a screening for the initial preventive physical examination

▶ ✳ **G0405**   Electrocardiogram, routine ECG with 12 leads; interpretation and report only, performed as a screening for the initial preventive physical examination

▶ ✳ **G0406**   Follow-up inpatient telehealth consultation, limited, physicians typically spend 15 minutes communicating with the patient via telehealth

▶ ✳ **G0407**   Follow-up inpatient telehealth consultation, intermediate, physicians typically spend 25 minutes communicating with the patient via telehealth

▶ ✳ **G0408**   Follow-up inpatient telehealth consultation, complex, physicians typically spend 35 minutes or more communicating with the patient via telehealth

▶ ✳ **G0409**   Social work and psychological services, directly relating to and/or furthering the patient's rehabilitation goals, each 15 minutes, face-to-face; individual (services provided by a CORF-qualified social worker or psychologist in a CORF)

▶ ✳ **G0410**   Group psychotherapy other than of a multiple-family group, in a partial hospitalization setting, approximately 45 to 50 minutes

▶ ✳ **G0411**   Interactive group psychotherapy, in a partial hospitalization setting, approximately 45 to 50 minutes

▶ ✳ **G0412**   Open treatment of iliac spine(s), tuberosity avulsion, or iliac wing fracture(s), unilateral or bilateral for pelvic bone fracture patterns which do not disrupt the pelvic ring includes internal fixation, when performed

▶ ✳ **G0413**   Percutaneous skeletal fixation of posterior pelvic bone fracture and/or dislocation, for fracture patterns which disrupt the pelvic ring, unilateral or bilateral, (includes ilium, sacroiliac joint and/or sacrum)

▶ ✳ **G0414**   Open treatment of anterior pelvic bone fracture and/or dislocation for fracture patterns which disrupt the pelvic ring, unilateral or bilateral, includes internal fixation when performed (includes pubic symphysis and/or superior/inferior rami)

▶ ✳ **G0415**   Open treatment of posterior pelvic bone fracture and/or dislocation, for fracture patterns which disrupt the pelvic ring, unilateral or bilateral, includes internal fixation, when performed (includes ilium, sacroiliac joint and/or sacrum)

▶ ✳ **G0416**   Surgical pathology, gross and microscopic examination for prostate needle saturation biopsy sampling, 1-20 specimens

▶ ✳ **G0417**   Surgical pathology, gross and microscopic examination for prostate needle saturation biopsy sampling, 21-40 specimens

▶ ✳ **G0418**   Surgical pathology, gross and microscopic examination for prostate needle saturation biopsy sampling, 41-60 specimens

▶ ✳ **G0419**   Surgical pathology, gross and microscopic examination for prostate needle saturation biopsy sampling, greater than 60 specimens

✳ **G3001**   Administration and supply of tositumomab, 450 mg

✳ **G8006**   Acute myocardial infarction: patient documented to have received aspirin at arrival

✳ **G8007**   Acute myocardial infarction: patient not documented to have received aspirin at arrival

✳ **G8008**   Clinician documented that acute myocardial infarction patient was not an eligible candidate to receive aspirin at arrival measure

---

◀▶ New   ←→ Revised   ✔ Reinstated   ✖ Deleted

○ Special coverage instructions   ◆ Not covered or valid by Medicare   ✳ Carrier discretion   ▶ ASC payment group

* **G8009** Acute myocardial infarction: patient documented to have received beta-blocker at arrival

* **G8010** Acute myocardial infarction: patient not documented to have received beta-blocker at arrival

* **G8011** Clinician documented that acute myocardial infarction patient was not an eligible candidate for beta-blocker at arrival measure

* **G8012** Pneumonia: patient documented to have received antibiotic within 4 hours of presentation

* **G8013** Pneumonia: patient not documented to have received antibiotic within 4 hours of presentation

* **G8014** Clinician documented that pneumonia patient was not an eligible candidate for antibiotic within 4 hours of presentation measure

* **G8015** Diabetic patient with most recent hemoglobin A1c level (within the last 6 months) documented as greater than 9%

* **G8016** Diabetic patient with most recent hemoglobin A1c level (within the last 6 months) documented as less than or equal to 9%

* **G8017** Clinician documented that diabetic patient was not eligible candidate for hemoglobin A1c measure

* **G8018** Clinician has not provided care for the diabetic patient for the required time for hemoglobin A1c measure (6 months)

* **G8019** Diabetic patient with most recent low-density lipoprotein (within the last 12 months) documented as greater than or equal to 100 mg/dl

* **G8020** Diabetic patient with most recent low-density lipoprotein (within the last 12 months) documented as less than 100 mg/dl

* **G8021** Clinician documented that diabetic patient was not eligible candidate for low-density lipoprotein measure

* **G8022** Clinician has not provided care for the diabetic patient for the required time for low-density lipoprotein measure (12 months)

* **G8023** Diabetic patient with most recent blood pressure (within the last 6 months) documented as equal to or greater than 140 systolic or equal to or greater than 80 mmHg diastolic

* **G8024** Diabetic patient with most recent blood pressure (within the last 6 months) documented as less than 140 systolic and less than 80 diastolic

* **G8025** Clinician documented that the diabetic patient was not eligible candidate for blood pressure measure

* **G8026** Clinician has not provided care for the diabetic patient for the required time for blood pressure measure (within the last 6 months)

* **G8027** Heart failure patient with left ventricular systolic dysfunction (LVSD) documented to be on either angiotensin-converting enzyme inhibitor or angiotensin-receptor blocker (ACE-I or ARB) therapy

* **G8028** Heart failure patient with left ventricular systolic dysfunction (LVSD) not documented to be on either angiotensin-converting enzyme inhibitor or angiotensin-receptor blocker (ACE-I or ARB) therapy

* **G8029** Clinician documented that heart failure patient was not an eligible candidate for either angiotensin-converting enzyme inhibitor or angiotensin-receptor blocker (ACE-I or ARB) therapy measure

* **G8030** Heart failure patient with left ventricular systolic dysfunction (LVSD) documented to be on beta-blocker therapy

* **G8031** Heart failure patient with left ventricular systolic dysfunction (LVSD) not documented to be on beta-blocker therapy

* **G8032** Clinician documented that heart failure patient was not eligible candidate for beta-blocker therapy measure

* **G8033** Prior myocardial infarction–coronary artery disease patient documented to be on beta-blocker therapy

* **G8034** Prior myocardial infarction–coronary artery disease patient not documented to be on beta-blocker therapy

* **G8035** Clinician documented that prior myocardial infarction–coronary artery disease patient was not eligible candidate for beta-blocker therapy measure

* **G8036** Coronary artery disease patient documented to be on antiplatelet therapy

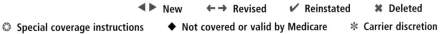

◀▶ New   ←→ Revised   ✔ Reinstated   ✖ Deleted
⊙ Special coverage instructions   ◆ Not covered or valid by Medicare   * Carrier discretion   ▶ ASC payment group

* **G8037** Coronary artery disease patient not documented to be on antiplatelet therapy

* **G8038** Clinician documented that coronary artery disease patient was not eligible candidate for antiplatelet therapy measure

* **G8039** Coronary artery disease – patient with low-density lipoprotein documented to be greater than 100 mg/dl

* **G8040** Coronary artery disease – patient with low-density lipoprotein documented to be less than or equal to 100 mg/dl

* **G8041** Clinician documented that coronary artery disease patient was not eligible candidate for low-density lipoprotein measure

* **G8051** Patient (female) documented to have been assessed for osteoporosis

* **G8052** Patient (female) not documented to have been assessed for osteoporosis

* **G8053** Clinician documented that (female) patient was not an eligible candidate for osteoporosis assessment measure

* **G8054** Patient not documented for the assessment for falls within last 12 months

* **G8055** Patient documented for the assessment for falls within last 12 months

* **G8056** Clinician documented that patient was not an eligible candidate for the falls assessment measure within the last 12 months

* **G8057** Patient documented to have received hearing assessment

* **G8058** Patient not documented to have received hearing assessment

* **G8059** Clinician documented that patient was not an eligible candidate for hearing assessment measure

* **G8060** Patient documented for the assessment of urinary incontinence

* **G8061** Patient not documented for the assessment of urinary incontinence

* **G8062** Clinician documented that patient was not an eligible candidate for urinary incontinence assessment measure

* **G8075** End-stage renal disease patient with documented dialysis dose of URR greater than or equal to 65% (or Kt/V greater than or equal to 1.2)

* **G8076** End-stage renal disease patient with documented dialysis dose of URR less than 65% (or Kt/V less than 1.2)

* **G8077** Clinician documented that end-stage renal disease patient was not an eligible candidate for URR or Kt/V measure

* **G8078** End-stage renal disease patient with documented hematocrit greater than or equal to 33 (or hemoglobin greater than or equal to 11)

* **G8079** End-stage renal disease patient with documented hematocrit less than 33 (or hemoglobin less than 11)

* **G8080** Clinician documented that end-stage renal disease patient was not an eligible candidate for hematocrit (hemoglobin) measure

* **G8081** End-stage renal disease patient requiring hemodialysis vascular access documented to have received autogenous AV fistula

* **G8082** End-stage renal disease patient requiring hemodialysis documented to have received vascular access other than autogenous AV fistula

* **G8085** End-stage renal disease patient requiring hemodialysis vascular access was not an eligible candidate for autogenous AV fistula

* **G8093** Newly diagnosed chronic obstructive pulmonary disease (COPD) patient documented to have received smoking cessation intervention, within 3 months of diagnosis

* **G8094** Newly diagnosed chronic obstructive pulmonary disease (COPD) patient not documented to have received smoking cessation intervention, within 3 months of diagnosis

* **G8099** Osteoporosis patient documented to have been prescribed calcium and vitamin D supplements

* **G8100** Clinician documented that osteoporosis patient was not an eligible candidate for calcium and vitamin D supplement measure

* **G8103** Newly diagnosed osteoporosis patient documented to have been treated with antiresorptive therapy and/or PTH within 3 months of diagnosis

* **G8104** Clinician documented that newly diagnosed osteoporosis patient was not an eligible candidate for antiresorptive therapy and/or PTH treatment measure within 3 months of diagnosis

---

◀ ▶ New   ←→ Revised   ✔ Reinstated   ✖ Deleted

⊙ Special coverage instructions   ◆ Not covered or valid by Medicare   ✳ Carrier discretion   ▶ ASC payment group

* **G8106** Within 6 months of suffering a nontraumatic fracture, female patient 65 years of age or older documented to have undergone bone mineral density testing or to have been prescribed a drug to treat or prevent osteoporosis

* **G8107** Clinician documented that female patient 65 years of age or older who suffered a nontraumatic fracture within the last 6 months was not an eligible candidate for measure to test bone mineral density or drug to treat or prevent osteoporosis

* **G8108** Patient documented to have received influenza vaccination during influenza season

* **G8109** Patient not documented to have received influenza vaccination during influenza season

* **G8110** Clinician documented that patient was not an eligible candidate for influenza vaccination measure

* **G8111** Patient (female) documented to have received a mammogram during the measurement year or prior year to the measurement year

* **G8112** Patient (female) not documented to have received a mammogram during the measurement year or prior year to the measurement year

* **G8113** Clinician documented that female patient was not an eligible candidate for mammography measure

* **G8114** Clinician did not provide care to patient for the required time of mammography measure (i.e., measurement year or prior year)

* **G8115** Patient documented to have received pneumococcal vaccination

* **G8116** Patient not documented to have received pneumococcal vaccination

* **G8117** Clinician documented that patient was not an eligible candidate for pneumococcal vaccination measure

* **G8126** Patient documented as being treated with antidepressant medication during the entire 12 week acute treatment phase

* **G8127** Patient not documented as being treated with antidepressant medication during the entire 12 weeks acute treatment phase

* **G8128** Clinician documented that patient was not an eligible candidate for antidepressant medication during the entire 12 week acute treatment phase measure

* **G8129** Patient documented as being treated with antidepressant medication for at least 6 months continuous treatment phase

* **G8130** Patient not documented as being treated with antidepressant medication for at least 6 months continuous treatment phase

* **G8131** Clinician documented that patient was not an eligible candidate for antidepressant medication for continuous treatment phase

* **G8152** Patient documented to have received antibiotic prophylaxis one hour prior to incision time (two hours for vancomycin)

* **G8153** Patient not documented to have received antibiotic prophylaxis one hour prior to incision time (two hours for vancomycin)

* **G8154** Clinician documented that patient was not an eligible candidate for antibiotic prophylaxis one hour prior to incision time (two hours for vancomycin) measure

* **G8155** Patient with documented receipt of thromboembolism prophylaxis

* **G8156** Patient without documented receipt of thromboembolism prophylaxis

* **G8157** Clinician documented that patient was not an eligible candidate for thromboembolism prophylaxis measure

* **G8159** Patient documented to have received coronary artery bypass graft without use of internal mammary artery

* **G8162** Patient with isolated coronary artery bypass graft not documented to have received pre-operative beta-blockade

* **G8164** Patient with isolated coronary artery bypass graft documented to have prolonged intubation

* **G8165** Patient with isolated coronary artery bypass graft not documented to have prolonged intubation

* **G8166** Patient with isolated coronary artery bypass graft documented to have required surgical re-exploration

◀▶ New   ←→ Revised   ✔ Reinstated   ✖ Deleted
☺ Special coverage instructions   ◆ Not covered or valid by Medicare   ✳ Carrier discretion   ▶ ASC payment group

* **G8167** Patient with isolated coronary artery bypass graft did not require surgical re-exploration

* **G8170** Patient with isolated coronary artery bypass graft documented to have been discharged on aspirin or clopidogrel

* **G8171** Patient with isolated coronary artery bypass graft not documented to have been discharged on aspirin or clopidogrel

* **G8172** Clinician documented that patient with isolated coronary artery bypass graft was not an eligible candidate for antiplatelet therapy at discharge measure

* **G8182** Clinician has not provided care for the cardiac patient for the required time for low-density lipoprotein measure (6 months)

* **G8183** Patient with heart failure and atrial fibrillation documented to be on warfarin therapy

* **G8184** Clinician documented that patient with heart failure and atrial fibrillation was not an eligible candidate for warfarin therapy measure

* **G8185** Patients diagnosed with symptomatic osteoarthritis with documented annual assessment of function and pain

* **G8186** Clinician documented that symptomatic osteoarthritis patient was not an eligible candidate for annual assessment of function and pain measure

* **G8193** Clinician did not document that an order for prophylactic antibiotic to be given within one hour (if vancomycin, two hours) prior to surgical incision (or start of procedure when no incision is required) was given

* **G8196** Clinician did not document a prophylactic antibiotic was administered within one hour (if vancomycin, two hours) prior to surgical incision (or start of procedure when no incision is required)

* **G8200** Order for cefazolin or cefuroxime for antimicrobial prophylaxis not documented

* **G8204** Clinician did not document an order was given to discontinue prophylactic antibiotics within 24 hours of surgical end time

* **G8209** Clinician did not document an order was given to discontinue prophylactic antibiotics within 48 hours of surgical end time

* **G8214** Clinician did not document an order was given for appropriate venous thromboembolism (VTE) prophylaxis to be given within 24 hrs prior to incision time or 24 hours after surgery end time

* **G8217** Patient not documented to have received DVT prophylaxis by end of hospital day 2

* **G8219** Patient documented to have received DVT prophylaxis by end of hospital day 2

* **G8220** Patient not documented to have received DVT prophylaxis by end of hospital day 2

* **G8221** Clinician documented that patient was not an eligible candidate for DVT prophylaxis by the end of hospital day 2, including physician documentation that patient is ambulatory

* **G8223** Patient not documented to have received prescription for antiplatelet therapy at discharge

* **G8226** Patient not documented to have received prescription for anticoagulant therapy at discharge

* **G8231** Patient not documented to have received T-PA or not documented to have been considered a candidate for T-PA administration

* **G8234** Patient not documented to have received dysphagia screening

* **G8238** Patient not documented to have received order for or consideration for rehabilitation services

* **G8240** Internal carotid stenosis patient in the 30-99% range, and no documentation of reference to measurements of distal internal carotid diameter as the denominator for stenosis measurement

* **G8243** Patient not documented to have received CT or MRI and the presence or absence of hemorrhage, mass lesion and acute infarction not documented in the final report

* **G8246** Patient was not an eligible candidate for medical history review with assessment of new or changing moles

* **G8248** Patient with at least one alarm symptom not documented to have had upper endoscopy or referral for upper endoscopy

* **G8251** Patient not documented to have received an esophageal biopsy when suspicion of Barrett's esophagus is indicated in the endoscopy report

* **G8254** Patient with no documentation order for barium swallow test

* **G8257** Clinician has not documented reconciliation of discharge medications with current medication list in medical record

* **G8260** Patient not documented to have surrogate decision maker or advance care plan in medical record

* **G8263** Patient not documented to have been assessed for presence or absence of urinary incontinence

* **G8266** Patient not documented to have received characterization of urinary incontinence

* **G8268** Patient not documented to have received plan of care for urinary incontinence

* **G8271** Patient with no documentation of screening for fall risks (2 or more falls in the past year or any fall with injury in the past year)

* **G8274** Clinician has not documented presence or absence of alarm symptoms

* **G8276** Patient not documented to have received medical history with assessment of new or changing moles

* **G8279** Patient not documented to have received a complete physical skin exam

* **G8282** Patient not documented to have received counseling to perform a self-examination

* **G8285** Patient not documented to have received pharmacologic therapy

* **G8289** Patient with no documentation of calcium and vitamin D use or counseling regarding both calcium and vitamin D use, or exercise

* **G8293** COPD patient without spirometry results documented

* **G8296** COPD patient not documented to have inhaled bronchodilator therapy prescribed

* **G8298** Patient documented to have received optic nerve head evaluation

* **G8299** Patient not documented to have received optic nerve head evaluation

* **G8302** Patient documented to have a specific target intraocular pressure range goal

* **G8303** Patient not documented to have a specific target intraocular pressure range goal

* **G8304** Clinician documented that patient was not an eligible candidate for a specific target intraocular pressure range goal

* **G8305** Clinician has not provided care for the primary open-angle glaucoma patient for the required time for treatment range goal documentation measurement

* **G8306** Primary open-angle glaucoma patient with intraocular pressure above the target range goal documented to have received plan of care

* **G8307** Primary open-angle glaucoma patient with intraocular pressure at or below goal, no plan of care necessary

* **G8308** Primary open-angle glaucoma patient with intraocular pressure above the target range goal, and not documented to have received plan of care during the reporting year

* **G8310** Patient not documented to have been prescribed/recommended at least one antioxidant vitamin or mineral supplement during the reporting year

* **G8314** Patient not documented to have received macular exam with documentation of presence or absence of macular thickening or hemorrhage and no documentation of level of macular degeneration severity

* **G8318** Patient documented not to have visual functional status assessed

* **G8322** Patient not documented to have had pre-surgical axial length, corneal power measurement and method of intraocular lens power calculation

* **G8326** Patient not documented to have received fundus evaluation within six months prior to cataract surgery

* **G8330** Patient not documented to have received dilated macular or fundus exam with level of severity of retinopathy and the presence or absence of macular edema not documented

◀▶ New   ←→ Revised   ✔ Reinstated   ✖ Deleted
◎ Special coverage instructions   ◆ Not covered or valid by Medicare   ＊ Carrier discretion   ▶ ASC payment group

* **G8334** Documentation of findings of macular or fundus exam not communicated to the physician managing the patient's ongoing diabetes care

* **G8338** Clinician has not documented that communication was sent to the physician managing ongoing care of patient that a fracture occurred and that the patient was or should be tested or treated for osteoporosis

* **G8341** Patient not documented to have had central DEXA measurement or pharmacologic therapy

* **G8345** Patient not documented to have had central DEXA measurement ordered or performed or pharmacologic therapy

* **G8351** Patient not documented to have had ECG

* **G8354** Patient not documented to have received or taken aspirin 24 hours before emergency department arrival or during emergency department stay

* **G8357** Patient not documented to have had ECG

* **G8360** Patient not documented to have vital signs recorded and reviewed

* **G8362** Patient not documented to have oxygen saturation assessed

* **G8365** Patient not documented to have mental status assessed

* **G8367** Patient not documented to have appropriate empiric antibiotic prescribed

* **G8370** Asthma patients with numeric frequency of symptoms or patient completion of an asthma assessment tool/survey/questionnaire not documented

* **G8371** Chemotherapy documented as not received or prescribed for stage III colon cancer patients

* **G8372** Chemotherapy documented as received or prescribed for stage III colon cancer patients

* **G8373** Chemotherapy plan documented prior to chemotherapy administration

* **G8374** Chemotherapy plan not documented prior to chemotherapy administration

* **G8375** Chronic lymphocytic leukemia (CLL) patient with no documentation of baseline flow cytometry performed

* **G8376** Clinician documentation that breast cancer patient was not eligible for tamoxifen or aromatase inhibitor therapy measure

* **G8377** Clinician documentation that colon cancer patient is not eligible for chemotherapy measure

* **G8378** Clinician documentation that patient was not an eligible candidate for radiation therapy measure

* **G8379** Documentation of radiation therapy recommended within 12 months of first office visit

* **G8380** For patients with ER or PR positive, stage IC-III breast cancer, clinician did not document that the patient received or was prescribed tamoxifen or aromatase inhibitor

* **G8381** For patients with ER or PR positive, stage IC-III breast cancer, clinician documented or prescribed that the patient is receiving tamoxifen or aromatase inhibitor

* **G8382** Multiple myeloma patients with no documentation of prescribed or received intravenous bisphosphonate therapy

* **G8383** No documentation of radiation therapy recommended within 12 months of first office visit

* **G8384** Baseline cytogenetic testing not performed in patients with myelodysplastic syndrome (MDS) or acute leukemias

* **G8385** Diabetic patients with no documentation of hemoglobin A1c level (within the last 12 months)

* **G8386** Diabetic patients with no documentation of low-density lipoprotein (within the last 12 months)

* **G8387** End-stage renal disease patient with a hematocrit or hemoglobin not documented

* **G8388** End-stage renal disease patient with URR or KT/V value not documented, but otherwise eligible for measure

* **G8389** Myelodysplastic syndrome (MDS) patients with no documentation of iron stores prior to receiving erythropoietin therapy

* **G8390** Diabetic patients with no documentation of blood pressure measurement (within the last 12 months)

◀▶ New   ←→ Revised   ✔ Reinstated   ✖ Deleted

⊙ Special coverage instructions   ◆ Not covered or valid by Medicare   * Carrier discretion   ▶ ASC payment group

* **G8391** Patients with persistent asthma, no documentation of preferred long term control medication or acceptable alternative treatment prescribed

* **G8395** Left ventricular ejection fraction (LVEF) $> = 40\%$ or documentation as normal or mildly depressed left ventricular systolic function

* **G8396** Left ventricular ejection fraction (LVEF) not performed or documented

* **G8397** Dilated macular or fundus exam performed, including documentation of the presence or absence of macular edema and level of severity of retinopathy

* **G8398** Dilated macular or fundus exam not performed

* **G8399** Patient with central dual-energy x-ray absorptiometry (DXA) results documented or ordered or pharmacologic therapy (other than minerals/vitamins) for osteoporosis prescribed)

* **G8400** Patient with central dual-energy x-ray absorptiometry (DXA) results not documented or not ordered or pharmacologic therapy (other than minerals/vitamins) for osteoporosis not prescribed

* **G8401** Clinician documented that patient was not an eligible candidate for screening or therapy for osteoporosis for women measure

* **G8402** Tobacco (smoke) use cessation intervention, counseling

* **G8403** Tobacco (smoke) use cessation intervention not counseled

* **G8404** Lower extremity neurological exam performed and documented

* **G8405** Lower extremity neurological exam not performed

* **G8406** Clinician documented that patient was not an eligible candidate for lower extremity neurological exam measure

* **G8407** ABI measured and documented

* **G8408** ABI measurement was not obtained

* **G8409** Clinician documented that patient was not an eligible candidate for ABI measurement measure

* **G8410** Footwear evaluation performed and documented

* **G8415** Footwear evaluation was not performed

* **G8416** Clinician documented that patient was not an eligible candidate for footwear evaluation measure

→ * **G8417** Calculated BMI above the upper parameter and a follow-up plan was documented in the medical record

→ * **G8418** Calculated BMI below the lower parameter and a follow-up plan was documented in the medical record

→ * **G8419** Calculated BMI outside normal parameters, no follow-up plan was documented in the medical record

→ * **G8420** Calculated BMI within normal parameters and documented

* **G8421** BMI not calculated

* **G8422** Patient not eligible for BMI calculation

* **G8423** Documented that patient was screened and either influenza vaccination status is current or patient was counseled

* **G8424** Influenza vaccine status was not screened

* **G8425** Influenza vaccine status screened, patient not current and counseling was not provided

* **G8426** Documented that patient was not appropriate for screening and/or counseling about the influenza vaccine (e.g., allergy to eggs)

→ * **G8427** List of current medications with dosages (includes prescription, over-the-counter, herbals, vitamin/mineral/dietary [nutritional] supplements) and verification with the patient or authorized representative documented by the provider

→ * **G8428** Provider documentation of current medications with dosages (includes prescription, over-the-counter, herbals, vitamin/mineral/dietary [nutritional] supplements) without documented patient verification

→ * **G8429** Incomplete or no provider documentation that patient's current medications with dosages (includes prescription, over-the-counter, herbals, vitamin/mineral/dietary [nutritional] supplements) were assessed

→ * **G8430** Provider documentation that patient is not eligible for medication assessment

---

◀▶ **New**   ←→ **Revised**   ✔ **Reinstated**   ✖ **Deleted**

⊗ **Special coverage instructions**   ◆ **Not covered or valid by Medicare**   * **Carrier discretion**   ▶ **ASC payment group**

→ * **G8431** Positive screen for clinical depression using a standardized tool and a follow-up plan documented

* **G8432** No documentation of clinical depression screening using a standardized tool

→ * **G8433** Screening for clinical depression using a standardized tool not documented, patient not eligible/appropriate

* **G8434** Documentation of cognitive impairment screening using a standardized tool

* **G8435** No documentation of cognitive impairment screening using a standardized tool

* **G8436** Patient not eligible/not appropriate for cognitive impairment screening

→ * **G8437** Documentation of clinician and patient involvement with the development of a plan of care including signature by the practitioner/therapist and either a co-signature by the patient or documented verbal agreement obtained from the patient or, when necessary, an authorized representative

→ * **G8438** No documentation of clinician and patient involvement with the development of a plan of care including signature by the practitioner/therapist and either a co-signature by the patient or documented verbal agreement obtained from the patient or, when necessary, an authorized representative

→ * **G8439** Documentation that patient is not eligible for co-developing a plan of care including signature by the practitioner/therapist and either a co-signature by the patient or documented verbal agreement obtained from the patient or, when necessary, an authorized representative

→ * **G8440** Documentation of pain assessment (including location, intensity and description) prior to initiation of treatment or documentation of the absence of pain as a result of assessment through discussion with the patient including the use of a standardized tool and a follow-up plan is documented

* **G8441** No documentation of pain assessment (including location, intensity and description) prior to initiation of treatment

* **G8442** Documentation that patient is not eligible for pain assessment

* **G8443** All prescriptions created during the encounter were generated using a qualified E-prescribing system

* **G8445** No prescriptions were generated during the encounter, provider does have access to a qualified E-prescribing system

→ * **G8446** Provider does have access to a qualified e-prescribing system and some or all of the prescriptions generated during the encounter were printed or phoned in as required by state or federal law or regulations, patient request or pharmacy system being unable to receive electronic transmission; or because they were for narcotics or other controlled substances

→ * **G8447** Patient encounter was documented using a CCHIT certified EHR

→ * **G8448** Patient encounter was documented using a (non-CCHIT certified) EHR

* **G8449** Patient encounter was not documented using an EMR due to system reasons such as, the system being inoperable at the time of the visit; use of this code implies that an EMR is in place and generally available

* **G8450** Beta-blocker therapy prescribed for patients with left ventricular ejection fraction (LVEF) <40% or documentation as moderately or severely depressed left ventricular systolic function

* **G8451** Clinician documented patient with left ventricular ejection fraction (LVEF) <40% or documentation as moderately or severely depressed left ventricular systolic function was not eligible candidate for beta-blocker therapy

* **G8452** Beta-blocker therapy not prescribed for patients with left ventricular ejection fraction (LVEF) <40% or documentation as moderately or severely depressed left ventricular systolic function

* **G8453** Tobacco use cessation intervention, counseling

◄► New   ←→ Revised   ✔ Reinstated   ✖ Deleted

⊘ Special coverage instructions   ◆ Not covered or valid by Medicare   * Carrier discretion   ▶ ASC payment group

* **G8454** Tobacco use cessation intervention not counseled, reason not specified

* **G8455** Current tobacco smoker

* **G8456** Current smokeless tobacco user

→ * **G8457** Current tobacco non-user

* **G8458** Clinician documented that patient is not an eligible candidate for genotype testing; patient not receiving antiviral treatment for hepatitis C

* **G8459** Clinician documented that patient is receiving antiviral treatment for hepatitis C

* **G8460** Clinician documented that patient is not an eligible candidate for quantitative RNA testing at week 12; patient not receiving antiviral treatment for hepatitis C

* **G8461** Patient receiving antiviral treatment for hepatitis C

* **G8462** Clinician documented that patient is not an eligible candidate for counseling regarding contraception prior to antiviral treatment; patient not receiving antiviral treatment for hepatitis C

* **G8463** Patient receiving antiviral treatment for hepatitis C documented

* **G8464** Clinician documented that prostate cancer patient is not an eligible candidate for adjuvant hormonal therapy; low or intermediate risk of recurrence or risk of recurrence not determined

* **G8465** High risk of recurrence of prostate cancer

* **G8466** Clinician documented that patient is not an eligible candidate for suicide risk assessment; major depressive disorder, in remission

* **G8467** Documentation of new diagnosis of initial or recurrent episode of major depressive disorder

* **G8468** Angiotensin converting enzyme (ACE) inhibitor or angiotensin receptor blocker (ARB) therapy prescribed for patients with a left ventricular ejection fraction (LVEF) <40% or documentation of moderately or severely depressed left ventricular systolic function

* **G8469** Clinician documented that patient with a left ventricular ejection fraction (LVEF) <40% or documentation of moderately or severely depressed left ventricular systolic function was not an eligible candidate for angiotensin converting enzyme (ACE) inhibitor or angiotensin receptor blocker (ARB) therapy

* **G8470** Patient with left ventricular ejection fraction (LVEF) > =40% or documentation as normal or mildly depressed left ventricular systolic function

* **G8471** Left ventricular ejection fraction (LVEF) was not performed or documented

* **G8472** Angiotensin converting enzyme (ACE) inhibitor or angiotensin receptor blocker (ARB) therapy not prescribed for patients with a left ventricular ejection fraction (LVEF) <40% or documentation of moderately or severely depressed left ventricular systolic function, reason not specified

* **G8473** Angiotensin converting enzyme (ACE) inhibitor or angiotensin receptor blocker (ARB) therapy prescribed

* **G8474** Angiotensin converting enzyme (ACE) inhibitor or angiotensin receptor blocker (ARB) therapy not prescribed for reasons documented by the clinician

* **G8475** Angiotensin converting enzyme (ACE) inhibitor or angiotensin receptor blocker (ARB) therapy not prescribed, reason not specified

* **G8476** Most recent blood pressure has a systolic measurement of <130 mm/Hg and a diastolic measurement of <80 mm/Hg

* **G8477** Most recent blood pressure has a systolic measurement of > =130 mm/Hg and/or a diastolic measurement of > =80 mm/Hg

* **G8478** Blood pressure measurement not performed or documented, reason not specified

* **G8479** Clinician prescribed angiotensin converting enzyme (ACE) inhibitor or angiotensin receptor blocker (ARB) therapy

---

◄ ► New   ←→ Revised   ✔ Reinstated   ✖ Deleted

⊗ Special coverage instructions   ◆ Not covered or valid by Medicare   * Carrier discretion   ▶ ASC payment group

* **G8480** Clinician documented that patient was not an eligible candidate for angiotensin converting enzyme (ACE) inhibitor or angiotensin receptor blocker (ARB) therapy

* **G8481** Clinician did not prescribe angiotensin converting enzyme (ACE) inhibitor or angiotensin receptor blocker (ARB) therapy, reason not specified

* **G8482** Influenza immunization was ordered or administered

* **G8483** Influenza immunization was not ordered or administered for reasons documented by clinician

* **G8484** Influenza immunization was not ordered or administered, reason not specified

▶ * **G8485** I intend to report the diabetes mellitus measures group

▶ * **G8486** I intend to report the preventive care measures group

▶ * **G8487** I intend to report the chronic kidney disease (CKD) measures group

▶ * **G8488** Clinician intends to report the end stage renal disease (ESRD) measure group

▶ * **G8489** I intend to report the coronary artery disease (CAD) measures group

▶ * **G8490** I intend to report the rheumatoid arthritis measures group

▶ * **G8491** I intend to report the HIV/AIDS measures group

▶ * **G8492** I intend to report the perioperative care measures group

▶ * **G8493** I intend to report the back pain measures group

▶ * **G8494** All quality actions for the applicable measures in the diabetes mellitus measures group have been performed for this patient

▶ * **G8495** All quality actions for the applicable measures in the CKD measures group have been performed for this patient

▶ * **G8496** All quality actions for the applicable measures in the preventive care measures group have been performed for this patient

▶ * **G8497** All quality actions for the applicable measures in the coronary artery bypass graft (CABG) measures group have been performed for this patient

▶ * **G8498** All quality actions for the applicable measures in the coronary artery disease (CAD) measures group have been performed for this patient

▶ * **G8499** All quality actions for the applicable measures in the rheumatoid arthritis measures group have been performed for this patient

▶ * **G8500** All quality actions for the applicable measures in the HIV/AIDS measures group have been performed for this patient

▶ * **G8501** All quality actions for the applicable measures in the perioperative care measures group have been performed for this patient

▶ * **G8502** All quality actions for the applicable measures in the back pain measures group have been performed for this patient

▶ * **G8503** Documentation that prophylactic antibiotic was given within one hour (if fluoroquinolone or vancomycin, two hours) prior to surgical incision (or start of procedure when no incision is required)

▶ * **G8504** Documentation of order for prophylactic antibiotics to be given within one hour (if fluoroquinolone or vancomycin, two hours) prior to surgical incision (or start of procedure when no incision is required)

▶ * **G8505** Documentation that prophylactic antibiotic was not given within one hour (if fluoroquinolone or vancomycin, two hours) prior to surgical incision (or start of procedure when no incision is required), reason not specified

▶ * **G8506** Patient receiving angiotensin converting enzyme (ACE) inhibitor or angiotensin receptor blocker (ARB) therapy

▶ * **G8507** Provider documentation that patient is not eligible for patient verification of current medications

▶ * **G8508** Documentation of pain assessment (including location, intensity and description) prior to initiation of treatment or documentation of the absence of pain as a result of assessment through discussion with the patient including the use of a standardized tool; no documentation of a follow-up plan, patient not eligible

▶ ✳ **G8509** Documentation of pain assessment (including location, intensity and description) prior to initiation of treatment or documentation of the absence of pain as a result of assessment through discussion with the patient including the use of a standardized tool; no documentation of a follow-up plan, reason not specified

▶ ✳ **G8510** Negative screen for clinical depression using a standardized tool, patient not eligible/appropriate for follow-up plan documented

▶ ✳ **G8511** Screen for clinical depression using a standardized tool documented, follow up plan not documented, reason not specified

▶ ✳ **G8512** Pain severity quantified; pain present

▶ ✳ **G8513** ABI measured and documented

▶ ✳ **G8514** Clinician documented that patient was not an eligible candidate for ABI measurement measure

▶ ✳ **G8515** ABI measurement was not obtained

▶ ✳ **G8516** Patient screened for future falls risk; documentation of two or more falls in the past year or any fall with injury in the past year

▶ ✳ **G8517** Patient screened for future fall risk; documentation of no falls in the past year or only one fall without injury in the past year

▶ ✳ **G8518** Clinical stage prior to surgery for lung cancer and esophageal cancer resection was recorded

▶ ✳ **G8519** Clinician documented that patient was not eligible for clinical stage prior to surgery for lung cancer and esophageal cancer resection measure

▶ ✳ **G8520** Clinician stage prior to surgery for lung cancer and esophageal cancer resection was not recorded, reason not specified

▶ ✳ **G8521** Antiplatelet therapy received (ASA [81-325 mg/day] and/or clopidogrel [75 mg/day]) within 48 hours of the initiation of surgery and at discharge

▶ ✳ **G8522** Clinician documented that patient was not an eligible candidate for antiplatelet therapy

▶ ✳ **G8523** Antiplatelet therapy not received 48 hours prior to CEA and at discharge, reason not specified

▶ ✳ **G8524** Patch closure used for patient undergoing conventional CEA

▶ ✳ **G8525** Clinician documented that patient did not receive conventional CEA

▶ ✳ **G8526** Patch closure not used for patient undergoing conventional CEA, reason not specified

▶ ✳ **G8527** Documentation of order for cefazolin or cefuroxime for antimicrobial prophylaxis

▶ ✳ **G8528** Clinician documented that patient was ineligible for prophylactic antibiotic selection measure

▶ ✳ **G8529** Order for cefazolin or cefuroxime for antimicrobial prophylaxis not documented, reason not specified

▶ ✳ **G8530** Autogenous AV fistula received

▶ ✳ **G8531** Clinician documented that patient was not an eligible candidate for autogenous AV fistula

▶ ✳ **G8532** Clinician documented that patient received vascular access other than autogenous AV fistula, reason not specified

▶ ✳ **G8533** Participation by a physician or other clinician in systematic clinical database registry that includes consensus-endorsed quality measures

▶ ✳ **G8534** Documentation of an elder maltreatment screen and follow-up plan

▶ ✳ **G8535** No documentation of an elder maltreatment screen, patient not eligible

▶ ✳ **G8536** No documentation of an elder maltreatment screen, reason not specified

▶ ✳ **G8537** Elder maltreatment screen documented, follow-up plan not documented, patient not eligible

▶ ✳ **G8538** Elder maltreatment screen documented, follow-up plan not documented, reason not specified

▶ ✳ **G8539** Documentation of a current functional outcome assessment using a standardized tool and care plan based on identified deficiencies

▶ ✳ **G8540** Documentation that the patient is not eligible for a functional outcome assessment using a standardized tool

▶ ✳ **G8541** No documentation of a current functional outcome assessment using a standardized tool, reason not specified

▶ ✳ **G8542** Documentation of a current functional outcome assessment using a standardized tool; no documentation of a care plan, patient not eligible

▶ ✳ **G8543** Documentation of a current functional outcome assessment using a standardized tool; no documentation of a care plan, reason not specified

▶ ✳ **G8544** I intend to report the coronary artery bypass graft (CABG) measures group

⊚ **G9001** Coordinated care fee, initial rate

⊚ **G9002** Coordinated care fee, maintenance rate

⊚ **G9003** Coordinated care fee, risk adjusted high, initial

⊚ **G9004** Coordinated care fee, risk adjusted low, initial

⊚ **G9005** Coordinated care fee, risk adjusted maintenance

⊚ **G9006** Coordinated care fee, home monitoring

⊚ **G9007** Coordinated care fee, scheduled team conference

⊚ **G9008** Coordinated care fee, physician coordinated care oversight services

⊚ **G9009** Coordinated care fee, risk adjusted maintenance, level 3

⊚ **G9010** Coordinated care fee, risk adjusted maintenance, level 4

⊚ **G9011** Coordinated care fee, risk adjusted maintenance, level 5

⊚ **G9012** Other specified case management services not elsewhere classified

◆ **G9013** ESRD demo basic bundle Level I

◆ **G9014** ESRD demo expanded bundle, including venous access and related services

◆ **G9016** Smoking cessation counseling, individual, in the absence of or in addition to any other evaluation and management service, per session (6-10 minutes) [demo project code only]

✳ **G9017** Amantadine hydrochloride, oral, per 100 mg (for use in a Medicare-approved demonstration project)

✳ **G9018** Zanamivir, inhalation powder, administered through inhaler, per 10 mg (for use in a Medicare-approved demonstration project)

✳ **G9019** Oseltamivir phosphate, oral, per 75 mg (for use in a Medicare-approved demonstration project)

✳ **G9020** Rimantadine hydrochloride, oral, per 100 mg (for use in a Medicare-approved demonstration project)

✳ **G9033** Amantadine hydrochloride, oral brand, per 100 mg (for use in a Medicare-approved demonstration project)

✳ **G9034** Zanamivir, inhalation powder, administered through inhaler, brand, per 10 mg (for use in a Medicare-approved demonstration project)

✳ **G9035** Oseltamivir phosphate, oral, brand, per 75 mg (for use in a Medicare-approved demonstration project)

Other: Tamiflu

✳ **G9036** Rimantadine hydrochloride, oral, brand, per 100 mg (for use in a Medicare-approved demonstration project)

✳ **G9041** Rehabilitation services for low vision by qualified occupational therapist, direct one-on-one contact, each 15 minutes

✳ **G9042** Rehabilitation services for low vision by certified orientation and mobility specialists, direct one-on-one contact, each 15 minutes

✳ **G9043** Rehabilitation services for low vision by certified low vision rehabilitation therapist, direct one-on-one contact, each 15 minutes

✳ **G9044** Rehabilitation services for low vision by certified low vision rehabilitation teacher, direct one-on-one contact, each 15 minutes

◆ **G9050** Oncology; primary focus of visit; work-up, evaluation, or staging at the time of cancer diagnosis or recurrence (for use in a Medicare-approved demonstration project)

◆ **G9051** Oncology; primary focus of visit; treatment decision-making after disease is staged or restaged, discussion of treatment options, supervising/coordinating active cancer directed therapy or managing consequences of cancer directed therapy (for use in a Medicare-approved demonstration project)

◆ **G9052** Oncology; primary focus of visit; surveillance for disease recurrence for patient who has completed definitive cancer-directed therapy and currently lacks evidence of recurrent disease; cancer directed therapy might be considered in the future (for use in a Medicare-approved demonstration project)

◀▶ New   ←→ Revised   ✔ Reinstated   ✖ Deleted

⊚ Special coverage instructions   ◆ Not covered or valid by Medicare   ✳ Carrier discretion   ▶ ASC payment group

◆ **G9053** Oncology; primary focus of visit; expectant management of patient with evidence of cancer for whom no cancer directed therapy is being administered or arranged at present; cancer directed therapy might be considered in the future (for use in a Medicare-approved demonstration project)

◆ **G9054** Oncology; primary focus of visit; supervising, coordinating or managing care of patient with terminal cancer or for whom other medical illness prevents further cancer treatment; includes symptom management, end-of-life care planning, management of palliative therapies (for use in a Medicare-approved demonstration project)

◆ **G9055** Oncology; primary focus of visit; other, unspecified service not otherwise listed (for use in a Medicare-approved demonstration project)

◆ **G9056** Oncology; practice guidelines; management adheres to guidelines (for use in a Medicare-approved demonstration project)

◆ **G9057** Oncology; practice guidelines; management differs from guidelines as a result of patient enrollment in an institutional review board approved clinical trial (for use in a Medicare-approved demonstration project)

◆ **G9058** Oncology; practice guidelines; management differs from guidelines because the treating physician disagrees with guideline recommendations (for use in a Medicare-approved demonstration project)

◆ **G9059** Oncology; practice guidelines; management differs from guidelines because the patient, after being offered treatment consistent with guidelines, has opted for alternative treatment or management, including no treatment (for use in a Medicare-approved demonstration project)

◆ **G9060** Oncology; practice guidelines; management differs from guidelines for reason(s) associated with patient comorbid illness or performance status not factored into guidelines (for use in a Medicare-approved demonstration project)

◆ **G9061** Oncology; practice guidelines; patient's condition not addressed by available guidelines (for use in a Medicare-approved demonstration project)

◆ **G9062** Oncology; practice guidelines; management differs from guidelines for other reason(s) not listed (for use in a Medicare-approved demonstration project)

* **G9063** Oncology; disease status; limited to non-small cell lung cancer; extent of disease initially established as stage I (prior to neo-adjuvant therapy, if any) with no evidence of disease progression, recurrence, or metastases (for use in a Medicare-approved demonstration project)

* **G9064** Oncology; disease status; limited to non-small cell lung cancer; extent of disease initially established as stage II (prior to neo-adjuvant therapy, if any) with no evidence of disease progression, recurrence, or metastases (for use in a Medicare-approved demonstration project)

* **G9065** Oncology; disease status; limited to non-small cell lung cancer; extent of disease initially established as stage IIIA (prior to neo-adjuvant therapy, if any) with no evidence of disease progression, recurrence, or metastases (for use in a Medicare-approved demonstration project)

* **G9066** Oncology; disease status; limited to non-small cell lung cancer; stage IIIB-IV at diagnosis, metastatic, locally recurrent, or progressive (for use in a Medicare-approved demonstration project)

* **G9067** Oncology; disease status; limited to non-small cell lung cancer; extent of disease unknown, staging in progress, or not listed (for use in a Medicare-approved demonstration project)

* **G9068** Oncology; disease status; limited to small cell and combined small cell/non-small cell; extent of disease initially established as limited with no evidence of disease progression, recurrence, or metastases (for use in a Medicare-approved demonstration project)

* **G9069** Oncology; disease status; small cell lung cancer, limited to small cell and combined small cell/non-small cell; extensive stage at diagnosis, metastatic, locally recurrent, or progressive (for use in a Medicare-approved demonstration project)

◀▶ New   ←→ Revised   ✔ Reinstated   ✖ Deleted

⊘ Special coverage instructions   ◆ Not covered or valid by Medicare   * Carrier discretion   ▶ ASC payment group

TEMPORARY PROCEDURES/PROFESSIONAL SERVICES

* **G9070** Oncology; disease status; small cell lung cancer, limited to small cell and combined small cell/non-small cell; extent of disease unknown, staging in progress, or not listed (for use in a Medicare-approved demonstration project)

* **G9071** Oncology; disease status; invasive female breast cancer (does not include ductal carcinoma in situ); adenocarcinoma as predominant cell type; stage I or stage IIA-IIB; or T3, N1, M0; and ER and/or PR positive; with no evidence of disease progression, recurrence, or metastases (for use in a Medicare-approved demonstration project)

* **G9072** Oncology; disease status; invasive female breast cancer (does not include ductal carcinoma in situ); adenocarcinoma as predominant cell type; stage I, or stage IIA-IIB; or T3, N1, M0; and ER and PR negative; with no evidence of disease progression, recurrence, or metastases (for use in a Medicare-approved demonstration project)

* **G9073** Oncology; disease status; invasive female breast cancer (does not include ductal carcinoma in situ); adenocarcinoma as predominant cell type; stage IIIA-IIIB; and not T3, N1, M0; and ER and/or PR positive; with no evidence of disease progression, recurrence, or metastases (for use in a Medicare-approved demonstration project)

* **G9074** Oncology; disease status; invasive female breast cancer (does not include ductal carcinoma in situ); adenocarcinoma as predominant cell type; stage IIIA-IIIB; and not T3, N1, M0; and ER and PR negative; with no evidence of disease progression, recurrence, or metastases (for use in a Medicare-approved demonstration project)

* **G9075** Oncology; disease status; invasive female breast cancer (does not include ductal carcinoma in situ); adenocarcinoma as predominant cell type; M1 at diagnosis, metastatic, locally recurrent, or progressive (for use in a Medicare-approved demonstration project)

* **G9077** Oncology; disease status; prostate cancer, limited to adenocarcinoma as predominant cell type; T1-T2c and Gleason 2-7 and PSA < or equal to 20 at diagnosis with no evidence of disease progression, recurrence, or metastases (for use in a Medicare-approved demonstration project)

* **G9078** Oncology; disease status; prostate cancer, limited to adenocarcinoma as predominant cell type; T2 or T3a Gleason 8-10 or PSA > 20 at diagnosis with no evidence of disease progression, recurrence, or metastases (for use in a Medicare-approved demonstration project)

* **G9079** Oncology; disease status; prostate cancer, limited to adenocarcinoma as predominant cell type; T3b-T4, any N; any T, N1 at diagnosis with no evidence of disease progression, recurrence, or metastases (for use in a Medicare-approved demonstration project)

* **G9080** Oncology; disease status; prostate cancer, limited to adenocarcinoma; after initial treatment with rising PSA or failure of PSA decline (for use in a Medicare-approved demonstration project)

* **G9083** Oncology; disease status; prostate cancer, limited to adenocarcinoma; extent of disease unknown, staging in progress, or not listed (for use in a Medicare-approved demonstration project)

* **G9084** Oncology; disease status; colon cancer, limited to invasive cancer, adenocarcinoma as predominant cell type; extent of disease initially established as T1-3, N0, M0 with no evidence of disease progression, recurrence, or metastases (for use in a Medicare-approved demonstration project)

* **G9085** Oncology; disease status; colon cancer, limited to invasive cancer, adenocarcinoma as predominant cell type; extent of disease initially established as T4, N0, M0 with no evidence of disease progression, recurrence, or metastases (for use in a Medicare-approved demonstration project)

◀▶ New   ←→ Revised   ✔ Reinstated   ✖ Deleted
○ Special coverage instructions   ◆ Not covered or valid by Medicare   ✱ Carrier discretion   ▶ ASC payment group

170

* **G9086** Oncology; disease status; colon cancer, limited to invasive cancer, adenocarcinoma as predominant cell type; extent of disease initially established as T1-4, N1-2, M0 with no evidence of disease progression, recurrence, or metastases (for use in a Medicare-approved demonstration project)

* **G9087** Oncology; disease status; colon cancer, limited to invasive cancer, adenocarcinoma as predominant cell type; M1 at diagnosis, metastatic, locally recurrent, or progressive with current clinical, radiologic, or biochemical evidence of disease (for use in a Medicare-approved demonstration project)

* **G9088** Oncology; disease status; colon cancer, limited to invasive cancer, adenocarcinoma as predominant cell type; M1 at diagnosis, metastatic, locally recurrent, or progressive without current clinical, radiologic, or biochemical evidence of disease (for use in a Medicare-approved demonstration project)

* **G9089** Oncology; disease status; colon cancer, limited to invasive cancer, adenocarcinoma as predominant cell type; extent of disease unknown, staging in progress, or not listed (for use in a Medicare-approved demonstration project)

* **G9090** Oncology; disease status; rectal cancer, limited to invasive cancer, adenocarcinoma as predominant cell type; extent of disease initially established as T1-2, N0, M0 (prior to neo-adjuvant therapy, if any) with no evidence of disease progression, recurrence, or metastases (for use in a Medicare-approved demonstration project)

* **G9091** Oncology; disease status; rectal cancer, limited to invasive cancer, adenocarcinoma as predominant cell type; extent of disease initially established as T3, N0, M0 (prior to neo-adjuvant therapy, if any) with no evidence of disease progression, recurrence, or metastases (for use in a Medicare-approved demonstration project)

* **G9092** Oncology; disease status; rectal cancer, limited to invasive cancer, adenocarcinoma as predominant cell type; extent of disease initially established as T1-3, N1-2, M0 (prior to neo-adjuvant therapy, if any) with no evidence of disease progression, recurrence or metastases (for use in a Medicare-approved demonstration project)

* **G9093** Oncology; disease status; rectal cancer, limited to invasive cancer, adenocarcinoma as predominant cell type; extent of disease initially established as T4, any N, M0 (prior to neo-adjuvant therapy, if any) with no evidence of disease progression, recurrence, or metastases (for use in a Medicare-approved demonstration project)

* **G9094** Oncology; disease status; rectal cancer, limited to invasive cancer, adenocarcinoma as predominant cell type; M1 at diagnosis, metastatic, locally recurrent, or progressive (for use in a Medicare-approved demonstration project)

* **G9095** Oncology; disease status; rectal cancer, limited to invasive cancer, adenocarcinoma as predominant cell type; extent of disease unknown, staging in progress, or not listed (for use in a Medicare-approved demonstration project)

* **G9096** Oncology; disease status; esophageal cancer, limited to adenocarcinoma or squamous cell carcinoma as predominant cell type; extent of disease initially established as T1-T3, N0-N1 or NX (prior to neo-adjuvant therapy, if any) with no evidence of disease progression, recurrence, or metastases (for use in a Medicare-approved demonstration project)

* **G9097** Oncology; disease status; esophageal cancer, limited to adenocarcinoma or squamous cell carcinoma as predominant cell type; extent of disease initially established as T4, any N, M0 (prior to neo-adjuvant therapy, if any) with no evidence of disease progression, recurrence, or metastases (for use in a Medicare-approved demonstration project)

◄► New   ←→ Revised   ✔ Reinstated   ✖ Deleted

☺ Special coverage instructions   ◆ Not covered or valid by Medicare   * Carrier discretion   ▶ ASC payment group

* **G9098**   Oncology; disease status; esophageal cancer, limited to adenocarcinoma or squamous cell carcinoma as predominant cell type; M1 at diagnosis, meta-static, locally recurrent, or progressive (for use in a Medicare-approved demonstration project)

* **G9099**   Oncology; disease status; esophageal cancer, limited to adenocarcinoma or squamous cell carcinoma as predominant cell type; extent of disease unknown, staging in progress, or not listed (for use in a Medicare-approved demonstration project)

* **G9100**   Oncology; disease status; gastric cancer, limited to adenocarcinoma as predominant cell type; post R0 resection (with or without neoadjuvant therapy) with no evidence of disease recurrence, progression, or metastases (for use in a Medicare-approved demonstration project)

* **G9101**   Oncology; disease status; gastric cancer, limited to adenocarcinoma as predominant cell type; post R1 or R2 resection (with or without neoadjuvant therapy) with no evidence of disease progression, or metastases (for use in a Medicare-approved demonstration project)

* **G9102**   Oncology; disease status; gastric cancer, limited to adenocarcinoma as predominant cell type; clinical or pathologic M0, unresectable with no evidence of disease progression, or metastases (for use in a Medicare-approved demonstration project)

* **G9103**   Oncology; disease status; gastric cancer, limited to adenocarcinoma as predominant cell type; clinical or pathologic M1 at diagnosis, metastatic, locally recurrent, or progressive (for use in a Medicare-approved demonstration project)

* **G9104**   Oncology; disease status; gastric cancer, limited to adenocarcinoma as predominant cell type; extent of disease unknown, staging in progress, or not listed (for use in a Medicare-approved demonstration project)

* **G9105**   Oncology; disease status; pancreatic cancer, limited to adenocarcinoma as predominant cell type; post R0 resection without evidence of disease progression, recurrence, or metastases (for use in a Medicare-approved demonstration project)

* **G9106**   Oncology; disease status; pancreatic cancer, limited to adenocarcinoma; post R1 or R2 resection with no evidence of disease progression or metastases (for use in a Medicare-approved demonstration project)

* **G9107**   Oncology; disease status; pancreatic cancer, limited to adenocarcinoma; unresectable at diagnosis, M1 at diagnosis, metastatic, locally recurrent, or progressive (for use in a Medicare-approved demonstration project)

* **G9108**   Oncology; disease status; pancreatic cancer, limited to adenocarcinoma; extent of disease unknown, staging in progress, or not listed (for use in a Medicare-approved demonstration project)

* **G9109**   Oncology; disease status; head and neck cancer, limited to cancers of oral cavity, pharynx and larynx with squamous cell as predominant cell type; extent of disease initially established as T1-T2 and N0, M0 (prior to neo-adjuvant therapy, if any) with no evidence of disease progression, recurrence, or metastases (for use in a Medicare-approved demonstration project)

* **G9110**   Oncology; disease status; head and neck cancer, limited to cancers of oral cavity, pharynx, and larynx with squamous cell as predominant cell type; extent of disease initially established as T3-4 and/ or N1-3, M0 (prior to neo-adjuvant therapy, if any) with no evidence of disease progression, recurrence, or metastases (for use in a Medicare-approved demonstration project)

* **G9111**   Oncology; disease status; head and neck cancer, limited to cancers of oral cavity, pharynx and larynx with squamous cell as predominant cell type; M1 at diagnosis, metastatic, locally recurrent, or progressive (for use in a Medicare-approved demonstration project)

* **G9112**   Oncology; disease status; head and neck cancer, limited to cancers of oral cavity, pharynx and larynx with squamous cell as predominant cell type; extent of disease unknown, staging in progress, or not listed (for use in a Medicare-approved demonstration project)

◄► New   ←→ Revised   ✔ Reinstated   ✖ Deleted

☺ Special coverage instructions   ◆ Not covered or valid by Medicare   ✳ Carrier discretion   ▶ ASC payment group

* **G9113** Oncology; disease status; ovarian cancer, limited to epithelial cancer; pathologic stage IA-B (grade 1) without evidence of disease progression, recurrence, or metastases (for use in a Medicare-approved demonstration project)

* **G9114** Oncology; disease status; ovarian cancer, limited to epithelial cancer; pathologic stage IA-B (grade 2-3); or stage IC (all grades); or stage II; without evidence of disease progression, recurrence, or metastases (for use in a Medicare-approved demonstration project)

* **G9115** Oncology; disease status; ovarian cancer, limited to epithelial cancer; pathologic stage III-IV; without evidence of progression, recurrence, or metastases (for use in a Medicare-approved demonstration project)

* **G9116** Oncology; disease status; ovarian cancer, limited to epithelial cancer; evidence of disease progression, or recurrence and/or platinum resistance (for use in a Medicare-approved demonstration project)

* **G9117** Oncology; disease status; ovarian cancer, limited to epithelial cancer; extent of disease unknown, staging in progress, or not listed (for use in a Medicare-approved demonstration project)

* **G9123** Oncology; disease status; chronic myelogenous leukemia, limited to Philadelphia chromosome positive and/or BCR-ABL positive; chronic phase not in hematologic, cytogenetic, or molecular remission (for use in a Medicare-approved demonstration project)

* **G9124** Oncology; disease status; chronic myelogenous leukemia, limited to Philadelphia chromosome positive and/or BCR-ABL positive; accelerated phase not in hematologic cytogenetic, or molecular remission (for use in a Medicare-approved demonstration project)

* **G9125** Oncology; disease status; chronic myelogenous leukemia, limited to Philadelphia chromosome positive and/or BCR-ABL positive; blast phase not in hematologic, cytogenetic, or molecular remission (for use in a Medicare-approved demonstration project)

* **G9126** Oncology; disease status; chronic myelogenous leukemia, limited to Philadelphia chromosome positive and/or BCR-ABL positive; in hematologic, cytogenetic, or molecular remission (for use in a Medicare-approved demonstration project)

G9128 Oncology: disease status; limited to multiple myeloma, systemic disease; smouldering, stage I (for use in a Medicare-approved demonstration project)

* **G9129** Oncology; disease status; limited to multiple myeloma, systemic disease; stage II or higher (for use in a Medicare-approved demonstration project)

* **G9130** Oncology; disease status; limited to multiple myeloma, systemic disease; extent of disease unknown, staging in progress, or not listed (for use in a Medicare-approved demonstration project)

* **G9131** Oncology; disease status; invasive female breast cancer (does not include ductal carcinoma in situ); adenocarcinoma as predominant cell type; extent of disease unknown, staging in progress, or not listed (for use in a Medicare-approved demonstration project)

* **G9132** Oncology; disease status; prostate cancer, limited to adenocarcinoma; hormone-refractory/androgen-independent (e.g., rising PSA on anti-androgen therapy or post-orchiectomy); clinical metastases (for use in a Medicare-approved demonstration project)

* **G9133** Oncology; disease status; prostate cancer, limited to adenocarcinoma; hormone-responsive; clinical metastases or M1 at diagnosis (for use in a Medicare-approved demonstration project)

* **G9134** Oncology; disease status; non-Hodgkin's lymphoma, any cellular classification; stage I, II at diagnosis, not relapsed, not refractory (for use in a Medicare-approved demonstration project)

* **G9135** Oncology; disease status; non-Hodgkin's lymphoma, any cellular classification; stage III, IV, not relapsed, not refractory (for use in a Medicare-approved demonstration project)

◄► New ←→ Revised ✔ Reinstated ✖ Deleted
☼ Special coverage instructions ◆ Not covered or valid by Medicare * Carrier discretion ▌ ASC payment group

* **G9136**   Oncology; disease status; non-Hodgkin's lymphoma, transformed from original cellular diagnosis to a second cellular classification (for use in a Medicare-approved demonstration project)

* **G9137**   Oncology; disease status; non-Hodgkin's lymphoma, any cellular classification; relapsed/refractory (for use in a Medicare-approved demonstration project)

* **G9138**   Oncology; disease status; non-Hodgkin's lymphoma, any cellular classification; diagnostic evaluation, stage not determined, evaluation of possible relapse or non-response to therapy, or not listed (for use in a Medicare-approved demonstration project)

* **G9139**   Oncology; disease status; chronic myelogenous leukemia, limited to Philadelphia chromosome positive and/or BCR-ABL positive; extent of disease unknown, staging in progress, not listed (for use in a Medicare-approved demonstration project)

* **G9140**   Frontier extended stay clinic demonstration; for a patient stay in a clinic approved for the CMS demonstration project; the following measures should be present: the stay must be equal to or greater than 4 hours; weather or other conditions must prevent transfer or the case falls into a category of monitoring and observation cases that are permitted by the rules of the demonstration; there is a maximum frontier extended stay clinic (FESC) visit of 48 hours, except in the case when weather or other conditions prevent transfer; payment is made on each period up to 4 hours, after the first 4 hours

◄▶ New   ←→ Revised   ✔ Reinstated   ✖ Deleted

⊘ Special coverage instructions   ◆ Not covered or valid by Medicare   * Carrier discretion   ▶ ASC payment group

BEHAVIORAL HEALTH AND/OR SUBSTANCE ABUSE TREATMENT SERVICES (H0001-H9999)

- ◆ **H0001** Alcohol and/or drug assessment
- ◆ **H0002** Behavioral health screening to determine eligibility for admission to treatment program
- ◆ **H0003** Alcohol and/or drug screening; laboratory analysis of specimens for presence of alcohol and/or drugs
- ◆ **H0004** Behavioral health counseling and therapy, per 15 minutes
- ◆ **H0005** Alcohol and/or drug services; group counseling by a clinician
- ◆ **H0006** Alcohol and/or drug services; case management
- ◆ **H0007** Alcohol and/or drug services; crisis intervention (outpatient)
- ◆ **H0008** Alcohol and/or drug services; sub-acute detoxification (hospital inpatient)
- ◆ **H0009** Alcohol and/or drug services; acute detoxification (hospital inpatient)
- ◆ **H0010** Alcohol and/or drug services; sub-acute detoxification (residential addiction program inpatient)
- ◆ **H0011** Alcohol and/or drug services; acute detoxification (residential addiction program inpatient)
- ◆ **H0012** Alcohol and/or drug services; sub-acute detoxification (residential addiction program outpatient)
- ◆ **H0013** Alcohol and/or drug services; acute detoxification (residential addiction program outpatient)
- ◆ **H0014** Alcohol and/or drug services; ambulatory detoxification
- ◆ **H0015** Alcohol and/or drug services; intensive outpatient (treatment program that operates at least 3 hours/day and at least 3 days/week and is based on an individualized treatment plan), including assessment, counseling; crisis intervention, and activity therapies or education
- ◆ **H0016** Alcohol and/or drug services; medical/somatic (medical intervention in ambulatory setting)
- ◆ **H0017** Behavioral health; residential (hospital residential treatment program), without room and board, per diem
- ◆ **H0018** Behavioral health; short-term residential (non-hospital residential treatment program), without room and board, per diem
- ◆ **H0019** Behavioral health; long-term residential (non-medical, non-acute care in a residential treatment program where stay is typically longer than 30 days), without room and board, per diem
- ◆ **H0020** Alcohol and/or drug services; methadone administration and/or service (provision of the drug by a licensed program)
- ◆ **H0021** Alcohol and/or drug training service (for staff and personnel not employed by providers)
- ◆ **H0022** Alcohol and/or drug intervention service (planned facilitation)
- ◆ **H0023** Behavioral health outreach service (planned approach to reach a targeted population)
- ◆ **H0024** Behavioral health prevention information dissemination service (one-way direct or non-direct contact with service audiences to affect knowledge and attitude)
- ◆ **H0025** Behavioral health prevention education service (delivery of services with target population to affect knowledge, attitude and/or behavior)
- ◆ **H0026** Alcohol and/or drug prevention process service, community-based (delivery of services to develop skills of impactors)
- ◆ **H0027** Alcohol and/or drug prevention environmental service (broad range of external activities geared toward modifying systems in order to mainstream prevention through policy and law)
- ◆ **H0028** Alcohol and/or drug prevention problem identification and referral service (e.g. student assistance and employee assistance programs), does not include assessment
- ◆ **H0029** Alcohol and/or drug prevention alternatives service (services for populations that exclude alcohol and other drug use e.g. alcohol-free social events)
- ◆ **H0030** Behavioral health hotline service
- ◆ **H0031** Mental health assessment, by non-physician
- ◆ **H0032** Mental health service plan development by non-physician
- ◆ **H0033** Oral medication administration, direct observation
- ◆ **H0034** Medication training and support, per 15 minutes
- ◆ **H0035** Mental health partial hospitalization, treatment, less than 24 hours

◀▶ New ←→ Revised ✔ Reinstated ✖ Deleted
⊕ Special coverage instructions ◆ Not covered or valid by Medicare ✳ Carrier discretion ▮ ASC payment group

◆ **H0036** Community psychiatric supportive treatment, face-to-face, per 15 minutes

◆ **H0037** Community psychiatric supportive treatment program, per diem

◆ **H0038** Self-help/peer services, per 15 minutes

◆ **H0039** Assertive community treatment, face-to-face, per 15 minutes

◆ **H0040** Assertive community treatment program, per diem

◆ **H0041** Foster care, child, non-therapeutic, per diem

◆ **H0042** Foster care, child, non-therapeutic, per month

◆ **H0043** Supported housing, per diem

◆ **H0044** Supported housing, per month

◆ **H0045** Respite care services, not in the home, per diem

◆ **H0046** Mental health services, not otherwise specified

◆ **H0047** Alcohol and/or other drug abuse services, not otherwise specified

◆ **H0048** Alcohol and/or other drug testing: collection and handling only, specimens other than blood

◆ **H0049** Alcohol and/or drug screening

◆ **H0050** Alcohol and/or drug services, brief intervention, per 15 minutes

◆ **H1000** Prenatal care, at-risk assessment

◆ **H1001** Prenatal care, at-risk enhanced service; antepartum management

◆ **H1002** Prenatal care, at-risk enhanced service; care coordination

◆ **H1003** Prenatal care, at-risk enhanced service; education

◆ **H1004** Prenatal care, at-risk enhanced service; follow-up home visit

◆ **H1005** Prenatal care, at-risk enhanced service package (includes H1001-H1004)

◆ **H1010** Non-medical family planning education, per session

◆ **H1011** Family assessment by licensed behavioral health professional for state defined purposes

◆ **H2000** Comprehensive multidisciplinary evaluation

◆ **H2001** Rehabilitation program, per 1/2 day

◆ **H2010** Comprehensive medication services, per 15 minutes

◆ **H2011** Crisis intervention service, per 15 minutes

◆ **H2012** Behavioral health day treatment, per hour

◆ **H2013** Psychiatric health facility service, per diem

◆ **H2014** Skills training and development, per 15 minutes

◆ **H2015** Comprehensive community support services, per 15 minutes

◆ **H2016** Comprehensive community support services, per diem

◆ **H2017** Psychosocial rehabilitation services, per 15 minutes

◆ **H2018** Psychosocial rehabilitation services, per diem

◆ **H2019** Therapeutic behavioral services, per 15 minutes

◆ **H2020** Therapeutic behavioral services, per diem

◆ **H2021** Community-based wrap-around services, per 15 minutes

◆ **H2022** Community-based wrap-around services, per diem

◆ **H2023** Supported employment, per 15 minutes

◆ **H2024** Supported employment, per diem

◆ **H2025** Ongoing support to maintain employment, per 15 minutes

◆ **H2026** Ongoing support to maintain employment, per diem

◆ **H2027** Psychoeducational service, per 15 minutes

◆ **H2028** Sexual offender treatment service, per 15 minutes

◆ **H2029** Sexual offender treatment service, per diem

◆ **H2030** Mental health clubhouse services, per 15 minutes

◆ **H2031** Mental health clubhouse services, per diem

◆ **H2032** Activity therapy, per 15 minutes

◆ **H2033** Multisystemic therapy for juveniles, per 15 minutes

◆ **H2034** Alcohol and/or drug abuse halfway house services, per diem

◆ **H2035** Alcohol and/or other drug treatment program, per hour

◆ **H2036** Alcohol and/or other drug treatment program, per diem

◆ **H2037** Developmental delay prevention activities, dependent child of client, per 15 minutes

◀▶ New	←→ Revised	✔ Reinstated	✖ Deleted
⊙ Special coverage instructions	◆ Not covered or valid by Medicare	✳ Carrier discretion	▶ ASC payment group

DRUGS OTHER THAN CHEMOTHERAPY
(J0100-J9999)

⚙ **J0120** Injection, tetracycline, **up to 250 mg**

Other: Achromycin, Ala-Tet, Brodspec, Panmycin, Sumycin, Tetra-Con

IOM: 100-02, 15, 50

✳ **J0128▌** Injection, abarelix, **10 mg**

Other: Plenaxis, Abarelix

✳ **J0129▌** Injection, abatacept, **10 mg**

Other: Orencia

⚙ **J0130▌** Injection, abciximab, **10 mg**

NDC: ReoPro

Other: Abciximab

IOM: 100-02, 15, 50

✳ **J0132▌** Injection, acetylcysteine, **100 mg**

Other: Acetadote, Acetylcysteine, Mucomyst (injection)

✳ **J0133** Injection, acyclovir, **5 mg**

NDC: Acyclovir Sodium

Other: Acyclovir, Zovirax

✳ **J0135▌** Injection, adalimumab, **20 mg**

NDC: Humira

Other: Adalimumab

IOM: 100-02, 15, 50

⚙ **J0150▌** Injection, adenosine, for therapeutic use, **6 mg** (not to be used to report any adenosine phosphate compounds, instead use A9270)

NDC: Adenocard

Other: Adenoscan, Adenosine

IOM: 100-02, 15, 50

✳ **J0152▌** Injection, adenosine, for diagnostic use, **30 mg** (not to be used to report any adenosine phosphate compounds; instead use A9270)

NDC: Adenoscan, Adenosine

⚙ **J0170** Injection, adrenalin, epinephrine, **up to 1 ml ampule**

NDC: Epinephrine HCl

Other: Adrenalin, Adrenalin Chloride, Epinephrine Hydrochloride, Epinephrine adrenalin, EpiPen, SusPhrine, Twinject

IOM: 100-02, 15, 50

✳ **J0180▌** Injection, agalsidase beta, **1 mg**

NDC: Fabrazyme

Other: Agalsidase Beta

IOM: 100-02, 15, 50

⚙ **J0190** Injection, biperiden lactate, **per 5 mg**

Other: Akineton, Biperiden lactate

IOM: 100-02, 15, 50

⚙ **J0200** Injection, alatrofloxacin mesylate, **100 mg**

Other: Alatrofloxacin mesylate, Trovan (Note: No longer available in the U.S.)

IOM: 100-02, 15, 50

⚙ **J0205▌** Injection, alglucerase, **per 10 units**

NDC: Ceredase

Other: Alglucerase

IOM: 100-02, 15, 50

⚙ **J0207▌** Injection, amifostine, **500 mg**

NDC: Ethyol

Other: Amifostine

IOM: 100-02, 15, 50

⚙ **J0210▌** Injection, methyldopate HCL, **up to 250 mg**

Other: Aldomet; Aldomet Ester HCl; Methyldopate HCl

IOM: 100-02, 15, 50

✳ **J0215▌** Injection, alefacept, **0.5 mg**

NDC: Amevive

Other: Alefacept

✳ **J0220▌** Injection, alglucosidase alfa, **10 mg**

Other: Myozyme; Alglucosidase; Alglucosidase alfa

⚙ **J0256▌** Injection, alpha 1 - proteinase inhibitor (human), **10 mg**

NDC: Aralast, Prolastin, Zemaira

Other: Alpha-1-proteinase inhibitor, human

IOM: 100-02, 15, 50

⚙ **J0270** Injection, alprostadil, **per 1.25 mcg** (Code may be used for Medicare when drug administered under the direct supervision of a physician, not for use when drug is self administered)

NDC: Caverject, Caverject Impulse, Edex; Prostin VR

Other: Alprostadil, PGE1, Prostaglandin E1, Prostin VR Pediatric, Prostaglandin, Prostin

IOM: 100-02, 15, 50

◀▶ New   ←→ Revised   ✔ Reinstated   ✖ Deleted

⚙ Special coverage instructions   ◆ Not covered or valid by Medicare   ✳ Carrier discretion   ▌ ASC payment group

177

⊗ **J0275**   Alprostadil urethral suppository (Code may be used for Medicare when drug administered under the direct supervision of a physician, not for use when drug is self administered)

NDC: Muse

Other: Alprostadil

IOM: 100-02, 15, 50

∗ **J0278**   Injection, amikacin sulfate, **100 mg**

Other: Amikin, Amikacin Sulfate, Amikin Pediatric, Amikacin Sulfate Pediatric

⊗ **J0280**   Injection, aminophylline, **up to 250 mg**

Other: Aminophylline, Aminophylline Anhydrous; Aminophylline Dihydrate

IOM: 100-02, 15, 50

⊗ **J0282**   Injection, amiodarone hydrochloride, **30 mg**

NDC: Cordarone IV

Other: Aminodarone HCl

IOM: 100-02, 15, 50

⊗ **J0285**   Injection, amphotericin B, **50 mg**

NDC: Amphocin; Fungizone

Other: Abelcet; ABLC; Amphotericin B; Fungizone for tissue culture

IOM: 100-02, 15, 50

⊗ **J0287▶**   Injection, amphotericin B lipid complex, **10 mg**

NDC: Abelcet

Other: Amphotericin B

IOM: 100-02, 15, 50

⊗ **J0288▶**   Injection, amphotericin B cholesteryl sulfate complex, **10 mg**

NDC: Amphotec

Other: Amphotericin B

IOM: 100-02, 15, 50

⊗ **J0289▶**   Injection, amphotericin B liposome, **10 mg**

NDC: AmBisome

Other: Amphotericin B

IOM: 100-02, 15, 50

⊗ **J0290**   Injection, ampicillin sodium, **500 mg**

Other: Ampicillin sodium, Omnipen-N, Polycillin-N, Totacillin-N, Omnipen-N sodium, Polycillin-N sodium, Totacillin-N sodium

IOM: 100-02, 15, 50

⊗ **J0295**   Injection, ampicillin sodium/sulbactam sodium, **per 1.5 gm**

NDC: Ampicillin-Sulbactam, Unasyn

Other: Omnipen-N sodium/sulbactam sodium; Polycillin-N sodium/sulbactam sodium; Totacillin-N sodium/sulbactam sodium

IOM: 100-02, 15, 50

⊗ **J0300**   Injection, amobarbital, **up to 125 mg**

NDC: Amytal sodium

Other: Amobarbital

IOM: 100-02, 15, 50

⊗ **J0330**   Injection, succinylcholine chloride, **up to 20 mg**

NDC: Anectine; Quelicin

Other: Sucostrin; Quelicin chloride; Succinylcholine

IOM: 100-02, 15, 50

→ ∗ **J0348▶**   Injection, anidulafungin, **1 mg**

Other: Anidulafungin; Eraxis

⊗ **J0350**   Injection, anistreplase, **per 30 units**

Other: Anistreplase, Eminase

IOM: 100-02, 15, 50

⊗ **J0360**   Injection, hydralazine hydrochloride, **up to 20 mg**

Other: Apresoline HCl, Hydralazine HCl

IOM: 100-02, 15, 50

∗ **J0364**   Injection, apomorphine hydrochloride, **1 mg**

NDC: Apokyn

Other: Apomorphine hydrochloride

⊗ **J0365▶**   Injection, aprotinin, **10,000 KIU**

NDC: Trasylol

Other: Aprotonin

IOM: 100-02, 15, 50

⊗ **J0380**   Injection, metaraminol bitartrate, **per 10 mg**

Other: Aramine; Metaraminol bitartrate

IOM: 100-02, 15, 50

⊗ **J0390**   Injection, chloroquine hydrochloride, **up to 250 mg**

Other: Aralen; Chloroquine HCl

(Benefit only for diagnosed malaria or amebiasis)

IOM: 100-02, 15, 50

⊗ **J0395**   Injection, arbutamine HCL, **1 mg**

Other: Arbutamine, GenESA

IOM: 100-02, 15, 50

◀▶ New   ←→ Revised   ✔ Reinstated   ✖ Deleted

⊗ Special coverage instructions   ◆ Not covered or valid by Medicare   ∗ Carrier discretion   ▶ ASC payment group

* **J0400** Injection, aripiprazole, intramuscular, **0.25 mg**

  Other: Abilify, Aripiprazole

☼ **J0456** Injection, azithromycin, **500 mg**

  NDC: Zithromax

  Other: Azithromycin

  IOM: 100-02, 15, 50

☼ **J0460** Injection, atropine sulfate, **up to 0.3 mg**

  Other: AtroPen, Atropine sulfate

  IOM: 100-02, 15, 50

☼ **J0470**▸ Injection, dimercaprol, **per 100 mg**

  NDC: BAL In Oil

  Other: Dimercaprol

  IOM: 100-02, 15, 50

☼ **J0475**▸ Injection, baclofen, **10 mg**

  NDC: Lioresal

  Other: Lioresal Intrathecal refill kit; Baclofen

  IOM: 100-02, 15, 50

☼ **J0476**▸ Injection, baclofen **50 mcg** for intrathecal trial

  NDC: Lioresal

  Other: Lioresal Intrathecal screening kit, Lioresal Intrathecal trial, Baclofen Intrathecal trial

  IOM: 100-02, 15, 50

☼ **J0480**▸ Injection, basiliximab, **20 mg**

  NDC: Simulect

  Other: Basiliximab

  IOM: 100-02, 15, 50

☼ **J0500** Injection, dicyclomine HCL, **up to 20 mg**

  NDC: Bentyl

  Other: Antispas, Dibent, Dicyclocot, Dilomine, Di-Spa; Neoquess; Spasmoject

  IOM: 100-02, 15, 50

☼ **J0515** Injection, benztropine mesylate, **per 1 mg**

  NDC: Cogentin

  Other: Benztropine mesylate

  IOM: 100-02, 15, 50

☼ **J0520** Injection, bethanechol chloride, myotonachol or urecholine, **up to 5 mg**

  Other: Bethanechol chloride; Urecholine

  IOM: 100-02, 15, 50

☼ **J0530** Injection, penicillin G benzathine and penicillin G procaine, **up to 600,000 units**

  NDC: Bicillin C-R (600000)

  Other: Penicillin G benzathine and penicillin G procaine

  IOM: 100-02, 15, 50

☼ **J0540** Injection, penicillin G benzathine and penicillin G procaine, **up to 1,200,000 units**

  NDC: Bicillin C-R, Bicillin C-R (1200000), Bicillin C-R 900/300, Bicillin C-R Pediatric, Bicillin C-R (600000)

  Other: Bicillin C-R 900/300 Pediatric; Penicillin G benzathine and penicillin G procaine

  IOM: 100-02, 15, 50

☼ **J0550**▸ Injection, penicillin G benzathine and penicillin G procaine, **up to 2,400,000 units**

  NDC: Bicillin C-R, Bicillin C-R 900/300, Bicillin C-R (1200000), Bicillin C-R (2400000), Bicillin CR Pediatric

  Other: Penicillin G benzathine and penicillin G procaine

  IOM: 100-02, 15, 50

☼ **J0560** Injection, penicillin G benzathine, **up to 600,000 units**

  NDC: Bicillin L-A

  Other: Permapen Isoject; Penicillin G benzathine; Permapen

  IOM: 100-02, 15, 50

☼ **J0570** Injection, penicillin G benzathine, **up to 1,200,000 units**

  NDC: Bicillin L-A

  Other: Permapen Isoject; Penicillin G benzathine; Permapen

  IOM: 100-02, 15, 50

☼ **J0580** Injection, penicillin G benzathine, **up to 2,400,000 units**

  NDC: Bicillin L-A

  Other: Permapen Isoject; Penicillin G benzathine; Permapen

  IOM: 100-02, 15, 50

* **J0583**▸ Injection, bivalirudin, **1 mg**

  NDC: Angiomax

  Other: Bivalirudin

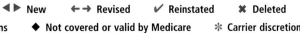

◀▶ New   ←→ Revised   ✔ Reinstated   ✘ Deleted

☼ Special coverage instructions   ◆ Not covered or valid by Medicare   * Carrier discretion   ▸ ASC payment group

DRUGS OTHER THAN CHEMOTHERAPY

☺ **J0585**▸ Botulinum toxin type A, **per unit**

NDC: Botox

Other: Botox Cosmetic, Botulinum toxin type A; Oculinum

(Bill per unit)

IOM: 100-02, 15, 50

☺ **J0587**▸ Botulinum toxin type B, **per 100 units**

NDC: Myobloc

Other: Botulinum toxin type B

IOM: 100-02, 15, 50

☺ **J0592** Injection, buprenorphine hydrochloride, **0.1 mg**

NDC: Buprenex

Other: Buprenorphine hydrochloride

IOM: 100-02, 15, 50

✳ **J0594**▸ Injection, busulfan, **1 mg**

Other: Busulfex, Busulfan

✳ **J0595** Injection, butorphanol tartrate, **1 mg**

NDC: Stadol, Stadol NS

Other: Butorphanol tartrate

☺ **J0600**▸ Injection, edetate calcium disodium, **up to 1000 mg**

NDC: Calcium Disodium Versenate

Other: Calcium EDTA, Edetate calcium disodium

IOM: 100-02, 15, 50

☺ **J0610** Injection, calcium gluconate, **per 10 ml**

Other: Calcium gluconate; Kaleinate

IOM: 100-02, 15, 50

☺ **J0620** Injection, calcium glycerophosphate and calcium lactate, **per 10 ml**

Other: Calcium glycerophosphate & calcium lactate; Calphosan

MCM 2049

IOM: 100-02, 15, 50

☺ **J0630**▸ Injection, calcitonin (salmon), **up to 400 units**

NDC: Miacalcin

Other: Calcitonin-salmon

IOM: 100-02, 15, 50

☺ **J0636** Injection, calcitriol, **0.1 mcg**

NDC: Calcijex

Other: Calcitriol

(non-dialysis use)

IOM: 100-02, 15, 50

✳ **J0637**▸ Injection, caspofungin acetate, **5 mg**

NDC: Cancidas

Other: Caspofungin acetate

☺ **J0640** Injection, leucovorin calcium, **per 50 mg**

Other: Leucovorin calcium; Wellcovorin

IOM: 100-02, 15, 50

▸☺ **J0641**▸ Injection, levoleucovorin calcium, **0.5 mg**

☺ **J0670** Injection, mepivacaine HCL, **per 10 ml**

NDC: Carbocaine, Polocaine; Polocaine-MPF

Other: Carbocaine HCL, Carbocaine with Neo-Cobefrin, Polocaine Dental, Isocaine HCl, Mepivacaine HCl, Scandonest

(Local anesthesia may not be billed with surgical procedure)

IOM: 100-02, 15, 50

☺ **J0690** Injection, cefezolin sodium, **500 mg**

NDC: Ancef; Cefazolin Sodium-Dextrose, Kefzol

IOM: 100-02, 15, 50

✳ **J0692** Injection, cefepime HCL, **500 mg**

NDC: Maxipime

Other: Cefepime hydrochloride

☺ **J0694** Injection, cefoxitin sodium, **1 gm**

NDC: Cefoxitin; Mefoxin In Dextrose

Other: Cefoxitin sodium

IOM: 100-02, 15, 50,

Cross Reference Q0090

☺ **J0696** Injection, ceftriaxone sodium, **per 250 mg**

NDC: Rocephin, Ceftriaxone, Ceftriaxone in D5W

Other: Ceftriaxone sodium

IOM: 100-02, 15, 50

☺ **J0697** Injection, sterile cefuroxime sodium, **per 750 mg**

NDC: Cefuroxime Sodium, Cefuroxime-Dextrose, Zinacef, Zinacef in D5W, Zinacef in Sterile Water

Other: Kefurox

IOM: 100-02, 15, 50

☺ **J0698** Injection, cefotaxime sodium, **per gm**

NDC: Claforan, Claforan in D5W

Other: Cefotaxime sodium

IOM: 100-02, 15, 50

◀▶ New   ←→ Revised   ✔ Reinstated   ✖ Deleted

☺ Special coverage instructions   ◆ Not covered or valid by Medicare   ✳ Carrier discretion   ▸ ASC payment group

⊕ **J0702**   Injection, betamethasone acetate **3 mg** and betamethasone sodium phosphate **3 mg**

NDC: Celestone Soluspan, Celestone Syrup

Other: Betamethasone acetate & betamethasone sodium phosphate

IOM: 100-02, 15, 50

⊕ **J0704**   Injection, betamethasone sodium phosphate, **per 4 mg**

Other: Celestone phosphate, Cel-U-Jec, Betameth, Betamethasone sodium phosphate, Selestoject

MCM 2049

IOM: 100-02, 15, 50

✳ **J0706**   Injection, caffeine citrate, **5 mg**

NDC: Cafcit

Other: Caffeine citrate, Ciprofloxacin

⊕ **J0710**   Injection, cephapirin sodium, **up to 1 gm**

Other: Cefadyl, Cephapirin sodium

IOM: 100-02, 15, 50

⊕ **J0713**   Injection, ceftazidime, **per 500 mg**

NDC: Ceptaz; Fortaz; Fortaz in D5W, Tazicef

Other: Ceftazidime, Tazidime, Tazidime Technetium TC Sestambi

IOM: 100-02, 15, 50

⊕ **J0715**   Injection, ceftizoxime sodium, **per 500 mg**

NDC: Cefizox In D5W

Other: Ceftizoxime sodium

IOM: 100-02, 15, 50

⊕ **J0720**   Injection, chloramphenicol sodium succinate, **up to 1 gm**

Other: Chloramphenicol sodium succinate, Chloromycetin Sodium Succinate

IOM: 100-02, 15, 50

⊕ **J0725**   Injection, chorionic gonadotropin, **per 1,000 USP units**

NDC: Pregnyl; Profasi HP, Profasi, Novarel,

Other: A.P.L., Chorex-5, Chorex-10, Choron-10, Chorignon, Chorionic gonadotropin, Corgonject-5, Gonic, Glukor

IOM: 100-02, 15, 50

⊕ **J0735)**   Injection, clonidine hydrochloride (HCL), **1 mg**

NDC: Duraclon

Other: Catapres, Clorpres, Clonidine HCl

IOM: 100-02, 15, 50

⊕ **J0740)**   Injection, cidofovir, **375 mg**

NDC: Vistide

Other: Cidofovir

IOM: 100-02, 15, 50

⊕ **J0743**   Injection, cilastatin sodium; imipenem, **per 250 mg**

NDC: Primaxin IV

Other: Cilastatin sodium, imipenem; Primaxin IM

IOM: 100-02, 15, 50

✳ **J0744**   Injection, ciprofloxacin for intravenous infusion, **200 mg**

NDC: Cipro, Cipro in D5W

⊕ **J0745**   Injection, codeine phosphate, **per 30 mg**

Other: Codeine phosphate

IOM: 100-02, 15, 50

⊕ **J0760**   Injection, colchicine, **per 1 mg**

Other: Colchicine

IOM: 100-02, 15, 50

⊕ **J0770**   Injection, colistimethate sodium, **up to 150 mg**

NDC: Colistimethate, Coly-Mycin M

IOM: 100-02, 15, 50

⊕ **J0780**   Injection, prochlorperazine, **up to 10 mg**

NDC: Compazine, Prochlorperazine Edisylate

Other: Cotolone, Cotranzine, Compa-Z, Edisylate, Prochlorperazine, Utrazine-10

IOM: 100-02, 15, 50

⊕ **J0795)**   Injection, corticorelin ovine triflutate, **1 microgram**

NDC: Acthrel

Other: Corticorelin ovine triflutate

IOM: 100-02, 15, 50

⊕ **J0800)**   Injection, corticotropin, **up to 40 units**

NDC: H.P Acthar,

Other: H.P. Acthar Gel, ACTH, Corticotropin

IOM: 100-02, 15, 50

◀▶ New   ←→ Revised   ✔ Reinstated   ✖ Deleted

⊕ Special coverage instructions   ◆ Not covered or valid by Medicare   ✳ Carrier discretion   ▶ ASC payment group

◎ **J0835** ▶ Injection, cosyntropin, **per 0.25 mg**

NDC: Cortrosyn

Other: Cosyntropin

IOM: 100-02, 15, 50

◎ **J0850** ▶ Injection, cytomegalovirus immune globulin intravenous (human), **per vial**

NDC: CytoGam

Other: Cytomegalovirum immune globulin IV (human)

IOM: 100-02, 15, 50

✳ **J0878** ▶ Injection, daptomycin, **1 mg**

NDC: Cubicin

Other: Daptomycin

◎ **J0881** ▶ Injection, darbepoetin alfa, **1 microgram** (non-ESRD use)

NDC: Aranesp

Other: Darbepoetin alfa

◎ **J0882** Injection, darbepoetin alfa, **1 microgram** (for ESRD on dialysis)

NDC: Aranesp

Other: Darbepoetin alfa

IOM: 100-02, 6, 10; 100-04, 4, 240

◎ **J0885** ▶ Injection, epoetin alfa, (for non-ESRD use), **1000 units**

NDC: Epogen; Procrit

Other: Aranesp

IOM: 100-02, 15, 50

◎ **J0886** Injection, epoetin alfa, **1000 units** (for ESRD on dialysis)

NDC: Epogen; Procrit

IOM: 100-02, 6, 10; 100-04, 4, 240

✳ **J0894** ▶ Injection, decitabine, **1 mg**

Other: Dacogen, Decitabine

◎ **J0895** Injection, deferoxamine mesylate, **500 mg**

NDC: Desferal

Other: Deferoxamine mesylate, Desferal mesylate

IOM: 100-02, 15, 50,

Cross Reference Q0087

◎ **J0900** Injection, testosterone enanthate and estradiol valerate, **up to 1 cc**

Other: Andrest 90-4, Andro-Estro 90-4, Androgyn L.A., Deladumone, Deladumone OB, Delatestadiol, Ditate-DS, Dua-Gen, L.A., Duoval PA, Estra-Testrin, TEEV, Testadiate, Valertest No. 1, Valertest No. 2, Testosterone enanthate and estradiol valerate, Testradiol 90/4

IOM: 100-02, 15, 50

◎ **J0945** Injection, brompheniramine maleate, **per 10 mg**

Other: B Lodrane, Brom-a-cot, Brompheniramine maleate, BroveX; BroveX CT; Codimal-A; Colhist, Cophene-B, Decongest, Dehist, B Lodrane 12 hour; Histaject; Histine B, Nasahist B, ND Stat, Oraminic II; Vazol; Sinusol-B

IOM: 100-02, 15, 50

◎ **J0970** Injection, estradiol valerate, **up to 40 mg**

NDC: Delestrogen

Other: Clinagen LA, Clinagen LA-10, Clinagen LA 20,Clinagen LA-40, Estradiol valerate, Gynogen LA-A40, Valergen 40

IOM: 100-02, 15, 50

◎ **J1000** Injection, depo-estradiol cypionate, **up to 5 mg**

NDC: Depo-Estradiol

Other:, Depogen, DepGynogen, Depo-Estradiol cypionate, Dura-Estrin, Estradiol Cypionate, Estra-D, Estrin, Estro-Cyp, Estro-LA, Estroject LA, Estronol-LA

IOM: 100-02, 15, 50

◎ **J1020** Injection, methylprednisolone acetate, **20 mg**

NDC: Depo-Medrol

Other: Depopred-40, Depopred-80, D-Med 80, Duralone-40, Duralone-80, Medralone-40, Medralone-80; Methylprednisolone acetate, M-Prednisol 40, M-Prednisol 80, Rep-Pred 40, Rep-Pred 80

IOM: 100-02, 15, 50

◎ **J1030** Injection, methylprednisolone acetate, **40 mg**

NDC: Depo-Medrol, Methylpred 40

Other: Dep-Medalone 40; Depoject, Methylprednisolone Acetate Micronized, M-Prednisol-40, Rep-Pred 40, Sano-Drol; Methylprenisolone acetate

IOM: 100-02, 15, 50

◎ **J1040** Injection, methylprednisolone acetate, **80 mg**

NDC: Depo-Medrol;

Other: Cortimed, Dep Medalone 80; Depoject 80; Depoject, Duro Cort, Medracone, Methylcotolone, M-Prednisol, Pri-Methylate, Rep-Pred 40, Sano-Drol; Methyprenisolone acetate; M-Prednisol 80, Rep-Pred 40

IOM: 100-02, 15, 50

◀ ▶ New ← → Revised ✔ Reinstated ✖ Deleted

◎ Special coverage instructions ◆ Not covered or valid by Medicare ✳ Carrier discretion ▶ ASC payment group

182

⊕ **J1051** Injection, medroxyprogesterone acetate, **50 mg**

NDC: Depo-Provera

Other: Depo-Subq Provera 104; Medroxyprogesterone acetate

IOM: 100-02, 15, 50

◆ **J1055** Injection, medroxyprogesterone acetate for contraceptive use, **150 mg**

Other: Depo-Provera Contraceptive; Medroxyprogesterone acetate

Medicare Statute 1862a1

✳ **J1056** Injection, medroxyprogesterone acetate/ estradiol cypionate, **5 mg/25 mg**

Other: Estradiol cypionate; Lunelle; Medroxyprogesterone acetate/estradiol cypionate

⊕ **J1060** Injection, testosterone cypionate and estradiol cypionate, **up to 1 ml**

NDC: Depo-Testadiol

Other: Andro/Fem, Duospan, Duospan II, De-Comberol, Depotestogen, Duratestin, Duratestrin, DepAndrogyn; Estradiol cypionate; Menoject LA; Monoject LA, Test-Estro Cypionates, Test-Estro-C, Valertest No. 1; Testosterone cypionate and estradiol cypionate

IOM: 100-02, 15, 50

⊕ **J1070** Injection, testosterone cypionate, **up to 100 mg**

NDC: Depo-Testosterone

Other: Andro-Cyp, Andro-Cyp 200, Andronaq-LA, Andronate-200, Andronate-100, DepoAndro, DepAndro 100, DepAndro 200, Depotest, Duratest-100, Duratest-200, Testa-C, Testadiate-Depo, Testoject-LA, Testaject-LA, Testosterone cypionate

IOM: 100-02, 15, 50

⊕ **J1080** Injection, testosterone cypionate, **1 cc, 200 mg**

NDC: Depo-Testosterone

Other: Andro-Cyp, Andro-Cyp 200, Andronate 200, Andronaq-LA, Andronate-100, DepAndro 100, DepAndro 200, Depotest, Depotestadiol, Duratest-100, Duratest-200, Testaject-LA, Virilon, Testa-C, Testadiate-Depo, Testoject-LA, Testosterone cypionate

IOM: 100-02, 15, 50

⊕ **J1094** Injection, dexamethasone acetate, **1 mg**

NDC: Dexasone L.A.; Dekasol LA

Other: Dexamethasone Acetat Micronized; Dexamethasone Acetate Anhydrous; Dexamethasone Micronized; Dexamethasone, Dexacen-LA-8, Delacone D.P., Cortastat LA; Cortastat; Dalalone; Dalalone LA; Decadron Phosphate, Decadrone LA, Decaject LA, Dexasone LA, Dexone-LA, Solurex LA, Hexadrol Phosphate

IOM: 100-02, 15, 50

⊕ **J1100** Injection, dexamethasone sodium phosphate, **1 mg**

DC: Dekasol, Dekasol-10

Other: Adrenocort, Cortastat, Dalalone, Decadron, Decadron Phosphate, Dalalone, Decaject, Dexasone, Dexamethasone, Dexamethasone sodium phosphate, Dexim, Dexone, Dexacen-4, Hexadrol Phosphate, Dekasol-10, Medidex, Primethasone, Solurex, Spectro-Dex

IOM: 100-02, 15, 50

⊕ **J1110** Injection, dihydroergotamine mesylate, **per 1 mg**

NNDC: D.H.E. 45

Other: Dihydroergotamine mesylate

IOM: 100-02, 15, 50

⊕ **J1120** Injection, acetazolamide sodium, **up to 500 mg**

Other: Diamox, Acetazolamid Sodium

IOM: 100-02, 15, 50

⊕ **J1160** Injection, digoxin, **up to 0.5 mg**

NDC: Digoxin, Lanoxin

IOM: 100-02, 15, 50

⊕ **J1162▶** Injection, digoxin immune Fab (ovine), **per vial**

NDC: Digibind; DigiFab

Other: Digoxin immune Fab (ovine)

IOM: 100-02, 15, 50

⊕ **J1165** Injection, phenytoin sodium, **per 50 mg**

Other: Dilantin; Phenytoin sodium

IOM: 100-02, 15, 50

⊕ **J1170** Injection, hydromorphone, **up to 4 mg**

NDC: Dilaudid, Hydromorphone HCl

Other: Dilaudid-5; Dilaudid-HP, Hydromorphone Hcl/Sodium Chloride

IOM: 100-02, 15, 50

◀ ▶ New	← → Revised	✔ Reinstated	✖ Deleted
⊕ Special coverage instructions	◆ Not covered or valid by Medicare	✳ Carrier discretion	▶ ASC payment group

⊗ **J1180**   Injection, dyphylline, **up to 500 mg**

Other: Dilor, Dyphylline, Lufyllin, Zinecard

IOM: 100-02, 15, 50

⊗ **J1190▸** Injection, dexrazoxane hydrochloride, **per 250 mg**

NDC: Zinecard, Dexrazoxane

Other: Dexrazoxane HCl

IOM: 100-02, 15, 50

⊗ **J1200**   Injection, diphenhydramine HCL, **up to 50 mg**

IOM: 100-02, 15, 50

⊗ **J1205▸** Injection, chlorothiazide sodium, **per 500 mg**

NDC: Diuril IV

Other: Chlorothiazide sodium; Diuril Sodium

IOM: 100-02, 15, 50

⊗ **J1212▸** Injection, DMSO, dimethyl sulfoxide, 50%, **50 ml**

NDC: Rimso-50

Other: DMSO dimethyl sulfoxide 50%

IOM: 100-02, 15, 50; 100-03, 4, 230.12

⊗ **J1230**   Injection, methadone HCL, **up to 10 mg**

Other: Dolophine HCl; Methadone HCl

MCM 2049

IOM: 100-02, 15, 50

⊗ **J1240**   Injection, dimenhydrinate, **up to 50 mg**

Other: Dimenhydrinate, Dinate, Dommanate, Dramanate, Dymenate, Hydrate, Dramamine, Dramoject, Dramilin, Dramocen, Dymenate, Marmine, Wehamine

IOM: 100-02, 15, 50

⊗ **J1245**   Injection, dipyridamole, **per 10 mg**

Other: Dipyridamole, Persantine IV

IOM: 100-04, 15, 50; 100-04, 12, 30.6

⊗ **J1250**   Injection, dobutamine HCL, **per 250 mg**

Other: Dextrose/Dobutamine, Dobutamine HCl, Dobutrex

IOM: 100-02, 15, 50

⊗ **J1260▸** Injection, dolasetron mesylate, **10 mg**

NDC: Anzemet

Other: Dolasetron mesylate (injection)

IOM: 100-02, 15, 50

✳ **J1265**   Injection, dopamine HCL, **40 mg**

Other: Dopamine, Dopamine in D5W, Dopamine HCl

▶ ✳ **J1267▸** Injection, doripenem, **10 mg**

✳ **J1270**   Injection, doxercalciferol, **1 mcg**

NDC: Hectorol

Other: Doxercalciferol

✳ **J1300▸** Injection, eculizumab, **10 mg**

Other: Eculizumab, Soliris

⊗ **J1320**   Injection, amitriptyline HCL, **up to 20 mg**

Other: Amitriptyline HCl; Elavil; Enovil; Vanatrip

IOM: 100-02, 15, 50

✳ **J1324**   Injection, enfuvirtide, **1 mg**

Other: Enfuvirtide, Fuzeon

⊗ **J1325**   Injection, epoprostenol, **0.5 mg**

NDC: Flolan

Other: Epoprostenol

IOM: 100-02, 15, 50

⊗ **J1327▸** Injection, eptifibatide, **5 mg**

NDC: Integrilin

Other: Eptifibatide (injection)

IOM: 100-02, 15, 50

⊗ **J1330**   Injection, ergonovine maleate, **up to 0.2 mg**

Other: Ergotrate, Ergonovine maleate (Benefit limited to obstetrical diagnosis)

IOM: 100-02, 15, 50

✳ **J1335**   Injection, ertapenem sodium, **500 mg**

NDC: Invanz

Other: Ertapenem sodium

⊗ **J1364**   Injection, erythromycin lactobionate, **per 500 mg**

NDC: Erythrocin

Other: Erthrocin, Erythromycin lactobionate

IOM: 100-02, 15, 50

◂ ▶ New   ←→ Revised   ✔ Reinstated   ✖ Deleted

⊗ Special coverage instructions   ◆ Not covered or valid by Medicare   ✳ Carrier discretion   ▸ ASC payment group

⊗ **J1380** Injection, estradiol valerate, **up to 10 mg**

NDC: Delestrogen,
Other: Dioval, Dioval XX, Dioval 40, Duragen-10, Duragen-20, Duragen-40, Estradiol L.A., Estradiol L.A. 20, Estradiol L.A. 40, Gynogen L.A. A10, Gynogen L.A. A20, Gynogen L.A. A40, Valergen, Valergen 10, Valergen 20, Valergen 40, Estra-L 20, Estra-L 40, L. A.E. 20, Estradiol valerate, Gynogen L.A.

IOM: 100-02, 15, 50

⊗ **J1390** Injection, estradiol valerate, **up to 20 mg**

NDC: Delestrogen
Other: Dioval, Dioval XX, Dioval 40, Duragen-10, Duragen-20, Duragen-40, Estradiol L.A., Estradiol L.A. 20, Estradiol L.A. 40, Estradiol valerate, Gynogen L.A. A10, Gynogen L.A. A20, Gynogen L.A. A40, Valergen, Valergen 10, Valergen 20, Valergen 40, Estra-L 20, Estra-L 40, L.A.E. 20

IOM: 100-02, 15, 50

⊗ **J1410▶** Injection, estrogen conjugated, **per 25 mg**

NDC: Premarin
Other: Estrogen conjugated, Premarin Intravenous, Primestrin Aqueous, Natural Estrogenic Substance, Premarin Aqueous

IOM: 100-02, 15, 50

⊗ **J1430▶** Injection, ethanolamine oleate, **100 mg**

NDC: Ethamolin
Other: Ethanolamine

IOM: 100-02, 15, 50

⊗ **J1435** Injection, estrone, **per 1 mg**

Other: Estrone Aqueous, Estragyn 5; Estro-A; Estronol, Estrone, Esrtone 5, Kestrone 5, Theelin, Theelin Aqueous

IOM: 100-02, 15, 50

⊗ **J1436▶** Injection, etidronate disodium, **per 300 mg**

Other: Didronel I.V., Etidronate disodium

IOM: 100-02, 15, 50

⊗ **J1438▶** Injection, etanercept, **25 mg** (Code may be used for Medicare when drug administered under the direct supervision of a physician, not for use when drug is self-administered.)

NDC: Enbrel
Other: Etanercept (injection)

IOM: 100-02, 15, 50

⊗ **J1440▶** Injection, filgrastim (G-CSF), **300 mcg**

NDC: Neupogen
Other: Filgrastim (G-CSF)

IOM: 100-02, 15, 50

⊗ **J1441▶** Injection, filgrastim (G-CSF), **480 mcg**

NDC: Neupogen
Other: Filgrastim (G-CSF)

IOM: 100-02, 15, 50

⊗ **J1450** Injection, fluconazole, **200 mg**

NDC: Diflucan IV, Diflucan In Sodium Choloride, Fluconazole In Sodium Chloride, Fluconazole In Dextrose
Other: Fluconazole

IOM: 100-02, 15, 50

⊗ **J1451▶** Injection, fomepizole, **15 mg**

NDC: Antizol
Other: Fomepizole

IOM: 100-02, 15, 50

⊗ **J1452** Injection, fomivirsen sodium, intraocular, **1.65 mg**

Other: Vitravene; Fomivirsen sodium

IOM: 100-02, 15, 50

▶ ✳ **J1453▶** Injection, fosaprepitant, **1 mg**

⊗ **J1455▶** Injection, foscarnet sodium, **per 1000 mg**

NDC: Foscavir
Other: Foscarnet sodium

IOM: 100-02, 15, 50

✳ **J1457▶** Injection, gallium nitrate, **1 mg**

NDC: Ganite
Other: Gallium nitrate

✳ **J1458▶** Injection, galsulfase, **1 mg**

NDC: Naglazyme
Other: Galsulfase

▶ ✳ **J1459▶** Injection, immune globulin (Privigen), intravenous, non-lyophilized (e.g., liquid), **500 mg**

⊗ **J1460▶** Injection, gamma globulin, intramuscular, **1 cc**

NDC: Baygam, Immune Globulin (Human), GamaSTAN S/D
Other: Gammar, Flebogamma, Gamastan, Gamma globulin

IOM: 100-02, 15, 50

◀ ▶ **New**   ←→ **Revised**   ✔ **Reinstated**   ✖ **Deleted**

⊗ **Special coverage instructions**   ◆ **Not covered or valid by Medicare**   ✳ **Carrier discretion**   ▶ **ASC payment group**

⊛ **J1470** Injection, gamma globulin, intramuscular, **2 cc**

NDC: Baygam, GamaSTAN S/D, Immune Globin (Human)

Other: Gammar, Gamastan, Gamma globulin

IOM: 100-02, 15, 50

⊛ **J1480** Injection, gamma globulin, intramuscular, **3 cc**

NDC: Baygam, Immune Globin (Human), GamaSTAN S/D

Other: Gammar, Gamastan, Gamma globulin

IOM: 100-02, 15, 50

⊛ **J1490** Injection, gamma globulin, intramuscular, **4 cc**

NDC: Baygam, Immune Globin (Human), GamaSTAN S/D

Other: Gammar, Gamastan, Gamma globulin

IOM: 100-02, 15, 50

⊛ **J1500** Injection, gamma globulin, intramuscular, **5 cc**

NDC: Baygam, Immune Globin (Human), GamaSTAN S/D

Other: Gammar, Gamastan, Gamma globulin

IOM: 100-02, 15, 50

⊛ **J1510** Injection, gamma globulin, intramuscular, **6 cc**

NDC: Baygam, Immune Globin (Human), GamaSTAN S/D

Other: Gammar, Gamastan, Gamma globulin

IOM: 100-02, 15, 50

⊛ **J1520** Injection, gamma globulin, intramuscular, **7 cc**

NDC: Baygam, Immune Globin (Human), GamaSTAN S/D

Other: Gamma, Gamastan, Gamma globulin

IOM: 100-02, 15, 50

⊛ **J1530** Injection, gamma globulin, intramuscular, **8 cc**

NDC: Baygam, Immune Globin (Human), GamaSTAN S/D

Other: Gammar, Gamastan, Gamma globulin

IOM: 100-02, 15, 50

⊛ **J1540** Injection, gamma globulin, intramuscular, **9 cc**

NDC: Baygam, Immune Globin (Human), GamaSTAN S/D

Other: Gammar, Gamastan, Gamma globulin

IOM: 100-02, 15, 50

⊛ **J1550** Injection, gamma globulin, intramuscular, **10 cc**

NDC: Baygam, Immune Globin (Humna), GamaSTAN S/D

Other: Gammar, Gamastan, Gamma globulin

IOM: 100-02, 15, 50

⊛ **J1560** Injection, gamma globulin, intramuscular, **over 10 cc**

NDC: Baygam, Immune Globin (Human), GamaSTAN S/D

Other: Gammar, Gamastan, Gamma globulin

IOM: 100-02, 15, 50

⊛ **J1561** Injection, immune globulin, (Gamunex), intravenous, non-lyophilized (e.g. liquid), **500 mg**

Other: Gamunex; Immune globulin (Gamunex)

IOM: 100-02, 15, 50

✳ **J1562** Injection, immune globulin (Vivaglobin), **100 mg**

Other: Immune globulin (Subcutaneous)

⊛ **J1565** Injection, respiratory syncytial virus immune globulin, intravenous, **50 mg**

Other: RespiGam; Respiratory syncytial virus immune globulin

IOM: 100-02, 15, 50

⊛ **J1566** Injection, immune globulin, intravenous, lyophilized (e.g., powder), not otherwise specified, **500 mg**

NDC: Carimune, Carimune Classic, Carimune NF, Gammagard S/D, Gammar-P IV, Iveegam EN, Panglobulin NF, Polygam S/D,

Other: Immune globulin (NOS)

IOM: 100-02, 15, 50

✳ **J1568** Injection, immune globulin, (Octagam), intravenous, non-lyophilized (e.g., liquid), **500 mg**

Other: Immune globulin (Octagam); Octagam

◀▶ New   ←→ Revised   ✔ Reinstated   ✖ Deleted

⊛ Special coverage instructions   ◆ Not covered or valid by Medicare   ✳ Carrier discretion   ▶ ASC payment group

186

✿ **J1569**▶ Injection, immune globulin, (Gammagard Liquid), intravenous, non-lyophilized, (e.g. liquid), **500 mg**

Other: Gammagard Liquid; Immune globulin (Gammagard Liquid)

IOM: 100-02, 15, 50

✿ **J1570** Injection, ganciclovir sodium, **500 mg**

NDC: Cytovene

Other: Ganciclovir sodium

IOM: 100-02, 15, 50

✿ **J1571**▶ Injection, hepatitis B immune globulin (HepaGam B), intramuscular, **0.5 ml**

Other: HepGam B; Immune globulin (HepaGam B)

IOM: 100-02, 15, 50

➙ ✿ **J1572**▶ Injection, immune globulin, (flebogamma/flebogamma DIF) intravenous, non-lyophilized (e.g. liquid), **500 mg**

Other: Flebogamma; Immune globulin (Flebogamma)

IOM: 100-02, 15, 50

✳ **J1573**▶ Injection, hepatitis B immune globulin (HepaGam B), intravenous, **0.5 ml**

Other: HepaGam B

✿ **J1580** Injection, Garamycin, gentamicin, **up to 80 mg**

NDC: Gentamicin Sulfate

Other: Jenamicin; Garamycin gentamicin

IOM: 100-02, 15, 50

✳ **J1590** Injection, gatifloxacin, **10 mg**

NDC: Tequin

Other: Gatifloxacin

✿ **J1595**▶ Injection, glatiramer acetate, **20 mg**

NDC: Copaxone

Other: Glatiramer acetate

IOM: 100-02, 15, 50

✿ **J1600** Injection, gold sodium thiomalate, **up to 50 mg**

NDC: Myochrysine

Other: Gold sodium thiomalate

IOM: 100-02, 15, 50

✿ **J1610**▶ Injection, glucagon hydrochloride, **per 1 mg**

NDC: GlucaGen, Glucagon Emergency, Glucagon Diagnostic

Other: GlucaGen Hypokit, Glucagon HCl

IOM: 100-02, 15, 50

✿ **J1620**▶ Injection, gonadorelin hydrochloride, **per 100 mcg**

Other: Factrel, Lutrepulse, Gonadorelin HCl

IOM: 100-02, 15, 50

✿ **J1626**▶ Injection, granisetron hydrochloride, **100 mcg**

NDC: Kytril

Other: Granisetron HCl (injection)

IOM: 100-02, 15, 50

✿ **J1630** Injection, haloperidol, **up to 5 mg**

NDC: Haldol, Haloperidol Lactate, Haloperidol

IOM: 100-02, 15, 50

✿ **J1631** Injection, haloperidol decanoate, **per 50 mg**

NDC: Haldol Decanoate

IOM: 100-02, 15, 50

✿ **J1640**▶ Injection, hemin, **1 mg**

NDC: Panhematin

Other: Hemin

IOM: 100-02, 15, 50

✿ **J1642** Injection, heparin sodium, (heparin lock flush), **per 10 units**

NDC: Hep-Lock; Hep-Lock Flush, Hep Flush-10; Heparin Sodium Lock Flush; Heparin (Porcine) Lock Flush; Hep-Lock PF; Heparin Sodium Flush; Heparine (Porcine) In Nacl; Heparine Combination; Vasceze

Other: Hep-Lock U/P; Hep-Lock 100; Hep-Pak; Heparin Lock Flush/Saline Flush; Monoject Prefill Heparin Lock Flush, Lok-Pak, Heparin Sodium (heparin lock flush)

IOM: 100-02, 15, 50

✿ **J1644** Injection, heparin sodium, **per 1000 units**

NDC: Heparin (Porcine) In Nacl; Heparin (Porcine) In D5W, Heparin Sodium (Bovine), Heparin Sodium (Procine)

Other: Heparin Sodium/Sodium Chloride; Dextrose/Heparin Sodium; Hep-Pak; Liqaumein Sodium; Heparin Sodium

IOM: 100-02, 15, 50

◀ ▶ New   ←→ Revised   ✔ Reinstated   ✖ Deleted

✿ **Special coverage instructions**   ◆ **Not covered or valid by Medicare**   ✳ **Carrier discretion**   ▶ **ASC payment group**

⊛ **J1645** Injection, dalteparin sodium, **per 2500 IU**

NDC: Fragmin

Other: Dalteparin sodium

IOM: 100-02, 15, 50

✳ **J1650** Injection, enoxaparin sodium, **10 mg**

NDC: Lovenox

Other: Enoxaparin sodium

⊛ **J1652▸** Injection, fondaparinux sodium, **0.5 mg**

NDC: Arixtra

Other: Fondaparinux sodium

IOM: 100-02, 15, 50

✳ **J1655** Injection, tinzaparin sodium, **1000 IU**

NDC: Innohep

Other: Tinzaparin

⊛ **J1670▸** Injection, tetanus immune globulin, human, **up to 250 units**

NDC: BayTet, Hypertet S/D

Other: Hyper-tet; Tetanus immune globulin (human)

IOM: 100-02, 15, 50

⊛ **J1675** Injection, histrelin acetate, **10 micrograms**

Other: Histrelin acetate

IOM: 100-02, 15, 50

⊛ **J1700** Injection, hydrocortisone acetate, **up to 25 mg**

Other: Cortef Acetate, Hydrocortone Acetate, Hydrocortisone acetate

IOM: 100-02, 15, 50

⊛ **J1710** Injection, hydrocortisone sodium phosphate, **up to 50 mg**

Other: A-hydroCort, Hydrocortone phosphate, Solu-Cortef, Hydrocortisone sodium phosphate

IOM: 100-02, 15, 50

⊛ **J1720** Injection, hydrocortisone sodium succinate, **up to 100 mg**

NDC: A-Hydrocort, Solu-Cortef, Hydrocortisone succinate sodium

IOM: 100-02, 15, 50

⊛ **J1730▸** Injection, diazoxide, **up to 300 mg**

Other: Diazoxide, Hyperstat IV

IOM: 100-02, 15, 50

✳ **J1740▸** Injection, ibandronate sodium, **1 mg**

Other: Boniva, Ibandronate sodium

⊛ **J1742▸** Injection, ibutilide fumarate, **1 mg**

NDC: Corvert

Other: Ibutilide fumarate

IOM: 100-02, 15, 50

✳ **J1743▸** Injection, idursulfase, **1 mg**

Other: Idursulfase

⊛ **J1745▸** Injection, infliximab, **10 mg**

NDC: Remicade

Other: Infliximab (injection)

IOM: 100-02, 15, 50

✔ ⊛ **J1750▸** Injection, iron dextran, **50 mg**

IOM: 100-02, 15, 50

~~J1751~~ ~~Injection, iron dextran 165, **50 mg**~~ ✖

~~J1752~~ ~~Injection, iron dextran 267, **50 mg**~~ ✖

✳ **J1756▸** Injection, iron sucrose, **1 mg**

NDC: Venofer

Other: Iron sucrose

⊛ **J1785▸** Injection, imiglucerase, **per unit**

NDC: Cerezyme

Other: Imiglucerase

IOM: 100-02, 15, 50

⊛ **J1790** Injection, droperidol, **up to 5 mg**

NDC: Inapsine

Other: Droperidol

IOM: 100-02, 15, 50

⊛ **J1800** Injection, propranolol HCL, **up to 1 mg**

NDC: Inderal

Other: Propranolol HCl

IOM: 100-02, 15, 50

⊛ **J1810** Injection, droperidol and fentanyl citrate, **up to 2 ml ampule**

Other: Droperidol and fentanyl citrate, Innovar

IOM: 100-02, 15, 50

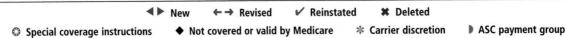

◀ ▶ New   ← → Revised   ✔ Reinstated   ✖ Deleted

⊛ Special coverage instructions   ◆ Not covered or valid by Medicare   ✳ Carrier discretion   ▸ ASC payment group

188

⊕ **J1815** Injection, insulin, **per 5 units**

NDC: Humalog, Humalog Mix 75/25, Humalog Mix 75/25 Pen, Humalog Pen, Humulin 50/50, Humulin 70/30, Humulin 70/30 Pen, Humulin L, Humulin N, Humulin N Pen, Humulin R, Humulin U, Iletin I NPH, Iletin I Regular, Lantus, Novolin 70/30, Novolin 70/30 Innolet, Novolin 70/30 Penfill, Novolin L, Novolin N, Novolin N Innolet, Novolin N Penfill, Novolin R, Novolin R Innolet, Novolin R Penfill, Novolog, Novolog Flexpen, Novolog Penfill, Novolog Mix 70/30, Novolog Mix 70/30 Flexpen, Novolog Mix 70/30 Penfill, Relion 70/30, Relion 70/30 Innolet, Relion N, Relion N Innolet, Relion R, Velosulin Br (RDNA)

Other: Relion/Novolin R; Insulin Human Regular; Insulin Lispo; Novo Nordsik; NPH; Insulin; Regular Insulin; Iletin; Iletin II Regular Port; Innolet, Novolin; Novo Nordsik; NPH; Humulin R U-500; Humulin; Relion; Apidra; Levemir

IOM: 100-02, 15, 50; 100-03, 4, 280.14

✳ **J1817** Insulin for administration through DME (i.e., insulin pump) **per 50 units**

NDC: Humalog, Humalog Mix 75/25, Humalog Mix 75/25 Pen, Humalog Pen, Humulin, 50/50, Humulin 70/30, Humulin 70/30 Pen, Humulin L, Humulin N, Humulin N Pen, Humulin R, Humulin U, Iletin I NPH, Iletin I Regular, Lantus, Novolin 70/30, Novolin 70/30 Innolet, Novolin 70/30 Penfill, Novolin L, Novolin N, Novolin N Innolet, Novolin N Penfill, Novolin R, Novolin R Innolet, Novolin R Penfill, Novolog, Novolog Flexpen, Novolog Mix 70/30, Novolog Mix 70/30 Flexpen, Novolog Mix 70/30 Penfill, Novolog Penfill, Relion 70/30, Relion 70/30 Innolet, Relion N, Relion N Innolet, Relion R, Velosulin Br (RDNA)

Other: Apidra, Humalog Mix 50/50; Humalog Mix 75/25 Pen; Iletin; Insulin Lispro; Lantus Solostar; Apidra; Novolin; regular insulin; Humalog; Novolog; Apidra; Relion/Novolin N; Novolin N Innolet; Novolin 70/30 Innolet; Novolog Mix 70/30; Humulin 70; Humulin; Relion Novolin N Innolet; Relion Novolin 70/30 Innolet; Relion; Vesolin BR; Lispro-PFC

◆ **J1825** Injection, interferon beta-1a, **33 mcg**

Other: Avonex; Rebif; Interferon beta-1a

⊕ **J1830▶** Injection interferon beta-1b, **0.25 mg** (Code may be used for Medicare when drug administered under the direct supervision of a physician, not for use when drug is self administered)

NDC: Betaseron

Other: Actimmune; Interferon beta-1b

IOM: 100-02, 15, 50

✳ **J1835▶** Injection, itraconazole, **50 mg**

NDC: Sporanox

Other: Itraconazole

⊕ **J1840** Injection, kanamycin sulfate, **up to 500 mg**

Other: Kantrex, Kanamycin sulfate; Klebcil

IOM: 100-02, 15, 50

⊕ **J1850** Injection, kanamycin sulfate, **up to 75 mg**

Other: Kantrex, Klebcil, Kanamycin sulfate

IOM: 100-02, 15, 50

⊕ **J1885** Injection, ketorolac tromethamine, **per 15 mg**

NDC: Toradol IM/IV; Toradol

Other: Ketorolac tromethamine

IOM: 100-02, 15, 50

⊕ **J1890** Injection, cephalothin sodium, **up to 1 gram**

Other: Cephalothin sodium, Keflin

IOM: 100-02, 15, 50

▶ ✳ **J1930▶** Injection, lanreotide, **1 mg**

✳ **J1931▶** Injection, laronidase, **0.1 mg**

NDC: Aldurazyme

Other: Laronidase

⊕ **J1940** Injection, furosemide, **up to 20 mg**

Other: Lasix, Furomide M.D., Furosemide

MCM 2049

IOM: 100-02, 15, 50

⊕ **J1945▶** Injection, lepirudin, **50 mg**

NDC: Refludan

Other: Lepirudin

IOM: 100-02, 15, 50

◀▶ New   ←→ Revised   ✔ Reinstated   ✖ Deleted

⊕ **Special coverage instructions**   ◆ **Not covered or valid by Medicare**   ✳ **Carrier discretion**   ▶ **ASC payment group**

⊛ **J1950**▶ Injection, leuprolide acetate (for depot suspension), **per 3.75 mg**

NDC: Lupron Depot; Lupron Depot-Ped

Other: Eliguard, Eliuard, Lupron; Lupron 3; Lupron 4; Leuprolide acetate (for depot suspension)

IOM: 100-02, 15, 50

▶ ✳ **J1953**▶ Injection, levetiracetam, **10 mg**

⊛ **J1955** Injection, levocarnitine, **per 1 gm**

NDC: Carnitor

Other: L-Carnitine; L-Carnitine Free Base; L-Carnitine Hydrachloride; Levocarnitine

IOM: 100-02, 15, 50

⊛ **J1956** Injection, levofloxacin, **250 mg**

NDC: Levaquin

Other: Levofloxacin

IOM: 100-02, 15, 50

⊛ **J1960** Injection, levorphanol tartrate, **up to 2 mg**

Other: Levo-Dromoran; Levorphanol tartrate

MCM 2049

IOM: 100-02, 15, 50

⊛ **J1980** Injection, hyoscyamine sulfate, **up to 0.25 mg**

NDC: Levsin

Other: Hyoscyamine sulfate

IOM: 100-02, 15, 50

⊛ **J1990** Injection, chlordiazepoxide HCL, **up to 100 mg**

NDC: Librium

Other: Chlordiazepoxide hydrochloride

IOM: 100-02, 15, 50

⊛ **J2001** Injection, lidocaine HCL for intravenous infusion, **10 mg**

NDC: Xylocaine (Cardiac), Lidocaine in D5W

Other: Caine-1; Caine-2; Dextrose/ Lidocaine Hcl; Dilocaine; L-Caine; Lidocaine HCl; Lidoject-1; Lidoject-2; Xylocaine-MPF; Sensi-Touch Lumbar Puncture Tray; Xylocaine Dental; Nervocaine 1%; Nervocaine 2%; Xylocaine HCl

IOM: 100-02, 15, 50

⊛ **J2010** Injection, lincomycin HCL, **up to 300 mg**

NDC: Lincocin;

Other: Lincomycin HCl

IOM: 100-02, 15, 50

✳ **J2020**▶ Injection, linezolid, **200 mg**

NDC: Zyvox

Other: Linezolid

⊛ **J2060** Injection, lorazepam, **2 mg**

NDC: Ativan

Other: Lorazepam

IOM: 100-02, 15, 50

⊛ **J2150** Injection, mannitol, **25% in 50 ml**

Other: Osmitrol; Mannitol

MCM 2049

IOM: 100-02, 15, 50

✳ **J2170** Injection, mecasermin, **1 mg**

Other: Increlex, Iplex; Mecasermin

⊛ **J2175** Injection, meperidine hydrochloride, **per 100 mg**

NDC: Demerol

Other: Demerol Hydrocholoride; Meperidine Hcl/Sodium Chloride; Meperidine HCl

IOM: 100-02, 15, 50

⊛ **J2180** Injection, meperidine and promethazine HCL, **up to 50 mg**

Other: Mepergan, Meprozine; Meperidine and promethazine HCl

IOM: 100-02, 15, 50

✳ **J2185** Injection, meropenem, **100 mg**

NDC: Merrem

Other: Meropenem

⊛ **J2210** Injection, methylergonovine maleate, **up to 0.2 mg**

NDC: Methergine

(Benefit limited to obstetrical diagnoses)

IOM: 100-02, 15, 50

✳ **J2248**▶ Injection, micafungin sodium, **1 mg**

Other: Mycamine; Micafungin sodium

⊛ **J2250** Injection, midazolam hydrochloride, **per 1 mg**

Other: Midazolam HCL, Versed

IOM: 100-02, 15, 50

◀▶ **New** ←→ **Revised** ✔ **Reinstated** ✖ **Deleted**

⊛ **Special coverage instructions** ◆ **Not covered or valid by Medicare** ✳ **Carrier discretion** ▶ **ASC payment group**

✷ **J2260** Injection, milrinone lactate, **5 mg**

NDC: Milrinone In Dextrose, Primacor, Primacor In Dextrose

Other: Dextrose/Milrinone Lactate; Milrinone lactate

IOM: 100-02, 15, 50

✷ **J2270** Injection, morphine sulfate, **up to 10 mg**

Other: Dextrose/Morphine Sulfate; Morphine Sulf; Morphine Sulfate/ Sodium Chloride, Infumorph, Duramorph, Depodur; Morphine sulfate

IOM: 100-02, 15, 50

✷ **J2271** Injection, morphine sulfate, **100 mg**

NDC: Morphine Sulfate In Dextrose

Other: Infumorph, Depodur; Morphine sulfate

IOM: 100-02, 15, 50; 100-03, 4, 280.14

✷ **J2275** Injection, morphine sulfate (preservative-free sterile solution), **per 10 mg**

NDC: Astramorph, Duramorph, Infumorph 200, Infumorph 500

Other: Astramorph PF, Infumorph, Morphine sulfate (preservative free)

IOM: 100-02, 15, 50; 100-03, 4, 280.14

✷ **J2278▸** Injection, ziconotide, **1 microgram**

NDC: Prialt

Other: Ziconotide

✳ **J2280** Injection, moxifloxacin, **100 mg**

NDC: Avelox

Other: Avelox IV; Moxifloxacin

✷ **J2300** Injection, nalbuphine hydrochloride, **per 10 mg**

NDC: Nubain

Other: Nalbuphine HCl; Nulicaine

IOM: 100-02, 15, 50

✷ **J2310** Injection, naloxone hydrochloride, **per 1 mg**

Other: Naloxone HCL, Narcan

IOM: 100-02, 15, 50

✳ **J2315▸** Injection, naltrexone, depot form, **1 mg**

Other: Vivitrol; ReVia; Naltrexone (depot form)

✷ **J2320** Injection, nandrolone decanoate, **up to 50 mg**

Other: Anabolin LA 100, Androlone-D 100, Deca-Durabolin, Decolone-50, Decolone-100, Hybolin Decanoate, Neo-Durabolic, Nandrobolic LA, Nandrolone decanoate

IOM: 100-02, 15, 50

✷ **J2321** Injection, nandrolone decanoate, **up to 100 mg**

Other: Deca-Durabolin; Hybolin Decanoate; Nandrolone decanoate

IOM: 100-02, 15, 50

✷ **J2322** Injection, nandrolone decanoate, **up to 200 mg**

Other: Deca-Durabolin; Pri-Andriol LA; Nandrolone decanoate

IOM: 100-02, 15, 50

✳ **J2323▸** Injection, natalizumab, **1 mg**

Other: Tysabri; Natalizumab

✷ **J2325▸** Injection, nesiritide, **0.1 mg**

NDC: Natrecor

Other: Nesiritide 0.1 mg

IOM: 100-02, 15, 50

✳ **J2353▸** Injection, octreotide, depot form for intramuscular injection, **1 mg**

NDC: Sandostatin LAR Depot

Other: Octreotide acetate (injection)

✳ **J2354** Injection, octreotide, non-depot form for subcutaneous or intravenous injection, **25 mcg**

NDC: Sandostatin, Octreotide Acetate

Injection, oprelvekin, 5 milligrams (mg)

✷ **J2355▸** Injection, oprelvekin, **5 mg**

NDC: Neumega

Other: Oprelvekin

IOM: 100-02, 15, 50

✳ **J2357▸** Injection, omalizumab, **5 mg**

NDC: Xolair

Other: Omalizumab

✷ **J2360** Injection, orphenadrine citrate, **up to 60 mg**

NDC: Norflex

Other: Banflex; Flexon Myolin, Neocyten, Flexoject, Flexon; K-Flex; O-Flex; Orphenadrine citrate; Orphenate

IOM: 100-02, 15, 50

| ◀▶ New | ←→ Revised | ✔ Reinstated | ✖ Deleted |

✷ Special coverage instructions ◆ Not covered or valid by Medicare ✳ Carrier discretion ▸ ASC payment group

DRUGS OTHER THAN CHEMOTHERAPY

J2260 – J2360

⊛ **J2370** Injection, phenylephrine HCL, **up to 1 ml**

NDC: Neo-Synephrine

Other: Phenylephrine HCl

IOM: 100-02, 15, 50

⊛ **J2400** Injection, chloroprocaine hydrochloride, **per 30 ml**

NDC: Nesacaine; Nesacaine-MPF

Other: Chloroprocaine HCl

IOM: 100-02, 15, 50

⊛ **J2405**▸ Injection, ondansetron hydrochloride, **per 1 mg**

NDC: Zofran

Other: Ondansetron and Dextrose; Ondansetron HCl

IOM: 100-02, 15, 50

⊛ **J2410** Injection, oxymorphone HCL, **up to 1 mg**

NDC: Numorphan, Opana

Other: Numorphan HP; Oxymorphone HCl

IOM: 100-02, 15, 50

✳ **J2425**▸ Injection, palifermin, **50 micrograms**

NDC: Kepivance

Other: Palifermin

⊛ **J2430**▸ Injection, pamidronate disodium, **per 30 mg**

NDC: Aredia

Other: Pamidronate disodium

IOM: 100-02, 15, 50

⊛ **J2440** Injection, papaverine HCL, **up to 60 mg**

Other: Pavagen TD; Papaverine HCl

IOM: 100-02, 15, 50

⊛ **J2460**▸ Injection, oxytetracycline HCL, **up to 50 mg**

Other: Terramycin IM; Oxytetracycline HCl

IOM: 100-02, 15, 50

✳ **J2469**▸ Injection, palonosetron HCL, **25 mcg**

NDC: Aloxi

Other: Palonosetron HCl

⊛ **J2501** Injection, paricalcitol, **1 mcg**

NDC: Zemplar

Other: Paricalcitol injection

IOM: 100-02, 15, 50

✳ **J2503**▸ Injection, pegaptanib sodium, **0.3 mg**

NDC: Macugen

Other: Pegaptanib

⊛ **J2504**▸ Injection, pegademase bovine, **25 IU**

NDC: Adagen

Other: Pegademase bovine

IOM: 100-02, 15, 50

✳ **J2505**▸ Injection, pegfilgrastim, **6 mg**

NDC: Neulasta

Other: Pegfilgrastim

⊛ **J2510** Injection, penicillin G procaine, aqueous, **up to 600,000 units**

NDC: Wycillin

Other: Duracillin AS, Pfizerpen AS, Crysticillin 300 A.S., Crysticillin 600 A.S.; Penicillin G procaine aqueous; Pfizerpen-AS

IOM: 100-02, 15, 50

⊛ **J2513**▸ Injection, pentastarch, 10% solution, **100 ml**

Other: Pentaspan; Pentastarch 10% solution

IOM: 100-02, 15, 50

⊛ **J2515**▸ Injection, pentobarbital sodium, **per 50 mg**

NDC: Nembutal

Other: Nembutal sodium solution; Pentobarbital sodium

IOM: 100-02, 15, 50

⊛ **J2540** Injection, penicillin G potassium, **up to 600,000 units**

NDC: Pfizerpen-G, Penicillin-G Pot In Dextrose

Other: Penicillin G potassium; Pfizerpen

IOM: 100-02, 15, 50

⊛ **J2543** Injection, piperacillin sodium/ tazobactam sodium, **1 gram/0.125 grams (1.125 grams)**

NDC: Zosyn

Other: Piperacillin/tazobactam sodium (injection)

IOM: 100-02, 15, 50

⊛ **J2545** Pentamidine isethionate, inhalation solution, FDA-approved final product, non-compounded, administered through DME, unit dose form, **per 300 mg**

NDC: Nebupent

Other: Pentacarinat, Pentam, Pentamidine isethionate

◀▶ New   ←→ Revised   ✔ Reinstated   ✖ Deleted

⊛ Special coverage instructions   ◆ Not covered or valid by Medicare   ✳ Carrier discretion   ▸ ASC payment group

⊛ **J2550** Injection, promethazine HCL, **up to 50 mg**

NDC: Phenergan, Prometh-50

Other: Anergan 25, Anergan 50, Phenazine 25, Phenazine 50, Porex, VGan 50, Promehazine HCl, Prorex 25, Prorex 50, Prothazine, VGan 25, VGan

IOM: 100-02, 15, 50

⊛ **J2560** Injection, phenobarbital sodium, **up to 120 mg**

NDC: Luminal

Other: Luminal Sodium; Phenobarbital sodium

IOM: 100-02, 15, 50

⊛ **J2590** Injection, oxytocin, **up to 10 units**

NDC: Pitocin

Other: Syntocinon; Oxytocin

IOM: 100-02, 15, 50

⊛ **J2597** Injection, desmopressin acetate, **per 1 mcg**

NDC: DDAVP

Other: Desmopressin acetate

IOM: 100-02, 15, 50

⊛ **J2650** Injection, prednisolone acetate, **up to 1 ml**

NDC: Cotolone, Predacort 50, Pred-Ject-50

Other: Key-Pred 25; Key-Pred 50, Predalone 50, Predcor 25, Predicort 50, Predoject 50, Prednisolone acetate

IOM: 100-02, 15, 50

⊛ **J2670** Injection, tolazoline HCL, **up to 25 mg**

Other: Priscoline Hydrochloride; Tolazoline HCl

IOM: 100-02, 15, 50

⊛ **J2675** Injection, progesterone, **per 50 mg**

Other: Progest, Gesterone, Gestrin, Gestrol 50, Progestaject, Progesterone

IOM: 100-02, 15, 50

⊛ **J2680** Injection, fluphenazine decanoate, **up to 25 mg**

Other: Prolixin Decanoate

MCM 2049

IOM: 100-02, 15, 50

⊛ **J2690** Injection, procainamide HCL, **up to 1 gm**

Other: Pronestyl; Pronestyl-SR, Procainamide HCl; Prostaphlin

(Benefit limited to obstetrical diagnoses)

IOM: 100-02, 15, 50

⊛ **J2700** Injection, oxacillin sodium, **up to 250 mg**

NDC: Bactocill In Dextrose

Other: Prostaphlin; Oxacillin sodium

IOM: 100-02, 15, 50

⊛ **J2710** Injection, neostigmine methylsulfate, **up to 0.5 mg**

Other: Prostigmin; Neostigmine methylsulfate

IOM: 100-02, 15, 50

⊛ **J2720** Injection, protamine sulfate, **per 10 mg**

Other: Protamine sulfate

IOM: 100-02, 15, 50

✳ **J2724▶** Injection, protein C concentrate, intravenous, human, **10 IU**

Other: Protein C concentrate

⊛ **J2725** Injection, protirelin, **per 250 mcg**

Other: Relefact TRH, Thypinone; Thyprel TRH, Thyrel TRH; Protirelin

IOM: 100-02, 15, 50

⊛ **J2730▶** Injection, pralidoxime chloride, **up to 1 gm**

NDC: Protopam Chloride

Other: Pralidoxime chloride

IOM: 100-02, 15, 50

⊛ **J2760** Injection, phentolamine mesylate, **up to 5 mg**

Other: Regitine; Phentolmine mesylate

IOM: 100-02, 15, 50

⊛ **J2765** Injection, metoclopramide HCL, **up to 10 mg**

NDC: Reglan

Other: Metoclopramide HCl

IOM: 100-02, 15, 50

⊛ **J2770▶** Injection, quinupristin/dalfopristin, **500 mg (150/350)**

NDC: Synercid

Other: Quinupristin/dalfopristin

IOM: 100-02, 15, 50

✳ **J2778▶** Injection, ranibizumab, **0.1 mg**

Other: Lucentis; Ranibizumab

⊛ **J2780** Injection, ranitidine hydrochloride, **25 mg**

NDC: Zantac, Zantac in NaCl

Other: Ranitidine HCl (injection)

IOM: 100-02, 15, 50

◀▶ New   ←→ Revised   ✔ Reinstated   ✖ Deleted

⊛ Special coverage instructions   ◆ Not covered or valid by Medicare   ✳ Carrier discretion   ▶ ASC payment group

DRUGS OTHER THAN CHEMOTHERAPY

J2783 – J2940

* **J2783** Injection, rasburicase, **0.5 mg**

NDC: Elitek

Other: Rasburicase

▶ * **J2785** Injection, regadenoson, **0.1 mg**

→ ⊙ **J2788** Injection, Rho D immune globulin, human, minidose, **50 mcg (250 IU)**

NDC: BayRHo-D, MicRhoGAM, MICRhoGAM, Ultra Filtered Plus

Other: HypRho-D, Ultra-Filtered, RhoGam

IOM: 100-02, 15, 50

→ ⊙ **J2790** Injection, Rho D immune globulin, human, full dose, **300 mcg (1500 IU)**

NDC: BayRHo-D, Hyperrho S/D, RhoGAM (Human), RhoGAM Ultra-Filtered Plus

Other: Gamulin Rh (immune globulin, human); HypRho-D; Rhesonativ; Rho(D) immune globulin (human)

(Benefit limited to obstetrical diagnoses)

IOM: 100-02, 15, 50

⊙ **J2791** Injection, Rho(D) immune globulin (human), (Rhophylac), intramuscular or intravenous, **100 IU**

Other: Gamulin RH (immune globulin), Immune globulin (Rhophylac); Rho(D) immune globulin; Rhophylac

IOM: 100-02, 15, 50

⊙ **J2792** Injection, Rho D immune globulin intravenous, human, solvent detergent, **100 IU**

NDC: WinRHo-SDF

Other: BayRHo-D, Hyperrho S/D, RHoPhylac, Gamulin RH (immune globulin, human, solvent detergent), Immune globulin (Rhophylac); Rho(D) immune globulin (human, solvent detergent), Win Rho SD

IOM: 100-02, 15, 50

* **J2794** Injection, risperidone, long acting, **0.5 mg**

NDC: Risperdal Costa

Other: Risperidone

* **J2795** Injection, ropivacaine hydrochloride, **1 mg**

NDC: Naropin

Other: Naropin SDV; Ropivacaine HCl

(Local anesthesia cannot be billed with surgical procedure)

⊙ **J2800** Injection, methocarbamol, **up to 10 ml**

NDC: Robaxin

Other: Methocarbamol

IOM: 100-02, 15, 50

* **J2805** Injection, sincalide, **5 micrograms**

Other: Kinevac; Sincalide

⊙ **J2810** Injection, theophylline, **per 40 mg**

NDC: Dextrose/Theophylline, Theophylline in D5W

Other: Salyrgan-Theophylline; Theophylline Anhydrous, Theophylline

IOM: 100-02, 15, 50

⊙ **J2820** Injection, sargramostim (GM-CSF), **50 mcg**

NDC: Leukine

Other: Prokine; Sargramostim (GM-CSF)

IOM: 100-02, 15, 50

⊙ **J2850** Injection, secretin, synthetic, human, **1 microgram**

Other: SecreFlo

IOM: 100-02, 15, 50

⊙ **J2910** Injection, aurothioglucose, **up to 50 mg**

Other: Solganal, Aurothioglucose

IOM: 100-02, 15, 50

⊙ **J2916** Injection, sodium ferric gluconate complex in sucrose injection, **12.5 mg**

NDC: Ferrlecit

Other: Sodium ferric gluconate in sucrose

IOM: 100-02, 15, 50

⊙ **J2920** Injection, methylprednisolone sodium succinate, **up to 40 mg**

NDC: A-MethaPred; Solu-Medrol

Other: Methylprednisolone sodium succinate

IOM: 100-02, 15, 50

⊙ **J2930** Injection, methylprednisolone sodium succinate, **up to 125 mg**

NDC: A-MethaPred, Solu-Medrol

Other: Methylprednisolone sodium succinate

IOM: 100-02, 15, 50

⊙ **J2940** Injection, somatrem, **1 mg**

Other: Protropin; Somatrem

IOM: 100-02, 15, 50,

Medicare Statute 1861s2b

◀▶ New   ←→ Revised   ✔ Reinstated   ✖ Deleted
⊙ Special coverage instructions   ◆ Not covered or valid by Medicare   * Carrier discretion   ▶ ASC payment group

⊛ **J2941** ▶ Injection, somatropin, **1 mg**

*NDC: Genotropin, Humatrope, Norditropin, Nutropin, Nutropin AQ, Nutropin AQ Pen, Nutropin Depot, Tev-Tropin, Saizen, **Serostim***

Other: Genotropin Nutropin, Genotropin Miniquick, Norditropin Nordiflex, Nutropin AQ Pen Cartridge, Saizen Click Easy Cartrdige, Zorbtive, Sazien Somatropin RDNA Origin, Serostim RDNA Origin; Somatropin

IOM: 100-02, 15, 50,

Medicare Statute 1861s2b

⊛ **J2950** Injection, promazine HCL, **up to 25 mg**

Other: Prorex-25, Prozine-50, Sparine, Promazine HCl

IOM: 100-02, 15, 50

⊛ **J2993** ▶ Injection, reteplase, **18.1 mg**

NDC: Retavase, Retavase Half-Kit

Other: Reteplase

IOM: 100-02, 15, 50

⊛ **J2995** ▶ Injection, streptokinase, **per 250,000 IU**

Other: Streptase, Kabikinase, Streptokinase

(Bill 1 unit for each 250,000 unit)

IOM: 100-02, 15, 50

⊛ **J2997** ▶ Injection, alteplase recombinant, **1 mg**

NDC: Activase, Cathflo Activase

Other: Alteplase recombinant

IOM: 100-02, 15, 50

⊛ **J3000** Injection, streptomycin, **up to 1 gm**

Other: Streptomycin Sulfate; Streptomycin

IOM: 100-02, 15, 50

⊛ **J3010** Injection, fentanyl citrate, **0.1 mg**

NDC: Sublimaze

Other: Fentanyl Citrate/Sodium Chloride; Fentanyl Citrate

IOM: 100-02, 15, 50

⊛ **J3030** ▶ Injection, sumatriptan succinate, **6 mg** (Code may be used for Medicare when drug administered under the direct supervision of a physician, not for use when drug is self administered)

NDC: Imitrex, Imitrex Statdose, Imitrex Statdose Pen

Other: Sumatriptan succinate

IOM: 100-02, 15, 150

⊛ **J3070** Injection, pentazocine, **30 mg**

NDC: Talwin, Talwin Lactate

Other: Pentazocine HCl

IOM: 100-02, 15, 50

~~J3100~~ ~~Injection, tenecteplase, 50 mg~~ ✖

▶ ✳ **J3101** ▶ Injection, tenecteplase, **1 mg**

⊛ **J3105** Injection, terbutaline sulfate, **up to 1 mg**

NDC: Brethine

Other: Bricanyl; Terbutaline sulfate

IOM: 100-02, 15, 50

⊛ **J3110** Injection, teriparatide, **10 mcg**

Other: Forteo; Teriparatide

⊛ **J3120** Injection, testosterone enanthate, **up to 100 mg**

NDC: Delatestryl

Other: Andro LA 200, Depo-Testosterone, Durathate-200, Andropository 100, Andryl 200, Delatest, Everone, Testone LA 100, Testrin PA, Testone LA 200, Testosterone enanthate

IOM: 100-02, 15, 50

⊛ **J3130** Injection, testosterone enanthate, **up to 200 mg**

NDC: Delatestryl

Other: Andro LA 200; Andropository 100, Andryl 200, Delatest, Durathate-200, Everone, Testro-L.A. 200, Testone LA 100, Testone LA 200, Testosterone enanthate, Testrin PA

IOM: 100-02, 15, 50

⊛ **J3140** Injection, testosterone suspension, **up to 50 mg**

Other: Adronaq-50, Testro AQ, Testosterone, Testosterone Micronized, Aqueous testosterone, Testaqua, Histerone-50, Histerone-100, Testoject-50, Testosterone suspension

IOM: 100-02, 15, 50

⊛ **J3150** Injection, testosterone propionate, **up to 100 mg**

Other: Bricanyl Subcutaneous, DepAndro 100, Testosterone Propionate Micronized, Testex, Testosterone propionate

IOM: 100-02, 15, 50

⊛ **J3230** Injection, chlorpromazine HCL, **up to 50 mg**

NDC: Thorazine

Other: Chlorpromazine HCl; Ormazine

IOM: 100-02, 15, 50

◀▶ New   ←→ Revised   ✔ Reinstated   ✖ Deleted

⊛ Special coverage instructions   ◆ Not covered or valid by Medicare   ✳ Carrier discretion   ▶ ASC payment group

⊛ **J3240▸** Injection, thyrotropin alfa, **0.9 mg provided in 1.1 mg vial**

NDC: Thyrogen

Other: Thyrotropin alfa (injection);

IOM: 100-02, 15, 50

✳ **J3243▸** Injection, tigecycline, **1 mg**

Other: Tygacil; Tigecycline

✳ **J3246▸** Injection, tirofiban HCL, **0.25 mg**

NDC: Aggrastat

Other: Tirofiban HCl

⊛ **J3250** Injection, trimethobenzamide HCL, **up to 200 mg**

NDC: Benzacot, Tigan

Other: Tiject 20, Arrestin, Tiject, Trimethobenzamide HCl

IOM: 100-02, 15, 50

⊛ **J3260** Injection, tobramycin sulfate, **up to 80 mg**

Other: Nebcin, Nebcin Pediatric, Tobramycin sulfate

IOM: 100-02, 15, 50

⊛ **J3265** Injection, torsemide, **10 mg/ml**

NDC: Demadex

Other: Torsemide

IOM: 100-02, 15, 50

⊛ **J3280** Injection, thiethylperazine maleate, **up to 10 mg**

Other: Torecan; Norzine (injection); Thiethylperazine maleate (injection)

IOM: 100-02, 15, 50

✳ **J3285▸** Injection, treprostinil, **1 mg**

NDC: Remodulin

Other: Treprostinil

▶⊛ **J3300** Injection, triamcinolone acetonide, preservative free, **1 mg**

→⊛ **J3301** Injection, triamcinolone acetonide, not otherwise specified, **10 mg**

NDC: Kenalog

Other: Cenacort A-40, Kenaject-40; Kenalog-10; Kenalog-40; Tac-3; Tach-40; Tri-Kort; Trilog; Triam A; Tramonide 40; Triamcinolone acetonide

IOM: 100-02, 15, 50

⊛ **J3302** Injection, triamcinolone diacetate, **per 5 mg**

NDC: Aristocort Forte; Clincacort, Aristocort Intralesional

Other: Aristocort, Cenacort Forte, Triam Forte Tristoject, Trilone, Amcort, Cinolene, Triamcinolone diacetate

IOM: 100-02, 15, 50

⊛ **J3303** Injection, triamcinolone hexacetonide, **per 5 mg**

NDC: Aristospan Intralesional, Aristospan Intra-Articular, Triamcinolone hexacetonide

IOM: 100-02, 15, 50

⊛ **J3305▸** Injection, trimetrexate glucuronate, **per 25 mg**

Other: NeuTrexin, Trimetrexate glucuronate

IOM: 100-02, 15, 50

⊛ **J3310** Injection, perphenazine, **up to 5 mg**

Other: Trilafon, Debioclip Kit, Perphenazine (injection)

IOM: 100-02, 15, 50

⊛ **J3315▸** Injection, triptorelin pamoate, **3.75 mg**

NDC: Trelstar Depot; Trelstar LA

Other: Triptorelin pamoate

IOM: 100-02, 15, 50

⊛ **J3320** Injection, spectinomycin dihydrochloride, **up to 2 gm**

Other: Trobicin; Spectinomycin dihydrochloride

IOM: 100-02, 15, 50

⊛ **J3350** Injection, urea, **up to 40 gm**

Other: Ureaphil, Urea

IOM: 100-02, 15, 50

⊛ **J3355▸** Injection, urofollitropin, **75 IU**

NDC: Bravelle

Other: Metrodin, Fertinex, Urofollitropin

IOM: 100-02, 15, 50

⊛ **J3360** Injection, diazepam, **up to 5 mg**

NDC: Valium

Other: Diastat, Dizac, Diazpam, Zetran

IOM: 100-02, 15, 50

⊛ **J3364** Injection, urokinase, **5000 IU vial**

NDC: Abbokinase

Other: Kinlytic, Urokinase

IOM: 100-02, 15, 50

◀▶ New   ←→ Revised   ✔ Reinstated   ✖ Deleted

⊛ Special coverage instructions   ◆ Not covered or valid by Medicare   ✳ Carrier discretion   ▸ ASC payment group

⊛ **J3365** Injection, IV, urokinase, **250,000 IU vial**

NDC: Abbokinase

Other: Kinlytic, Urokinase

IOM: 100-02, 15, 50,

Cross Reference Q0089

⊛ **J3370** Injection, vancomycin HCL, **500 mg**

NDC: Vancocin HCl

Other: Vancoled, Vancocin, Vancomycin HCl

IOM: 100-02, 15, 50; 100-03, 4, 280.14

⊛ **J3396** Injection, verteporfin, **0.1 mg**

NDC: Visudyne

Other: Verteporfin

IOM: 100-03, 1, 80.2; 100-03, 1, 80.3

⊛ **J3400** Injection, triflupromazine HCL, **up to 20 mg**

Other: Vesprin; Triflupromazine HCl

IOM: 100-02, 15, 50

⊛ **J3410** Injection, hydroxyzine HCL, **up to 25 mg**

NDC: Restall, Vistaril, Vistacot

Other: Hydroxyzine HCl, Hyzine, Hyzine-50, Vistaject 25

IOM: 100-02, 15, 50

✳ **J3411** Injection, thiamine HCL, **100 mg**

Other: Vitamin B1; Thiamine HCl

✳ **J3415** Injection, pyridoxine HCL, **100 mg**

Other: Vitamin B6; Pyridoxine HCl

⊛ **J3420** Injection, vitamin B-12 cyanocobalamin, **up to 1000 mcg**

NDC: Nervidox S; Neuro B-12 S; Tia-Doce S; Neuro B-12 Forte S; Cyanocobalamin; Nervidox-6 S; Cobal-1000

Other: Hydroxocobalamin; Cyomin; Depo-Cobolin; LA-12., Cobex, Sytobex, Redisol, Rubramin PC, Betalin 12, Berubigen, Crystal B-12, Cyano, Nutri-twelve, Vitamin B-12 (Cyanocobalamin)

IOM: 100-02, 15, 50; 100-03, 2, 150.6

⊛ **J3430** Injection, phytonadione (vitamin K), **per 1 mg**

NDC: Aqua-Mephyton; Vitamin K1

Other: Menadione, Konakion, Phytonadione (Vitamin K), Synkavite, Vitamin K (Phytonadione menadion, menadiol sodium diphosphate)

IOM: 100-02, 15, 50

⊛ **J3465** Injection, voriconazole, **10 mg**

NDC: VFEND IV

Other: Voriconazole

IOM: 100-02, 15, 50

⊛ **J3470** Injection, hyaluronidase, **up to 150 units**

NDC: Amphadase

Other: Hyaluronidase, Hydase, Hylenex, Vitrase, Wydase

IOM: 100-02, 15, 50

⊛ **J3471** Injection, hyaluronidase, ovine, preservative free, **per 1 USP unit (up to 999 USP units)**

NDC: Vitrase

Other: Hyaluronidase (ovine)

⊛ **J3472** Injection, hyaluronidase, ovine, preservative free, **per 1000 USP units**

NDC: Vitrase

Other: Hyaluronidase (ovine)

⊛ **J3473** Injection, hyaluronidase, recombinant, **1 USP unit**

Other: Hyaluronidase (recombinant); Hylenex

IOM: 100-02, 15, 50

⊛ **J3475** Injection, magnesium sulfate, **per 500 mg**

Other:, Epsom Salt, Magnes Sulf, Sulfa Mag; Magnesium sulfate

IOM: 100-02, 15, 50

⊛ **J3480** Injection, potassium chloride, **per 2 meq**

Other: Potassium chloride

IOM: 100-02, 15, 50

⊛ **J3485** Injection, zidovudine, **10 mg**

NDC: Retrovir

Other: Zidovudine

IOM: 100-02, 15, 50

✳ **J3486** Injection, ziprasidone mesylate, **10 mg**

NDC: Geodon

Other: Ziprasidone mesylate

✳ **J3487** Injection, zoledronic acid (Zometa), **1 mg**

NDC: Zometa

Other: Zoledronic acid

⊛ **J3488** Injection, zoledronic acid (Reclast), **1 mg**

NDC: Reclast

◄ ▶ New　　←→ Revised　　✔ Reinstated　　✖ Deleted

⊛ Special coverage instructions　　◆ Not covered or valid by Medicare　　✳ Carrier discretion　　▶ ASC payment group

◎ **J3490**   Unclassified drugs

Other: Acthib; Altima; Amicar; Aminocaproic Acid; Azactam; Baci-RX; Baciim; Bacitracin; Bayhep; Bayhep B; Bretylium; Brevital Sodium; Bumetanide; Bupivacaine; Cefotan; Cimetidine HCL; Cleocin Phosphate; Clindamycin Phosphate; Cortisone Acetate; Diprivan; Engerix-B; Engerix-B Pediatric;; Famotidine; Ganirelix acetate; Glofil-125; Gonal-F; Granite; Hibtiter; Hyaluronic Acid; Hylutin; Hyperhep B; Inamrinone Lactate; Kineret; Marcaine; Metronidazole; Nabi-HB; Nafcillin Sodium; Nafcillin; Pegasys; Peg-Intron; Pepcid;; Pridoxine HCL; Propofol; Ovidrel; Raptiva; Recombivax; Rifadin; Sensorcaine; Septra Infusion; Smz-TMP; Sufenta; Sufentanil Citrate; Timentin; Tosylate; Twinrix; NOC drugs; Unclassified drugs

(Bill on paper. Bill one unit. Identify drug and total dosage in "Remarks" field.)

IOM: 100-02, 15, 50

◆ **J3520**   Edetate disodium, **per 150 mg**

Other: Endrate, Disotate, Meritate, Chealamide, Edetate disodium, Endrate ethylenediamine-tetra-acetic

IOM: 100-03, 1, 20.21; 100-03, 1, 20.22

◎ **J3530**   Nasal vaccine inhalation

Other: Nasal vaccine inhalation

IOM: 100-02, 15, 50

◆ **J3535**   Drug administered through a metered dose inhaler

Other: Drug administered through a metered dose inhaler

IOM: 100-02, 15, 50

◆ **J3570**   Laetrile, amygdalin, vitamin B-17

Other: Amygdalin17; Laetril amygdalin vitamin B-17

IOM: 100-03, 1, 30.7

✳ **J3590**   Unclassified biologics

Other: Norplant System

(Bill on paper. Bill one unit. Identify drug and total dosage in "Remarks" field.)

Miscellaneous Drugs and Solutions

◎ **J7030**   Infusion, normal saline solution , **1000 cc**

NDC: Sodium Chloride

Other: Saline Solution 5% Dextrose (infusion)

IOM: 100-02, 15, 50

◎ **J7040**   Infusion, normal saline solution, sterile **(500 ml=1 unit)**

NDC: Sodium Chloride

Other: Saline solution (sterile)

IOM: 100-02, 15, 50

◎ **J7042**   5% dextrose/normal saline **(500 ml = 1 unit)**

NDC: Dextrose-Nacl

Other: Dextrose/Sodium Chloride, Dextrose 5% Saline solution

IOM: 100-02, 15, 50

◎ **J7050**   Infusion, normal saline solution , **250 cc**

NDC: Sodium Chloride

Other: Saline Solution 5% Dextrose (infusion)

IOM: 100-02, 15, 50

◎ **J7060**   5% dextrose/water **(500 ml = 1 unit)**

Other: Dextrose/water 5%

IOM: 100-02, 15, 50

◎ **J7070**   Infusion, D 5 W, **1000 cc**

NDC: Dextrose

Other: D-5-W (infusion)

IOM: 100-02, 15, 50

◎ **J7100**   Infusion, dextran 40, **500 ml**

NDC: LMD In NACL, Rheomacrodex In NACL, Dextran 40 in D5W, Dextran 40 in NaCl, Centran 40 in D5W, Gentran 40 in NaCl

Other: Centran 40, Gentran, LMD (10%), Rheomacrodex

IOM: 100-02, 15, 50

◎ **J7110**   Infusion, dextran 75, **500 ml**

NDC: Gentran 75 In NACL, Dextran 70 w/NACL, Dextran 75 in NaCl, Dextran 75 in D5W

Other: Gendex 75, Gentran 75

IOM: 100-02, 15, 50

◀▶ New   ←→ Revised   ✔ Reinstated   ✖ Deleted

◎ Special coverage instructions   ◆ Not covered or valid by Medicare   ✳ Carrier discretion   ▶ ASC payment group

⊕ **J7120** Ringer's lactate infusion, **up to 1000 cc**

Other: Potassium Chloride Solution, Ringers Injection, Ringer's lactate infusion

IOM: 100-02, 15, 50

⊕ **J7130** Hypertonic saline solution, **50 or 100 meq, 20 cc vial**

MCM 2049

IOM: 100-02, 15, 50

▶ ⊕ **J7186▶** Injection, antihemophilic factor VIII/ von Willebrand factor complex (human), **per factor VIII IU**

IOM: 100-02, 15, 50

⊕ **J7187▶** Injection, von Willebrand factor complex (HUMATE-P), **per IU VWF: RCO**

NDC: Humate-P

Other: Von Willebrand factor complex (human)

IOM: 100-02, 15, 50

⊕ **J7189▶** Factor VIIa (antihemophilic factor, recombinant), **per 1 microgram**

NDC: NovoSeven

Other: Factor VIIa (antihemophilic factor, recombinant)

IOM: 100-02, 15, 50

⊕ **J7190▶** Factor VIII anti hemophilic factor, human, **per IU**

NDC: Alphanate; Hemofil M; Koate DVI; Monarc-M; Monoclate-P

Other: Factor VIII anti-hemophilic factor (human); Koate-HP (anti-hemophilic factor, human); Kogenate; Monarc; Recombinate (anti-hemophilic factor, human)

IOM: 100-02, 15, 50

⊕ **J7191▶** Factor VIII, anti hemophilic factor (porcine), **per IU**

Other: Hyate C; Factor VII anti-hemophilic factor (porcine); Koate-HP (anti-hemophilic factor, porcine); Recombinate (anti-hemophilic factor, porcine)

IOM: 100-02, 15, 50

⊕ **J7192▶** Factor VIII (anti hemophilic factor, recombinant) **per IU**

NDC: Advate, Helixate FS, Kogenate FS, Kogenate FS Bio-Set, Recombinate, Refacto

Other: Bicclate, Bioclate, Genarc, Bioclate,Method M Monoclonal Purified, Factor VIII anti-hemophilic factor (recombinant); Koate-HP (anti-hemophilic factor, recombinant); Kogenate

IOM: 100-02, 15, 50

⊕ **J7193▶** Factor IX (anti-hemophilic factor, purified, non-recombinant) **per IU**

NDC: AlphaNine SD; Mononine

Othe: Profilnine-SD; Factor IX (anti-hemophilic factor, purified, non-recombinant)

IOM: 100-02, 15, 50

⊕ **J7194▶** Factor IX, complex, **per IU**

NDC: Bebulin VH; Proplex T, Factor IX Complex, Profilnine SD,

Other: AlphaNine SD, Konyne-80, Proplex SX-T, Profilnine Heat-treated, Factor IX (complex)

IOM: 100-02, 15, 50

⊕ **J7195▶** Factor IX (anti-hemophilic factor, recombinant) **per IU**

NDC: Benefix

Other: Konyne 80, Profilnine SD; Proplex T; Factor IX (anti-hemophilic factor, recombinant)

IOM: 100-02, 15, 50

⊕ **J7197** Anti-thrombin III (human), **per IU**

NDC: Thrombate III

Other: ATnativ, Antithrombin III

IOM: 100-02, 15, 50

⊕ **J7198▶** Anti-inhibitor, **per IU**

NDC: Autoplex T, Feiba VH Immuno

Other: Anti-inhibitor; Hemophilia clotting factors (e.g., anti-inhibitors)

IOM: 100-02, 15, 50; 100-03, 2, 110.3

⊕ **J7199** Hemophilia clotting factor, not otherwise classified

Other: Hemophilia clotting factors (NOC)

IOM: 100-02, 15, 50; 100-03, 2, 110.3

◀ ▶ New   ← → Revised   ✔ Reinstated   ✘ Deleted

⊕ Special coverage instructions   ◆ Not covered or valid by Medicare   ✳ Carrier discretion   ▶ ASC payment group

◆ **J7300** Intrauterine copper contraceptive

Other: ParaGard T38OH, Para Gard, Copper contraceptive, Intrauterine copper contraceptive, Paragar T 380 A

(Report IVD insertion with 58300. Bill usual and customary charge.)

Medicare Statute 1862a1

◆ **J7302** Levonorgestrel-releasing intrauterine contraceptive system, **52 mg**

Other: Mirena; Levonorgestrel-releasing intrauterine contraceptive

Medicare Statute 1862a1

◆ **J7303** Contraceptive supply, hormone containing vaginal ring, each

Other: NuvaRing

Medicare Statute 1862.1

◆ **J7304** Contraceptive supply, hormone containing patch, each

Other: Ortho Evra

(Only billed by Family Planning Clinics)

Medicare Statute 1862.1

◆ **J7306** Levonorgestrel (contraceptive) implant system, including implants and supplies

Other: Norplant II; Levonorgestrel implant

◆ **J7307** Etonogestrel (contraceptive) implant system, including implant and supplies

Other: Implanon; Etonogestrel implant

❋ **J7308▶** Aminolevulinic acid HCL for topical administration, 20%, single unit dosage form **(354 mg)**

NDC: Levulan Kerastick

Other: Aminolevulinic acid HCl

⊙ **J7310▶** Ganciclovir, **4.5 mg,** long-acting implant

NDC: Vitrasert

Other: Ganciclovir (implant)

IOM: 100-02, 15, 50

❋ **J7311▶** Fluocinolone acetonide, intravitreal implant

Other: Retisert; Flucinolone

❋ **J7321▶** Hyaluronan or derivative, Hyalgan or Supartz, for intra-articular injection, **per dose**

Other: Hyalgan; Sodium Hyaluronate (Hyalgan); Sodium Hyaluronate (Supartz); Supartz

❋ **J7322▶** Hyaluronan or derivative, Synvisc, for intra-articular injection, **per dose**

Other: Hylan G-F 20; Synvisc

❋ **J7323▶** Hyaluronan or derivative, Euflexxa, for intra-articular injection, **per dose**

Other: Euflexxa; Sodium Hyaluronate (Euflexxa)

❋ **J7324▶** Hyaluronan or derivative, Orthovisc, for intra-articular injection, **per dose**

Other: Sodium Hyaluronate (Orthovisc)

❋ **J7330** Autologous cultured chondrocytes, **implant**

NDC: Carticel

Other: Autologous cultured chondrocytes; Orthovisc

~~J7340~~ ~~Dermal and epidermal, (substitute)~~ ✖ ~~tissue of human origin, with or without bioengineered or processed elements, with metabolically active elements,~~ ~~**per square centimeter**~~

~~J7341~~ ~~Dermal (substitute) tissue of non-~~ ✖ ~~human origin, with or without other bioengineered or processed elements, with metabolically active elements,~~ ~~**per square centimeter**~~

~~J7342~~ ~~Dermal (substitute) tissue of~~ ✖ ~~human origin, with or without other bioengineered or processed elements, with metabolically active elements,~~ ~~**per square centimeter**~~

~~J7343~~ ~~Dermal and epidermal, (substitute)~~ ✖ ~~tissue of non-human origin, with or without other bioengineered or processed elements, without metabolically active elements,~~ ~~**per square centimeter**~~

~~J7344~~ ~~Dermal (substitute) tissue of~~ ✖ ~~human origin, with or without other bioengineered or processed elements, without metabolically active elements,~~ ~~**per square centimeter**~~

~~J7346~~ ~~Dermal (substitute) tissue of~~ ✖ ~~human origin, injectable, with or without other bioengineered or processed elements, but without metabolically active elements,~~ ~~**1 cc**~~

~~J7347~~ ~~Dermal (substitute) tissue of non-~~ ✖ ~~human origin, with or without other bioengineered or processed elements, without metabolically active elements (Integra Matrix),~~ ~~**per square centimeter**~~

~~J7348~~ ~~Dermal (substitute) tissue of non-~~ ✖ ~~human origin, with or without other bioengineered or processed elements, without metabolically active elements (TissueMend),~~ ~~**per square centimeter**~~

◄ ▶ **New**   ←→ **Revised**   ✔ **Reinstated**   ✖ **Deleted**

⊙ **Special coverage instructions**   ◆ **Not covered or valid by Medicare**   ❋ **Carrier discretion**   ▶ **ASC payment group**

J7349   Dermal (substitute) tissue of non- ✖
~~human origin, with or without other bioengineered or processed elements, without metabolically active elements (PriMatrix),~~ **per square centimeter**

Immunosuppressive Drugs (Includes Non-injectibles)

⊘ **J7500**   Azathioprine, oral, **50 mg**
NDC: Azasan; Imuran; Azathioprine
IOM: 100-02, 15, 50

⊘ **J7501**▶   Azathioprine, parenteral, **100 mg**
NDC: Imuran
Other: Azathioprine
IOM: 100-02, 15, 50

⊘ **J7502**▶   Cyclosporine, oral, **100 mg**
NDC: Gengraf; Neoral; Sandimmune
Other: Sangcya, Cyclosporine
IOM: 100-02, 15, 50

⊘ **J7504**▶   Lymphocyte immune globulin, antithymocyte globulin, equine, parenteral, **250 mg**
NDC: Atgam
Other: Lymphocyte immune globulin (anti-thymocyte globulin, equine)
IOM: 100-02, 15, 50; 100-03, 2, 110.3

⊘ **J7505**▶   Muromonab-CD3, parenteral, **5 mg**
NDC: Orthoclone OKT3
Other: Monoclonal antibodies (parenteral); Muromonab-CD
IOM: 100-02, 15, 50

⊘ **J7506**   Prednisone, oral, **per 5 mg**
NDC: Deltasone; Liquid Pred; Sterapred; Sterapred DS, Prednisone Intensol
Other: Meticorten; Orasong; Prednicen-M; Prednicot; Predone, Prednisone
IOM: 100-02, 15, 50

⊘ **J7507**▶   Tacrolimus, oral, **per 1 mg**
NDC: Prograf
Other: Tacrolimus
IOM: 100-02, 15, 50

⊘ **J7509**   Methylprednisolone oral, **per 4 mg**
NDC: Medrol, Medrol (Pak)
Other: Methylpred DP; Methylprednisolone oral
IOM: 100-02, 15, 50

⊘ **J7510**   Prednisolone oral, **per 5 mg**
Other: Delta-Cortef, Orapred ODT, Pediapred; Prelone, Cotolone, Prednoral; Prednisolone
IOM: 100-02, 15, 50

✳ **J7511**▶   Lymphocyte immune globulin, antithymocyte globulin, rabbit, parenteral, **25 mg**
NDC: Thymoglobulin
Other: Lymphocyte immune globulin (anti-thymocyte globulin, rabbit)

⊘ **J7513**▶   Daclizumab, parenteral, **25 mg**
NDC: Zenapax
Other: Daclizumab
IOM: 100-02, 15, 50

✳ **J7515**   Cyclosporine, oral, **25 mg**
NDC: Gengraf; Neoral; Sandimmune
Other: Sangcya, Cyclosporine

✳ **J7516**▶   Cyclosporin, parenteral, **250 mg**
NDC: Sandimmune
Other: Neoral, Gengraf, Sangcya, Cyclosporin (parental)

✳ **J7517**▶   Mycophenolate mofetil, oral, **250 mg**
NDC: CellCept
Other: Mycophenolate mofetil

⊘ **J7518**▶   Mycophenolic acid, oral, **180 mg**
NDC: Myfortic
Other: Mycophenolic acid
IOM: 100-04, 4, 240; 100-4, 17, 80.3.1

⊘ **J7520**▶   Sirolimus, oral, **1 mg**
NDC: Rapamune
Other: Sirolimus
IOM: 100-02, 15, 50

⊘ **J7525**▶   Tacrolimus, parenteral, **5 mg**
NDC: Prograf
Other: Tacrolimus (parenteral)
IOM: 100-02, 15, 50

⊘ **J7599**   Immunosuppressive drug, not otherwise classified
Other: Immunosuppressive drug (not otherwise classified); NOC drugs (immunosuppressive)
(Bill on paper. Bill one unit. Identify drug and total dosage in "Remarks" field.)
IOM: 100-02, 15, 50

◀▶ New   ←→ Revised   ✔ Reinstated   ✖ Deleted
⊘ Special coverage instructions   ◆ Not covered or valid by Medicare   ✳ Carrier discretion   ▶ ASC payment group

Inhalation Solutions

J7602 ~~Albuterol, all formulations including~~ ✖
~~separated isomers, inhalation solution,~~
~~FDA-approved final product, non-~~
~~compounded, administered through~~
~~DME, concentrated form,~~ **per 1 mg**
~~(albuterol) or~~ **per 0.5 mg** ~~(levalbuterol)~~

J7603 ~~Albuterol, all formulations including~~ ✖
~~separated isomers, inhalation solution,~~
~~FDA-approved final product, non-~~
~~compounded, administered through~~
~~DME, unit dose,~~ **per 1 mg** ~~(albuterol)~~
~~or~~ **per 0.5 mg** ~~(levalbuterol)~~

✳ **J7604** Acetylcysteine, inhalation solution,
compounded product, administered
through DME, unit dose form, **per
gram**

*Other: Acetylcysteine; Mucomyst (unit
dose form)*

✳ **J7605** Arformoterol, inhalation solution, FDA
approved final product, non-
compounded, administered through
DME, unit dose form, **15 micrograms**

Other: Arformoterol tartrate

▶ ✳ **J7606** Formoterol fumarate, inhalation
solution, FDA approved final product,
non-compounded, administered
through DME, unit dose form, **20
micrograms**

✳ **J7607** Levalbuterol, inhalation solution,
compounded product, administered
through DME, concentrated form,
0.5 mg

*Other: Xopenex; Levalbuterol HCl
(concentrated form)*

☺ **J7608** Acetylcysteine, inhalation solution,
FDA-approved final product, non-
compounded, administered through
DME, unit dose form, **per gram**

*Other: Mucomyst, Mucomyst-10;
Mucomyst-20, Mucosil, Acetadote,
Acetylcysteine, Mucosol*

✳ **J7609** Albuterol, inhalation solution,
compounded product, administered
through DME, unit dose, **1 mg**

Other: Albuterol

✳ **J7610** Albuterol, inhalation solution,
compounded product, administered
through DME, concentrated form, **1 mg**

Other: Albuterol

✔ ◆ **J7611** Albuterol, inhalation solution, FDA-
approved final product, non-
compounded, administered through
DME, concentrated form, **1 mg**

✔ ◆ **J7612** Levalbuterol, inhalation solution, FDA-
approved final product, non-
compounded, administered through
DME, concentrated form, **0.5 mg**

✔ ◆ **J7613** Albuterol, inhalation solution, FDA-
approved final product, non-
compounded, administered through
DME, unit dose, **1 mg**

✔ ◆ **J7614** Levalbuterol, inhalation solution, FDA-
approved final product, non-
compounded, administered through
DME, unit dose, **0.5 mg**

✳ **J7615** Levalbuterol, inhalation solution,
compounded product, administered
through DME, unit dose, **0.5 mg**

Other: Levalbuterol HCl (unit form)

☺ **J7620** Albuterol, **up to 2.5 mg** and
ipratropium bromide, **up to 0.5 mg,**
FDA-approved final product, non-
compounded, administered through
DME

NDC: DuoNeb

*Other: Albuterol, Combivent; Combivent,
ipratropium; DuoNeb, albuterol;
DuoNeb, ipratropium*

✳ **J7622** Beclomethasone, inhalation solution,
compounded product, administered
through DME, unit dose form, **per
milligram**

*Other: Beclovent; Beconase; Qvar;
Vancenase; Vanceril*

✳ **J7624** Betamethasone, inhalation solution,
compounded product, administered
through DME, unit dose form, **per mg**

*Other: Celestone Phosphate;
Beclomethason inhalation solution;
Betamethasone inhalation solution*

✳ **J7626** Budesonide inhalation solution, FDA-
approved final product, non-
compounded, administered through
DME, unit dose form, **up to 0.5 mg**

NDC: Pulmicort

*Other: Budesonide inhalation solution,
Pulmicort Respules, Pulmicort Flexhaler,
Pulmicort Respulses (non-compounded,
concentrated)*

✳ **J7627** Budesonide, inhalation solution,
compounded product, administered
through DME, unit dose form, **up to
0.5 mg**

*Other: Budesonide inhalation solution,
Pulmicort Respulses*

◄ ▶ New   ← → Revised   ✔ Reinstated   ✖ Deleted

☺ Special coverage instructions   ◆ Not covered or valid by Medicare   ✳ Carrier discretion   ▶ ASC payment group

✿ **J7628** Bitolterol mesylate, inhalation solution, compounded product, administered through DME, concentrated form, **per milligram**

Other: Bitolterol mesylate; Tornalate

✿ **J7629** Bitolterol mesylate, inhalation solution, compounded product, administered through DME, unit dose form, **per milligram**

Other: Bitolterol mesylate, Tornalate

✿ **J7631** Cromolyn sodium, inhalation solution, FDA-approved final product, non-compounded, administered through DME, unit dose form, **per 10 milligrams**

NDC: Intal

Other: Gastrocrom, Nasalcrom, Cromolyn sodium

✳ **J7632** Cromolyn sodium, inhalation solution, compounded product, administered through DME, unit dose form, **per 10 milligrams**

Other: Cromolyn sodium

✳ **J7633** Budesonide, inhalation solution, FDA-approved final product, non-compounded, administered through DME, concentrated form, **per 0.25 milligram**

Other: Budesonide inhalation solution, Pulmicort, Pulmicort Flexhaler, Pulmicort Respules

✳ **J7634** Budesonide, inhalation solution, compounded product, administered through DME, concentrated form, **per 0.25 milligram**

Other: Budesonide inhalation solution

✿ **J7635** Atropine, inhalation solution, compounded product, administered through DME, concentrated form, **per milligram**

Other: Atropine

✿ **J7636** Atropine, inhalation solution, compounded product, administered through DME, unit dose form, **per milligram**

Other: Atropine

✿ **J7637** Dexamethasone, inhalation solution, compounded product, administered through DME, concentrated form, **per milligram**

Other: Dexamethasone (concentrated form)

✿ **J7638** Dexamethasone, inhalation solution, compounded product, administered through DME, unit dose form, **per milligram**

Other: Dexamethasone (unit form)

➜✿ **J7639** Dornase alfa, inhalation solution, FDA-approved final product, non-compounded, administered through DME, unit dose form, **per milligram**

NDC: Pulmozyme

Other: Dornase alpha (unit dose form)

✳ **J7640** Formoterol, inhalation solution, compounded product, administered through DME, unit dose form, **12 micrograms**

Other: Foradil Aerolizer; Formoterol

✳ **J7641** Flunisolide, inhalation solution, compounded product, administered through DME, unit dose, **per milligram**

Other: AeroBid; AeroBid-M; Flunisolide inhalation solution (unit dose form)

✿ **J7642** Glycopyrrolate, inhalation solution, compounded product, administered through DME, concentrated form, **per milligram**

Other: Glycopyrrolate (concentrated form)

✿ **J7643** Glycopyrrolate, inhalation solution, compounded product, administered through DME, unit dose form, **per milligram**

Other: Robinul; Glycopyrrolate (unit dose form)

✿ **J7644** Ipratropium bromide, inhalation solution, FDA-approved final product, non-compounded, administered through DME, unit dose form, **per milligram**

NDC: Atrovent

Other: Ipratropium bromide (unit dose form)

✳ **J7645** Ipratropium bromide, inhalation solution, compounded product, administered through DME, unit dose form, **per milligram**

Other: Ipratropium bromide (unit dose form)

✳ **J7647** Isoetharine HCL, inhalation solution, compounded product, administered through DME, concentrated form, **per milligram**

Other: Bronkosol; Isoetharine HCl (concentrated form)

⌬ **J7648** Isoetharine HCL, inhalation solution, FDA-approved final product, non-compounded, administered through DME, concentrated form, **per milligram**

Other: Beta-2, Bronkosol; Isoetharine HCl (concentrated form)

⌬ **J7649** Isoetharine HCL, inhalation solution, FDA-approved final product, non-compounded, administered through DME, unit dose form, **per milligram**

Other: Bronkosol; Isoetharine HCl (unit dose form)

✳ **J7650** Isoetharine HCL, inhalation solution, compounded product, administered through DME, unit dose form, **per milligram**

Other: Bronkosol; Isoetharine HCl (unit dose form)

✳ **J7657** Isoproterenol HCL, inhalation solution, compounded product, administered through DME, concentrated form, **per milligram**

Other: Isoproterenol HCl (concentrated form); Isuprel (concentrated form)

⌬ **J7658** Isoproterenol HCL inhalation solution, FDA-approved final product, non-compounded, administered through DME, concentrated form, **per milligram**

Other: Isoproterenol HCl (concentrated form); Isuprel (concentrated form)

⌬ **J7659** Isoproterenol HCL, inhalation solution, FDA-approved final product, non-compounded, administered through DME, unit dose form, **per milligram**

Other: Isoproterenol HCl (unit dose form); Isuprel (unit dose form)

✳ **J7660** Isoproterenol HCL, inhalation solution, compounded product, administered through DME, unit dose form, **per milligram**

Other: Isuprel (unit dose form); Isoproterenol HCl (unit dose form)

✳ **J7667** Metaproterenol sulfate, inhalation solution, compounded product, concentrated form, **per 10 milligrams**

Other: Metaprel (concentrated form); Metaproterenol sulfate (concentrated form)

⌬ **J7668** Metaproterenol sulfate, inhalation solution, FDA-approved final product, non-compounded, administered through DME, concentrated form, **per 10 milligrams**

Other: Metaprel (concentrated form); Metaproterenol sulfate (concentrated form)

⌬ **J7669** Metaproterenol sulfate, inhalation solution, FDA-approved final product, non-compounded, administered through DME, unit dose form, **per 10 milligrams**

NDC: Alupent

Other: Metaprel (unit dose form); Metaproterenol sulfate (unit dose form)

✳ **J7670** Metaproterenol sulfate, inhalation solution, compounded product, administered through DME, unit dose form, **per 10 milligrams**

Other: Metaprel (unit dose form); Metaproterenol sulfate (unit dose form)

✳ **J7674** Methacholine chloride administered as inhalation solution through a nebulizer, **per 1 mg**

NDC: Provocholine

Other: Methacholine chloride

✳ **J7676** Pentamidine isethionate, inhalation solution, compounded product, administered through DME, unit dose form, **per 300 mg**

Other: Pentamidine isethionate

⌬ **J7680** Terbutaline sulfate, inhalation solution, compounded product, administered through DME, concentrated form, **per milligram**

Other: Brethine, Bricanyl, Terbutaline sulfate (concentrated form)

⌬ **J7681** Terbutaline sulfate, inhalation solution, compounded product, administered through DME, unit dose form, **per milligram**

Other: Brethine, Terbutaline sulfate (unit dose form)

⌬ **J7682** Tobramycin, inhalation solution, FDA-approved final product, non-compounded unit dose form, administered through DME, **per 300 milligrams**

NDC: Tobi

Other: Nebcin; Tobramycin (inhalation solution)

◀▶ New   ←→ Revised   ✔ Reinstated   ✖ Deleted

⌬ Special coverage instructions   ◆ Not covered or valid by Medicare   ✳ Carrier discretion   ▶ ASC payment group

⚙ **J7683** Triamcinolone, inhalation solution, compounded product, administered through DME, concentrated form, **per milligram**

Other: Azmacort; Triamcinolone (concentrated form)

⚙ **J7684** Triamcinolone, inhalation solution, compounded product, administered through DME, unit dose form, **per milligram**

Other: Azmacort; Triamcinolone (unit dose form)

✳ **J7685** Tobramycin, inhalation solution, compounded product, administered through DME, unit dose form, **per 300 milligrams**

Other: Tobramycin (inhalation solution)

⚙ **J7699** NOC drugs, inhalation solution administered through DME

Other: Acetylcysteine; Brovana; Cromolyn Sodium; Gentamicin Sulfate (inhalation solution); N-Acetyl-L-Cysteine, NebuPent, Pentam; Pentamidine Isethionate; Sodium Chloride, NOC drugs (INH, administered through DME)

⚙ **J7799** NOC drugs, other than inhalation drugs, administered through DME

Other: Dextrose; Dextrose Hypertonic; Dextrose/Sodium Chloride; Epinephrine; Epinephrine HCL; Epinephrine (other), Mannitol;Osmitrol, Phenylephrine HCL; Resectisol; Sodium Chloride, NOC drugs (other than INH, administered through DME)

(Bill on paper. Bill one unit and identify drug and total dosage in the "Remark" field.)

IOM: 100-02, 15, 110.3

Other

⚙ **J8498** Antiemetic drug, rectal/suppository, not otherwise specified Medicare Statute 1861(s)2t

Other: Compazine, Compro; Phenadoz; Phenergan; Prochlorperazine; Prochlorperazine HCL; Promethazine; Promethazine HCL; Promethegan; Thorazine

◆ **J8499** Prescription drug, oral, non chemotherapeutic, NOS

Other: Acyclovir; Zovirax; NOC drugs (non-chemotherapeutic); Prescription (non-chemotherapeutic, NOS)

IOM: 100-02, 15, 50

⚙ **J8501**▶ Aprepitant, oral, **5 mg**

NDC: Emend, Emend Tri-Fold

⚙ **J8510**▶ Busulfan; oral, **2 mg**

NDC: Myleran

Other: Busulfex; Busulfan

IOM 100-02, 15, 50; 100-04, 4, 240; 100-04, 17, 80.1.1

◆ **J8515** Cabergoline, oral, **0.25 mg**

Other: Cabergoline, Dostinex

IOM: 100-02, 15, 50; 100-04, 4, 240

⚙ **J8520**▶ Capecitabine, oral, **150 mg**

NDC: Xeloda

Other: Capecitabine

IOM: 100-02, 15, 50; 100-04, 4, 240; 100-04, 17, 80.1.1

⚙ **J8521**▶ Capecitabine, oral, **500 mg**

NDC: Xeloda

Other: Capecitabine

IOM: 100-02, 15, 50; 100-04, 4, 240; 100-04, 17, 80.1.1

⚙ **J8530** Cyclophosphamide; oral, **25 mg**

NDC: Cytoxan (oral)

Other: Cyclophosphamide (oral)

IOM: 100-02, 15, 50; 100-04, 4, 240; 100-04, 17, 80.1.1

⚙ **J8540** Dexamethasone, oral, **0.25 mg**

Other: Decadron, Dexpak JR Taperpak, Dexamethasone, Dexone

Medicare Statute 1861(s)2t

⚙ **J8560**▶ Etoposide; oral, **50 mg**

NDC: VePesid

Other: Etoposide

IOM: 100-02, 15, 50; 100-04, 4, 230.1; 100-04, 4, 240; 100-04, 17, 80.1.1

◆ **J8565** Gefitinib, oral, **250 mg**

Other: Iressa; Gefitinib

⚙ **J8597** Antiemetic drug, oral, not otherwise specified

Medicare Statute 1861(s)2t

◀▶ New   ←→ Revised   ✔ Reinstated   ✖ Deleted
⚙ Special coverage instructions   ◆ Not covered or valid by Medicare   ✳ Carrier discretion   ▶ ASC payment group

⊛ **J8600** Melphalan; oral, **2 mg**

Other: Alkeran; Melphalan (oral)

IOM: 100-02, 15, 50; 100-04, 4, 240; 100-04, 17, 80.1.1

⊛ **J8610** Methotrexate; oral, **2.5 mg**

NDC: Rheumatrex, Trexall

Other: Rheumatrex Dose Pack; Methotrexate

IOM: 100-02, 15, 50; 100-04, 4, 240; 100-04, 17, 80.1.1

✳ **J8650)** Nabilone, oral, **1 mg**

Other: Cesamet; Nabilone

⊛ **J8700)** Temozolomide, oral, **5 mg**

NDC: Temodar

Other: Temozolomide

IOM: 100-02, 15, 50; 100-04, 4, 240

▶ ✳ **J8705)** Topotecan, oral, **0.25 mg**

⊛ **J8999** Prescription drug, oral, chemotherapeutic, NOS

Other: Arimidex; Aromasin; Ceenu; Droxia; Flutamide; Flutamide Citrate; Hydrea; Hydroxyurea; Leukeran; Malulane; Megace; Megestrol Acetate; Mercaptopurine; Nolvadex; Soltamox; Tamoxifen Citrate; NOC drugs (chemotherapeutic); Prescription (chemotherapeutic, NOS)

IOM: 100-02, 15, 50; 100-04, 4, 250; 100-04, 17, 80.1.1; 100-04, 17, 80.1.2

CHEMOTHERAPY DRUGS (J9000-J9999)

NOTE: These codes cover the cost of the chemotherapy drug only, not to include the administration

→ ⊛ **J9000** Injection, doxorubicin hydrochloride, **10 mg**

NDC: Adriamycin

Other: Adriamycin PFS; Adriamycin RDF, Rubex; Adriamycin Sulfate; Doxorubicin HCl

IOM: 100-02, 15, 50

→ ⊛ **J9001)** Injection, doxorubicin hydrochloride, all lipid formulations, **10 mg**

NDC: Doxil

Other: Doxorubicin HCl (all lipid)

IOM: 100-02, 15, 50

→ ⊛ **J9010)** Injection, alemtuzumab, **10 mg**

NDC: Campath

Other: Alemtuzumab

Medicare Statute 1833(t)

→ ⊛ **J9015)** Injection, aldesleukin, **per single use vial**

NDC: Proleukin

Other: Aldesleukin; IL-2, Interleukin

IOM: 100-02, 15, 50

→ ✳ **J9017)** Injection, arsenic trioxide, **1 mg**

NDC: Trisenox

Other: Arsenic trioxide

→ ⊛ **J9020)** Injection, asparaginase, **10,000 units**

NDC: Elspar

Other: Asparaginase

IOM: 100-02, 15, 50

✳ **J9025)** Injection, azacitidine, **1 mg**

Other: Azacitidine, Vidaza

✳ **J9027)** Injection, clofarabine, **1 mg**

NDC: Clolar

Other: Clofarabine

⊛ **J9031)** BCG (intravesical), **per instillation**

NDC: TheraCys; Tice BCG

Other: Pacis, BCG (live)

IOM: 100-02, 15, 50

▶ ✳ **J9033)** Injection, bendamustine HCL, **1 mg**

✳ **J9035)** Injection, bevacizumab, **10 mg**

NDC: Avastin

Other: Bevacizumab

→ ⊛ **J9040** Injection, bleomycin sulfate, **15 units**

NDC: Blenoxane

Other: Bleomycin sulfate

IOM: 100-02, 15, 50

✳ **J9041)** Injection, bortezomib, **0.1 mg**

NDC: Velcade

Other: Bortezomib

→ ⊛ **J9045** Injection, carboplatin, **50 mg**

NDC: Paraplatin

Other: Carboplantin

IOM: 100-02, 15, 50

→ ⊛ **J9050)** Injection, carmustine, **100 mg**

NDC: BiCNU

Other: Carmustine

IOM: 100-02, 15, 50

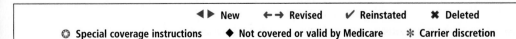

◀ ▶ New   ← → Revised   ✔ Reinstated   ✖ Deleted

⊛ Special coverage instructions   ◆ Not covered or valid by Medicare   ✳ Carrier discretion   ▶ ASC payment group

✳ **J9055** ▸ Injection, cetuximab, **10 mg**

NDC: Erbitux

Other: Cetuximab

❂ **J9060** Cisplatin, powder or solution, **per 10 mg**

NDC: Plantinol AQ

Other: Cisplatin

IOM: 100-02, 15, 50

❂ **J9062** Cisplatin, **50 mg**

NDC: Plantinol AQ

Other: Cisplatin

IOM: 100-02, 15, 50

❂ **J9065** ▸ Injection, cladribine, **per 1 mg**

NDC: Leustatin

Other: Cladribine

IOM: 100-02, 15, 50

❂ **J9070** Cyclophosphamide, **100 mg**

NDC: Cytoxan

Other: Neosar, Endoxan-Asta, Cyclophosphamide

IOM: 100-02, 15, 50

❂ **J9080** Cyclophosphamide, **200 mg**

NDC: Cytoxan

Other: Neosar, Cyclophosphamide

IOM: 100-02, 15, 50

❂ **J9090** Cyclophosphamide, **500 mg**

NDC: Cytoxan

Other: Neosar, Cyclophosphamide

IOM: 100-02, 15, 50

❂ **J9091** Cyclophosphamide, **1 gram**

NDC: Cytoxan

Other: Neosar, Cyclophosphamide

IOM: 100-02, 15, 50

❂ **J9092** Cyclophosphamide, **2 gram**

NDC: Cytoxan

Other: Neosar, Cyclophosphamide

IOM: 100-02, 15, 50

❂ **J9093** Cyclophosphamide, lyophilized, **100 mg**

NDC: Cytoxan Lyophilized

Other: Neosar; Lyophilized Cytoxan, Cyclophosphamide Lyophilized; Lyophilized

IOM: 100-02, 15, 50

❂ **J9094** Cyclophosphamide, lyophilized, **200 mg**

NDC: Cytoxan Lyophilized

Other: Neosar; Lyophilized Cytoxan, Cyclophosphamide Lyphilized; Lyophilized

IOM: 100-02, 15, 50

❂ **J9095** Cyclophosphamide, lyophilized, **500 mg**

NDC: Cytoxan Lyophilized

Other: Cytoxan; Neosar; Lyophilized Cytoxan, Cyclophosphamide Lymphilized; Lyophilized

IOM: 100-02, 15, 50

❂ **J9096** Cyclophosphamide, lyophilized, **1.0 gram**

NDC: Cytoxan Lyophilized

Other: Cytoxan; Neosar; Lyophilized Cytoxan, Cyclophosphamide Lymphilized; Lyophilized

IOM: 100-02, 15, 50

❂ **J9097** Cyclophosphamide, lyophilized, **2.0 gram**

NDC: Cytoxan Lyophilized

Other: Cytoxan; Neosar; Lyophilized Cytoxan, Cyclophosphamide Lymphilized; Lyophilized

IOM: 100-02, 15, 50

→ ✳ **J9098** ▸ Injection, cytarabine liposome, **10 mg**

NDC: DepoCyt

Other: Cytarabine liposome

→ ❂ **J9100** Injection, cytarabine, **100 mg**

Other: Cytosar-U, Ara-C, Tarabin CFS, Cytarabine

IOM: 100-02, 15, 50

→ ❂ **J9110** Injection, cytarabine, **500 mg**

Other: Cytosar-U, Cytarabine

IOM: 100-02, 15, 50

→ ❂ **J9120** ▸ Injection, dactinomycin, **0.5 mg**

NDC: Cosmegen

Other: Actinomycin D, Dactinomycin

IOM: 100-02, 15, 50

❂ **J9130** Dacarbazine, **100 mg**

NDC: DTIC-Dome

Other: Dacarbazine

IOM: 100-02, 15, 50

❂ **J9140** Dacarbazine, **200 mg**

Other: DTIC-Dome, Dacarbazine

IOM: 100-02, 15, 50

◀▶ New   ←→ Revised   ✔ Reinstated   ✖ Deleted

❂ Special coverage instructions   ◆ Not covered or valid by Medicare   ✳ Carrier discretion   ▸ ASC payment group

→ ⊕ **J9150**〗 Injection, daunorubicin, **10 mg**
NDC: Cerubidine
Other: Daunomycin, Daunorubicin HCl,
Rubidomycin
IOM: 100-02, 15, 50

→ ⊕ **J9151**〗 Injection, daunorubicin citrate,
liposomal formulation, **10 mg**
NDC: Daunoxome
Other: Daunorubicin citrate (liposomal formulation)
IOM: 100-02, 15, 50

→ ✳ **J9160**〗 Injection, denileukin diftitox, **300 micrograms**
NDC: Ontak
Other: Denileukin diftitox

→ ⊕ **J9165**〗 Injection, diethylstilbestrol
diphosphate, **250 mg**
Other: Diethylstilbestrol disphosphate, Stilphostrol
IOM: 100-02, 15, 50

→ ⊕ **J9170**〗 Injection, docetaxel, **20 mg**
NDC: Taxotere
Other: Docetaxel
IOM: 100-02, 15, 50

⊕ **J9175** Injection, Elliott's B solution, **1 ml**
Other: Elliott's b solution
IOM: 100-02, 15, 50

✳ **J9178**〗 Injection, epirubicin HCL, **2 mg**
NDC: Ellence
Other: Epirubicin HCl

→ ⊕ **J9181** Injection, etoposide, **10 mg**
NDC: Etopophos; VePesid
Other: Etoposide; Toposar
IOM: 100-02, 15, 50

J9182 ~~Etoposide, **100 mg**~~ ✖

→ ⊕ **J9185**〗 Injection, fludarabine phosphate, **50 mg**
NDC: Fludara
Other: Fludarabine phosphate
IOM: 100-02, 15, 50

→ ⊕ **J9190** Injection, fluorouracil, **500 mg**
NDC: Adrucil
Other: Fluorouracil
IOM: 100-02, 15, 50

→ ⊕ **J9200**〗 Injection, floxuridine, **500 mg**
Other: FUDR, Floxuridine
IOM: 100-02, 15, 50

→ ⊕ **J9201**〗 Injection, gemcitabine hydrochloride, **200 mg**
NDC: Gemzar
Other: Gemcitabine HCl
IOM: 100-02, 15, 50

⊕ **J9202**〗 Goserelin acetate implant, **per 3.6 mg**
NDC: Zoladex
Other: Goserelin acetate implant
IOM: 100-02, 15, 50

→ ⊕ **J9206**〗 Injection, irinotecan, **20 mg**
NDC: Camptosar
Other: Comptosar; Irinotecan
IOM: 100-02, 15, 50

▶ ✳ **J9207**〗 Injection, ixabepilone, **1 mg**

→ ⊕ **J9208**〗 Injection, ifosfamide, **1 gm**
NDC: Ifex
Other: Mitoxana; Ifosfamide
IOM: 100-02, 15, 50

→ ⊕ **J9209**〗 Injection, mesna, **200 mg**
NDC: Mesnex
Other: Mesna
IOM: 100-02, 15, 50

→ ⊕ **J9211**〗 Injection, idarubicin hydrochloride, **5 mg**
NDC: Idamycin PFS
Other: Idamycin; Idarubicin HCl
IOM: 100-02, 15, 50

→ ⊕ **J9212** Injection, interferon alfacon-1, recombinant, **1 mcg**
NDC: Infergen
Other: Interferon alfacon-1 (recombinant)
IOM: 100-02, 15, 50

→ ⊕ **J9213**〗 Injection, interferon, alfa-2a, recombinant,
3 million units
NDC: Roferon-A
IOM: 100-02, 15, 50

→ ⊕ **J9214**〗 Injection, interferon, alfa-2b, recombinant,
1 million units
NDC: Intron-A
Other: Rebetron Kit, Interferon alfa-2b (recombinant)
IOM: 100-02, 15, 50

◀ ▶ New   ←→ Revised   ✔ Reinstated   ✖ Deleted

⊕ **Special coverage instructions**   ◆ **Not covered or valid by Medicare**   ✳ **Carrier discretion**   〗 **ASC payment group**

→ ۞ **J9215)** Interferon, alfa-n3 (human leukocyte derived), **250,000 IU**

Other: Alferon N; Interferon alfa-n3 (human leukocyte derived)

IOM: 100-02, 15, 50

→ ۞ **J9216)** Injection, interferon, gamma-1B, **3 million units**

NDC: Actimmune

Other: Interferon gamma-1b

IOM: 100-02, 15, 50

۞ **J9217)** Leuprolide acetate (for depot suspension), **7.5 mg**

NDC: Lupon Depot; Lupon Depot-Ped, Eligard

Other: Leuprolide acetate (for depot suspension); Lupron

IOM: 100-02, 15, 50

۞ **J9218)** Leuprolide acetate, **per 1 mg**

NDC: Lupron

Other: Leuprolide acetate

IOM: 100-02, 15, 50

۞ **J9219)** Leuprolide acetate implant, **65 mg**

NDC: Viadur

Other: Lupron Implant; Leuprolide acetate implant

IOM: 100-02, 15, 50

۞ **J9225)** Histrelin implant (Vantas), **50 mg**

Other: Supprelin LA; Histrelin implant

IOM: 100-02, 15, 50

۞ **J9226)** Histrelin implant (Supprelin LA), **50 mg**

IOM: 100-02, 15, 50

→ ۞ **J9230)** Injection, mechlorethamine hydrochloride, (nitrogen mustard), **10 mg**

NDC: Mustargen

Other: Mechlorethamine HCl (nitrogen mustard, HN)

IOM: 100-02, 15, 50

۞ **J9245)** Injection, melphalan hydrochloride, **50 mg**

NDC: Alkeran

Other: L-phenylalanine mustard; Melphalan HCl

IOM: 100-02, 15, 50

۞ **J9250** Methotrexate sodium, **5 mg**

Other: Rheumatrex; Trexall, Methotrexate LPF, Folex, Folex PFS; Methotrexate sodium

IOM: 100-02, 15, 50

۞ **J9260** Methotrexate sodium, **50 mg**

Other: Rheumatrex; Trexall, Methotrexate LPF, Folex, Folex PFS; Methotrexate sodium

IOM: 100-02, 15, 50

✳ **J9261)** Injection, nelarabine, **50 mg**

NDC: Arranon

Other: Nelarabine

✳ **J9263)** Injection, oxaliplatin, **0.5 mg**

NDC: Eloxatin

Other: Oxaliplatin

✳ **J9264)** Injection, paclitaxel protein-bound particles, **1 mg**

NDC: Abraxane

Other: Paclitaxel protein-bound particles

→ ۞ **J9265)** Injection, paclitaxel, **30 mg**

NDC: Onxol; Taxol

Other: Nov-Onxol; Paclitaxel 30 mg

IOM: 100-02, 15, 50

→ ۞ **J9266)** Injection, pegaspargase, **per single dose vial**

NDC: Oncaspar

Other: Pegaspargase

IOM: 100-02, 15, 50

→ ۞ **J9268)** Injection, pentostatin, **10 mg**

NDC: Nipent

Other: Pentostatin

IOM: 100-02, 15, 50

→ ۞ **J9270)** Injection, plicamycin, **2.5 mg**

Other: Mithracin, Mithramycin, Plicamycin

IOM: 100-02, 15, 50

۞ **J9280)** Mitomycin, **5 mg**

NDC: Mutamycin

Other: Mitomycin

IOM: 100-02, 15, 50

۞ **J9290)** Mitomycin, **20 mg**

NDC: Mutamycin

Other: Mitomycin

IOM: 100-02, 15, 50

◄▶ **New**   ←→ **Revised**   ✔ **Reinstated**   ✖ **Deleted**

۞ **Special coverage instructions**   ◆ **Not covered or valid by Medicare**   ✳ **Carrier discretion**   ▶ **ASC payment group**

⊛ **J9291)** Mitomycin, **40 mg**
NDC: Mutamycin
Other: Mitomycin
IOM: 100-02, 15, 50

⊛ **J9293)** Injection, mitoxantrone hydrochloride, **per 5 mg**
NDC: Novantrone
Other: Mitoxantrone HCl
IOM: 100-02, 15, 50

→ ✳ **J9300)** Injection, gemtuzumab ozogamicin, **5 mg**
NDC: Mylotarg
Other: Gemtuzumab ozogamicin

✳ **J9303)** Injection, panitumumab, **10 mg**
Other: Vectibix; Panitumumab

✳ **J9305)** Injection, pemetrexed, **10 mg**
NDC: Alimta
Other: Pemetrexed

→ ⊛ **J9310)** Injection, rituximab, **100 mg**
NDC: RituXan
Other: Rituximab
IOM: 100-02, 15, 50

→ ⊛ **J9320)** Injection, streptozocin, **1 gram**
NDC: Zanosar
Other: Streptozocin
IOM: 100-02, 15, 50

▶ ✳ **J9330)** Injection, temsirolimus, **1 mg**

→ ⊛ **J9340)** Injection, thiotepa, **15 mg**
Other: Thioplex, Triethylenethosphoramide, Thiotepa
IOM: 100-02, 15, 50

→ ⊛ **J9350)** Injection, topotecan, **4 mg**
NDC: Hycamtin
Other: Topotecan
IOM: 100-02, 15, 50

→ ✳ **J9355)** Injection, trastuzumab, **10 mg**
NDC: Herceptin
Other: Trastuzumab

→ ⊛ **J9357)** Injection, valrubicin, intravesical, **200 mg**
Other: Valstar; Valrubicin (intravesical)
IOM: 100-02, 15, 50

→ ⊛ **J9360** Injection, vinblastine sulfate, **1 mg**
Other: Alkaban-AQ; Velban; Velsar; Vinblastine sulfate
IOM: 100-02, 15, 50

⊛ **J9370** Vincristine sulfate, **1 mg**
NDC: Vincasar PFS
Other: Oncovin; Vincristine sulfate
IOM: 100-02, 15, 50

⊛ **J9375** Vincristine sulfate, **2 mg**
NDC: Vincasar PFS
Other: Oncovin; Vincristine sulfate
IOM: 100-02, 15, 50

⊛ **J9380** Vincristine sulfate, **5 mg**
NDC: Vincasar PFS
Other: Oncovin; Vincristine sulfate
IOM: 100-02, 15, 50

→ ⊛ **J9390)** Injection, vinorelbine tartrate, **10 mg**
NDC: Navelbine
Other: Vinorelbine tartrate
IOM: 100-02, 15, 50

✳ **J9395)** Injection, fulvestrant, **25 mg**
NDC: Faslodex
Other: Fulvestrant

→ ⊛ **J9600)** Injection, porfimer sodium, **75 mg**
NDC: Photofrin
Other: Porfimer sodium
IOM: 100-02, 15, 50

⊛ **J9999** Not otherwise classified, antineoplastic drugs
Other: Allopurinol Sodium; Aloprim; Ifex/Mesnex; NOC drugs (antineoplastic)
(Bill on paper, bill one unit, and identify drug and total dosage in "Remarks" field. Include invoice of cost or NDC number in "Remarks" field.)
IOM: 100-02, 15, 50; 100-03, 2, 110.2

◀ ▶ New   ←→ Revised   ✔ Reinstated   ✖ Deleted

⊛ Special coverage instructions   ◆ Not covered or valid by Medicare   ✳ Carrier discretion   ▶ ASC payment group

210

TEMPORARY CODES ASSIGNED TO DME REGIONAL CARRIERS (K0000-K9999)

Wheelchairs and Accessories

NOTE: This section contains national codes assigned by CMS on a temporary basis and for the exclusive use of the durable medical equipment regional carriers (DMERC).

* ✳ **K0001**   Standard wheelchair
* ✳ **K0002**   Standard hemi (low seat) wheelchair
* ✳ **K0003**   Lightweight wheelchair
* ✳ **K0004**   High strength, lightweight wheelchair
* ✳ **K0005**   Ultralightweight wheelchair
* ✳ **K0006**   Heavy duty wheelchair
* ✳ **K0007**   Extra heavy duty wheelchair
* ✳ **K0009**   Other manual wheelchair/base
* ✳ **K0010**   Standard - weight frame motorized/power wheelchair
* ✳ **K0011**   Standard - weight frame motorized/power wheelchair with programmable control parameters for speed adjustment, tremor dampening, acceleration control and braking
* ✳ **K0012**   Lightweight portable motorized/power wheelchair
* ✳ **K0014**   Other motorized/power wheelchair base
* ✳ **K0015**   Detachable, non-adjustable height armrest, each
* ✳ **K0017**   Detachable, adjustable height armrest, base, each
* ✳ **K0018**   Detachable, adjustable height armrest, upper portion, each
* ✳ **K0019**   Arm pad, each
* ✳ **K0020**   Fixed, adjustable height armrest, pair
* ✳ **K0037**   High mount flip-up footrest, each
* ✳ **K0038**   Leg strap, each
* ✳ **K0039**   Leg strap, H style, each
* ✳ **K0040**   Adjustable angle footplate, each
* ✳ **K0041**   Large size footplate, each
* ✳ **K0042**   Standard size footplate, each
* ✳ **K0043**   Footrest, lower extension tube, each
* ✳ **K0044**   Footrest, upper hanger bracket, each
* ✳ **K0045**   Footrest, complete assembly
* ✳ **K0046**   Elevating legrest, lower extension tube, each
* ✳ **K0047**   Elevating legrest, upper hanger bracket, each
* ✳ **K0050**   Ratchet assembly

* ✳ **K0051**   Cam release assembly, footrest or legrests, each
* ✳ **K0052**   Swing-away, detachable footrests, each
* ✳ **K0053**   Elevating footrests, articulating (telescoping), each
* ✳ **K0056**   Seat height less than 17″ or equal to or greater than 21″ for a high strength, lightweight, or ultralightweight wheelchair
* ✳ **K0065**   Spoke protectors, each
* ✳ **K0069**   Rear wheel assembly, complete, with solid tire, spokes or molded, each
* ✳ **K0070**   Rear wheel assembly, complete, with pneumatic tire, spokes or molded, each
* ✳ **K0071**   Front caster assembly, complete, with pneumatic tire, each
* ✳ **K0072**   Front caster assembly, complete, with semi-pneumatic tire, each
* ✳ **K0073**   Caster pin lock, each
* ✳ **K0077**   Front caster assembly, complete, with solid tire, each
* ✳ **K0098**   Drive belt for power wheelchair
* ✳ **K0105**   IV hanger, each
* ✳ **K0108**   Wheelchair component or accessory, not otherwise specified
* ◎ **K0195**   Elevating leg rests, pair (for use with capped rental wheelchair base)
  IOM: 100-03, 4, 280.1
* ◎ **K0455**   Infusion pump used for uninterrupted parenteral administration of medication (e.g., epoprostenol or treprostinol)
  IOM: 100-03, 1, 50.3
* ◎ **K0462**   Temporary replacement for patient owned equipment being repaired, any type
  IOM: 100-04, 20, 40.1
* ◎ **K0552**   Supplies for external drug infusion pump, syringe type cartridge, sterile, each
  IOM: 100-03, 1, 50.3
* ✳ **K0601**   Replacement battery for external infusion pump owned by patient, silver oxide, 1.5 volt, each
* ✳ **K0602**   Replacement battery for external infusion pump owned by patient, silver oxide, 3 volt, each
* ✳ **K0603**   Replacement battery for external infusion pump owned by patient, alkaline, 1.5 volt, each

◀▶ New	←→ Revised	✔ Reinstated	✖ Deleted
◎ Special coverage instructions	◆ Not covered or valid by Medicare	✳ Carrier discretion	▶ ASC payment group

* **K0604** Replacement battery for external infusion pump owned by patient, lithium, 3.6 volt, each

* **K0605** Replacement battery for external infusion pump owned by patient, lithium, 4.5 volt, each

* **K0606** Automatic external defibrillator, with integrated electrocardiogram analysis, garment type

* **K0607** Replacement battery for automated external defibrillator, garment type only, each

* **K0608** Replacement garment for use with automated external defibrillator, each

* **K0609** Replacement electrodes for use with automated external defibrillator, garment type only, each

→ * **K0669** Wheelchair accessory, wheelchair seat or back cushion, does not meet specific code criteria or no written coding verification from DME PDAC

▶ * **K0672** Addition to lower extremity orthosis, removable soft interface, all components, replacement only, each

* **K0730** Controlled dose inhalation drug delivery system

* **K0733** Power wheelchair accessory, 12 to 24 amp hour sealed lead acid battery, each (e.g., gel cell, absorbed glassmat)

* **K0734** Skin protection wheelchair seat cushion, adjustable, width less than 22 inches, any depth

* **K0735** Skin protection wheelchair seat cushion, adjustable, width 22 inches or greater, any depth

* **K0736** Skin protection and positioning wheelchair seat cushion, adjustable, width less than 22 inches, any depth

* **K0737** Skin protection and positioning wheelchair seat cushion, adjustable, width 22 inches or greater, any depth

* **K0738** Portable gaseous oxygen system, rental; home compressor used to fill portable oxygen cylinders; includes portable containers, regulator, flowmeter, humidifier, cannula or mask, and tubing

* **K0800** Power operated vehicle, group 1 standard, patient weight capacity up to and including 300 pounds

* **K0801** Power operated vehicle, group 1 heavy duty, patient weight capacity 301 to 450 pounds

* **K0802** Power operated vehicle, group 1 very heavy duty, patient weight capacity 451 to 600 pounds

* **K0806** Power operated vehicle, group 2 standard, patient weight capacity up to and including 300 pounds

* **K0807** Power operated vehicle, group 2 heavy duty, patient weight capacity 301 to 450 pounds

* **K0808** Power operated vehicle, group 2 very heavy duty, patient weight capacity 451 to 600 pounds

* **K0812** Power operated vehicle, not otherwise classified

* **K0813** Power wheelchair, group 1 standard, portable, sling/solid seat and back, patient weight capacity up to and including 300 pounds

* **K0814** Power wheelchair, group 1 standard, portable, captains chair, patient weight capacity up to and including 300 pounds

* **K0815** Power wheelchair, group 1 standard, sling/solid seat and back, patient weight capacity up to and including 300 pounds

* **K0816** Power wheelchair, group 1 standard, captains chair, patient weight capacity up to and including 300 pounds

* **K0820** Power wheelchair, group 2 standard, portable, sling/solid seat/back, patient weight capacity up to and including 300 pounds

* **K0821** Power wheelchair, group 2 standard, portable, captains chair, patient weight capacity up to and including 300 pounds

* **K0822** Power wheelchair, group 2 standard, sling/solid seat/back, patient weight capacity up to and including 300 pounds

* **K0823** Power wheelchair, group 2 standard, captains chair, patient weight capacity up to and including 300 pounds

* **K0824** Power wheelchair, group 2 heavy duty, sling/solid seat/back, patient weight capacity 301 to 450 pounds

* **K0825** Power wheelchair, group 2 heavy duty, captains chair, patient weight capacity 301 to 450 pounds

* **K0826** Power wheelchair, group 2 very heavy duty, sling/solid seat/back, patient weight capacity 451 to 600 pounds

◀▶ New   ←→ Revised   ✔ Reinstated   ✖ Deleted

☉ Special coverage instructions   ◆ Not covered or valid by Medicare   * Carrier discretion   ▶ ASC payment group

＊ **K0827** Power wheelchair, group 2 very heavy duty, captains chair, patient weight capacity 451 to 600 pounds

＊ **K0828** Power wheelchair, group 2 extra heavy duty, sling/solid seat/back, patient weight capacity 601 pounds or more

＊ **K0829** Power wheelchair, group 2 extra heavy duty, captains chair, patient weight 601 pounds or more

＊ **K0830** Power wheelchair, group 2 standard, seat elevator, sling/solid seat/back, patient weight capacity up to and including 300 pounds

＊ **K0831** Power wheelchair, group 2 standard, seat elevator, captains chair, patient weight capacity up to and including 300 pounds

＊ **K0835** Power wheelchair, group 2 standard, single power option, sling/solid seat/back, patient weight capacity up to and including 300 pounds

＊ **K0836** Power wheelchair, group 2 standard, single power option, captains chair, patient weight capacity up to and including 300 pounds

＊ **K0837** Power wheelchair, group 2 heavy duty, single power option, sling/solid seat/back, patient weight capacity 301 to 450 pounds

＊ **K0838** Power wheelchair, group 2 heavy duty, single power option, captains chair, patient weight capacity 301 to 450 pounds

＊ **K0839** Power wheelchair, group 2 very heavy duty, single power option sling/solid seat/back, patient weight capacity 451 to 600 pounds

＊ **K0840** Power wheelchair, group 2 extra heavy duty, single power option, sling/solid seat/back, patient weight capacity 601 pounds or more

＊ **K0841** Power wheelchair, group 2 standard, multiple power option, sling/solid seat/back, patient weight capacity up to and including 300 pounds

＊ **K0842** Power wheelchair, group 2 standard, multiple power option, captains chair, patient weight capacity up to and including 300 pounds

＊ **K0843** Power wheelchair, group 2 heavy duty, multiple power option, sling/solid seat/back, patient weight capacity 301 to 450 pounds

＊ **K0848** Power wheelchair, group 3 standard, sling/solid seat/back, patient weight capacity up to and including 300 pounds

＊ **K0849** Power wheelchair, group 3 standard, captains chair, patient weight capacity up to and including 300 pounds

＊ **K0850** Power wheelchair, group 3 heavy duty, sling/solid seat/back, patient weight capacity 301 to 450 pounds

＊ **K0851** Power wheelchair, group 3 heavy duty, captains chair, patient weight capacity 301 to 450 pounds

＊ **K0852** Power wheelchair, group 3 very heavy duty, sling/solid seat/back, patient weight capacity 451 to 600 pounds

＊ **K0853** Power wheelchair, group 3 very heavy duty, captains chair, patient weight capacity 451 to 600 pounds

＊ **K0854** Power wheelchair, group 3 extra heavy duty, sling/solid seat/back, patient weight capacity 601 pounds or more

＊ **K0855** Power wheelchair, group 3 extra heavy duty, captains chair, patient weight capacity 601 pounds or more

＊ **K0856** Power wheelchair, group 3 standard, single power option, sling/solid seat/back, patient weight capacity up to and including 300 pounds

＊ **K0857** Power wheelchair, group 3 standard, single power option, captains chair, patient weight capacity up to and including 300 pounds

＊ **K0858** Power wheelchair, group 3 heavy duty, single power option, sling/solid seat/back, patient weight 301 to 450 pounds

＊ **K0859** Power wheelchair, group 3 heavy duty, single power option, captains chair, patient weight capacity 301 to 450 pounds

＊ **K0860** Power wheelchair, group 3 very heavy duty, single power option, sling/solid seat/back, patient weight capacity 451 to 600 pounds

＊ **K0861** Power wheelchair, group 3 standard, multiple power option, sling/solid seat/back, patient weight capacity up to and including 300 pounds

＊ **K0862** Power wheelchair, group 3 heavy duty, multiple power option, sling/solid seat/back, patient weight capacity 301 to 450 pounds

＊ **K0863** Power wheelchair, group 3 very heavy duty, multiple power option, sling/solid seat/back, patient weight capacity 451 to 600 pounds

＊ **K0864** Power wheelchair, group 3 extra heavy duty, multiple power option, sling/solid seat/back, patient weight capacity 601 pounds or more

◀▶ New   ←→ Revised   ✔ Reinstated   ✖ Deleted

⊙ Special coverage instructions   ◆ Not covered or valid by Medicare   ＊ Carrier discretion   ▶ ASC payment group

* **K0868** Power wheelchair, group 4 standard, sling/solid seat/back, patient weight capacity up to and including 300 pounds

* **K0869** Power wheelchair, group 4 standard, captains chair, patient weight capacity up to and including 300 pounds

* **K0870** Power wheelchair, group 4 heavy duty, sling/solid seat/back, patient weight capacity 301 to 450 pounds

* **K0871** Power wheelchair, group 4 very heavy duty, sling/solid seat/back, patient weight capacity 451 to 600 pounds

* **K0877** Power wheelchair, group 4 standard, single power option, sling/solid seat/back, patient weight capacity up to and including 300 pounds

* **K0878** Power wheelchair, group 4 standard, single power option, captains chair, patient weight capacity up to and including 300 pounds

* **K0879** Power wheelchair, group 4 heavy duty, single power option, sling/solid seat/back, patient weight capacity 301 to 450 pounds

* **K0880** Power wheelchair, group 4 very heavy duty, single power option, sling/solid seat/back, patient weight 451 to 600 pounds

* **K0884** Power wheelchair, group 4 standard, multiple power option, sling/solid seat/back, patient weight capacity up to and including 300 pounds

* **K0885** Power wheelchair, group 4 standard, multiple power option, captains chair, patient weight capacity up to and including 300 pounds

* **K0886** Power wheelchair, group 4 heavy duty, multiple power option, sling/solid seat/back, patient weight capacity 301 to 450 pounds

* **K0890** Power wheelchair, group 5 pediatric, single power option, sling/solid seat/back, patient weight capacity up to and including 125 pounds

* **K0891** Power wheelchair, group 5 pediatric, multiple power option, sling/solid seat/back, patient weight capacity up to and including 125 pounds

* **K0898** Power wheelchair, not otherwise classified

→ * **K0899** Power mobility device, not coded by DME PDAC or does not meet criteria

◄▶ New   ←→ Revised   ✔ Reinstated   ✖ Deleted
☺ Special coverage instructions   ◆ Not covered or valid by Medicare   ✳ Carrier discretion   ▶ ASC payment group

ORTHOTICS (L0100-L4999)

Orthotic Devices: Spinal

Cervical

❋ **L0112** Cranial cervical orthosis, congenital torticollis type, with or without soft interface material, adjustable range of motion joint, custom fabricated

▶ ❋ **L0113** Cranial cervical orthosis, torticollis type, with or without joint, with or without soft interface material, prefabricated, includes fitting and adjustment

❋ **L0120** Cervical, flexible, non-adjustable (foam collar)

❋ **L0130** Cervical, flexible, thermoplastic collar, molded to patient

❋ **L0140** Cervical, semi-rigid, adjustable (plastic collar)

❋ **L0150** Cervical, semi-rigid, adjustable molded chin cup (plastic collar with mandibular/occipital piece)

❋ **L0160** Cervical, semi-rigid, wire frame occipital/mandibular support

❋ **L0170** Cervical, collar, molded to patient model

❋ **L0172** Cervical, collar, semi-rigid thermoplastic foam, two piece

❋ **L0174** Cervical, collar, semi-rigid, thermoplastic foam, two piece with thoracic extension

Multiple Post Collar

❋ **L0180** Cervical, multiple post collar, occipital/mandibular supports, adjustable

❋ **L0190** Cervical, multiple post collar, occipital/mandibular supports, adjustable cervical bars (SOMI, Guilford, Taylor types)

❋ **L0200** Cervical, multiple post collar, occipital/mandibular supports, adjustable cervical bars, and thoracic extension

Thoracic

❋ **L0210** Thoracic, rib belt

❋ **L0220** Thoracic, rib belt, custom fabricated

Thoracic-Lumbar-Sacral

Anterior-Posterior-Lateral Rotary-Control

❋ **L0430** Spinal orthosis, anterior-posterior-lateral control, with interface material, custom fitted (Dewall posture protector only)

❋ **L0450** TLSO, flexible, provides trunk support, upper thoracic region, produces intracavitary pressure to reduce load on the intevertebral disks with rigid stays or panel(s), includes shoulder straps and closures, prefabricated, includes fitting and adjustment

❋ **L0452** TLSO, flexible, provides trunk support, upper thoracic region, produces intracavitary pressure to reduce load on the intervertebral disks with rigid stays or panel(s), includes shoulder straps and closures, custom fabricated

❋ **L0454** TLSO flexible, provides trunk support, extends from sacrococcygeal junction to above T-9 vertebra, restricts gross trunk motion in the sagittal plane, produces intracavitary pressure to reduce load on the intervertebral disks with rigid stays or panel(s), includes shoulder straps and closures, prefabricated, includes fitting and adjustment

❋ **L0456** TLSO, flexible, provides trunk support, thoracic region, rigid posterior panel and soft anterior apron, extends from the sacrococcygeal junction and terminates just inferior to the scapular spine, restricts gross trunk motion in the sagittal plane, produces intracavitary pressure to reduce load on the intervertebral disks, includes straps and closures, prefabricated, includes fitting and adjustment

❋ **L0458** TLSO, triplanar control, modular segmented spinal system, two rigid plastic shells, posterior extends from the sacrococcygeal junction and terminates just inferior to the scapular spine, anterior extends from the symphysis pubis to the xiphoid, soft liner, restricts gross trunk motion in the sagittal, coronal, and transverse planes, lateral strength is provided by overlapping plastic and stabilizing closures, includes straps and closures, prefabricated, includes fitting and adjustment

* **L0460** TLSO, triplanar control, modular segmented spinal system, two rigid plastic shells, posterior extends from the sacrococcygeal junction and terminates just inferior to the scapular spine, anterior extends from the symphysis pubis to the sternal notch, soft liner, restricts gross trunk motion in the sagittal, coronal, and transverse planes, lateral strength is provided by overlapping plastic and stabilizing closures, includes straps and closures, prefabricated, includes fitting and adjustment

* **L0462** TLSO, triplanar control, modular segmented spinal system, three rigid plastic shells, posterior extends from the sacrococcygeal junction and terminates just inferior to the scapular spine, anterior extends from the symphysis pubis to the sternal notch, soft liner, restricts gross trunk motion in the sagittal, coronal, and transverse planes, lateral strength is provided by overlapping plastic and stabilizing closures, includes straps and closures, prefabricated, includes fitting and adjustment

* **L0464** TLSO, triplanar control, modular segmented spinal system, four rigid plastic shells, posterior extends from sacrococcygeal junction and terminates just inferior to scapular spine, anterior extends from symphysis pubis to the sternal notch, soft liner, restricts gross trunk motion in sagittal, coronal, and transverse planes, lateral strength is provided by overlapping plastic and stabilizing closures, includes straps and closures, prefabricated, includes fitting and adjustment

* **L0466** TLSO, sagittal control, rigid posterior frame and flexible soft anterior apron with straps, closures and padding, restricts gross trunk motion in sagittal plane, produces intracavitary pressure to reduce load on intervertebral disks, includes fitting and shaping the frame, prefabricated, includes fitting and adjustment

* **L0468** TLSO, sagittal-coronal control, rigid posterior frame and flexible soft anterior apron with straps, closures and padding, extends from sacrococcygeal junction over scapulae, lateral strength provided by pelvic, thoracic, and lateral frame pieces, restricts gross trunk motion in sagittal, and coronal planes, produces intracavitary pressure to reduce load on intervertebral disks, includes fitting and shaping the frame, prefabricated, includes fitting and adjustment

* **L0470** TLSO, triplanar control, rigid posterior frame and flexible soft anterior apron with straps, closures and padding, extends from sacrococcygeal junction to scapula, lateral strength provided by pelvic, thoracic, and lateral frame pieces, rotational strength provided by subclavicular extensions, restricts gross trunk motion in sagittal, coronal, and transverse planes, produces intracavitary pressure to reduce load on the intervertebral disks, includes fitting and shaping the frame, prefabricated, includes fitting and adjustment

* **L0472** TLSO, triplanar control, hyperextension, rigid anterior and lateral frame extends from symphysis pubis to sternal notch with two anterior components (one pubic and one sternal), posterior and lateral pads with straps and closures, limits spinal flexion, restricts gross trunk motion in sagittal, coronal, and transverse planes, includes fitting and shaping the frame, prefabricated, includes fitting and adjustment

* **L0480** TLSO, triplanar control, one piece rigid plastic shell without interface liner, with multiple straps and closures, posterior extends from sacrococcygeal junction and terminates just inferior to scapular spine, anterior extends from symphysis pubis to sternal notch, anterior or posterior opening, restricts gross trunk motion in sagittal, coronal, and transverse planes, includes a carved plaster or CAD-CAM model, custom fabricated

◀ ▶ **New**   ← → **Revised**   ✔ **Reinstated**   ✖ **Deleted**

⊙ **Special coverage instructions**   ◆ **Not covered or valid by Medicare**   ✳ **Carrier discretion**   ▶ **ASC payment group**

* **L0482** TLSO, triplanar control, one piece rigid plastic shell with interface liner, multiple straps and closures, posterior extends from sacrococcygeal junction and terminates just inferior to scapular spine, anterior extends from symphysis pubis to sternal notch, anterior or posterior opening, restricts gross trunk motion in sagittal, coronal, and transverse planes, includes a carved plaster or CAD-CAM model, custom fabricated

* **L0484** TLSO, triplanar control, two piece rigid plastic shell without interface liner, with multiple straps and closures, posterior extends from sacrococcygeal junction and terminates just inferior to scapular spine, anterior extends from symphysis pubis to sternal notch, lateral strength is enhanced by overlapping plastic, restricts gross trunk motion in the sagittal, coronal, and transverse planes, includes a carved plaster or CAD-CAM model, custom fabricated

* **L0486** TLSO, triplanar control, two piece rigid plastic shell with interface liner, multiple straps and closures, posterior extends from sacrococcygeal junction and terminates just inferior to scapular spine, anterior extends from symphysis pubis to sternal notch, lateral strength is enhanced by overlapping plastic, restricts gross trunk motion in the sagittal, coronal, and transverse planes, includes a carved plaster or CAD-CAM model, custom fabricated

* **L0488** TLSO, triplanar control, one piece rigid plastic shell with interface liner, multiple straps and closures, posterior extends from sacrococcygeal junction and terminates just inferior to scapular spine, anterior extends from symphysis pubis to sternal notch, anterior or posterior opening, restricts gross trunk motion in sagittal, coronal, and transverse planes, prefabricated, includes fitting and adjustment

* **L0490** TLSO, sagittal-coronal control, one piece rigid plastic shell, with overlapping reinforced anterior, with multiple straps and closures, posterior extends from sacrococcygeal junction and terminates at or before the T-9 vertebra, anterior extends from symphysis pubis to xiphoid, anterior opening, restricts gross trunk motion in sagittal and coronal planes, prefabricated, includes fitting and adjustment

* **L0491** TLSO, sagittal-coronal control, modular segmented spinal system, two rigid plastic shells, posterior extends from the sacrococcygeal junction and terminates just inferior to the scapular spine, anterior extends from the symphysis pubis to the xiphoid, soft liner, restricts gross trunk motion in the sagittal and coronal planes, lateral strength is provided by overlapping plastic and stabilizing closures, includes straps and closures, prefabricated, includes fitting and adjustment

* **L0492** TLSO, sagittal-coronal control, modular segmented spinal system, three rigid plastic shells, posterior extends from the sacrococcygeal junction and terminates just inferior to the scapular spine, anterior extends from the symphysis pubis to the xiphoid, soft liner, restricts gross trunk motion in the sagittal and coronal planes, lateral strength is provided by overlapping plastic and stabilizing closures, includes straps and closures, prefabricated, includes fitting and adjustment

Sacroilliac, Lumbar, Sacral Orthosis

* **L0621** Sacroiliac orthosis, flexible, provides pelvic-sacral support, reduces motion about the sacroiliac joint, includes straps, closures, may include pendulous abdomen design, prefabricated, includes fitting and adjustment

* **L0622** Sacroiliac orthosis, flexible, provides pelvic-sacral support, reduces motion about the sacroiliac joint, includes straps, closures, may include pendulous abdomen design, custom fabricated

* **L0623** Sacroiliac orthosis, provides pelvic-sacral support, with rigid or semi-rigid panels over the sacrum and abdomen, reduces motion about the sacroiliac joint, includes straps, closures, may include pendulous abdomen design, prefabricated, includes fitting and adjustment

* **L0624** Sacroiliac orthosis, provides pelvic-sacral support, with rigid or semi-rigid panels placed over the sacrum and abdomen, reduces motion about the sacroiliac joint, includes straps, closures, may include pendulous abdomen design, custom fabricated

* **L0625** Lumbar orthosis, flexible, provides lumbar support, posterior extends from L-1 to below L-5 vertebra, produces intracavitary pressure to reduce load on the intervertebral discs, includes straps, closures, may include pendulous abdomen design, shoulder straps, stays, prefabricated, includes fitting and adjustment

* **L0626** Lumbar orthosis, sagittal control, with rigid posterior panel(s), posterior extends from L-1 to below L-5 vertebra, produces intracavitary pressure to reduce load on the intervertebral discs, includes straps, closures, may include padding, stays, shoulder straps, pendulous abdomen design, prefabricated, includes fitting and adjustment

* **L0627** Lumbar orthosis, sagittal control, with rigid anterior and posterior panels, posterior extends from L-1 to below L-5 vertebra, produces intracavitary pressure to reduce load on the intervertebral discs, includes straps, closures, may include padding, shoulder straps, pendulous abdomen design, prefabricated, includes fitting and adjustment

* **L0628** Lumbar-sacral orthosis, flexible, provides lumbo-sacral support, posterior extends from sacrococcygeal junction to T-9 vertebra, produces intracavitary pressure to reduce load on the intervertebral discs, includes straps, closures, may include stays, shoulder straps, pendulous abdomen design, prefabricated, includes fitting and adjustment

* **L0629** Lumbar-sacral orthosis, flexible, provides lumbo-sacral support, posterior extends from sacrococcygeal junction to T-9 vertebra, produces intracavitary pressure to reduce load on the intervertebral discs, includes straps, closures, may include stays, shoulder straps, pendulous abdomen design, custom fabricated

* **L0630** Lumbar-sacral orthosis, sagittal control, with rigid posterior panel(s), posterior extends from sacrococcygeal junction to T-9 vertebra, produces intracavitary pressure to reduce load on the intervertebral discs, includes straps, closures, may include padding, stays, shoulder straps, pendulous abdomen design, prefabricated, includes fitting and adjustment

* **L0631** Lumbar-sacral orthosis, sagittal control, with rigid anterior and posterior panels, posterior extends from sacrococcygeal junction to T-9 vertebra, produces intracavitary pressure to reduce load on the intervertebral discs, includes straps, closures, may include padding, shoulder straps, pendulous abdomen design, prefabricated, includes fitting and adjustment

* **L0632** Lumbar-sacral orthosis, sagittal control, with rigid anterior and posterior panels, posterior extends from sacrococcygeal junction to T-9 vertebra, produces intracavitary pressure to reduce load on the intervertebral discs, includes straps, closures, may include padding, shoulder straps, pendulous abdomen design, custom fabricated

* **L0633** Lumbar-sacral orthosis, sagittal-coronal control, with rigid posterior frame/panel(s), posterior extends from sacrococcygeal junction to T-9 vertebra, lateral strength provided by rigid lateral frame/panels, produces intracavitary pressure to reduce load on intervertebral discs, includes straps, closures, may include padding, stays, shoulder straps, pendulous abdomen design, prefabricated, includes fitting and adjustment

* **L0634** Lumbar-sacral orthosis, sagittal-coronal control, with rigid posterior frame/panel(s), posterior extends from sacrococcygeal junction to T-9 vertebra, lateral strength provided by rigid lateral frame/panel(s), produces intracavitary pressure to reduce load on intervertebral discs, includes straps, closures, may include padding, stays, shoulder straps, pendulous abdomen design, custom fabricated

* **L0635** Lumbar-sacral orthosis, sagittal-coronal control, lumbar flexion, rigid posterior frame/panel(s), lateral articulating design to flex the lumbar spine, posterior extends from sacrococcygeal junction to T-9 vertebra, lateral strength provided by rigid lateral frame/panel(s), produces intracavitary pressure to reduce load on intervertebral discs, includes straps, closures, may include padding, anterior panel, pendulous abdomen design, prefabricated, includes fitting and adjustment

◄▶ New ←→ Revised ✔ Reinstated ✖ Deleted

○ Special coverage instructions ◆ Not covered or valid by Medicare * Carrier discretion ▶ ASC payment group

* **L0636** Lumbar sacral orthosis, sagittal-coronal control, lumbar flexion, rigid posterior frame/panels, lateral articulating design to flex the lumbar spine, posterior extends from sacrococcygeal junction to T-9 vertebra, lateral strength provided by rigid lateral frame/panels, produces intracavitary pressure to reduce load on intervertebral discs, includes straps, closures, may include padding, anterior panel, pendulous abdomen design, custom fabricated

* **L0637** Lumbar-sacral orthosis, sagittal-coronal control, with rigid anterior and posterior frame/panels, posterior extends from sacrococcygeal junction to T-9 vertebra, lateral strength provided by rigid lateral frame/panels, produces intracavitary pressure to reduce load on intervertebral discs, includes straps, closures, may include padding, shoulder straps, pendulous abdomen design, prefabricated, includes fitting and adjustment

* **L0638** Lumbar-sacral orthosis, sagittal-coronal control, with rigid anterior and posterior frame/panels, posterior extends from sacrococcygeal junction to T-9 vertebra, lateral strength provided by rigid lateral frame/panels, produces intracavitary pressure to reduce load on intervertebral discs, includes straps, closures, may include padding, shoulder straps, pendulous abdomen design, custom fabricated

* **L0639** Lumbar-sacral orthosis, sagittal-coronal control, rigid shell(s)/panel(s), posterior extends from sacrococcygeal junction to T-9 vertebra, anterior extends from symphysis pubis to xyphoid, produces intracavitary pressure to reduce load on the intervertebral discs, overall strength is provided by overlapping rigid material and stabilizing closures, includes straps, closures may include soft interface, pendulous abdomen design, prefabricated, includes fitting and adjustment

* **L0640** Lumbar-sacral orthosis, sagittal-coronal control, rigid shell(s)/panel(s), posterior extends from sacrococcygeal junction to T-9 vertebra, anterior extends from symphysis pubis to xyphoid, produces intracavitary pressure to reduce load on the intervertebral discs, overall strength is provided by overlapping rigid material and stabilizing closures, includes straps, closures, may include soft interface, pendulous abdomen design, custom fabricated

Cervical-Thoracic-Lumbar-Sacral

Anterior-Posterior-Lateral Control

* **L0700** Cervical-thoracic-lumbar-sacral-orthoses (CTLSO), anterior-posterior-lateral control, molded to patient model, (Minerva type)

* **L0710** CTLSO, anterior-posterior-lateral-control, molded to patient model, with interface material, (Minerva type)

HALO Procedure

* **L0810** HALO procedure, cervical halo incorporated into jacket vest

* **L0820** HALO procedure, cervical halo incorporated into plaster body jacket

* **L0830** HALO procedure, cervical halo incorporated into Milwaukee type orthosis

* **L0859** Addition to HALO procedure, magnetic resonance image compatible systems, rings and pins, any material

* **L0861** Addition to HALO procedure, replacement liner/interface material

Additions to Spinal Orthoses

* **L0970** TLSO, corset front
* **L0972** LSO, corset front
* **L0974** TLSO, full corset
* **L0976** LSO, full corset
* **L0978** Axillary crutch extension
* **L0980** Peroneal straps, pair
* **L0982** Stocking supporter grips, set of four (4)
* **L0984** Protective body sock, each
* **L0999** Addition to spinal orthosis, not otherwise specified

---

◀▶ New   ←→ Revised   ✔ Reinstated   ✖ Deleted
☉ Special coverage instructions   ◆ Not covered or valid by Medicare   ✳ Carrier discretion   ▶ ASC payment group

Orthotic Devices: Scoliosis Procedures (L1000-L1499)

NOTE: Orthotic care of scoliosis differs from other orthotic care in that the treatment is more dynamic in nature and uses ongoing continual modification of the orthosis to the patient's changing condition. This coding structure uses the proper names, or eponyms, of the procedures because they have historic and universal acceptance in the profession. It should be recognized that variations to the basic procedures described by the founders/developers are accepted in various medical and orthotic practices throughout the country. All procedures include a model of patient when indicated.

Scoliosis: Cervical-Thoracic-Lumbar-Sacral (CTLSO) (Milwaukee)

* **L1000**   Cervical-thoracic-lumbar-sacral orthosis (CTLSO) (Milwaukee), inclusive of furnishing initial orthosis, including model

* **L1001**   Cervical thoracic lumbar sacral orthosis, immobilizer, infant size, prefabricated, includes fitting and adjustment

* **L1005**   Tension based scoliosis orthosis and accessory pads, includes fitting and adjustment

* **L1010**   Addition to cervical-thoracic-lumbar-sacral orthosis (CTLSO) or scoliosis orthosis, axilla sling

Correction Pads

* **L1020**   Addition to CTLSO or scoliosis orthosis, kyphosis pad

* **L1025**   Addition to CTLSO or scoliosis orthosis, kyphosis pad, floating

* **L1030**   Addition to CTLSO or scoliosis orthosis, lumbar bolster pad

* **L1040**   Addition to CTLSO or scoliosis orthosis, lumbar or lumbar rib pad

* **L1050**   Addition to CTLSO or scoliosis orthosis, sternal pad

* **L1060**   Addition to CTLSO or scoliosis orthosis, thoracic pad

* **L1070**   Addition to CTLSO or scoliosis orthosis, trapezius sling

* **L1080**   Addition to CTLSO or scoliosis orthosis, outrigger

* **L1085**   Addition to CTLSO or scoliosis orthosis, outrigger, bilateral with vertical extensions

* **L1090**   Addition to CTLSO or scoliosis orthosis, lumbar sling

* **L1100**   Addition to CTLSO or scoliosis orthosis, ring flange, plastic or leather

* **L1110**   Addition to CTLSO or scoliosis orthosis, ring flange, plastic or leather, molded to patient model

* **L1120**   Addition to CTLSO, scoliosis orthosis, cover for upright, each

Scoliosis: Thoracic-Lumbar-Sacral (Low Profile)

* **L1200**   Thoracic-lumbar-sacral-orthosis (TLSO), inclusive of furnishing initial orthosis only

* **L1210**   Addition to TLSO, (low profile), lateral thoracic extension

* **L1220**   Addition to TLSO, (low profile), anterior thoracic extension

* **L1230**   Addition to TLSO, (low profile), Milwaukee type superstructure

* **L1240**   Addition to TLSO, (low profile), lumbar derotation pad

* **L1250**   Addition to TLSO, (low profile), anterior ASIS pad

* **L1260**   Addition to TLSO, (low profile), anterior thoracic derotation pad

* **L1270**   Addition to TLSO, (low profile), abdominal pad

* **L1280**   Addition to TLSO, (low profile), rib gusset (elastic), each

* **L1290**   Addition to TLSO, (low profile), lateral trochanteric pad

Other Scoliosis Procedures

* **L1300**   Other scoliosis procedure, body jacket molded to patient model

* **L1310**   Other scoliosis procedure, postoperative body jacket

* **L1499**   Spinal orthosis, not otherwise specified

Scoliosis: Thoracic-Hip-Knee-Ankle (THKA)

* **L1500**   Thoracic-hip-knee-ankle orthosis (THKAO), mobility frame (Newington, Parapodium types)

◀▶ New   ←→ Revised   ✔ Reinstated   ✖ Deleted

☺ Special coverage instructions   ◆ Not covered or valid by Medicare   * Carrier discretion   ▶ ASC payment group

＊ **L1510**   THKAO, standing frame, with or without tray and accessories

＊ **L1520**   THKAO, swivel walker

Orthotic Devices: Lower Limb

NOTE: the procedures in L1600-L2999 are considered as *base* or *basic procedures* and may be modified by listing procedure from the Additions Sections and adding them to the base procedure.

Hip: Flexible

＊ **L1600**   Hip orthosis (HO), abduction control of hip joints, flexible, Frejka type with cover, prefabricated, includes fitting and adjustment

＊ **L1610**   Hip orthosis, abduction control of hip joints, flexible, (Frejka cover only) prefabricated, includes fitting and adjustment

＊ **L1620**   Hip orthosis, abduction control of hip joints, flexible, (Pavlik harness), prefabricated, includes fitting and adjustment

＊ **L1630**   Hip orthosis, abduction control of hip joints, semi-flexible (Von Rosen type), custom-fabricated

＊ **L1640**   Hip orthosis, abduction control of hip joints, static, pelvic band or spreader bar, thigh cuffs, custom-fabricated

＊ **L1650**   Hip orthosis, abduction control of hip joints, static, adjustable, (Ilfled type), prefabricated, includes fitting and adjustment

＊ **L1652**   Hip orthosis, bilateral thigh cuffs with adjustable abductor spreader bar, adult size, prefabricated, includes fitting and adjustment, any type

＊ **L1660**   Hip orthosis, abduction control of hip joints, static, plastic, prefabricated, includes fitting and adjustment

＊ **L1680**   Hip orthosis, abduction control of hip joints, dynamic, pelvic control, adjustable hip motion control, thigh cuffs (Rancho hip action type), custom fabrication

＊ **L1685**   Hip orthosis, abduction control of hip joint, postoperative hip abduction type, custom fabricated

＊ **L1686**   Hip orthosis, abduction control of hip joint, postoperative hip abduction type, prefabricated, includes fitting and adjustment

＊ **L1690**   Combination, bilateral, lumbo-sacral, hip, femur orthosis providing adduction and internal rotation control, prefabricated, includes fitting and adjustment

Legg Perthes

＊ **L1700**   Legg-Perthes orthosis, (Toronto type), custom-fabricated

＊ **L1710**   Legg-Perthes orthosis, (Newington type), custom-fabricated

＊ **L1720**   Legg-Perthes orthosis, trilateral, (Tachdjian type), custom-fabricated

＊ **L1730**   Legg-Perthes orthosis, (Scottish Rite type), custom-fabricated

＊ **L1755**   Legg-Perthes orthosis, (Patten bottom type), custom-fabricated

Knee (KO)

＊ **L1800**   Knee orthosis (KO), elastic with stays, prefabricated, includes fitting and adjustment

＊ **L1810**   Knee orthosis, elastic with joints, prefabricated, includes fitting and adjustment

＊ **L1815**   Knee orthosis, elastic or other elastic type material with condylar pad(s), prefabricated, includes fitting and adjustment

＊ **L1820**   Knee orthosis, elastic with condylar pads and joints, with or without patellar control, prefabricated, includes fitting and adjustment

＊ **L1825**   Knee orthosis, elastic kneecap, prefabricated, includes fitting and adjustment

＊ **L1830**   Knee orthosis, immobilizer, canvas longitudinal, prefabricated, includes fitting and adjustment

＊ **L1831**   Knee orthosis, locking knee joint(s), positional orthosis, prefabricated, includes fitting and adjustment

＊ **L1832**   Knee orthrosis, adjustable knee joints (unicentric or polycentric), positional orthosis, rigid support, prefabricated, includes fitting and adjustment

＊ **L1834**   Knee orthosis, without knee joint, rigid, custom-fabricated

---

◀▶ New   ←→ Revised   ✔ Reinstated   ✖ Deleted

⊙ Special coverage instructions   ◆ Not covered or valid by Medicare   ＊ Carrier discretion   ▶ ASC payment group

✳ **L1836** Knee orthosis, rigid, without joint(s), includes soft interface material, prefabricated, includes fitting and adjustment

✳ **L1840** Knee orthosis, derotation, medial-lateral, anterior cruciate ligament, custom fabricated

✳ **L1843** Knee orthosis, single upright, thigh and calf, with adjustable flexion and extension joint (unicentric or polycentric), medial-lateral and rotation control, with or without varus/valgus adjustment; prefabricated, includes fitting and adjustment

✳ **L1844** Knee orthosis, single upright, thigh and calf, with adjustable flexion and extension joint (unicentric or polycentric), medial-lateral and rotation control, with or without varus/valgus adjustment, custom fabricated

✳ **L1845** Knee orthrosis, double upright, thigh and calf, with adjustable flexion and extension joint (unicentric or polycentric), medial-lateral and rotation control, with or without varus/valgus adjustment, prefabricated, includes fitting and adjustment

✳ **L1846** Knee orthrosis, double upright, thigh and calf, with adjustable flexion and extension joint (unicentric or polycentric), medial-lateral and rotation control, with or without varus/valgus adjustment, custom fabricated

✳ **L1847** Knee orthosis, double upright with adjustable joint, with inflatable air support chambers, prefabricated, includes fitting and adjustment

✳ **L1850** Knee orthosis, Swedish type, prefabricated, includes fitting and adjustment

✳ **L1860** Knee orthosis, modification of supracondylar prosthetic socket, custom fabricated (SK)

Ankle-Foot (AFO)

✳ **L1900** Ankle foot orthosis (AFO), spring wire, dorsiflexion assist calf band, custom-fabricated

✳ **L1901** Ankle orthosis, elastic, prefabricated, includes fitting and adjustment (e.g. neoprene, Lycra)

✳ **L1902** Ankle foot orthosis, ankle gauntlet, prefabricated, includes fitting and adjustment

✳ **L1904** Ankle foot orthosis, molded ankle gauntlet, custom-fabricated

✳ **L1906** Ankle-foot orthosis, multiligamentus ankle support, prefabricated, includes fitting and adjustment

✳ **L1907** AFO, supramalleolar with straps, with or without interface/pads, custom fabricated

✳ **L1910** Ankle foot orthosis, posterior, single bar, clasp attachment to shoe counter, prefabricated, includes fitting and adjustment

✳ **L1920** Ankle foot orthosis, single upright with static or adjustable stop (Phelps or Perlstein type), custom-fabricated

✳ **L1930** Ankle-foot orthosis, plastic or other material, prefabricated, includes fitting and adjustment

✳ **L1932** AFO, rigid anterior tibial section, total carbon fiber or equal material, prefabricated, includes fitting and adjustment

✳ **L1940** Ankle foot orthosis, plastic or other material, custom-fabricated

✳ **L1945** Ankle foot orthosis, plastic, rigid anterior tibial section (floor reaction), custom-fabricated

✳ **L1950** Ankle foot orthosis, spiral, (Institute of Rehabilitation Medicine type), plastic, custom-fabricated

✳ **L1951** Ankle foot orthosis, spiral, (Institute of Rehabilitative Medicine type), plastic or other material, prefabricated, includes fitting and adjustment

✳ **L1960** Ankle foot orthosis, posterior solid ankle, plastic, custom-fabricated

✳ **L1970** Ankle foot orthosis, plastic, with ankle joint, custom-fabricated

✳ **L1971** Ankle foot orthosis, plastic or other material with ankle joint, prefabricated, includes fitting and adjustment

✳ **L1980** Ankle foot orthosis, single upright free plantar dorsiflexion, solid stirrup, calf band/cuff (single bar 'BK' orthosis), custom-fabricated

✳ **L1990** Ankle foot orthosis, double upright free plantar dorsiflexion, solid stirrup, calf band/cuff (double bar 'BK' orthosis), custom-fabricated

◄▶ New   ←→ Revised   ✔ Reinstated   ✘ Deleted

☺ Special coverage instructions   ◆ Not covered or valid by Medicare   ✳ Carrier discretion   ▶ ASC payment group

Hip-Knee-Ankle-Foot (or Any Combination)

NOTE: L2000, L2020, and L2036 are base procedures to be used with any knee joint. L2010 and L2030 are to be used only with no knee joint.

✳ **L2000** Knee ankle foot orthosis, single upright, free knee, free ankle, solid stirrup, thigh and calf bands/cuffs (single bar 'AK' orthosis), custom-fabricated

✳ **L2005** Knee ankle foot orthosis, any material, single or double upright, stance control, automatic lock and swing phase release, mechanical activation; includes ankle joint, any type, custom fabricated

✳ **L2010** Knee ankle foot orthosis, single upright, free ankle, solid stirrup, thigh and calf bands/cuffs (single bar 'AK' orthosis), without knee joint, custom-fabricated

✳ **L2020** Knee ankle foot orthosis, double upright, free knee, free ankle, solid stirrup, thigh and calf bands/cuffs (double bar 'AK' orthosis), custom-fabricated

✳ **L2030** Knee ankle foot orthosis, double upright, free ankle, solid stirrup, thigh and calf bands/cuffs (double bar 'AK' orthosis), without knee joint, custom fabricated

✳ **L2034** Knee ankle foot orthosis, full plastic, single upright, with or without free motion knee, medial lateral rotation control, with or without free motion ankle, custom fabricated

✳ **L2035** Knee ankle foot orthosis, full plastic, static (pediatric size), without free motion ankle, prefabricated, includes fitting and adjustment

✳ **L2036** Knee ankle foot orthosis, full plastic, double upright, with or without free motion knee, with or without free motion ankle, custom fabricated

✳ **L2037** Knee ankle foot orthosis, full plastic, single upright, with or without free motion knee, with or without free motion ankle, custom fabricated

✳ **L2038** Knee ankle foot orthosis, full plastic, with or without free motion knee, multi-axis ankle, custom fabricated

Torsion Control

✳ **L2040** Hip knee ankle foot orthosis, torsion control, bilateral rotation straps, pelvic band/belt, custom fabricated

✳ **L2050** Hip knee ankle foot orthosis, torsion control, bilateral torsion cables, hip joint, pelvic band/belt, custom-fabricated

✳ **L2060** Hip knee ankle foot orthosis, torsion control, bilateral torsion cables, ball bearing hip joint, pelvic band/belt, custom-fabricated

✳ **L2070** Hip knee ankle foot orthosis, torsion control, unilateral rotation straps, pelvic band/belt, custom-fabricated

✳ **L2080** Hip knee ankle foot orthosis, torsion control, unilateral torsion cable, hip joint, pelvic band/belt, custom-fabricated

✳ **L2090** Hip knee ankle foot orthosis, torsion control, unilateral torsion cable, ball bearing hip joint, pelvic band/belt, custom-fabricated

Fracture Orthoses

✳ **L2106** Ankle foot orthosis, fracture orthosis, tibial fracture cast orthosis, thermoplastic type casting material, custom-fabricated

✳ **L2108** Ankle foot orthosis, fracture orthosis, tibial fracture cast orthosis, custom-fabricated

✳ **L2112** Ankle foot orthosis, fracture orthosis, tibial fracture orthosis, soft, prefabricated, includes fitting and adjustment

✳ **L2114** Ankle foot orthosis, fracture orthosis, tibial fracture orthosis, semi-rigid, prefabricated, includes fitting and adjustment

✳ **L2116** Ankle foot orthosis, fracture orthosis, tibial fracture orthosis, rigid, prefabricated, includes fitting and adjustment

✳ **L2126** Knee ankle foot orthosis, fracture orthosis, femoral fracture cast orthosis, thermoplastic type casting material, custom-fabricated

✳ **L2128** Knee ankle foot orthosis, fracture orthosis, femoral fracture cast orthosis, custom-fabricated

✳ **L2132** KAFO, femoral fracture cast orthosis, soft, prefabricated, includes fitting and adjustment

✳ **L2134** KAFO, femoral fracture cast orthosis, semi-rigid, prefabricated, includes fitting and adjustment

◀▶ New   ←→ Revised   ✔ Reinstated   ✖ Deleted

⊙ Special coverage instructions   ◆ Not covered or valid by Medicare   ✳ Carrier discretion   ▶ ASC payment group

ORTHOTICS

* **L2136** KAFO, fracture orthosis, femoral fracture cast orthosis, rigid, prefabricated, includes fitting and adjustment

Additions to Fracture Orthosis

* **L2180** Addition to lower extremity fracture orthosis, plastic shoe insert with ankle joints

* **L2182** Addition to lower extremity fracture orthosis, drop lock knee joint

* **L2184** Addition to lower extremity fracture orthosis, limited motion knee joint

* **L2186** Addition to lower extremity fracture orthosis, adjustable motion knee joint, Lerman type

* **L2188** Addition to lower extremity fracture orthosis, quadrilateral brim

* **L2190** Addition to lower extremity fracture orthosis, waist belt

* **L2192** Addition to lower extremity fracture orthosis, hip joint, pelvic band, thigh flange, and pelvic belt

Additions to Lower Extremity Orthosis

Shoe-Ankle-Shin-Knee

* **L2200** Addition to lower extremity, limited ankle motion, each joint

* **L2210** Addition to lower extremity, dorsiflexion assist (plantar flexion resist), each joint

* **L2220** Addition to lower extremity, dorsiflexion and plantar flexion assist/resist, each joint

* **L2230** Addition to lower extremity, split flat caliper stirrups and plate attachment

* **L2232** Addition to lower extremity orthosis, rocker bottom for total contact ankle foot orthosis, for custom fabricated orthosis only

* **L2240** Addition to lower extremity, round caliper and plate attachment

* **L2250** Addition to lower extremity, foot plate, molded to patient model, stirrup attachment

* **L2260** Addition to lower extremity, reinforced solid stirrup (Scott-Craig type)

* **L2265** Addition to lower extremity, long tongue stirrup

* **L2270** Addition to lower extremity, varus/valgus correction ('T') strap, padded/lined or malleolus pad

* **L2275** Addition to lower extremity, varus/valgus correction, plastic modification, padded/lined

* **L2280** Addition to lower extremity, molded inner boot

* **L2300** Addition to lower extremity, abduction bar (bilateral hip involvement), jointed, adjustable

* **L2310** Addition to lower extremity, abduction bar-straight

* **L2320** Addition to lower extremity, non-molded lacer, for custom fabricated orthosis only

* **L2330** Addition to lower extremity, lacer molded to patient model, for custom fabricated orthosis only

* **L2335** Addition to lower extremity, anterior swing band

* **L2340** Addition to lower extremity, pre-tibial shell, molded to patient model

* **L2350** Addition to lower extremity, prosthetic type, (BK) socket, molded to patient model, (used for 'PTB' and 'AFO' orthoses)

* **L2360** Addition to lower extremity, extended steel shank

* **L2370** Addition to lower extremity, Patten bottom

* **L2375** Addition to lower extremity, torsion control, ankle joint and half solid stirrup

* **L2380** Addition to lower extremity, torsion control, straight knee joint, each joint

* **L2385** Addition to lower extremity, straight knee joint, heavy duty, each joint

* **L2387** Addition to lower extremity, polycentric knee joint, for custom fabricated knee ankle foot orthosis, each joint

* **L2390** Addition to lower extremity, offset knee joint, each joint

* **L2395** Addition to lower extremity, offset knee joint, heavy duty, each joint

* **L2397** Addition to lower extremity orthosis, suspension sleeve

Additions to Straight Knee or Offset Knee Joints

* **L2405** Addition to knee joint, drop lock, each

◄▶ **New**   ←→ **Revised**   ✔ **Reinstated**   ✘ **Deleted**
☺ **Special coverage instructions**   ◆ **Not covered or valid by Medicare**   * **Carrier discretion**   ▶ **ASC payment group**

L2136 – L2405

224

* **L2415** Addition to knee lock with integrated release mechanism (bail, cable, or equal), any material, each joint

* **L2425** Addition to knee joint, disc or dial lock for adjustable knee flexion, each joint

* **L2430** Addition to knee joint, ratchet lock for active and progressive knee extension, each joint

* **L2492** Addition to knee joint, lift loop for drop lock ring

Additions to Thigh/Weight Bearing

Gluteal/Ischial Weight Bearing

* **L2500** Addition to lower extremity, thigh/weight bearing, gluteal/ischial weight bearing, ring

* **L2510** Addition to lower extremity, thigh/weight bearing, quadri-lateral brim, molded to patient model

* **L2520** Addition to lower extremity, thigh/weight bearing, quadri-lateral brim, custom fitted

* **L2525** Addition to lower extremity, thigh/weight bearing, ischial containment/narrow M-L brim molded to patient model

* **L2526** Addition to lower extremity, thigh/weight bearing, ischial containment/narrow M-L brim, custom fitted

* **L2530** Addition to lower extremity, thigh-weight bearing, lacer, non-molded

* **L2540** Addition to lower extremity, thigh/weight bearing, lacer, molded to patient model

* **L2550** Addition to lower extremity, thigh/weight bearing, high roll cuff

Additions to Pelvic and Thoracic Control

* **L2570** Addition to lower extremity, pelvic control, hip joint, Clevis type two position joint, each

* **L2580** Addition to lower extremity, pelvic control, pelvic sling

* **L2600** Addition to lower extremity, pelvic control, hip joint, Clevis type, or thrust bearing, free, each

* **L2610** Addition to lower extremity, pelvic control, hip joint, Clevis or thrust bearing, lock, each

* **L2620** Addition to lower extremity, pelvic control, hip joint, heavy duty, each

* **L2622** Addition to lower extremity, pelvic control, hip joint, adjustable flexion, each

* **L2624** Addition to lower extremity, pelvic control, hip joint, adjustable flexion, extension, abduction control, each

* **L2627** Addition to lower extremity, pelvic control, plastic, molded to patient model, reciprocating hip joint and cables

* **L2628** Addition to lower extremity, pelvic control, metal frame, reciprocating hip joint and cables

* **L2630** Addition to lower extremity, pelvic control, band and belt, unilateral

* **L2640** Addition to lower extremity, pelvic control, band and belt, bilateral

* **L2650** Addition to lower extremity, pelvic and thoracic control, gluteal pad, each

* **L2660** Addition to lower extremity, thoracic control, thoracic band

* **L2670** Addition to lower extremity, thoracic control, paraspinal uprights

* **L2680** Addition to lower extremity, thoracic control, lateral support uprights

General Additions

* **L2750** Addition to lower extremity orthosis, plating chrome or nickel, per bar

* **L2755** Addition to lower extremity orthosis, high strength, lightweight material, all hybrid lamination/prepreg composite, per segment, for custom fabricated orthosis only

* **L2760** Addition to lower extremity orthosis, extension, per extension, per bar (for lineal adjustment for growth)

* **L2768** Orthotic side bar disconnect device, per bar

* **L2770** Addition to lower extremity orthosis, any material - per bar or joint

* **L2780** Addition to lower extremity orthosis, non-corrosive finish, per bar

* **L2785** Addition to lower extremity orthosis, drop lock retainer, each

* **L2795** Addition to lower extremity orthosis, knee control, full kneecap

* **L2800** Addition to lower extremity orthosis, knee control, knee cap, medial or lateral pull, for use with custom fabricated orthosis only

* **L2810** Addition to lower extremity orthosis, knee control, condylar pad

◄► New   ←→ Revised   ✔ Reinstated   ✖ Deleted
✪ Special coverage instructions   ◆ Not covered or valid by Medicare   ✳ Carrier discretion   ▶ ASC payment group

L2820 Addition to lower extremity orthosis, soft interface for molded plastic, below knee section

L2830 Addition to lower extremity orthosis, soft interface for molded plastic, above knee section

L2840 Addition to lower extremity orthosis, tibial length sock, fracture or equal, each

L2850 Addition to lower extremity orthosis, femoral length sock, fracture or equal, each

L2860 Addition to lower extremity joint, knee or ankle, concentric adjustable torsion style mechanism, each ✖

L2999 Lower extremity orthoses, not otherwise specified

Foot (Orthopedic Shoes)

Insert, Removable, Molded to Patient Model

L3000 Foot, insert, removable, molded to patient model, 'UCB' type, Berkeley shell, each
IOM: 100-02, 15, 290

L3001 Foot, insert, removable, molded to patient model, Spenco, each
IOM: 100-02, 15, 290

L3002 Foot, insert, removable, molded to patient model, Plastazote or equal, each
IOM: 100-02, 15, 290

L3003 Foot, insert, removable, molded to patient model, silicone gel, each
IOM: 100-02, 15, 290

L3010 Foot, insert, removable, molded to patient model, longitudinal arch support, each
IOM: 100-02, 15, 290

L3020 Foot, insert, removable, molded to patient model, longitudinal/ metatarsal support, each
IOM: 100-02, 15, 290

L3030 Foot, insert, removable, formed to patient foot, each
IOM: 100-02, 15, 290

L3031 Foot, insert/plate, removable, addition to lower extremity orthosis, high strength, lightweight material, all hybrid lamination/prepreg composite, each

Arch Support, Removable, Premolded

L3040 Foot, arch support, removable, premolded, longitudinal, each
IOM: 100-02, 15, 290

L3050 Foot, arch support, removable, premolded, metatarsal, each
IOM: 100-02, 15, 290

L3060 Foot, arch support, removable, premolded, longitudinal/ metatarsal, each
IOM: 100-02, 15, 290

Arch Support, Non-removable, Attached to Shoe

L3070 Foot, arch support, non-removable attached to shoe, longitudinal, each
IOM: 100-02, 15, 290

L3080 Foot, arch support, non-removable attached to shoe, metatarsal, each
IOM: 100-02, 15, 290

L3090 Foot, arch support, non-removable attached to shoe, longitudinal/ metatarsal, each
IOM: 100-02, 15, 290

L3100 Hallus-valgus night dynamic splint
IOM: 100-02, 15, 290

Abduction and Rotation Bars

L3140 Foot, abduction rotation bar, including shoes
IOM: 100-02, 15, 290

L3150 Foot, abduction rotation bar, without shoes
IOM: 100-02, 15, 290

L3160 Foot, adjustable shoe-styled positioning device

L3170 Foot, plastic, silicone or equal, heel stabilizer, each
IOM: 100-02, 15, 290

Orthopedic Footwear

L3201 Orthopedic shoe, oxford with supinator or pronator, infant
IOM: 100-02, 15, 290

L3202 Orthopedic shoe, oxford with supinator or pronator, child
IOM: 100-02, 15, 290

◄► New   ←→ Revised   ✔ Reinstated   ✖ Deleted

⊕ Special coverage instructions   ◆ Not covered or valid by Medicare   ✳ Carrier discretion   ▶ ASC payment group

⊗ **L3203** Orthopedic shoe, oxford with supinator or pronator, junior
IOM: 100-02, 15, 290

⊗ **L3204** Orthopedic shoe, hightop with supinator or pronator, infant
IOM: 100-02, 15, 290

⊗ **L3206** Orthopedic shoe, hightop with supinator or pronator, child
IOM: 100-02, 15, 290

⊗ **L3207** Orthopedic shoe, hightop with supinator or pronator, junior
IOM: 100-02, 15, 290

⊗ **L3208** Surgical boot, infant, each
IOM: 100-02, 15, 100

⊗ **L3209** Surgical boot, each, child
IOM: 100-02, 15, 100

⊗ **L3211** Surgical boot, each, junior
IOM: 100-02, 15, 100

⊗ **L3212** Benesch boot, pair, infant
IOM: 100-02, 15, 100

⊗ **L3213** Benesch boot, pair, child
IOM: 100-02, 15, 100

⊗ **L3214** Benesch boot, pair, junior
IOM: 100-02, 15, 100

◆ **L3215** Orthopedic footwear, ladies shoe, oxford, each
Medicare Statute 1862a8

◆ **L3216** Orthopedic footwear, ladies shoe, depth inlay, each
Medicare Statute 1862a8

◆ **L3217** Orthopedic footwear, ladies shoe, hightop, depth inlay, each
Medicare Statute 1862a8

◆ **L3219** Orthopedic footwear, mens shoe, oxford, each
Medicare Statute 1862a8

◆ **L3221** Orthopedic footwear, mens shoe, depth inlay, each
Medicare Statute 1862a8

◆ **L3222** Orthopedic footwear, mens shoe, hightop, depth inlay, each
Medicare Statute 1862a8

⊗ **L3224** Orthopedic footwear, ladies shoe, oxford, used as an integral part of a brace (orthosis)
IOM: 100-02, 15, 290

⊗ **L3225** Orthopedic footwear, mens shoe, oxford, used as an integral part of a brace (orthosis)
IOM: 100-02, 15, 290

⊗ **L3230** Orthopedic footwear, custom shoe, depth inlay, each
IOM: 100-02, 15, 290

⊗ **L3250** Orthopedic footwear, custom molded shoe, removable inner mold, prosthetic shoe, each
IOM: 100-02, 15, 290

⊗ **L3251** Foot, shoe molded to patient model, silicone shoe, each
IOM: 100-02, 15, 290

⊗ **L3252** Foot, shoe molded to patient model, Plastazote (or similar), custom fabricated, each
IOM: 100-02, 15, 290

⊗ **L3253** Foot, molded shoe Plastazote (or similar), custom fitted, each
IOM: 100-02, 15, 290

⊗ **L3254** Non-standard size or width
IOM: 100-02, 15, 290

⊗ **L3255** Non-standard size or length
IOM: 100-02, 15, 290

⊗ **L3257** Orthopedic footwear, additional charge for split size
IOM: 100-02, 15, 290

⊗ **L3260** Surgical boot/shoe, each
IOM: 100-02, 15, 100

✳ **L3265** Plastazote sandal, each

Shoe Modifications

Lifts

⊗ **L3300** Lift, elevation, heel, tapered to metatarsals, per inch
IOM: 100-02, 15, 290

⊗ **L3310** Lift, elevation, heel and sole, Neoprene, per inch
IOM: 100-02, 15, 290

⊗ **L3320** Lift, elevation, heel and sole, cork, per inch
IOM: 100-02, 15, 290

⊗ **L3330** Lift, elevation, metal extension (skate)
IOM: 100-02, 15, 290

◄▶ New   ←→ Revised   ✔ Reinstated   ✖ Deleted
⊗ Special coverage instructions   ◆ Not covered or valid by Medicare   ✳ Carrier discretion   ▶ ASC payment group

ORTHOTICS

⊕ **L3332** Lift, elevation, inside shoe, tapered, up to one-half inch
IOM: 100-02, 15, 290

⊕ **L3334** Lift, elevation, heel, per inch
IOM: 100-02, 15, 290

Wedges

⊕ **L3340** Heel wedge, SACH
IOM: 100-02, 15, 290

⊕ **L3350** Heel wedge
IOM: 100-02, 15, 290

⊕ **L3360** Sole wedge, outside sole
IOM: 100-02, 15, 290

⊕ **L3370** Sole wedge, between sole
IOM: 100-02, 15, 290

⊕ **L3380** Clubfoot wedge
IOM: 100-02, 15, 290

⊕ **L3390** Outflare wedge
IOM: 100-02, 15, 290

⊕ **L3400** Metatarsal bar wedge, rocker
IOM: 100-02, 15, 290

⊕ **L3410** Metatarsal bar wedge, between sole
IOM: 100-02, 15, 290

⊕ **L3420** Full sole and heel wedge, between sole
IOM: 100-02, 15, 290

Heels

⊕ **L3430** Heel, counter, plastic reinforced
IOM: 100-02, 15, 290

⊕ **L3440** Heel, counter, leather reinforced
IOM: 100-02, 15, 290

⊕ **L3450** Heel, SACH cushion type
IOM: 100-02, 15, 290

⊕ **L3455** Heel, new leather, standard
IOM: 100-02, 15, 290

⊕ **L3460** Heel, new rubber, standard
IOM: 100-02, 15, 290

⊕ **L3465** Heel, Thomas with wedge
IOM: 100-02, 15, 290

⊕ **L3470** Heel, Thomas extended to ball
IOM: 100-02, 15, 290

⊕ **L3480** Heel, pad and depression for spur
IOM: 100-02, 15, 290

⊕ **L3485** Heel, pad, removable for spur
IOM: 100-02, 15, 290

Additions to Orthopedic Shoes

⊕ **L3500** Orthopedic shoe addition, insole, leather
IOM: 100-02, 15, 290

⊕ **L3510** Orthopedic shoe addition, insole, rubber
IOM: 100-02, 15, 290

⊕ **L3520** Orthopedic shoe addition, insole, felt covered with leather
IOM: 100-02, 15, 290

⊕ **L3530** Orthopedic shoe addition, sole, half
IOM: 100-02, 15, 290

⊕ **L3540** Orthopedic shoe addition, sole, full
IOM: 100-02, 15, 290

⊕ **L3550** Orthopedic shoe addition, toe tap standard
IOM: 100-02, 15, 290

⊕ **L3560** Orthopedic shoe addition, toe tap, horseshoe
IOM: 100-02, 15, 290

⊕ **L3570** Orthopedic shoe addition, special extension to instep (leather with eyelets)
IOM: 100-02, 15, 290

⊕ **L3580** Orthopedic shoe addition, convert instep to Velcro closure
IOM: 100-02, 15, 290

⊕ **L3590** Orthopedic shoe addition, convert firm shoe counter to soft counter
IOM: 100-02, 15, 290

⊕ **L3595** Orthopedic shoe addition, March bar
IOM: 100-02, 15, 290

Transfer or Replacement

⊕ **L3600** Transfer of an orthosis from one shoe to another, caliper plate, existing
IOM: 100-02, 15, 290

⊕ **L3610** Transfer of an orthosis from one shoe to another, caliper plate, new
IOM: 100-02, 15, 290

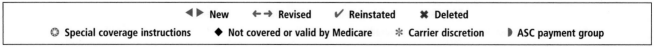

◀▶ New   ←→ Revised   ✔ Reinstated   ✖ Deleted
⊕ Special coverage instructions   ◆ Not covered or valid by Medicare   ✳ Carrier discretion   ▶ ASC payment group

L3332 – L3610

☺ **L3620** Transfer of an orthosis from one shoe to another, solid stirrup, existing

IOM: 100-02, 15, 290

☺ **L3630** Transfer of an orthosis from one shoe to another, solid stirrup, new

IOM: 100-02, 15, 290

☺ **L3640** Transfer of an orthosis from one shoe to another, Dennis Browne splint (Riveton), both shoes

IOM: 100-02, 15, 290

☺ **L3649** Orthopedic shoe, modification, addition or transfer, not otherwise specified

IOM: 100-02, 15, 290

Orthotic Devices: Upper Limb

NOTE: The procedures in this section are considered as *base* or *basic procedures* and may be modified by listing procedures from the Additions section and adding them to the base procedure.

Shoulder

✳ **L3650** Shoulder orthosis, (SO), figure of eight design abduction restrainer, prefabricated, includes fitting and adjustment

✳ **L3651** Shoulder orthosis, single shoulder, elastic, prefabricated, includes fitting and adjustment (e.g. neoprene, Lycra)

✳ **L3652** Shoulder orthosis, double shoulder, elastic, prefabricated, includes fitting and adjustment (e.g. neoprene, Lycra)

✳ **L3660** Shoulder orthosis, figure of eight design abduction restrainer, canvas and webbing, prefabricated, includes fitting and adjustment

✳ **L3670** Shoulder orthosis, acromio/clavicular (canvas and webbing type), prefabricated, includes fitting and adjustment

✳ **L3671** Shoulder orthosis, shoulder cap design, without joints, may include soft interface, straps, custom fabricated, includes fitting and adjustment

✳ **L3672** Shoulder orthosis, abduction positioning (airplane design), thoracic component and support bar, without joints, may include soft interface, straps, custom fabricated, includes fitting and adjustment

✳ **L3673** Shoulder orthosis, abduction positioning (airplane design), thoracic component and support bar, includes nontorsion joint/turnbuckle, may include soft interface, straps, custom fabricated, includes fitting and adjustment

✳ **L3675** Shoulder orthosis, vest type abduction restrainer, canvas webbing type or equal, prefabricated, includes fitting and adjustment

☺ **L3677** Shoulder orthosis, hard plastic, shoulder stabilizer, pre-fabricated, includes fitting and adjustment

Elbow

✳ **L3700** Elbow orthosis (EO), elastic with stays, prefabricated, includes fitting and adjustment

✳ **L3701** Elbow orthosis, elastic, prefabricated, includes fitting and adjustment (e.g. neoprene, Lycra)

✳ **L3702** Elbow orthosis, without joints, may include soft interface, straps, custom fabricated, includes fitting and adjustment

✳ **L3710** Elbow orthosis, elastic with metal joints, prefabricated, includes fitting and adjustment

✳ **L3720** Elbow orthosis, double upright with forearm/arm cuffs, free motion, custom-fabricated

✳ **L3730** Elbow orthosis, double upright with forearm/arm cuffs, extension/flexion assist, custom-fabricated

✳ **L3740** Elbow orthosis, double upright with forearm/arm cuffs, adjustable position lock with active control, custom-fabricated

✳ **L3760** Elbow orthosis, with adjustable position locking joint(s), prefabricated, includes fitting and adjustments, any type

✳ **L3762** Elbow orthosis, rigid, without joints, includes soft interface material, prefabricated, includes fitting and adjustment

✳ **L3763** Elbow wrist hand orthosis, rigid, without joints, may include soft interface, straps, custom fabricated, includes fitting and adjustment

---

◄► New ← → Revised ✔ Reinstated ✖ Deleted

☺ Special coverage instructions ◆ Not covered or valid by Medicare ✳ Carrier discretion ▶ ASC payment group

* **L3764**   Elbow wrist hand orthosis, includes one or more nontorsion joints, elastic bands, turnbuckles, may include soft interface, straps, custom fabricated, includes fitting and adjustment

* **L3765**   Elbow wrist hand finger orthosis, rigid, without joints, may include soft interface, straps, custom fabricated, includes fitting and adjustment

* **L3766**   Elbow wrist hand finger orthosis, includes one or more nontorsion joints, elastic bands, turnbuckles, may include soft interface, straps, custom fabricated, includes fitting and adjustment

Wrist-Hand-Finger Orthosis (WHFO)

* **L3806**   Wrist hand finger orthosis, includes one or more nontorsion joint(s), turnbuckles, elastic bands/springs, may include soft interface material, straps, custom fabricated, includes fitting and adjustment

* **L3807**   Wrist hand finger orthosis, without joint(s), prefabricated, includes fitting and adjustments, any type

* **L3808**   Wrist hand finger orthosis, rigid without joints, may include soft interface material; straps, custom fabricated, includes fitting and adjustment

Additions and Extensions

~~**L3890**   Addition to upper extremity joint, wrist or elbow, concentric adjustable torsion style mechanism, each~~   ✖

* **L3900**   Wrist hand finger orthosis, dynamic flexor hinge, reciprocal wrist extension/flexion, finger flexion/extension, wrist or finger driven, custom-fabricated

* **L3901**   Wrist hand finger orthosis, dynamic flexor hinge, reciprocal wrist extension/flexion, finger flexion/extension, cable driven, custom-fabricated

External Power

* **L3904**   Wrist hand finger orthosis, external powered, electric, custom-fabricated

* **L3905**   Wrist hand orthosis, includes one or more nontorsion joints, elastic bands, turnbuckles, may include soft interface, straps, custom fabricated, includes fitting and adjustment

Other Wrist-Hand-Finger Orthoses: Custom Fitted

* **L3906**   Wrist hand orthosis, without joints, may include soft interface, straps, custom fabricated, includes fitting and adjustment

* **L3908**   Wrist hand orthosis, wrist extension control cock-up, non molded, prefabricated, includes fitting and adjustment

* **L3909**   Wrist orthosis, elastic, prefabricated, includes fitting and adjustment (e.g. neoprene, Lycra)

* **L3911**   Wrist hand finger orthosis, elastic, prefabricated, includes fitting and adjustment (e.g. neoprene, Lycra)

* **L3912**   Hand finger orthosis, flexion glove with elastic finger control, prefabricated, includes fitting and adjustment

* **L3913**   Hand finger orthosis, without joints, may include soft interface, straps, custom fabricated, includes fitting and adjustment

* **L3915**   Wrist hand orthosis, includes one or more nontorsion joint(s), elastic bands, turnbuckles, may include soft interface, straps, prefabricated, includes fitting and adjustment

* **L3917**   Hand orthosis, metacarpal fracture orthosis, prefabricated, includes fitting and adjustment

* **L3919**   Hand orthosis, without joints, may include soft interface, straps, custom fabricated, includes fitting and adjustment

* **L3921**   Hand finger orthosis, includes one or more nontorsion joints, elastic bands, turnbuckles, may include soft interface, straps, custom fabricated, includes fitting and adjustment

* **L3923**   Hand finger orthosis, without joints, may include soft interface, straps, prefabricated, includes fitting and adjustments

* **L3925** Finger orthosis, proximal interphalangeal (PIP)/distal interphalangeal (DIP), non torsion joint/spring, extension/flexion, may include soft interface material, prefabricated, includes fitting and adjustment

* **L3927** Finger orthosis, proximal interphalangeal (PIP)/distal interphalangeal (DIP), without joint/spring, extension/flexion (e.g. static or ring type), may include soft interface material, prefabricated, includes fitting and adjustment

* **L3929** Hand finger orthosis, includes one or more nontorsion joint(s), turnbuckles, elastic bands/springs, may include soft interface material, straps, prefabricated, includes fitting and adjustment

* **L3931** Wrist hand finger orthosis, includes one or more nontorsion joint(s), turnbuckles, elastic bands/springs, may include soft interface material, straps, prefabricated, includes fitting and adjustment

* **L3933** Finger orthosis, without joints, may include soft interface, custom fabricated, includes fitting and adjustment

* **L3935** Finger orthosis, nontorsion joint, may include soft interface, custom fabricated, includes fitting and adjustment

* **L3956** Addition of joint to upper extremity orthosis, any material, per joint

Shoulder-Elbow-Wrist-Hand Orthosis (SEWHO)

Abduction Positioning: Custom Fitted

* **L3960** Shoulder elbow wrist hand orthosis, abduction positioning, airplane design, prefabricated, includes fitting and adjustment

* **L3961** Shoulder elbow wrist hand orthosis, shoulder cap design, without joints, may include soft interface, straps, custom fabricated, includes fitting and adjustment

* **L3962** Shoulder elbow wrist hand orthosis, abduction positioning, Erbs palsy design, prefabricated, includes fitting and adjustment

* **L3964** Shoulder elbow orthosis, mobile arm support attached to wheelchair, balanced, adjustable, prefabricated, includes fitting and adjustment

* **L3965** Shoulder elbow orthosis, mobile arm support attached to wheelchair, balanced, adjustable Rancho type, prefabricated, includes fitting and adjustment

* **L3966** Shoulder elbow orthosis, mobile arm support attached to wheelchair, balanced, reclining, prefabricated, includes fitting and adjustment

* **L3967** Shoulder elbow wrist hand orthosis, abduction positioning (airplane design), thoracic component and support bar, without joints, may include soft interface, straps, custom fabricated, includes fitting and adjustment

* **L3968** Shoulder elbow orthosis, mobile arm support attached to wheelchair, balanced, friction arm support (friction dampening to proximal and distal joints), prefabricated, includes fitting and adjustment

* **L3969** Shoulder elbow orthosis, mobile arm support, monosuspension arm and hand support, overhead elbow forearm hand sling support, yoke type suspension support, prefabricated, includes fitting and adjustment

Additions to Mobile Arm Supports and SEWHO

* **L3970** SEO, addition to mobile arm support, elevating proximal arm

* **L3971** Shoulder elbow wrist hand orthosis, shoulder cap design, includes one or more nontorsion joints, elastic bands, turnbuckles, may include soft interface, straps, custom fabricated, includes fitting and adjustment

* **L3972** SEO, addition to mobile arm support, offset or lateral rocker arm with elastic balance control

* **L3973** Shoulder elbow wrist hand orthosis, abduction positioning (airplane design), thoracic component and support bar, includes one or more nontorsion joints, elastic bands, turnbuckles, may include soft interface, straps, custom fabricated, includes fitting and adjustment

* **L3974** SEO, addition to mobile arm support, supinator

◀▶ New   ←→ Revised   ✔ Reinstated   ✖ Deleted
☺ Special coverage instructions   ◆ Not covered or valid by Medicare   * Carrier discretion   ▶ ASC payment group

ORTHOTICS

* **L3975** Shoulder elbow wrist hand finger orthosis, shoulder cap design, without joints, may include soft interface, straps, custom fabricated, includes fitting and adjustment

* **L3976** Shoulder elbow wrist hand finger orthosis, abduction positioning (airplane design), thoracic component and support bar, without joints, may include soft interface, straps, custom fabricated, includes fitting and adjustment

* **L3977** Shoulder elbow wrist hand finger orthosis, shoulder cap design, includes one or more nontorsion joints, elastic bands, turnbuckles, may include soft interface, straps, custom fabricated, includes fitting and adjustment

* **L3978** Shoulder elbow wrist hand finger orthosis, abduction positioning (airplane design), thoracic component and support bar, includes one or more nontorsion joints, elastic bands, turnbuckles, may include soft interface, straps, custom fabricated, includes fitting and adjustment

Fracture Orthoses

* **L3980** Upper extremity fracture orthosis, humeral, prefabricated, includes fitting and adjustment

* **L3982** Upper extremity fracture orthosis, radius/ulnar, prefabricated, includes fitting and adjustment

* **L3984** Upper extremity fracture orthosis, wrist, prefabricated, includes fitting and adjustment

* **L3995** Addition to upper extremity orthosis, sock, fracture or equal, each

* **L3999** Upper limb orthosis, not otherwise specified

Specific Repair

* **L4000** Replace girdle for spinal orthosis (CTLSO or SO)

* **L4002** Replacement strap, any orthosis, includes all components, any length, any type

* **L4010** Replace trilateral socket brim

* **L4020** Replace quadrilateral socket brim, molded to patient model

* **L4030** Replace quadrilateral socket brim, custom fitted

* **L4040** Replace molded thigh lacer, for custom fabricated orthosis only

* **L4045** Replace non-molded thigh lacer, for custom fabricated orthosis only

* **L4050** Replace molded calf lacer, for custom fabricated orthosis only

* **L4055** Replace non-molded calf lacer, for custom fabricated orthosis only

* **L4060** Replace high roll cuff

* **L4070** Replace proximal and distal upright for KAFO

* **L4080** Replace metal bands KAFO, proximal thigh

* **L4090** Replace metal bands KAFO-AFO, calf or distal thigh

* **L4100** Replace leather cuff KAFO, proximal thigh

* **L4110** Replace leather cuff KAFO-AFO, calf or distal thigh

* **L4130** Replace pretibial shell

Repairs

⊘ **L4205** Repair of orthotic device, labor component, per 15 minutes

  IOM: 100-02, 15, 110.2

⊘ **L4210** Repair of orthotic device, repair or replace minor parts

  IOM: 100-02, 15, 110.2; 100-02, 15, 120

Ancillary Orthotic Services

* **L4350** Ankle control orthosis, stirrup style, rigid, includes any type interface (e.g., pneumatic, gel), prefabricated, includes fitting and adjustment

→ * **L4360** Walking boot, pneumatic, and/or vacuum, with or without joints, with or without interface material, prefabricated, includes fitting and adjustment

* **L4370** Pneumatic full leg splint, prefabricated, includes fitting and adjustment

* **L4380** Pneumatic knee splint, prefabricated, includes fitting and adjustment

* **L4386** Walking boot, non-pneumatic, with or without joints, with or without interface material, prefabricated, includes fitting and adjustment

* **L4392** Replacement, soft interface material, static AFO

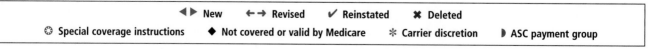

◀▶ New   ←→ Revised   ✔ Reinstated   ✖ Deleted
⊘ Special coverage instructions   ◆ Not covered or valid by Medicare   * Carrier discretion   ▶ ASC payment group

* **L4394** Replace soft interface material, foot drop splint

* **L4396** Static ankle foot orthosis, including soft interface material, adjustable for fit, for positioning, pressure reduction, may be used for minimal ambulation, prefabricated, includes fitting and adjustment

* **L4398** Foot drop splint, recumbent positioning device, prefabricated, includes fitting and adjustment

PROSTHETICS (L5000-L9999)

Lower Limb (L5000-L5999)

NOTE: The procedures in this sections are considered as *base* or *basic procedures* and may be modified by listing items/procedures or special materials from the Additions section and adding them to the base procedure.

Partial Foot

⊚ **L5000** Partial foot, shoe insert with longitudinal arch, toe filler
IOM: 100-02, 15, 290

⊚ **L5010** Partial foot, molded socket, ankle height, with toe filler
IOM: 100-02, 15, 290

⊚ **L5020** Partial foot, molded socket, tibial tubercle height, with toe filler
IOM: 100-02, 15, 290

Ankle

* **L5050** Ankle, Symes, molded socket, SACH foot

* **L5060** Ankle, Symes, metal frame, molded leather socket, articulated ankle/foot

Below Knee

* **L5100** Below knee, molded socket, shin, SACH foot

* **L5105** Below knee, plastic socket, joints and thigh lacer, SACH foot

Knee Disarticulation

* **L5150** Knee disarticulation (or through knee), molded socket, external knee joints, shin, SACH foot

* **L5160** Knee disarticulation (or through knee), molded socket, bent knee configuration, external knee joints, shin, SACH foot

Above Knee

* **L5200** Above knee, molded socket, single axis constant friction knee, shin, SACH foot

* **L5210** Above knee, short prosthesis, no knee joint ('stubbies'), with foot blocks, no ankle joints, each

* **L5220** Above knee, short prosthesis, no knee joint ('stubbies'), with articulated ankle/foot, dynamically aligned, each

* **L5230** Above knee, for proximal femoral focal deficiency, constant friction knee, shin, SACH foot

Hip Disarticulation

* **L5250** Hip disarticulation, Canadian type; molded socket, hip joint, single axis constant friction knee, shin, SACH foot

* **L5270** Hip disarticulation, tilt table type; molded socket, locking hip joint, single axis constant friction knee, shin, SACH foot

Hemipelvectomy

* **L5280** Hemipelvectomy, Canadian type; molded socket, hip joint, single axis constant friction knee, shin, SACH foot

Endoskeleton: Below Knee

* **L5301** Below knee, molded socket, shin, SACH foot, endoskeletal system

Endoskeletal: Knee Disarticulation

* **L5311** Knee disarticulation (or through knee), molded socket, external knee joints, shin, SACH foot, endoskeletal system

Endoskeletal: Above Knee

* **L5321** Above knee, molded socket, open end, SACH foot, endoskeletal system, single axis knee

L4394 – L5321

Endoskeletal: Hip Disarticulation

* **L5331**   Hip disarticulation, Canadian type, molded socket, endoskeletal system, hip joint, single axis knee, SACH foot

Endoskeletal: Hemipelvectomy

* **L5341**   Hemipelvectomy, Canadian type, molded socket, endoskeletal system, hip joint, single axis knee, SACH foot

Immediate Postsurgical or Early Fitting Procedures

* **L5400**   Immediate post surgical or early fitting, application of initial rigid dressing, including fitting, alignment, suspension, and one cast change, below knee

* **L5410**   Immediate post surgical or early fitting, application of initial rigid dressing, including fitting, alignment and suspension, below knee, each additional cast change and realignment

* **L5420**   Immediate post surgical or early fitting, application of initial rigid dressing, including fitting, alignment and suspension and one cast change 'AK' or knee disarticulation

* **L5430**   Immediate postsurgical or early fitting, application of initial rigid dressing, including fitting, alignment, and suspension, 'AK' or knee disarticulation, each additional cast change and realignment

* **L5450**   Immediate post surgical or early fitting, application of non-weight bearing rigid dressing, below knee

* **L5460**   Immediate post surgical or early fitting, application of non-weight bearing rigid dressing, above knee

Initial Prosthesis

* **L5500**   Initial, below knee 'PTB' type socket, non-alignable system, pylon, no cover, SACH foot, plaster socket, direct formed

* **L5505**   Initial, above knee–knee disarticulation, ischial level socket, non-alignable system, pylon, no cover, SACH foot, plaster socket, direct formed

Preparatory Prosthesis

* **L5510**   Preparatory, below knee 'PTB' type socket, non-alignable system, pylon, no cover, SACH foot, plaster socket, molded to model

* **L5520**   Preparatory, below knee 'PTB' type socket, non-alignable system, pylon, no cover, SACH foot, thermoplastic or equal, direct formed

* **L5530**   Preparatory, below knee 'PTB' type socket, non-alignable system, pylon, no cover, SACH foot, thermoplastic or equal, molded to model

* **L5535**   Preparatory, below knee 'PTB' type socket, non-alignable system, no cover, SACH foot, prefabricated, adjustable open end socket

* **L5540**   Preparatory, below knee 'PTB' type socket, non-alignable system, pylon, no cover, SACH foot, laminated socket, molded to model

* **L5560**   Preparatory, above knee - knee disarticulation, ischial level socket, non-alignable system, pylon, no cover, SACH foot, plaster socket, molded to model

* **L5570**   Preparatory, above knee - knee disarticulation, ischial level socket, non-alignable system, pylon, no cover, SACH foot, thermoplastic or equal, direct formed

* **L5580**   Preparatory, above knee - knee disarticulation, ischial level socket, non-alignable system, pylon, no cover, SACH foot, thermoplastic or equal, molded to model

* **L5585**   Preparatory, above knee - knee disarticulation, ischial level socket, non-alignable system, pylon, no cover, SACH foot, prefabricated adjustable open end socket

* **L5590**   Preparatory, above knee - knee disarticulation, ischial level socket, non-alignable system, pylon, no cover, SACH foot, laminated socket, molded to model

* **L5595**   Preparatory, hip disarticulation-hemipelvectomy, pylon, no cover, SACH foot, thermoplastic or equal, molded to patient model

* **L5600**   Preparatory, hip disarticulation-hemipelvectomy, pylon, no cover, SACH foot, laminated socket, molded to patient model

◀▶ New   ←→ Revised   ✔ Reinstated   ✖ Deleted
○ Special coverage instructions   ◆ Not covered or valid by Medicare   * Carrier discretion   ▶ ASC payment group

Additions to Lower Extremity

✳ **L5610** Addition to lower extremity, endoskeletal system, above knee, hydracadence system

✳ **L5611** Addition to lower extremity, endoskeletal system, above knee-knee disarticulation, 4 bar linkage, with friction swing phase control

✳ **L5613** Addition to lower extremity, endoskeletal system, above knee-knee disarticulation, 4 bar linkage, with hydraulic swing phase control

✳ **L5614** Addition to lower extremity, exoskeletal system, above knee-knee disarticulation, 4 bar linkage, with pneumatic swing phase control

✳ **L5616** Addition to lower extremity, endoskeletal system, above knee, universal multiplex system, friction swing phase control

✳ **L5617** Addition to lower extremity, quick change self-aligning unit, above knee or below knee, each

Additions to Test Sockets

✳ **L5618** Addition to lower extremity, test socket, Symes

✳ **L5620** Addition to lower extremity, test socket, below knee

✳ **L5622** Addition to lower extremity, test socket, knee disarticulation

✳ **L5624** Addition to lower extremity, test socket, above knee

✳ **L5626** Addition to lower extremity, test socket, hip disarticulation

✳ **L5628** Addition to lower extremity, test socket, hemipelvectomy

✳ **L5629** Addition to lower extremity, below knee, acrylic socket

Additions to Socket Variations

✳ **L5630** Addition to lower extremity, Symes type, expandable wall socket

✳ **L5631** Addition to lower extremity, above knee or knee disarticulation, acrylic socket

✳ **L5632** Addition to lower extremity, Symes type, 'PTB' brim design socket

✳ **L5634** Addition to lower extremity, Symes type, posterior opening (Canadian) socket

✳ **L5636** Addition to lower extremity, Symes type, medial opening socket

✳ **L5637** Addition to lower extremity, below knee, total contact

✳ **L5638** Addition to lower extremity, below knee, leather socket

✳ **L5639** Addition to lower extremity, below knee, wood socket

✳ **L5640** Addition to lower extremity, knee disarticulation, leather socket

✳ **L5642** Addition to lower extremity, above knee, leather socket

✳ **L5643** Addition to lower extremity, hip disarticulation, flexible inner socket, external frame

✳ **L5644** Addition to lower extremity, above knee, wood socket

✳ **L5645** Addition to lower extremity, below knee, flexible inner socket, external frame

✳ **L5646** Addition to lower extremity, below knee, air, fluid, gel or equal, cushion socket

✳ **L5647** Addition to lower extremity, below knee, suction socket

✳ **L5648** Addition to lower extremity, above knee, air, fluid, gel or equal, cushion socket

✳ **L5649** Addition to lower extremity, ischial containment/narrow M-L socket

✳ **L5650** Additions to lower extremity, total contact, above knee or knee disarticulation socket

✳ **L5651** Addition to lower extremity, above knee, flexible inner socket, external frame

✳ **L5652** Addition to lower extremity, suction suspension, above knee or knee disarticulation socket

✳ **L5653** Addition to lower extremity, knee disarticulation, expandable wall socket

Additions to Socket Insert and Suspension

✳ **L5654** Addition to lower extremity, socket insert, Symes, (Kemblo, Pelite, Aliplast, Plastazote or equal)

✳ **L5655** Addition to lower extremity, socket insert, below knee (Kemblo, Pelite, Aliplast, Plastazote or equal)

✳ **L5656** Addition to lower extremity, socket insert, knee disarticulation (Kemblo, Pelite, Aliplast, Plastazote or equal)

◄ ▶ **New**   ← → **Revised**   ✔ **Reinstated**   ✖ **Deleted**
⊙ **Special coverage instructions**   ◆ **Not covered or valid by Medicare**   ✳ **Carrier discretion**   ▶ **ASC payment group**

* **L5658** Addition to lower extremity, socket insert, above knee (Kemblo, Pelite, Aliplast, Plastazote or equal)

* **L5661** Addition to lower extremity, socket insert, multi-durometer Symes

* **L5665** Addition to lower extremity, socket insert, multi-durometer, below knee

* **L5666** Addition to lower extremity, below knee, cuff suspension

* **L5668** Addition to lower extremity, below knee, molded distal cushion

* **L5670** Addition to lower extremity, below knee, molded supracondylar suspension ('PTS' or similar)

* **L5671** Addition to lower extremity, below knee/above knee suspension locking mechanism (shuttle, lanyard or equal), excludes socket insert

* **L5672** Addition to lower extremity, below knee, removable medial brim suspension

* **L5673** Addition to lower extremity, below knee/above knee, custom fabricated from existing mold or prefabricated, socket insert, silicone gel, elastomeric or equal, for use with locking mechanism

* **L5676** Additions to lower extremity, below knee, knee joints, single axis, pair

* **L5677** Additions to lower extremity, below knee, knee joints, polycentric, pair

* **L5678** Additions to lower extremity, below knee, joint covers, pair

* **L5679** Addition to lower extremity, below knee/above knee, custom fabricated from existing mold or prefabricated, socket insert, silicone gel, elastomeric or equal, not for use with locking mechanism

* **L5680** Addition to lower extremity, below knee, thigh lacer, nonmolded

* **L5681** Addition to lower extremity, below knee/above knee, custom fabricated socket insert for congenital or atypical traumatic amputee, silicone gel, elastomeric or equal, for use with or without locking mechanism, initial only (for other than initial, use code L5673 or L5679)

* **L5682** Addition to lower extremity, below knee, thigh lacer, gluteal/ischial, molded

* **L5683** Addition to lower extremity, below knee/above knee, custom fabricated socket insert for other than congenital or atypical traumatic amputee, silicone gel, elastomeric, or equal, for use with or without locking mechanism, initial only (for other than initial, use code L5673 or L5679)

* **L5684** Addition to lower extremity, below knee, fork strap

* **L5685** Addition to lower extremity prosthesis, below knee, suspension/sealing sleeve, with or without valve, any material, each

* **L5686** Addition to lower extremity, below knee, back check (extension control)

* **L5688** Addition to lower extremity, below knee, waist belt, webbing

* **L5690** Addition to lower extremity, below knee, waist belt, padded and lined

* **L5692** Addition to lower extremity, above knee, pelvic control belt, light

* **L5694** Addition to lower extremity, above knee, pelvic control belt, padded and lined

* **L5695** Addition to lower extremity, above knee, pelvic control, sleeve suspension, neoprene or equal, each

* **L5696** Addition to lower extremity, above knee or knee disarticulation, pelvic joint

* **L5697** Addition to lower extremity, above knee or knee disarticulation, pelvic band

* **L5698** Addition to lower extremity, above knee or knee disarticulation, Silesian bandage

* **L5699** All lower extremity prostheses, shoulder harness

Additions/Replacements to Feet-Ankle Units

* **L5700** Replacement, socket, below knee, molded to patient model

* **L5701** Replacement, socket, above knee/knee disarticulation, including attachment plate, molded to patient model

* **L5702** Replacement, socket, hip disarticulation, including hip joint, molded to patient model

* **L5703** Ankle, Symes, molded to patient model, socket without solid ankle cushion heel (SACH) foot, replacement only

* **L5704** Custom shaped protective cover, below knee

* **L5705** Custom shaped protective cover, above knee

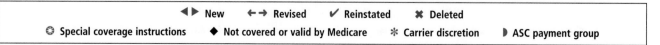

◄► New   ←→ Revised   ✔ Reinstated   ✖ Deleted
⊙ Special coverage instructions   ◆ Not covered or valid by Medicare   ✳ Carrier discretion   ▶ ASC payment group

* **L5706** Custom shaped protective cover, knee disarticulation

* **L5707** Custom shaped protective cover, hip disarticulation

Additions to Exoskeletal–Knee-Shin System

* **L5710** Addition, exoskeletal knee-shin system, single axis, manual lock

* **L5711** Additions exoskeletal knee-shin system, single axis, manual lock, ultra-light material

* **L5712** Addition, exoskeletal knee-shin system, single axis, friction swing and stance phase control (safety knee)

* **L5714** Addition, exoskeletal knee-shin system, single axis, variable friction swing phase control

* **L5716** Addition, exoskeletal knee-shin system, polycentric, mechanical stance phase lock

* **L5718** Addition, exoskeletal knee-shin system, polycentric, friction swing and stance phase control

* **L5722** Addition, exoskeletal knee-shin system, single axis, pneumatic swing, friction stance phase control

* **L5724** Addition, exoskeletal knee-shin system, single axis, fluid swing phase control

* **L5726** Addition, exoskeletal knee-shin system, single axis, external joints, fluid swing phase control

* **L5728** Addition, exoskeletal knee-shin system, single axis, fluid swing and stance phase control

* **L5780** Addition, exoskeletal knee-shin system, single axis, pneumatic/hydra pneumatic swing phase control

* **L5781** Addition to lower limb prosthesis, vacuum pump, residual limb volume management and moisture evacuation system

* **L5782** Addition to lower limb prosthesis, vacuum pump, residual limb volume management and moisture evacuation system, heavy duty

Component Modification

* **L5785** Addition, exoskeletal system, below knee, ultra-light material (titanium, carbon fiber, or equal)

* **L5790** Addition, exoskeletal system, above knee, ultra-light material (titanium, carbon fiber, or equal)

* **L5795** Addition, exoskeletal system, hip disarticulation, ultra-light material (titanium, carbon fiber, or equal)

Endoskeletal

* **L5810** Addition, endoskeletal knee-shin system, single axis, manual lock

* **L5811** Addition, endoskeletal knee-shin system, single axis, manual lock, ultralight material

* **L5812** Addition, endoskeletal knee-shin system, single axis, friction swing and stance phase control (safety knee)

* **L5814** Addition, endoskeletal knee-shin system, polycentric, hydraulic swing phase control, mechanical stance phase lock

* **L5816** Addition, endoskeletal knee-shin system, polycentric, mechanical stance phase lock

* **L5818** Addition, endoskeletal knee-shin system, polycentric, friction swing, and stance phase control

* **L5822** Addition, endoskeletal knee-shin system, single axis, pneumatic swing, friction stance phase control

* **L5824** Addition, endoskeletal knee-shin system, single axis, fluid swing phase control

* **L5826** Addition, endoskeletal knee-shin system, single axis, hydraulic swing phase control, with miniature high activity frame

* **L5828** Addition, endoskeletal knee-shin system, single axis, fluid swing and stance phase control

* **L5830** Addition, endoskeletal knee-shin system, single axis, pneumatic/swing phase control

* **L5840** Addition, endoskeletal knee/shin system, 4-bar linkage or multiaxial, pneumatic swing phase control

* **L5845** Addition, endoskeletal, knee-shin system, stance flexion feature, adjustable

* **L5848** Addition to endoskeletal, knee-shin system, fluid stance extension, dampening feature, with or without adjustability

* **L5850** Addition, endoskeletal system, above knee or hip disarticulation, knee extension assist

---

◀ ▶ New   ← → Revised   ✔ Reinstated   ✖ Deleted
◎ Special coverage instructions   ◆ Not covered or valid by Medicare   ✳ Carrier discretion   ▶ ASC payment group

ORTHOTICS

* **L5855** Addition, endoskeletal system, hip disarticulation, mechanical hip extension assist

* **L5856** Addition to lower extremity prosthesis, endoskeletal knee-shin system, microprocessor control feature, swing and stance phase; includes electronic sensor(s), any type

* **L5857** Addition to lower extremity prosthesis, endoskeletal knee-shin system, microprocessor control feature, swing phase only; includes electronic sensor(s), any type

* **L5858** Addition to lower extremity prosthesis, endoskeletal knee shin system, microprocessor control feature, stance phase only, includes electronic sensor(s), any type

* **L5910** Addition, endoskeletal system, below knee, alignable system

* **L5920** Addition, endoskeletal system, above knee or hip disarticulation, alignable system

* **L5925** Addition, endoskeletal system, above knee, knee disarticulation or hip disarticulation, manual lock

* **L5930** Addition, endoskeletal system, high activity knee control frame

* **L5940** Addition, endoskeletal system, below knee, ultra-light material (titanium, carbon fiber or equal)

* **L5950** Addition, endoskeletal system, above knee, ultra-light material (titanium, carbon fiber or equal)

* **L5960** Addition, endoskeletal system, hip disarticulation, ultra-light material (titanium, carbon fiber, or equal)

* **L5962** Addition, endoskeletal system, below knee, flexible protective outer surface covering system

* **L5964** Addition, endoskeletal system, above knee, flexible protective outer surface covering system

* **L5966** Addition, endoskeletal system, hip disarticulation, flexible protective outer surface covering system

* **L5968** Addition to lower limb prosthesis, multiaxial ankle with swing phase active dorsiflexion feature

* **L5970** All lower extremity prostheses, foot, external keel, SACH foot

* **L5971** All lower extremity prosthesis, solid ankle cushion keel (SACH) foot, replacement only

* **L5972** All lower extremity prostheses, flexible heel foot (Safe, Sten, Bock Dynamic or equal)

* **L5974** All lower extremity prostheses, foot, single axis ankle/foot

* **L5975** All lower extremity prostheses, combination single axis ankle and flexible keel foot

* **L5976** All lower extremity prostheses, energy storing foot (Seattle Carbon Copy II or equal)

* **L5978** All lower extremity prostheses, foot, multiaxial ankle/foot

* **L5979** All lower extremity prostheses, multiaxial ankle, dynamic response foot, one piece system

* **L5980** All lower extremity prostheses, flex foot system

* **L5981** All lower extremity prostheses, flexwalk system or equal

* **L5982** All exoskeletal lower extremity prostheses, axial rotation unit

* **L5984** All endoskeletal lower extremity prostheses, axial rotation unit, with or without adjustability

* **L5985** All endoskeletal lower extremity prostheses, dynamic prosthetic pylon

* **L5986** All lower extremity prostheses, multiaxial rotation unit ('MCP' or equal)

* **L5987** All lower extremity prostheses, shank foot system with vertical loading pylon

* **L5988** Addition to lower limb prosthesis, vertical shock reducing pylon feature

* **L5990** Addition to lower extremity prosthesis, user adjustable heel height

~~L5993~~ ~~Addition to lower extremity prosthesis, heavy duty feature, foot only, (for patient weight greater than 300 lbs)~~ ✖

~~L5994~~ ~~Addition to lower extremity prosthesis, heavy duty feature, knee only, (for patient weight greater than 300 lbs)~~ ✖

~~L5995~~ ~~Addition to lower extremity prosthesis, heavy duty feature other than foot or knee, (for patient weight greater than 300 lbs)~~ ✖

* **L5999** Lower extremity prosthesis, not otherwise specified

L5855 – L5999

◀▶ **New**   ←→ **Revised**   ✔ **Reinstated**   ✖ **Deleted**
⊙ **Special coverage instructions**   ◆ **Not covered or valid by Medicare**   ✳ **Carrier discretion**   ▶ **ASC payment group**

Upper Limb

NOTE: The procedures in L6000-L6599 are considered as base or basic procedures and may be modified by listing procedures from the additions sections. The base procedures include only standard friction wrist and control cable system unless otherwise specified.

Partial Hand

∗ **L6000** Partial hand, Robin-Aids, thumb remaining (or equal)

∗ **L6010** Partial hand, Robin-Aids, little and/or ring finger remaining (or equal)

∗ **L6020** Partial hand, Robin-Aids, no finger remaining (or equal)

∗ **L6025** Transcarpal/metacarpal or partial hand disarticulation prosthesis, external power, self-suspended, inner socket with removable forearm section, electrodes and cables, two batteries, charger, myoelectric control of terminal device

Wrist Disarticulation

∗ **L6050** Wrist disarticulation, molded socket, flexible elbow hinges, triceps pad

∗ **L6055** Wrist disarticulation, molded socket with expandable interface, flexible elbow hinges, triceps pad

Below Elbow

∗ **L6100** Below elbow, molded socket, flexible elbow hinge, triceps pad

∗ **L6110** Below elbow, molded socket, (Muenster or Northwestern suspension types)

∗ **L6120** Below elbow, molded double wall split socket, step-up hinges, half cuff

∗ **L6130** Below elbow, molded double wall split socket, stump activated locking hinge, half cuff

Elbow Disarticulation

∗ **L6200** Elbow disarticulation, molded socket, outside locking hinge, forearm

∗ **L6205** Elbow disarticulation, molded socket with expandable interface, outside locking hinges, forearm

Above Elbow

∗ **L6250** Above elbow, molded double wall socket, internal locking elbow, forearm

Shoulder Disarticulation

∗ **L6300** Shoulder disarticulation, molded socket, shoulder bulkhead, humeral section, internal locking elbow, forearm

∗ **L6310** Shoulder disarticulation, passive restoration (complete prosthesis)

∗ **L6320** Shoulder disarticulation, passive restoration (shoulder cap only)

Interscapular Thoracic

∗ **L6350** Interscapular thoracic, molded socket, shoulder bulkhead, humeral section, internal locking elbow, forearm

∗ **L6360** Interscapular thoracic, passive restoration (complete prosthesis)

∗ **L6370** Interscapular thoracic, passive restoration (shoulder cap only)

Immediate and Early Postsurgical Procedures

∗ **L6380** Immediate post surgical or early fitting, application of initial rigid dressing, including fitting alignment and suspension of components, and one cast change, wrist disarticulation or below elbow

∗ **L6382** Immediate post surgical or early fitting, application of initial rigid dressing including fitting alignment and suspension of components, and one cast change, elbow disarticulation or above elbow

∗ **L6384** Immediate post surgical or early fitting, application of initial rigid dressing including fitting alignment and suspension of components, and one cast change, shoulder disarticulation or interscapular thoracic

∗ **L6386** Immediate post surgical or early fitting, each additional cast change and realignment

∗ **L6388** Immediate post surgical or early fitting, application of rigid dressing only

◄► New　←→ Revised　✔ Reinstated　✖ Deleted
⊗ Special coverage instructions　◆ Not covered or valid by Medicare　∗ Carrier discretion　▶ ASC payment group

ORTHOTICS

Endoskeletal: Below Elbow

* **L6400**   Below elbow, molded socket, endoskeletal system, including soft prosthetic tissue shaping

Endoskeletal: Elbow Disarticulation

* **L6450**   Elbow disarticulation, molded socket, endoskeletal system, including soft prosthetic tissue shaping

Endoskeletal: Above Elbow

* **L6500**   Above elbow, molded socket, endoskeletal system, including soft prosthetic tissue shaping

Endoskeletal: Shoulder Disarticulation

* **L6550**   Shoulder disarticulation, molded socket, endoskeletal system, including soft prosthetic tissue shaping

Endoskeletal: Interscapular Thoracic

* **L6570**   Interscapular thoracic, molded socket, endoskeletal system, including soft prosthetic tissue shaping

* **L6580**   Preparatory, wrist disarticulation or below elbow, single wall plastic socket, friction wrist, flexible elbow hinges, figure of eight harness, humeral cuff, Bowden cable control, USMC or equal pylon, no cover, molded to patient model

* **L6582**   Preparatory, wrist disarticulation or below elbow, single wall socket, friction wrist, flexible elbow hinges, figure of eight harness, humeral cuff, Bowden cable control, USMC or equal pylon, no cover, direct formed

* **L6584**   Preparatory, elbow disarticulation or above elbow, single wall plastic socket, friction wrist, locking elbow, figure of eight harness, fair lead cable control, USMC or equal pylon, no cover, molded to patient model

* **L6586**   Preparatory, elbow disarticulation or above elbow, single wall socket, friction wrist, locking elbow, figure of eight harness, fair lead cable control, USMC or equal pylon, no cover, direct formed

* **L6588**   Preparatory, shoulder disarticulation or interscapular thoracic, single wall plastic socket, shoulder joint, locking elbow, friction wrist, chest strap, fair lead cable control, USMC or equal pylon, no cover, molded to patient model

* **L6590**   Preparatory, shoulder disarticulation or interscapular thoracic, single wall socket, shoulder joint, locking elbow, friction wrist, chest strap, fair lead cable control, USMC or equal pylon, no cover, direct formed

Additions to Upper Limb

NOTE: The following procedures/modifications/components may be added to other base procedures. The items in this section should reflect the additional complexity of each modification procedure, in addition to base procedure, at the time of the original order.

* **L6600**   Upper extremity additions, polycentric hinge, pair

* **L6605**   Upper extremity additions, single pivot hinge, pair

* **L6610**   Upper extremity additions, flexible metal hinge, pair

* **L6611**   Addition to upper extremity prosthesis, external powered, additional switch, any type

* **L6615**   Upper extremity addition, disconnect locking wrist unit

* **L6616**   Upper extremity addition, additional disconnect insert for locking wrist unit, each

* **L6620**   Upper extremity addition, flexion/extension wrist unit, with or without friction

* **L6621**   Upper extremity prosthesis addition, flexion/extension wrist with or without friction, for use with external powered terminal device

* **L6623**   Upper extremity addition, spring assisted rotational wrist unit with latch release

* **L6624**   Upper extremity addition, flexion/extension and rotation wrist unit

* **L6625**   Upper extremity addition, rotation wrist unit with cable lock

* **L6628**   Upper extremity addition, quick disconnect hook adapter, Otto Bock or equal

---

◄► New   ←→ Revised   ✔ Reinstated   ✖ Deleted

Ⓢ Special coverage instructions   ◆ Not covered or valid by Medicare   * Carrier discretion   ▶ ASC payment group

L6400 – L6628

* **L6629** Upper extremity addition, quick disconnect lamination collar with coupling piece, Otto Bock or equal

* **L6630** Upper extremity addition, stainless steel, any wrist

* **L6632** Upper extremity addition, latex suspension sleeve, each

* **L6635** Upper extremity addition, lift assist for elbow

* **L6637** Upper extremity addition, nudge control elbow lock

* **L6638** Upper extremity addition to prosthesis, electric locking feature, only for use with manually powered elbow

* **L6639** Upper extremity addition, heavy duty feature, any elbow

* **L6640** Upper extremity additions, shoulder abduction joint, pair

* **L6641** Upper extremity addition, excursion amplifier, pulley type

* **L6642** Upper extremity addition, excursion amplifier, lever type

* **L6645** Upper extremity addition, shoulder flexion-abduction joint, each

* **L6646** Upper extremity addition, shoulder joint, multipositional locking, flexion, adjustable abduction friction control, for use with body powered or external powered system

* **L6647** Upper extremity addition, shoulder lock mechanism, body powered actuator

* **L6648** Upper extremity addition, shoulder lock mechanism, external powered actuator

* **L6650** Upper extremity addition, shoulder universal joint, each

* **L6655** Upper extremity addition, standard control cable, extra

* **L6660** Upper extremity addition, heavy duty control cable

* **L6665** Upper extremity addition, Teflon, or equal, cable lining

* **L6670** Upper extremity addition, hook to hand, cable adapter

* **L6672** Upper extremity addition, harness, chest or shoulder, saddle type

* **L6675** Upper extremity addition, harness, (e.g. figure of eight type), single cable design

* **L6676** Upper extremity addition, harness, (e.g. figure of eight type), dual cable design

* **L6677** Upper extremity addition, harness, triple control, simultaneous operation of terminal device and elbow

* **L6680** Upper extremity addition, test socket, wrist disarticulation or below elbow

* **L6682** Upper extremity addition, test socket, elbow disarticulation or above elbow

* **L6684** Upper extremity addition, test socket, shoulder disarticulation or interscapular thoracic

* **L6686** Upper extremity addition, suction socket

* **L6687** Upper extremity addition, frame type socket, below elbow or wrist disarticulation

* **L6688** Upper extremity addition, frame type socket, above elbow or elbow disarticulation

* **L6689** Upper extremity addition, frame type socket, shoulder disarticulation

* **L6690** Upper extremity addition, frame type socket, interscapular-thoracic

* **L6691** Upper extremity addition, removable insert, each

* **L6692** Upper extremity addition, silicone gel insert or equal, each

* **L6693** Upper extremity addition, locking elbow, forearm counterbalance

* **L6694** Addition to upper extremity prosthesis, below elbow/above elbow, custom fabricated from existing mold or prefabricated, socket insert, silicone gel, elastomeric or equal, for use with locking mechanism

* **L6695** Addition to upper extremity prosthesis, below elbow/above elbow, custom fabricated from existing mold or prefabricated, socket insert, silicone gel, elastomeric or equal, not for use with locking mechanism

* **L6696** Addition to upper extremity prosthesis, below elbow/above elbow, custom fabricated socket insert for congenital or atypical traumatic amputee, silicone gel, elastomeric or equal, for use with or without locking mechanism, initial only (for other than initial, use code L6694 or L6695)

* **L6697** Addition to upper extremity prosthesis, below elbow/above elbow, custom fabricated socket insert for other than congenital or atypical traumatic amputee, silicone gel, elastomeric or equal, for use with or without locking mechanism, initial only (for other than initial, use code L6694 or L6695)

* **L6698** Addition to upper extremity prosthesis, below elbow/above elbow, lock mechanism, excludes socket insert

◀▶ New   ←→ Revised   ✔ Reinstated   ✖ Deleted
⊙ Special coverage instructions   ◆ Not covered or valid by Medicare   ✳ Carrier discretion   ▶ ASC payment group

L6629 – L6698

241

Terminal Devices

Hooks

* **L6703**   Terminal device, passive hand/mitt, any material, any size

* **L6704**   Terminal device, sport/recreational/work attachment, any material, any size

* **L6706**   Terminal device, hook, mechanical, voluntary opening, any material, any size, lined or unlined

* **L6707**   Terminal device, hook, mechanical, voluntary closing, any material, any size, lined or unlined

* **L6708**   Terminal device, hand, mechanical, voluntary opening, any material, any size

* **L6709**   Terminal device, hand, mechanical, voluntary closing, any material, any size

▶ * **L6711**   Terminal device, hook, mechanical, voluntary opening, any material, any size, lined or unlined, pediatric

▶ * **L6712**   Terminal device, hook, mechanical, voluntary closing, any material, any size, lined or unlined, pediatric

▶ * **L6713**   Terminal device, hand, mechanical, voluntary opening, any material, any size, pediatric

▶ * **L6714**   Terminal device, hand, mechanical, voluntary closing, any material, any size, pediatric

▶ * **L6721**   Terminal device, hook or hand, heavy duty, mechanical, voluntary opening, any material, any size, lined or unlined

▶ * **L6722**   Terminal device, hook or hand, heavy duty, mechanical, voluntary closing, any material, any size, lined or unlined

☺ **L6805**   Addition to terminal device, modifier wrist unit

   IOM: 100-02, 15, 120; 100-04, 3, 10.4

☺ **L6810**   Addition to terminal device, precision pinch device

   IOM: 100-02, 15, 120; 100-04, 3, 10.4

Hands

* **L6881**   Automatic grasp feature, addition to upper limb electric prosthetic terminal device

☺ **L6882**   Microprocessor control feature, addition to upper limb prosthetic terminal device

   IOM: 100-02, 15, 120; 100-04, 3, 10.4

Replacement Sockets

* **L6883**   Replacement socket, below elbow/wrist disarticulation, molded to patient model, for use with or without external power

* **L6884**   Replacement socket, above elbow/elbow disarticulation, molded to patient model, for use with or without external power

* **L6885**   Replacement socket, shoulder disarticulation/interscapular thoracic, molded to patient model, for use with or without external power

Gloves for Above Hands

* **L6890**   Addition to upper extremity prosthesis, glove for terminal device, any material, prefabricated, includes fitting and adjustment

* **L6895**   Addition to upper extremity prosthesis, glove for terminal device, any material, custom fabricated

Hand Restoration

* **L6900**   Hand restoration (casts, shading and measurements included), partial hand, with glove, thumb or one finger remaining

* **L6905**   Hand restoration (casts, shading and measurements included), partial hand, with glove, multiple fingers remaining

* **L6910**   Hand restoration (casts, shading and measurements included), partial hand, with glove, no fingers remaining

* **L6915**   Hand restoration (shading, and measurements included), replacement glove for above

External Power

Base Devices

* **L6920**   Wrist disarticulation, external power, self-suspended inner socket, removable forearm shell, Otto Bock or equal switch, cables, two batteries and one charger, switch control of terminal device

* **L6925**   Wrist disarticulation, external power, self-suspended inner socket, removable forearm shell, Otto Bock or equal electrodes, cables, two batteries and one charger, myoelectronic control of terminal device

---

◄▶ New   ←→ Revised   ✔ Reinstated   ✖ Deleted

☺ Special coverage instructions   ◆ Not covered or valid by Medicare   ✱ Carrier discretion   ▶ ASC payment group

✳ **L6930** Below elbow, external power, self-suspended inner socket, removable forearm shell, Otto Bock or equal switch, cables, two batteries and one charger, switch control of terminal device

✳ **L6935** Below elbow, external power, self-suspended inner socket, removable forearm shell, Otto Bock or equal electrodes, cables, two batteries and one charger, myoelectronic control of terminal device

✳ **L6940** Elbow disarticulation, external power, molded inner socket, removable humeral shell, outside locking hinges, forearm, Otto Bock or equal switch, cables, two batteries and one charger, switch control of terminal device

✳ **L6945** Elbow disarticulation, external power, molded inner socket, removable humeral shell, outside locking hinges, forearm, Otto Bock or equal electrodes, cables, two batteries and one charger, myoelectronic control of terminal device

✳ **L6950** Above elbow, external power, molded inner socket, removable humeral shell, internal locking elbow, forearm, Otto Bock or equal switch, cables, two batteries and one charger, switch control of terminal device

✳ **L6955** Above elbow, external power, molded inner socket, removable humeral shell, internal locking elbow, forearm, Otto Bock or equal electrodes, cables, two batteries and one charger, myoelectronic control of terminal device

✳ **L6960** Shoulder disarticulation, external power, molded inner socket, removable shoulder shell, shoulder bulkhead, humeral section, mechanical elbow, forearm, Otto Bock or equal switch, cables, two batteries and one charger, switch control of terminal device

✳ **L6965** Shoulder disarticulation, external power, molded inner socket, removable shoulder shell, shoulder bulkhead, humeral section, mechanical elbow, forearm, Otto Bock or equal electrodes, cables, two batteries and one charger, myoelectronic control of terminal device

✳ **L6970** Interscapular-thoracic, external power, molded inner socket, removable shoulder shell, shoulder bulkhead, humeral section, mechanical elbow, forearm, Otto Bock or equal switch, cables, two batteries and one charger, switch control of terminal device

✳ **L6975** Interscapular-thoracic, external power, molded inner socket, removable shoulder shell, shoulder bulkhead, humeral section, mechanical elbow, forearm, Otto Bock or equal electrodes, cables, two batteries and one charger, myoelectronic control of terminal device

Terminal Devices

✳ **L7007** Electric hand, switch or myoelectric controlled, adult

✳ **L7008** Electric hand, switch or myoelectric controlled, pediatric

✳ **L7009** Electric hook, switch or myoelectric controlled, adult

✳ **L7040** Prehensile actuator, switch controlled

✳ **L7045** Electric hook, switch or myoelectric controlled, pediatric

Elbow

✳ **L7170** Electronic elbow, Hosmer or equal, switch controlled

✳ **L7180** Electronic elbow, microprocessor sequential control of elbow and terminal device

✳ **L7181** Electronic elbow, microprocessor simultaneous control of elbow and terminal device

✳ **L7185** Electronic elbow, adolescent, Variety Village or equal, switch controlled

✳ **L7186** Electronic elbow, child, Variety Village or equal, switch controlled

✳ **L7190** Electronic elbow, adolescent, Variety Village or equal, myoelectronically controlled

✳ **L7191** Electronic elbow, child, Variety Village or equal, myoelectronically controlled

✳ **L7260** Electronic wrist rotator, Otto Bock or equal

✳ **L7261** Electronic wrist rotator, for Utah arm

✳ **L7266** Servo control, Steeper or equal

✳ **L7272** Analogue control, UNB or equal

✳ **L7274** Proportional control, 6-12 volt, Liberty, Utah or equal

Battery Components

✳ **L7360** Six volt battery, each

✳ **L7362** Battery charger, six volt, each

◀▶ New   ←→ Revised   ✔ Reinstated   ✖ Deleted

♺ Special coverage instructions   ◆ Not covered or valid by Medicare   ✳ Carrier discretion   ▶ ASC payment group

* **L7364** Twelve volt battery, each

* **L7366** Battery charger, twelve volt, each

* **L7367** Lithium ion battery, replacement

* **L7368** Lithium ion battery charger

Other/Repair

* **L7400** Addition to upper extremity prosthesis, below elbow/wrist disarticulation, ultralight material (titanium, carbon fiber or equal)

* **L7401** Addition to upper extremity prosthesis, above elbow disarticulation, ultralight material (titanium, carbon fiber or equal)

* **L7402** Addition to upper extremity prosthesis, shoulder disarticulation/interscapular thoracic, ultralight material (titanium, carbon fiber or equal)

* **L7403** Addition to upper extremity prosthesis, below elbow/wrist disarticulation, acrylic material

* **L7404** Addition to upper extremity prosthesis, above elbow disarticulation, acrylic material

* **L7405** Addition to upper extremity prosthesis, shoulder disarticulation/interscapular thoracic, acrylic material

* **L7499** Upper extremity prosthesis, not otherwise specified

⊗ **L7500** Repair of prosthetic device, hourly rate (excludes V5335 repair of oral or laryngeal prosthesis or artificial larynx)

IOM: 100-02, 15, 110.2; 100-02, 15, 120; 100-04, 32, 100

⊗ **L7510** Repair of prosthetic device, repair or replace minor parts

IOM: 100-02, 15, 110.2; 100-02, 15, 120; 100-04, 32, 100

* **L7520** Repair prosthetic device, labor component, per 15 minutes

◆ **L7600** Prosthetic donning sleeve, any material, each

Medicare Statute 1862(1)(a)

L7611 Terminal device, hook, mechanical, voluntary opening, any material, any size, lined or unlined, pediatric ✖
Cross Reference L6711

L7612 Terminal device, hook, mechanical, voluntary closing, any material, any size, lined or unlined, pediatric ✖
Cross Reference L6712

L7613 Terminal device, hand, mechanical, voluntary opening, any material, any size, pediatric ✖
Cross Reference L6713

L7614 Terminal device, hand, mechanical, voluntary closing, any material, any size, pediatric ✖
Cross Reference L6714

L7621 Terminal device, hook or hand, heavy duty, mechanical, voluntary opening, any material, any size, lined or unlined ✖
Cross Reference L6721

L7622 Terminal device, hook or hand, heavy duty, mechanical, voluntary closing, any material, any size, lined or unlined ✖
Cross Reference L6722

General

* **L7900** Male vacuum erection system

Breast Prostheses

⊗ **L8000** Breast prosthesis, mastectomy bra
IOM: 100-02, 15, 120

⊗ **L8001** Breast prosthesis, mastectomy bra, with integrated breast prosthesis form, unilateral
IOM: 100-02, 15, 120

⊗ **L8002** Breast prosthesis, mastectomy bra, with integrated breast prosthesis form, bilateral
IOM: 100-02, 15, 120

⊗ **L8010** Breast prosthesis, mastectomy sleeve
IOM: 100-02, 15, 120

⊗ **L8015** External breast prosthesis garment, with mastectomy form, post mastectomy
IOM: 100-02, 15, 120

⊗ **L8020** Breast prosthesis, mastectomy form
IOM: 100-02, 15, 120

⊗ **L8030** Breast prosthesis, silicone or equal
IOM: 100-02, 15, 120

⊗ **L8035** Custom breast prosthesis, post mastectomy, molded to patient model
IOM: 100-02, 15, 120

* **L8039** Breast prosthesis, not otherwise specified

◀▶ New	←→ Revised	✔ Reinstated	✖ Deleted
⊗ Special coverage instructions	◆ Not covered or valid by Medicare	* Carrier discretion	▸ ASC payment group

Nasal, Orbital, Auricular Prosthesis

✳ **L8040**   Nasal prosthesis, provided by a non-physician

✳ **L8041**   Midfacial prosthesis, provided by a non-physician

✳ **L8042**   Orbital prosthesis, provided by a non-physician

✳ **L8043**   Upper facial prosthesis, provided by a non-physician

✳ **L8044**   Hemi-facial prosthesis, provided by a non-physician

✳ **L8045**   Auricular prosthesis, provided by a non-physician

✳ **L8046**   Partial facial prosthesis, provided by a non-physician

✳ **L8047**   Nasal septal prosthesis, provided by a non-physician

✳ **L8048**   Unspecified maxillofacial prosthesis, by report, provided by a non-physician

✳ **L8049**   Repair or modification of maxillofacial prosthesis, labor component, 15 minute increments, provided by a non-physician

Trusses

⊛ **L8300**   Truss, single with standard pad
IOM: 100-02, 15, 120; 100-03, 4, 280.11; 100-03, 4, 280.12; 100-04, 4, 240

⊛ **L8310**   Truss, double with standard pads
IOM: 100-02, 15, 120; 100-03, 4, 280.11; 100-03, 4, 280.12; 100-04, 4, 240

⊛ **L8320**   Truss, addition to standard pad, water pad
IOM: 100-02, 15, 120; 100-03, 4, 280.11; 100-03, 4, 280.12; 100-04, 4, 240

⊛ **L8330**   Truss, addition to standard pad, scrotal pad
IOM: 100-02, 15, 120; 100-03, 4, 280.11; 100-03, 4, 280.12; 100-04, 4, 240

Prosthetic Socks

⊛ **L8400**   Prosthetic sheath, below knee, each
IOM: 100-02, 15, 200

⊛ **L8410**   Prosthetic sheath, above knee, each
IOM: 100-02, 15, 200

⊛ **L8415**   Prosthetic sheath, upper limb, each
IOM: 100-02, 15, 200

✳ **L8417**   Prosthetic sheath/sock, including a gel cushion layer, below knee or above knee, each

⊛ **L8420**   Prosthetic sock, multiple ply, below knee, each
IOM: 100-02, 15, 200

⊛ **L8430**   Prosthetic sock, multiple ply, above knee, each
IOM: 100-02, 15, 200

⊛ **L8435**   Prosthetic sock, multiple ply, upper limb, each
IOM: 100-02, 15, 200

⊛ **L8440**   Prosthetic shrinker, below knee, each
IOM: 100-02, 15, 200

⊛ **L8460**   Prosthetic shrinker, above knee, each
IOM: 100-02, 15, 200

⊛ **L8465**   Prosthetic shrinker, upper limb, each
IOM: 100-02, 15, 200

⊛ **L8470**   Prosthetic sock, single ply, fitting, below knee, each
IOM: 100-02, 15, 200

⊛ **L8480**   Prosthetic sock, single ply, fitting, above knee, each
IOM: 100-02, 15, 200

⊛ **L8485**   Prosthetic sock, single ply, fitting, upper limb, each
IOM: 100-02, 15, 200

✳ **L8499**   Unlisted procedure for miscellaneous prosthetic services

Prosthetic Implants

Integumentary System

⊛ **L8500**   Artificial larynx, any type
IOM: 100-02, 15, 120; 100-03, 1, 50.2; 100-04, 4, 240

⊛ **L8501**   Tracheostomy speaking valve
IOM: 100-03, 1, 50.4

✳ **L8505**   Artificial larynx replacement battery / accessory, any type

✳ **L8507**   Tracheo-esophageal voice prosthesis, patient inserted, any type, each

✳ **L8509**   Tracheo-esophageal voice prosthesis, inserted by a licensed health care provider, any type

⊛ **L8510**   Voice amplifier
IOM: 100-03, 1, 50.2

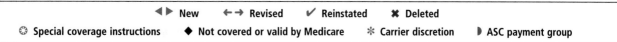

◄▶ New   ←→ Revised   ✔ Reinstated   ✖ Deleted

⊛ Special coverage instructions   ◆ Not covered or valid by Medicare   ✳ Carrier discretion   ▶ ASC payment group

* **L8511** Insert for indwelling tracheoesophageal prosthesis, with or without valve, replacement only, each

* **L8512** Gelatin capsules or equivalent, for use with tracheoesophageal voice prosthesis, replacement only, per 10

* **L8513** Cleaning device used with tracheoesophageal voice prosthesis, pipet, brush, or equal, replacement only, each

* **L8514** Tracheoesophageal puncture dilator, replacement only, each

* **L8515** Gelatin capsule, application device for use with tracheoesophageal voice prosthesis, each

⊙ **L8600** Implantable breast prosthesis, silicone or equal

IOM: 100-02, 15, 120; 100-3, 2, 140.2

Urinary System

⊙ **L8603** Injectable bulking agent, collagen implant, urinary tract, 2.5 ml syringe, includes shipping and necessary supplies

(Bill on paper, acquisition cost invoice required)

IOM: 100-03, 4, 280.1

▶ * **L8604** Injectable bulking agent, dextranomer/ hyaluronic acid copolymer implant, urinary tract, 1 ml, includes shipping and necessary supplies

⊙ **L8606** Injectable bulking agent, synthetic implant, urinary tract, 1 ml syringe, includes shipping and necessary supplies

(Bill on paper, acquisition cost invoice required)

IOM: 100-03, 4, 280.1

Head (Skull, Facial Bones, and Temporomandibular Joint)

* **L8609** Artificial cornea

⊙ **L8610** Ocular implant

IOM: 100-02, 15, 120

⊙ **L8612** Aqueous shunt

IOM: 100-02, 15, 120,
Cross Reference Q0074

⊙ **L8613** Ossicula implant

IOM: 100-02, 15, 120

⊙ **L8614** Cochlear device, includes all internal and external components

IOM: 100-02, 15, 120; 100-03, 1, 50.3

⊙ **L8615** Headset/headpiece for use with cochlear implant device, replacement

IOM: 100-03, 1, 50.3

⊙ **L8616** Microphone for use with cochlear implant device, replacement

IOM: 100-03, 1, 50.3

⊙ **L8617** Transmitting coil for use with cochlear implant device, replacement

IOM: 100-03, 1, 50.3

⊙ **L8618** Transmitter cable for use with cochlear implant device, replacement

IOM: 100-03, 1, 50.3

⊙ **L8619** Cochlear implant external speech processor, replacement

IOM: 100-03, 1, 50.3

* **L8621** Zinc air battery for use with cochlear implant device, replacement, each

* **L8622** Alkaline battery for use with cochlear implant device, any size, replacement, each

* **L8623** Lithium ion battery for use with cochlear implant device speech processor, other than ear level, replacement, each

* **L8624** Lithium ion battery for use with cochlear implant device speech processor, ear level, replacement, each

Upper Extremity

⊙ **L8630** Metacarpophalangeal joint implant

IOM: 100-02, 15, 120

⊙ **L8631** Metacarpal phalangeal joint replacement, two or more pieces, metal (e.g., stainless steel or cobalt chrome), ceramic-like material (e.g., pyrocarbon), for surgical implantation (all sizes, includes entire system)

IOM: 100-02, 15, 120

Lower Extremity (Joint: Knee, Ankle, Toe)

⊙ **L8641** Metatarsal joint implant

IOM: 100-02, 15, 120

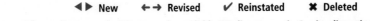

◀▶ New ←→ Revised ✔ Reinstated ✖ Deleted
⊙ Special coverage instructions ◆ Not covered or valid by Medicare * Carrier discretion ▶ ASC payment group

⊗ **L8642** Hallux implant

(May be billed by ambulatory surgical center or surgeon)

IOM: 100-02, 15, 120,

Cross Reference CPT Q0073

Miscellaneous Muscular-Skeletal

⊗ **L8658** Interphalangeal joint spacer, silicone or equal, each

IOM: 100-02, 15, 120

⊗ **L8659** Interphalangeal finger joint replacement, 2 or more pieces, metal (e.g., stainless steel or cobalt chrome), ceramic-like material (e.g., pyrocarbon) for surgical implantation, any size

IOM: 100-02, 15, 120

Cardiovascular System

⊗ **L8670** Vascular graft material, synthetic, implant

IOM: 100-02, 15, 120

Neurostimulator

⊗ **L8680** Implantable neurostimulator electrode, each

IOM: 100-03, 4, 280.4

→ ⊗ **L8681** Patient programmer (external) for use with implantable programmable neurostimulator pulse generator, replacement only

IOM: 100-03, 4, 280.4

⊗ **L8682** Implantable neurostimulator radiofrequency receiver

IOM: 100-03, 4, 280.4

⊗ **L8683** Radiofrequency transmitter (external) for use with implantable neurostimulator radiofrequency receiver

IOM: 100-03, 4, 280.4

⊗ **L8684** Radiofrequency transmitter (external) for use with implantable sacral root neurostimulator receiver for bowel and bladder management, replacement

IOM: 100-03, 4, 280.4

⊗ **L8685** Implantable neurostimulator pulse generator, single array, rechargeable, includes extension

IOM: 100-03, 4, 280.4

⊗ **L8686** Implantable neurostimulator pulse generator, single array, non-rechargeable, includes extension

IOM: 100-03, 4, 280.4

⊗ **L8687** Implantable neurostimulator pulse generator, dual array, rechargeable, includes extension

IOM: 100-03, 4, 280.4

⊗ **L8688** Implantable neurostimulator pulse generator, dual array, non-rechargeable, includes extension

IOM: 100-03, 4, 280.4

→ ⊗ **L8689** External recharging system for battery (internal) for use with implantable neurostimulator, replacement only

IOM: 100-03, 4, 280.4

✳ **L8690** Auditory osseointegrated device, includes all internal and external components

✳ **L8691** Auditory osseointegrated device, external sound processor, replacement

→ ⊗ **L8695** External recharging system for battery (external) for use with implantable neurostimulator, replacement only

IOM: 100-03, 4, 280.4

Genital

✳ **L8699** Prosthetic implant, not otherwise specified

✳ **L9900** Orthotic and prosthetic supply, accessory, and/or service component of another HCPCS "L" code

---

◀▶ **New**   ←→ **Revised**   ✔ **Reinstated**   ✖ **Deleted**

⊗ **Special coverage instructions**   ◆ **Not covered or valid by Medicare**   ✳ **Carrier discretion**   ▶ **ASC payment group**

OTHER MEDICAL SERVICES (M0000-M9999)

✪ **M0064** Brief office visit for the sole purpose of monitoring or changing drug prescriptions used in the treatment of mental psychoneurotic and personality disorders

IOM: 100-04, 12, 210.1

◆ **M0075** Cellular therapy

IOM: 100-03, 1, 30.8

◆ **M0076** Prolotherapy

IOM: 100-03, 2, 150.7

◆ **M0100** Intragastric hypothermia using gastric freezing

IOM: 100-03, 4, 250.1

◆ **M0300** IV chelation therapy (chemical endarterectomy)

(Bill on paper. Identify name, total dosage of chelating agent given in the "Remarks" field.)

IOM: 100-03, 1, 20.21

◆ **M0301** Fabric wrapping of abdominal aneurysm

IOM: 100-03, 1, 20.23

◀ ▶ **New**   ← → **Revised**   ✔ **Reinstated**   ✖ **Deleted**

✪ **Special coverage instructions**   ◆ **Not covered or valid by Medicare**   ✳ **Carrier discretion**   ▶ **ASC payment group**

LABORATORY SERVICES (P0000-P9999)

Chemistry and Toxicology Tests

⊕ **P2028** Cephalin floculation, blood
IOM: 100-03, 4, 300.1

⊕ **P2029** Congo red, blood
IOM: 100-03, 4, 300.1

◆ **P2031** Hair analysis (excluding arsenic)
IOM: 100-03, 4, 300.1

⊕ **P2033** Thymol turbidity, blood
IOM: 100-03, 4, 300.1

⊕ **P2038** Mucoprotein, blood (seromucoid) (medical necessity procedure)
IOM: 100-03, 4, 300.1

Pathology Screening Tests

⊕ **P3000** Screening Papanicolaou smear, cervical or vaginal, up to three smears, by technician under physician supervision
IOM: 100-03, 3, 190.2,

Laboratory Certification: Cytology

⊕ **P3001** Screening Papanicolaou smear, cervical or vaginal, up to three smears, requiring interpretation by physician
IOM: 100-03, 3, 190.2,

Laboratory Certification: Cytology

Microbiology Tests

◆ **P7001** Culture, bacterial, urine; quantitative, sensitivity study Cross Reference CPT, Laboratory Certification: Bacteriology

Miscellaneous Pathology

⊕ **P9010** Blood (whole), for transfusion, per unit
IOM: 100-01, 3, 20.5; 100-02, 1, 10

⊕ **P9011** Blood, split unit
IOM: 100-01, 3, 20.5; 100-02, 1, 10

⊕ **P9012** Cryoprecipitate, each unit
IOM: 100-01, 3, 20.5; 100-02, 1, 10

⊕ **P9016** Red blood cells, leukocytes reduced, each unit
IOM: 100-01, 3, 20.5; 100-02, 1, 10

⊕ **P9017** Fresh frozen plasma (single donor), frozen within 8 hours of collection, each unit
IOM: 100-01, 3, 20.5; 100-02, 1, 10

⊕ **P9019** Platelets, each unit
IOM: 100-01, 3, 20.5; 100-02, 1, 10

⊕ **P9020** Platelet rich plasma, each unit
IOM: 100-01, 3, 20.5; 100-02, 1, 10

⊕ **P9021** Red blood cells, each unit
IOM: 100-01, 3, 20.5; 100-02, 1, 10

⊕ **P9022** Red blood cells, washed, each unit
IOM: 100-01, 3, 20.5; 100-02, 1, 10

⊕ **P9023** Plasma, pooled multiple donor, solvent/detergent treated, frozen, each unit
Other: Plas+SD; Plasma (pooled multiple donor, frozen)
IOM: 100-01, 3, 20.5; 100-02, 1, 10

⊕ **P9031** Platelets, leukocytes reduced, each unit
IOM: 100-01, 3, 20.5; 100-02, 1, 10

⊕ **P9032** Platelets, irradiated, each unit
IOM: 100-01, 3, 20.5; 100-02, 1, 10

⊕ **P9033** Platelets, leukocytes reduced, irradiated, each unit
IOM: 100-01, 3, 20.5; 100-02, 1, 10

⊕ **P9034** Platelets, pheresis, each unit
IOM: 100-01, 3, 20.5; 100-02, 1, 10

⊕ **P9035** Platelets, pheresis, leukocytes reduced, each unit
IOM: 100-01, 3, 20.5; 100-02, 1, 10

⊕ **P9036** Platelets, pheresis, irradiated, each unit
IOM: 100-01, 3, 20.5; 100-02, 1, 10

⊕ **P9037** Platelets, pheresis, leukocytes reduced, irradiated, each unit
IOM: 100-01, 3, 20.5; 100-02, 1, 10

⊕ **P9038** Red blood cells, irradiated, each unit
IOM: 100-01, 3, 20.5; 100-02, 1, 10

⊕ **P9039** Red blood cells, deglycerolized, each unit
IOM: 100-01, 3, 20.5; 100-02, 1, 10

⊕ **P9040** Red blood cells, leukocytes reduced, irradiated, each unit
IOM: 100-01, 3, 20.5; 100-02, 1, 10

✳ **P9041**▶ Infusion, albumin (human), 5%, 50 ml

⊕ **P9043** Infusion, plasma protein fraction (human), 5%, 50 ml
IOM: 100-01, 3, 20.5; 100-02, 1, 10

◀▶ **New**   ←→ **Revised**   ✔ **Reinstated**   ✖ **Deleted**

⊕ **Special coverage instructions**   ◆ **Not covered or valid by Medicare**   ✳ **Carrier discretion**   ▶ **ASC payment group**

LABORATORY SERVICES

⊛ **P9044** Plasma, cryoprecipitate reduced, each unit

Other: Plasma (cryoprecipitate reduced)

IOM: 100-01, 3, 20.5; 100-02, 1, 10

✳ **P9045▶** Infusion, albumin (human), 5%, 250 ml

✳ **P9046▶** Infusion, albumin (human), 25%, 20 ml

✳ **P9047▶** Infusion, albumin (human), 25%, 50 ml

✳ **P9048** Infusion, plasma protein fraction (human), 5%, 250 ml

✳ **P9050** Granulocytes, pheresis, each unit

⊛ **P9051** Whole blood or red blood cells, leukocytes reduced, CMV-negative, each unit

Medicare Statute 1833(t)

⊛ **P9052** Platelets, HLA-matched leukocytes reduced, apheresis/pheresis, each unit

Medicare Statute 1833(t)

⊛ **P9053** Platelets, pheresis, leukocytes reduced, CMV-negative, irradiated, each unit

Medicare Statute 1833(t)

⊛ **P9054** Whole blood or red blood cells, leukocytes reduced, frozen, deglycerol, washed, each unit

Medicare Statute 1833(t)

⊛ **P9055** Platelets, leukocytes reduced, CMV-negative, apheresis/pheresis, each unit

Medicare Statute 1833(t)

⊛ **P9056** Whole blood, leukocytes reduced, irradiated, each unit

Medicare Statute 1833(t)

⊛ **P9057** Red blood cells, frozen/deglycerolized/washed, leukocytes reduced, irradiated, each unit

Medicare Statute 1833(t)

⊛ **P9058** Red blood cells, leukocytes reduced, CMV-negative, irradiated, each unit

Medicare Statute 1833(t)

⊛ **P9059** Fresh frozen plasma between 8-24 hours of collection, each unit

Medicare Statute 1833(t)

⊛ **P9060** Fresh frozen plasma, donor retested, each unit

Medicare Statute 1833(t)

⊛ **P9603** Travel allowance one way in connection with medically necessary laboratory specimen collection drawn from home bound or nursing home bound patient; prorated miles actually traveled

IOM: 100-04, 16, 60

⊛ **P9604** Travel allowance one way in connection with medically necessary laboratory specimen collection drawn from home bound or nursing home bound patient; prorated trip charge

IOM: 100-04, 16, 60

⊛ **P9612** Catheterization for collection of specimen, single patient, all places of service

IOM: 100-04, 16, 60

⊛ **P9615** Catheterization for collection of specimen(s) (multiple patients)

IOM: 100-04, 16, 60

◀▶ New   ←→ Revised   ✔ Reinstated   ✖ Deleted

⊛ Special coverage instructions   ◆ Not covered or valid by Medicare   ✳ Carrier discretion   ▶ ASC payment group

TEMPORARY CODES ASSIGNED BY CMS (Q0000-Q9999)

⚙ **Q0035** Cardiokymography

IOM: 100-03, 1, 20.24

⚙ **Q0081** Infusion therapy, using other than chemotherapeutic drugs, per visit

(Bill on paper. Requires a report.)

IOM: 100-03, 4, 280.14

✳ **Q0083** Chemotherapy administration by other than infusion technique only (eg, subcutaneous, intramuscular, push), per visit

⚙ **Q0084** Chemotherapy administration by infusion technique only, per visit

IOM: 100-03, 4, 280.14

✳ **Q0085** Chemotherapy administration by both infusion technique and other technique(s) (eg. subcutaneous, intramuscular, push), per visit

⚙ **Q0091** Screening Papanicolaou smear; obtaining, preparing and conveyance of cervical or vaginal smear to laboratory

IOM: 100-03, 3, 190.2

⚙ **Q0092** Set-up portable x-ray equipment

IOM: 100-04, 13, 90

✳ **Q0111** Wet mounts, including preparations of vaginal, cervical or skin specimens Laboratory Certification: Bacteriology, Mycology, Parasitology

✳ **Q0112** All potassium hydroxide (KOH) preparations Laboratory Certification: Mycology

✳ **Q0113** Pinworm examinations Laboratory Certification: Parasitology

✳ **Q0114** Fern test Laboratory certification: Routine chemistry

✳ **Q0115** Post-coital direct, qualitative examinations of vaginal or cervical mucous Laboratory Certification: Hematology

◆ **Q0144** Azithromycin dihydrate, oral, capsules/powder, 1 gm

Other: Azithromycin, Zithromax, Z-Max

⚙ **Q0163** Diphenhydramine hydrochloride, 50 mg, oral, FDA approved prescription anti-emetic, for use as a complete therapeutic substitute for an IV anti-emetic at time of chemotherapy treatment not to exceed a 48 hour dosage regimen

NDC: Dytuss, Compoz, Truxadryl

Other: Aler-Dryl, Miles Nervine, Anti-Hist, Banophen, Sleep Tabs, Allermax, Sleep-ettes D, Benadryl Allergy, Nytol Quickgels, Nytol Quickcaps, Aller-Med, Benadryl, Ben-Allergein-50, Benylin Decongestant Cough, Decongest, Good Sense Sleep Aid Softgels, Good Sense Antihistamine Allergy Relief, Good Sense Sleep, Good Sense Nighttime Sleep Aid, Hydramine, Q-Dryl, Nighttime Sleep Aid, Genahist, Children's Pedia Care, Diphenhist, Quenalin, Twilite, Rite Aid Allergy, Allergy Relief Medicine, Antihistamine, Complete Allergy Medication, Complete Allergy Relief, Serabrina La France, Diphedryl, Diphedryl Children's, Diphedryl Allergy, Dihydrex, Sleeping Aid, Sleep Tablets, Dormin Sleep Aid, Sleep Formula, Alertab, Diphen, Diphenacen-50, Diphenhydramine HCl, Valu-Dryl Allergy, Valu-Dryl Allergy Children's, Medicine Shoppe Nite Time Sleep, The Medicine Shoppe Medi-Phedryl, Hydramine, Sleepinal, Simply Sleep, Family Pharmacy Allergy, Sominex, Siladryl Allergy, Silphen, Geridryl, Altaryl, Altaryl Children's, Diphenyl, Diphenyl Elixir, Diphen AF, Mediphedryl, Quality Choice Sleep Aid, Allergy Relief Intense Strength, Quality Choice Rest Simply, Allergy Children's, Quality Choice Dye-Free Allergy Medicine, Health Care America Sleep-Ex, Health Care America Total Allergy, Unisom Sleep Gels Maximum Strength

Medicare Statute 4557

⚙ **Q0164** Prochlorperazine maleate, 5 mg, oral, FDA approved prescription anti-emetic, for use as a complete therapeutic substitute for an IV anti-emetic at the time of chemotherapy treatment, not to exceed a 48 hour dosage regimen

NDC: Compazine

Other: Prochlorperazine maleate

Medicare Statute 4557

◀▶ **New**   ←→ **Revised**   ✔ **Reinstated**   ✖ **Deleted**

⚙ **Special coverage instructions**   ◆ **Not covered or valid by Medicare**   ✳ **Carrier discretion**   ▶ **ASC payment group**

⊙ **Q0165** Prochlorperazine maleate, 10 mg, oral, FDA approved prescription anti-emetic, for use as a complete therapeutic substitute for an IV anti-emetic at the time of chemotherapy treatment, not to exceed a 48 hour dosage regimen

NDC: Compazine, Compazine Syrup

Other: Prochlorperazine maleate

Medicare Statute 4557

⊙ **Q0166▶** Granisetron hydrochloride, 1 mg, oral, FDA approved prescription anti-emetic, for use as a complete therapeutic substitute for an IV anti-emetic at the time of chemotherapy treatment, not to exceed a 24 hour dosage regimen

NDC: Kytril

Other: Granisetron HCl

Medicare Statute 4557

⊙ **Q0167** Dronabinol, 2.5 mg, oral, FDA approved prescription anti-emetic, for use as a complete therapeutic substitute for an IV anti-emetic at the time of chemotherapy treatment, not to exceed a 48 hour dosage regimen

NDC: Marinol

Other: Dronabinol

Medicare Statute 4557

⊙ **Q0168** Dronabinol, 5 mg, oral, FDA approved prescription anti-emetic, for use as a complete therapeutic substitute for an IV anti-emetic at the time of chemotherapy treatment, not to exceed a 48 hour dosage regimen

NDC: Marinol

Other: Dronabinol

Medicare Statute 4557

⊙ **Q0169** Promethazine hydrochloride, 12.5 mg, oral, FDA approved prescription anti-emetic, for use as a complete therapeutic substitute for an IV anti-emetic at the time of chemotherapy treatment, not to exceed a 48 hour dosage regimen

NDC: Phenergan

Other: Amgen, Anergan 25, Anergan 50, Phenazine 25, Phenzine 50, Promethazine HCl, Prorex-25, Prothazine, V-Gan 25, V-Gan 50

Medicare Statute 4557

⊙ **Q0170** Promethazine hydrochloride, 25 mg, oral, FDA approved prescription anti-emetic, for use as a complete therapeutic substitute for an IV anti-emetic at the time of chemotherapy treatment, not to exceed a 48 hour dosage regimen

NDC: Phenergan

Other: Anergan 25, Anergan 50, Phenazine 25, Phenazine 50, Promethazine HCl, Prorex-25, Prothazine, V-Gan 25, V-Gan 50

Medicare Statute 4557

⊙ **Q0171** Chlorpromazine hydrochloride, 10 mg, oral, FDA approved prescription anti-emetic, for use as a complete therapeutic substitute for an IV anti-emetic at the time of chemotherapy treatment, not to exceed a 48 hour dosage regimen

Other: Chlorpromazine HCl; Ormazine; Thorazine

Medicare Statute 4557

⊙ **Q0172** Chlorpromazine hydrochloride, 25 mg, oral, FDA approved prescription anti-emetic, for use as a complete therapeutic substitute for an IV anti-emetic at the time of chemotherapy treatment, not to exceed a 48 hour dosage regimen

Other: Chlorpromazine HCl; Ormazine; Thorazine

Medicare Statute 4557

⊙ **Q0173** Trimethobenzamide hydrochloride, 250 mg, oral, FDA approved prescription anti-emetic, for use as a complete therapeutic substitute for an IV anti-emetic at the time of chemotherapy treatment, not to exceed a 48 hour dosage regimen

Other: Arrestin, Tigan, Ticon, Trimethobenzamide HCl

Medicare Statute 4557

⊙ **Q0174** Thiethylperazine maleate, 10 mg, oral, FDA approved prescription anti-emetic, for use as a complete therapeutic substitute for an IV anti-emetic at the time of chemotherapy treatment, not to exceed a 48 hour dosage regimen

Other: Torecan; Norzine (oral); Thiethylperazine maleate (oral)

Medicare Statute 4557

◀▶ New   ←→ Revised   ✔ Reinstated   ✖ Deleted

⊙ Special coverage instructions   ◆ Not covered or valid by Medicare   ✳ Carrier discretion   ▶ ASC payment group

⊗ **Q0175** Perphenazine, 4 mg, oral, FDA approved prescription anti-emetic, for use as a complete therapeutic substitute for an IV anti-emetic at the time of chemotherapy treatment, not to exceed a 48 hour dosage regimen

Other: Trilafon; Perphenazine (tablets)

Medicare Statute 4557

⊗ **Q0176** Perphenazine, 8mg, oral, FDA approved prescription anti-emetic, for use as a complete therapeutic substitute for an IV anti-emetic at the time of chemotherapy treatment, not to exceed a 48 hour dosage regimen

Other: Trilafon; Perphenazine (tablets)

Medicare Statute 4557

⊗ **Q0177** Hydroxyzine pamoate, 25 mg, oral, FDA approved prescription anti-emetic, for use as a complete therapeutic substitute for an IV anti-emetic at the time of chemotherapy treatment, not to exceed a 48 hour dosage regimen

NDC: Vistaril

Other: Hydroxyzine pamoate

Medicare Statute 4557

⊗ **Q0178** Hydroxyzine pamoate, 50 mg, oral, FDA approved prescription anti-emetic, for use as a complete therapeutic substitute for an IV anti-emetic at the time of chemotherapy treatment, not to exceed a 48 hour dosage regimen

NDC: Vistaril

Other: Hydroxyzine pamoate

Medicare Statute 4557

⊗ **Q0179**▶ Ondansetron hydrochloride, 8 mg, oral, FDA approved prescription anti-emetic, for use as a complete therapeutic substitute for an IV anti-emetic at the time of chemotherapy treatment, not to exceed a 48 hour dosage regimen

NDC: Zofran, Zofran ODT

Other: Ondansetron HCl

Medicare Statute 4557

⊗ **Q0180**▶ Dolasetron mesylate, 100 mg, oral, FDA approved prescription anti-emetic, for use as a complete therapeutic substitute for an IV anti-emetic at the time of chemotherapy treatment, not to exceed a 24 hour dosage regimen

NDC: Anzemet

Other: Dolasetron mesylate (tablets)

Medicare Statute 4557

⊗ **Q0181** Unspecified oral dosage form, FDA approved prescription anti-emetic, for use as a complete therapeutic substitute for a IV anti-emetic at the time of chemotherapy treatment, not to exceed a 48 hour dosage regimen

Other: Unspecified oral antiemetic

Medicare Statute 4557

⊗ **Q0480** Driver for use with pneumatic ventricular assist device, replacement only

⊗ **Q0481** Microprocessor control unit for use with electric ventricular assist device, replacement only

⊗ **Q0482** Microprocessor control unit for use with electric/pneumatic combination ventricular assist device, replacement only

⊗ **Q0483** Monitor/display module for use with electric ventricular assist device, replacement only

⊗ **Q0484** Monitor/display module for use with electric or electric/pneumatic ventricular assist device, replacement only

⊗ **Q0485** Monitor control cable for use with electric ventricular assist device, replacement only

⊗ **Q0486** Monitor control cable for use with electric/pneumatic ventricular assist device, replacement only

⊗ **Q0487** Leads (pneumatic/electrical) for use with any type electric/pneumatic ventricular assist device, replacement only

⊗ **Q0488** Power pack base for use with electric ventricular assist device, replacement only

⊗ **Q0489** Power pack base for use with electric/ pneumatic ventricular assist device, replacement only

⊗ **Q0490** Emergency power source for use with electric ventricular assist device, replacement only

⊗ **Q0491** Emergency power source for use with electric/pneumatic ventricular assist device, replacement only

⊗ **Q0492** Emergency power supply cable for use with electric ventricular assist device, replacement only

⊗ **Q0493** Emergency power supply cable for use with electric/pneumatic ventricular assist device, replacement only

---

◄▶ New   ←→ Revised   ✔ Reinstated   ✘ Deleted

⊗ Special coverage instructions   ◆ Not covered or valid by Medicare   ✳ Carrier discretion   ▶ ASC payment group

⊘ **Q0494** Emergency hand pump for use with electric or electric/pneumatic ventricular assist device, replacement only

⊘ **Q0495** Battery/power pack charger for use with electric or electric/pneumatic ventricular assist device, replacement only

⊘ **Q0496** Battery for use with electric or electric/ pneumatic ventricular assist device, replacement only

⊘ **Q0497** Battery clips for use with electric or electric/pneumatic ventricular assist device, replacement only

⊘ **Q0498** Holster for use with electric or electric/ pneumatic ventricular assist device, replacement only

⊘ **Q0499** Belt/vest for use with electric or electric/pneumatic ventricular assist device, replacement only

⊘ **Q0500** Filters for use with electric or electric/ pneumatic ventricular assist device, replacement only

⊘ **Q0501** Shower cover for use with electric or electric/pneumatic ventricular assist device, replacement only

⊘ **Q0502** Mobility cart for pneumatic ventricular assist device, replacement only

⊘ **Q0503** Battery for pneumatic ventricular assist device, replacement only, each

⊘ **Q0504** Power adapter for pneumatic ventricular assist device, replacement only, vehicle type

⊘ **Q0505** Miscellaneous supply or accessory for use with ventricular assist device

⊘ **Q0510** Pharmacy supply fee for initial immunosuppressive drug(s), first month following transplant

⊘ **Q0511** Pharmacy supply fee for oral anti-cancer, oral anti-emetic or immunosuppressive drug(s); for the first prescription in a 30-day period

→ ⊘ **Q0512** Pharmacy supply fee for oral anti-cancer, oral anti-emetic or immunosuppressive drug(s); for a subsequent prescription in a 30-day period

⊘ **Q0513** Pharmacy dispensing fee for inhalation drug(s); per 30 days

⊘ **Q0514** Pharmacy dispensing fee for inhalation drug(s); per 90 days

⊘ **Q0515▷** Injection, sermorelin acetate, 1 microgram

NDC: Geref Diagnostic

Other: Sermorelin acetate

IOM: 100-02, 15, 50

✳ **Q1003▷** New technology intraocular lens category 3 (reduced spherical aberration)

⊘ **Q1004** New technology intraocular lens category 4 as defined in Federal Register notice

⊘ **Q1005** New technology intraocular lens category 5 as defined in Federal Register notice

⊘ **Q2004** Irrigation solution for treatment of bladder calculi, for example renacidin, per 500 ml

Other: Renacidin; Irrigation solution for Tx of bladder calculi

IOM: 100-02, 15, 50,

Medicare Statute 1861S2B

⊘ **Q2009** Injection, fosphenytoin, 50 mg

NDC: Cerebyx

Other: Fosphenytoin

IOM: 100-02, 15, 50,

Medicare Statute 1861S2B

⊘ **Q2017▷** Injection, teniposide, 50 mg

NDC: Vumon

Other: Teniposide

IOM: 100-02, 15, 50

Medicare Statute 1861S2B

⊘ **Q3001** Radioelements for brachytherapy, any type, each

IOM: 100-04, 12, 70; 100-04, 13, 20

✳ **Q3014** Telehealth originating site facility fee

⊘ **Q3025▷** Injection, interferon beta-1a, 11 mcg for intramuscular use

NDC: Avonex

Other: Interferon beta-1a

IOM: 100-02, 15, 50

◆ **Q3026** Injection, interferon beta-1a, 11 mcg for subcutaneous use

Other: Rebif

Other: Interferon beta-1a

⊘ **Q3031** Collagen skin test

IOM: 100-03, 4, 280.1

✳ **Q4001** Casting supplies, body cast adult, with or without head, plaster

---

◀▶ **New**   ←→ **Revised**   ✔ **Reinstated**   ✘ **Deleted**

⊘ **Special coverage instructions**   ◆ **Not covered or valid by Medicare**   ✳ **Carrier discretion**   ▷ **ASC payment group**

* **Q4002** Cast supplies, body cast adult, with or without head, fiberglass

* **Q4003** Cast supplies, shoulder cast, adult (11 years +), plaster

* **Q4004** Cast supplies, shoulder cast, adult (11 years +), fiberglass

* **Q4005** Cast supplies, long arm cast, adult (11 years +), plaster

* **Q4006** Cast supplies, long arm cast, adult (11 years +), fiberglass

* **Q4007** Cast supplies, long arm cast, pediatric (0-10 years), plaster

* **Q4008** Cast supplies, long arm cast, pediatric (0-10 years), fiberglass

* **Q4009** Cast supplies, short arm cast, adult (11 years +), plaster

* **Q4010** Cast supplies, short arm cast, adult (11 years +), fiberglass

* **Q4011** Cast supplies, short arm cast, pediatric (0-10 years), plaster

* **Q4012** Cast supplies, short arm cast, pediatric (0-10 years), fiberglass

* **Q4013** Cast supplies, gauntlet cast (includes lower forearm and hand), adult (11 years +), plaster

* **Q4014** Cast supplies, gauntlet cast (includes lower forearm and hand), adult (11 years +), fiberglass

* **Q4015** Cast supplies, gauntlet cast (includes lower forearm and hand), pediatric (0-10 years), plaster

* **Q4016** Cast supplies, gauntlet cast (includes lower forearm and hand), pediatric (0-10 years), fiberglass

* **Q4017** Cast supplies, long arm splint, adult (11 years +), plaster

* **Q4018** Cast supplies, long arm splint, adult (11 years +), fiberglass

* **Q4019** Cast supplies, long arm splint, pediatric (0-10 years), plaster

* **Q4020** Cast supplies, long arm splint, pediatric (0-10 years), fiberglass

* **Q4021** Cast supplies, short arm splint, adult (11 years +), plaster

* **Q4022** Cast supplies, short arm splint, adult (11 years +), fiberglass

* **Q4023** Cast supplies, short arm splint, pediatric (0-10 years), plaster

* **Q4024** Cast supplies, short arm splint, pediatric (0-10 years), fiberglass

* **Q4025** Cast supplies, hip spica (one or both legs), adult (11 years +), plaster

* **Q4026** Cast supplies, hip spica (one or both legs), adult (11 years +), fiberglass

* **Q4027** Cast supplies, hip spica (one or both legs), pediatric (0-10 years), plaster

* **Q4028** Cast supplies, hip spica (one or both legs), pediatric (0-10 years), fiberglass

* **Q4029** Cast supplies, long leg cast, adult (11 years +), plaster

* **Q4030** Cast supplies, long leg cast, adult (11 years +), fiberglass

* **Q4031** Cast supplies, long leg cast, pediatric (0-10 years), plaster

* **Q4032** Cast supplies, long leg cast, pediatric (0-10 years), fiberglass

* **Q4033** Cast supplies, long leg cylinder cast, adult (11 years +), plaster

* **Q4034** Cast supplies, long leg cylinder cast, adult (11 years +), fiberglass

* **Q4035** Cast supplies, long leg cylinder cast, pediatric (0-10 years), plaster

* **Q4036** Cast supplies, long leg cylinder cast, pediatric (0-10 years), fiberglass

* **Q4037** Cast supplies, short leg cast, adult (11 years +), plaster

* **Q4038** Cast supplies, short leg cast, adult (11 years +), fiberglass

* **Q4039** Cast supplies, short leg cast, pediatric (0-10 years), plaster

* **Q4040** Cast supplies, short leg cast, pediatric (0-10 years), fiberglass

* **Q4041** Cast supplies, long leg splint, adult (11 years +), plaster

* **Q4042** Cast supplies, long leg splint, adult (11 years +), fiberglass

* **Q4043** Cast supplies, long leg splint, pediatric (0-10 years), plaster

* **Q4044** Cast supplies, long leg splint, pediatric (0-10 years), fiberglass

* **Q4045** Cast supplies, short leg splint, adult (11 years +), plaster

* **Q4046** Cast supplies, short leg splint, adult (11 years +), fiberglass

* **Q4047** Cast supplies, short leg splint, pediatric (0-10 years), plaster

* **Q4048** Cast supplies, short leg splint, pediatric (0-10 years), fiberglass

* **Q4049** Finger splint, static

* **Q4050** Cast supplies, for unlisted types and materials of casts

* **Q4051** Splint supplies, miscellaneous (includes thermoplastics, strapping, fasteners, padding and other supplies)

◀▶ New ←→ Revised ✔ Reinstated ✖ Deleted
⊙ Special coverage instructions ◆ Not covered or valid by Medicare * Carrier discretion ▶ ASC payment group

* **Q4080** Iloprost, inhalation solution, FDA-approved final product, non-compounded, administered through DME, unit dose form, 20 micrograms

NDC: Ventavis

☉ **Q4081** Injection, epoetin alfa, 100 units (for ESRD on dialysis)

NDC: Epogen, Procrit

* **Q4082** Drug or biological, not otherwise classified, Part B drug competitive acquisition program (CAP)

~~**Q4096**~~ ~~Injection, von Willebrand factor complex, human, ristocetin cofactor (not otherwise specified), per I.U. VWF: RCO~~ ✖

~~**Q4097**~~ ~~Injection, immune globulin (Privigen), intravenous, non-lyophilized (e.g. liquid), 500 mg~~ ✖

Cross reference J1459

~~**Q4098**~~ ~~Injection, iron dextran, 50 mg~~ ✖

Cross reference J1750

~~**Q4099**~~ ~~Formoterol fumarate, inhalation solution, FDA approved final product, non-compounded, administered through DME, unit dose form, 20 micrograms~~ ✖

Cross reference J7606

▶ * **Q4100** Skin substitute, not otherwise specified

▶ * **Q4101**▶ Skin substitute, Apligraf, per square centimeter

▶ * **Q4102**▶ Skin substitute, Oasis Wound Matrix, per square centimeter

▶ * **Q4103**▶ Skin substitute, Oasis Burn Matrix, per square centimeter

▶ * **Q4104**▶ Skin substitute, Integra Bilayer Matrix Wound Dressing (BMWD), per square centimeter

▶ * **Q4105**▶ Skin substitute, Integra Dermal Regeneration Template (DRT), per square centimeter

▶ * **Q4106**▶ Skin substitute, Dermagraft, per square centimeter

▶ * **Q4107**▶ Skin substitute, Graftjacket, per square centimeter

▶ * **Q4108**▶ Skin substitute, Integra Matrix, per square centimeter

▶ * **Q4109** Skin substitute, TissueMend, per square centimeter

▶ * **Q4110**▶ Skin substitute, Primatrix, per square centimeter

▶ * **Q4111**▶ Skin substitute, GammaGraft, per square centimeter

▶ * **Q4112**▶ Allograft, Cymetra, injectable, 1cc

▶ * **Q4113**▶ Allograft, GraftJacket Express, injectable, 1cc

▶ * **Q4114**▶ Allograft, Integra Flowable Wound Matrix, injectable, 1cc

☉ **Q5001** Hospice care provided in patient's home/residence

☉ **Q5002** Hospice care provided in assisted living facility

☉ **Q5003** Hospice care provided in nursing long term care facility (LTC) or non-skilled nursing facility (NF)

☉ **Q5004** Hospice care provided in skilled nursing facility (SNF)

☉ **Q5005** Hospice care provided in inpatient hospital

☉ **Q5006** Hospice care provided in inpatient hospice facility

☉ **Q5007** Hospice care provided in long term care facility

☉ **Q5008** Hospice care provided in inpatient psychiatric facility

☉ **Q5009** Hospice care provided in place not otherwise specified (NOS)

Contrast

☉ **Q9951** Low osmolar contrast material, 400 or greater mg/ml iodine concentration, per ml

IOM: 100-04, 12, 70; 100-04, 13, 20; 100-04, 13, 90

☉ **Q9953** Injection, iron-based magnetic resonance contrast agent, per ml

NDC: Feridex IV

IOM: 100-04, 12, 70; 100-04, 13, 20; 100-04, 13, 90

☉ **Q9954** Oral magnetic resonance contrast agent, per 100 ml

NDC: Gastromark

IOM: 100-04, 12, 70; 100-04, 13, 20; 100-04, 13, 90

* **Q9955** Injection, perflexane lipid microspheres, per ml

* **Q9956** Injection, octafluoropropane microspheres, per ml

NDC: Optison

◀ ▶ **New**   ← → **Revised**   ✔ **Reinstated**   ✖ **Deleted**

☉ **Special coverage instructions**   ◆ **Not covered or valid by Medicare**   * **Carrier discretion**   ▶ **ASC payment group**

✳ **Q9957** Injection, perflutren lipid microspheres, per ml

NDC: Definity

✪ **Q9958** High osmolar contrast material, up to 149 mg/ml iodine concentration, per ml

NDC: Cystografin, Reno-30, Reno-Dip, Cystografin-Dilute, Hypaque Sodium Oral, Cysto-Conray LI, Conray 30

IOM: 100-04, 12, 70; 100-04, 13, 20; 100-04, 13, 90

✪ **Q9959** High osmolar contrast material, 150-199 mg/ml iodine concentration, per ml

IOM: 100-04, 12, 70; 100-04, 13, 20; 100-04, 13, 90

✪ **Q9960** High osmolar contrast material, 200-249 mg/ml iodine concentration, per ml

NDC: Conray 43

IOM: 100-04, 12, 70; 100-04, 13, 20; 100-04, 13, 90

✪ **Q9961** High osmolar contrast material, 250-299 mg/ml iodine concentration, per ml

NDC: Cholografin Meglumine, Reno-M60, Reno 60, Renografin-60, Hypaque, Conray

IOM: 100-04, 12, 70; 100-04, 13, 20; 100-04, 13, 90

✪ **Q9962** High osmolar contrast material, 300-349 mg/ml iodine concentration, per ml

IOM: 100-04, 12, 70; 100-04, 13, 20; 100-04, 13, 90

✪ **Q9963** High osmolar contrast material, 350-399 mg/ml iodine concentration, per ml

NDC: Gastrografin, Sinografin, Renocal-76, Md-76R, Hypaque, Md Gastroview

IOM: 100-04, 12, 70; 100-04, 13, 20; 100-04, 13, 90

✪ **Q9964** High osmolar contrast material, 400 or greater mg/ml iodine concentration, per ml

NDC: Conray 400

IOM: 100-04, 12, 70; 100-04, 13, 20; 100-04, 13, 90

✪ **Q9965** Low osmolar contrast material, 100-199 mg/ml iodine concentration, per ml

NDC: Ultravist 150, Omnipaque 180, Omnipaque 140, Optiray 160

IOM: 100-04, 12, 70; 100-04, 13, 20; 100-04, 13, 90

✪ **Q9966** Low osmolar contrast material, 200-299 mg/ml iodine concentration, per ml

NDC: Ultravist 240, Isovue-200, Isovue-250, Isovue-M-200, Omnipaque 240, Visipaque 270, Optiray 240

Other: Ultravist 300

IOM: 100-04, 12, 70; 100-04, 13, 20; 100-04, 13, 90

✪ **Q9967** Low osmolar contrast material, 300-399 mg/ml iodine concentration, per ml

NDC: Ultravist 300, Ultravist 370, Isovue-300, Isovue-370, Isovue-M-300, Omnipaque 300, Omnipaque 350, Vispaque 320, Oxilan 300, Oxilan 350, Optiray 300, Optiray 320, Optiray 350, Hexabrix 320

IOM: 100-04, 12, 70; 100-04, 13, 20; 100-04, 13, 90

DIAGNOSTIC RADIOLOGY SERVICES (R0000-R9999)

Transportation/Setup of Portable Equipment

⊗ **R0070** Transportation of portable x-ray equipment and personnel to home or nursing home, per trip to facility or location, one patient seen

IOM: 100-04, 13, 90; 100-04, 13, 90.3

⊗ **R0075** Transportation of portable x-ray equipment and personnel to home or nursing home, per trip to facility or location, more than one patient seen

IOM: 100-04, 13, 90; 100-04, 13, 90.3

⊗ **R0076** Transportation of portable ECG to facility or location, per patient

IOM: 100-01, 5, 90.2; 100-02, 15, 80; 100-03, 1, 20.15; 100-04, 13, 90; 100-04, 16, 10; 100-04, 16, 110.4

◀▶ New   ←→ Revised   ✔ Reinstated   ✖ Deleted

⊗ Special coverage instructions   ◆ Not covered or valid by Medicare   ✳ Carrier discretion   ▶ ASC payment group

TEMPORARY NATIONAL CODES ESTABLISHED BY PRIVATE PAYERS (S0009-S9999)

◆ **S0012** Butorphanol tartrate, nasal spray, 25 mg

Other: Stadol NS, Sadol NS, Stadol

◆ **S0014** Tacrine hydrochloride, 10 mg

◆ **S0017** Injection, aminocaproic acid, 5 grams

Other: Amicar

◆ **S0020** Injection, bupivacaine hydrochloride, 30 ml

◆ **S0021** Injection, cefoperazone sodium, 1 gram

Other: Cefobid

◆ **S0023** Injection, cimetidine hydrochloride, 300 mg

Other: Tagamet

◆ **S0028** Injection, famotidine, 20 mg

◆ **S0030** Injection, metronidazole, 500 mg

Other: Flagyl I.V. RtU

◆ **S0032** Injection, nafcillin sodium, 2 grams

Other: Nallpen, Unipen

◆ **S0034** Injection, ofloxacin, 400 mg

Other: Floxin IV

◆ **S0039** Injection, sulfamethoxazole and tri-methoprim, 10 ml

Other: Bactrim IV, Septra IV, Sulfatrim

◆ **S0040** Injection, ticarcillin disodium and clavulanate potassium, 3.1 grams

◆ **S0073** Injection, aztreonam, 500 mg

◆ **S0074** Injection, cefotetan disodium, 500 mg

◆ **S0077** Injection, clindamycin phosphate, 300 mg

◆ **S0078** Injection, fosphenytoin sodium, 750 mg

Other: Cerebyx

◆ **S0080** Injection, pentamidine isethionate, 300 mg

Other: Pentam 300, Pentacarinat, NebuPent

◆ **S0081** Injection, piperacillin sodium, 500 mg

Other: Pipracil

→ ◆ **S0088** Imatinib, 100 mg

Other: Gleevec

◆ **S0090** Sildenafil citrate, 25 mg

Other: Viagra

◆ **S0091** Granisetron hydrochloride, 1mg (for circumstances falling under the Medicare statute, use Q0166)

Other: Kytril

◆ **S0092** Injection, hydromorphone hydrochloride, 250 mg (loading dose for infusion pump)

Other: Dilaudid

◆ **S0093** Injection, morphine sulfate, 500 mg (loading dose for infusion pump)

Other: Duramorph

◆ **S0104** Zidovudine, oral, 100 mg

◆ **S0106** Bupropion HCl sustained release tablet, 150 mg, per bottle of 60 tablets

Other: Wellbutrin SR tablets

◆ **S0108** Mercaptopurine, oral, 50 mg

Other: Purinethol

◆ **S0109** Methadone, oral, 5 mg

Other: Dolophine

◆ **S0117** Tretinoin, topical, 5 grams

◆ **S0122** Injection, menotropins, 75 IU

Other: Humegon, Pergonal, Repronex

◆ **S0126** Injection, follitropin alfa, 75 IU

◆ **S0128** Injection, follitropin beta, 75 IU

Other: Follistim

◆ **S0132** Injection, ganirelix acetate, 250 mcg

Other: Antagon

◆ **S0136** Clozapine, 25 mg

Other: Clozaril

◆ **S0137** Didanosine (DDI), 25 mg

Other: Videx

◆ **S0138** Finasteride, 5 mg

Other: Propecia (oral), Proscar (oral)

◆ **S0139** Minoxidil, 10 mg

Other: Loniten (oral)

◆ **S0140** Saquinavir, 200 mg

Other: Fortovase (oral), Invirase (oral)

~~**S0141** Zalcitabine (DDC), 0.375 mg~~ ✖

◆ **S0142** Colistimethate sodium, inhalation solution administered through DME, concentrated form, per mg

Other: Colistimethate sodium

~~**S0143** Aztreonam, inhalation solution administered through DME, concentrated form, per gram~~ ✖

◀ ▶ New   ← → Revised   ✔ Reinstated   ✖ Deleted
 Special coverage instructions   ◆ Not covered or valid by Medicare   ✳ Carrier discretion   ▶ ASC payment group

◆ **S0145** Injection, pegylated interferon alfa-2a, 180 mcg per ml

◆ **S0146** Injection, pegylated interferon alfa-2b, 10 mcg per 0.5 ml

◆ **S0155** Sterile dilutant for epoprostenol, 50ml

◆ **S0156** Exemestane, 25 mg

◆ **S0157** Becaplermin gel 0.01%, 0.5 gm

Other: Regranex Gel

◆ **S0160** Dextroamphetamine sulfate, 5 mg

◆ **S0161** Calcitrol, 0.25 mg

◆ **S0162** Injection, efalizumab, 125 mg

◆ **S0164** Injection, pantoprazole sodium, 40 mg

Other: Protonix IV

◆ **S0166** Injection, olanzapine, 2.5 mg

Other: Zyprexa

◆ **S0170** Anastrozole, oral, 1mg

◆ **S0171** Injection, bumetanide, 0.5 mg

Other: Bumex

◆ **S0172** Chlorambucil, oral, 2mg

◆ **S0174** Dolasetron mesylate, oral 50mg (for circumstances falling under the Medicare statute, use Q0180)

Other: Anzemet

◆ **S0175** Flutamide, oral, 125mg

Other: Eulexin

◆ **S0176** Hydroxyurea, oral, 500mg

Other: Mylocel

◆ **S0177** Levamisole hydrochloride, oral, 50mg

Other: Ergamisol

◆ **S0178** Lomustine, oral, 10mg

◆ **S0179** Megestrol acetate, oral, 20mg

◆ **S0181** Ondansetron hydrochloride, oral, 4mg (for circumstances falling under the Medicare statute, use Q0179)

Other: Zofran

◆ **S0182** Procarbazine hydrochloride, oral, 50 mg

◆ **S0183** Prochlorperazine maleate, oral, 5mg (for circumstances falling under the Medicare statute, use Q0164-Q0165)

Other: Compazine; Prochlorperazine maleate

◆ **S0187** Tamoxifen citrate, oral, 10mg

◆ **S0189** Testosterone pellet, 75mg

◆ **S0190** Mifepristone, oral, 200 mg

Other: Mifoprex 200 mg oral

◆ **S0191** Misoprostol, oral 200 mcg

◆ **S0194** Dialysis/stress vitamin supplement, oral, 100 capsules

◆ **S0195** Pneumococcal conjugate vaccine, polyvalent, intramuscular, for children from five years to nine years of age who have not previously received the vaccine

Other: Pneumorax II

◆ **S0196** Injectable poly-l-lactic acid, restorative implant, 1 ml, face (deep dermis, subcutaneous layers)

◆ **S0197** Prenatal vitamins, 30-day supply

◆ **S0199** Medically induced abortion by oral ingestion of medication including all associated services and supplies (e.g., patient counseling, office visits, confirmation of pregnancy by HCG, ultrasound to confirm duration of pregnancy, ultrasound to confirm completion of abortion) except drugs

◆ **S0201** Partial hospitalization services, less than 24 hours, per diem

◆ **S0207** Paramedic intercept, non-hospital-based ALS service (non-voluntary), non-transport

◆ **S0208** Paramedic intercept, hospital-based ALS service (non-voluntary), non-transport

◆ **S0209** Wheelchair van, mileage, per mile

◆ **S0215** Non-emergency transportation; mileage per mile

◆ **S0220** Medical conference by a physician with interdisciplinary team of health professionals or representatives of community agencies to coordinate activities of patient care (patient is present); approximately 30 minutes

◆ **S0221** Medical conference by a physician with interdisciplinary team of health professionals or representatives of community agencies to coordinate activities of patient care (patient is present); approximately 60 minutes

◆ **S0250** Comprehensive geriatric assessment and treatment planning performed by assessment team

◆ **S0255** Hospice referral visit (advising patient and family of care options) performed by nurse, social worker, or other designated staff

◀▶ New   ←→ Revised   ✔ Reinstated   ✖ Deleted
✺ Special coverage instructions   ◆ Not covered or valid by Medicare   ✳ Carrier discretion   ▶ ASC payment group

◆ **S0257** Counseling and discussion regarding advance directives or end of life care planning and decisions, with patient and/or surrogate (list separately in addition to code for appropriate evaluation and management service)

◆ **S0260** History and physical (outpatient or office) related to surgical procedure (list separately in addition to code for appropriate evaluation and management service)

◆ **S0265** Genetic counseling, under physician supervision, each 15 minutes

◆ **S0270** Physician management of patient home care, standard monthly case rate (per 30 days)

◆ **S0271** Physician management of patient home care, hospice monthly case rate (per 30 days)

◆ **S0272** Physician management of patient home care, episodic care monthly case rate (per 30 days)

◆ **S0273** Physician visit at member's home, outside of a capitation arrangement

◆ **S0274** Nurse practitioner visit at member's home, outside of a capitation arrangement

◆ **S0302** Completed Early Periodic Screening Diagnosis and Treatment (EPSDT) service (list in addition to code for appropriate evaluation and management service)

◆ **S0310** Hospitalist services (list separately in addition to code for appropriate evaluation and management service)

◆ **S0315** Disease management program; initial assessment and initiation of the program

◆ **S0316** Disease management program; follow-up/reassessment

◆ **S0317** Disease management program; per diem

◆ **S0320** Telephone calls by a registered nurse to a disease management program member for monitoring purposes; per month

◆ **S0340** Lifestyle modification program for management of coronary artery disease, including all supportive services; first quarter / stage

◆ **S0341** Lifestyle modification program for management of coronary artery disease, including all supportive services; second or third quarter / stage

◆ **S0342** Lifestyle modification program for management of coronary artery disease, including all supportive services; fourth quarter / stage

◆ **S0345** Electrocardiographic monitoring utilizing a home computerized telemetry station with automatic activation and real-time notification of monitoring station, 24-hour attended monitoring, including recording, monitoring, receipt of transmissions, analysis, and physician review and interpretation; per 24-hour period

◆ **S0346** Electrocardiographic monitoring utilizing a home computerized telemetry station with automatic activation and real-time notification of monitoring station, 24-hour attended monitoring, including recording, monitoring, receipt of transmissions, and analysis; per 24-hour period

◆ **S0347** Electrocardiographic monitoring utilizing a home computerized telemetry station with automatic activation and real-time notification of monitoring station, 24-hour attended monitoring, including physician review and interpretation; 24-hour period

◆ **S0390** Routine foot care; removal and/or trimming of corns, calluses and/or nails and preventive maintenance in specific medical conditions (e.g. diabetes), per visit

◆ **S0395** Impression casting of a foot performed by a practitioner other than the manufacturer of the orthotic

◆ **S0400** Global fee for extracorporeal shock wave lithotripsy treatment of kidney stone(s)

◆ **S0500** Disposable contact lens, per lens

◆ **S0504** Single vision prescription lens (safety, athletic, or sunglass), per lens

◆ **S0506** Bifocal vision prescription lens (safety, athletic, or sunglass), per lens

◆ **S0508** Trifocal vision prescription lens (safety, athletic, or sunglass), per lens

◆ **S0510** Non-prescription lens (safety, athletic, or sunglass), per lens

◆ **S0512** Daily wear specialty contact lens, per lens

◆ **S0514** Color contact lens, per lens

◆ **S0515** Scleral lens, liquid bandage device, per lens

◆ **S0516** Safety eyeglass frames

◆ **S0518** Sunglasses frames

◀▶ New ←→ Revised ✔ Reinstated ✖ Deleted
○ Special coverage instructions ◆ Not covered or valid by Medicare ✳ Carrier discretion ▶ ASC payment group

◆ **S0580** Polycarbonate lens (list this code in addition to the basic code for the lens)

◆ **S0581** Nonstandard lens (list this code in addition to the basic code for the lens)

◆ **S0590** Integral lens service, miscellaneous services reported separately

◆ **S0592** Comprehensive contact lens evaluation

◆ **S0595** Dispensing new spectacle lenses for patient supplied frame

◆ **S0601** Screening proctoscopy

◆ **S0605** Digital rectal examination, annual

◆ **S0610** Annual gynecological examination, new patient

◆ **S0612** Annual gynecological examination, established patient

◆ **S0613** Annual gynecological examination; clinical breast examination without pelvic evaluation

◆ **S0618** Audiometry for hearing aid evaluation to determine the level and degree of hearing loss

◆ **S0620** Routine ophthalmological examination including refraction; new patient

◆ **S0621** Routine ophthalmological examination including refraction; established patient

◆ **S0622** Physical exam for college, new or established patient (list separately) in addition to appropriate evaluation and management code

◆ **S0625** Retinal telescreening by digital imaging of multiple different fundus areas to screen for vision-threatening conditions, including imaging, interpretation and report

◆ **S0630** Removal of sutures; by a physician other than the physician who originally closed the wound

◆ **S0800** Laser in situ keratomileusis (LASIK)

◆ **S0810** Photorefractive keratectomy (PRK)

◆ **S0812** Phototherapeutic keratectomy (PTK)

◆ **S1001** Deluxe item, patient aware (list in addition to code for basic item)

◆ **S1002** Customized item (list in addition to code for basic item)

◆ **S1015** IV tubing extension set

◆ **S1016** Non-PVC (polyvinyl chloride) intravenous administration set, for use with drugs that are not stable in PVC e.g. paclitaxel

◆ **S1030** Continuous noninvasive glucose monitoring device, purchase (for physician interpretation of data, use CPT code)

◆ **S1031** Continuous noninvasive glucose monitoring device, rental, including sensor, sensor replacement, and download to monitor (for physician interpretation of data, use CPT code)

◆ **S1040** Cranial remolding orthosis, pediatric, rigid, with soft interface material, custom fabricated, includes fitting and adjustment(s)

◆ **S2053** Transplantation of small intestine and liver allografts

◆ **S2054** Transplantation of multivisceral organs

◆ **S2055** Harvesting of donor multivisceral organs, with preparation and maintenance of allografts; from cadaver donor

◆ **S2060** Lobar lung transplantation

◆ **S2061** Donor lobectomy (lung) for transplantation, living donor

◆ **S2065** Simultaneous pancreas kidney transplantation

◆ **S2066** Breast reconstruction with gluteal artery perforator (GAP) flap, including harvesting of the flap, microvascular transfer, closure of donor site and shaping the flap into a breast, unilateral

◆ **S2067** Breast reconstruction of a single breast with "stacked" deep inferior epigastric perforator (diep) flap(s) and/or gluteal artery perforator (GAP) flap(s), including harvesting of the flap(s), microvascular transfer, closure of donor site(s) and shaping the flap into a breast, unilateral

◆ **S2068** Breast reconstruction with deep inferior epigastric perforator (DIEP) flap, or superficial inferior epigastric artery (SIEA) flap, including harvesting of the flap, microvascular transfer, closure of donor site and shaping the flap into a breast, unilateral

◆ **S2070** Cystourethroscopy, with ureteroscopy and/or pyeloscopy; with endoscopic laser treatment of ureteral calculi (includes ureteral catheterization)

~~**S2075** Laparoscopy, surgical; repair incisional or ventral hernia~~ ✖

~~**S2076** Laparoscopy, surgical; repair umbilical hernia~~ ✖

~~**S2077** Laparoscopy, surgical; implantation of mesh or other prosthesis for incisional or ventral hernia repair (list separately in addition to code for incisional or ventral hernia repair)~~ ✖

◆ **S2079** Laparoscopic esophagomyotomy (Heller type)

◀▶ New   ←→ Revised   ✔ Reinstated   ✖ Deleted

☉ Special coverage instructions   ◆ Not covered or valid by Medicare   ✳ Carrier discretion   ▶ ASC payment group

◆ **S2080** Laser-assisted uvulopalatoplasty (LAUP)

◆ **S2083** Adjustment of gastric band diameter via subcutaneous port by injection or aspiration of saline

◆ **S2095** Transcatheter occlusion or embolization for tumor destruction, percutaneous, any method, using yttrium-90 microspheres

◆ **S2102** Islet cell tissue transplant from pancreas; allogeneic

◆ **S2103** Adrenal tissue transplant to brain

◆ **S2107** Adoptive immunotherapy i.e. development of specific anti-tumor reactivity (e.g. tumor-infiltrating lymphocyte therapy) per course of treatment

◆ **S2112** Arthroscopy, knee, surgical for harvesting of cartilage (chondrocyte cells)

◆ **S2115** Osteotomy, periacetabular, with internal fixation

◆ **S2117** Arthroereisis, subtalar

→◆ **S2118** Metal-on-metal total hip resurfacing, including acetabular and femoral components

◆ **S2120** Low density lipoprotein (LDL) apheresis using heparin-induced extracorporeal LDL precipitation

~~**S2135**   Neurolysis, by injection, of metatarsal neuroma/interdigital neuritis, any interspace of the foot~~   ✖

◆ **S2140** Cord blood harvesting for transplantation, allogeneic

◆ **S2142** Cord blood-derived stem cell transplantation, allogeneic

◆ **S2150** Bone marrow or blood-derived stem cells (peripheral or umbilical), allogeneic or autologous, harvesting, transplantation, and related complications; including: pheresis and cell preparation/storage; marrow ablative therapy; drugs, supplies, hospitalization with outpatient follow-up; medical/surgical, diagnostic, emergency, and rehabilitative services; and the number of days of pre- and post-transplant care in the global definition

◆ **S2152** Solid organ(s), complete or segmental, single organ or combination of organs; deceased or living donor(s), procurement, transplantation, and related complications; including: drugs; supplies; hospitalization with outpatient follow-up; medical/surgical, diagnostic, emergency, and rehabilitative services, and the number of days of pre- and post-transplant care in the global definition

◆ **S2202** Echosclerotherapy

◆ **S2205** Minimally invasive direct coronary artery bypass surgery involving mini-thoracotomy or mini-sternotomy surgery, performed under direct vision; using arterial graft(s), single coronary arterial graft

◆ **S2206** Minimally invasive direct coronary artery bypass surgery involving mini-thoracotomy or mini-sternotomy surgery, performed under direct vision; using arterial graft(s), two coronary arterial grafts

◆ **S2207** Minimally invasive direct coronary artery bypass surgery involving mini-thoracotomy or mini-sternotomy surgery, performed under direct vision; using venous graft only, single coronary venous graft

◆ **S2208** Minimally invasive direct coronary artery bypass surgery involving mini-thoracotomy or mini-sternotomy surgery, performed under direct vision; using single arterial and venous graft(s), single venous graft

◆ **S2209** Minimally invasive direct coronary artery bypass surgery involving mini-thoracotomy or mini-sternotomy surgery, performed under direct vision; using two arterial grafts and single venous graft

◆ **S2225** Myringotomy, laser-assisted

◆ **S2230** Implantation of magnetic component of semi-implantable hearing device on ossicles in middle ear

◆ **S2235** Implantation of auditory brain stem implant

◆ **S2260** Induced abortion, 17 to 24 weeks

◆ **S2265** Induced abortion, 25 to 28 weeks

◆ **S2266** Induced abortion, 29 to 31 weeks

◆ **S2267** Induced abortion, 32 weeks or greater

▶◆ **S2270** Insertion of vaginal cylinder for application of radiation source or clinical brachytherapy (report separately in addition to radiation source delivery)

◀▶ New   ←→ Revised   ✔ Reinstated   ✖ Deleted
⊘ Special coverage instructions   ◆ Not covered or valid by Medicare   ✳ Carrier discretion   ▌ ASC payment group

◆ **S2300** Arthroscopy, shoulder, surgical; with thermally-induced capsulorrhaphy

◆ **S2325** Hip core decompression

◆ **S2340** Chemodenervation of abductor muscle(s) of vocal cord

◆ **S2341** Chemodenervation of adductor muscle(s) of vocal cord

◆ **S2342** Nasal endoscopy for post-operative debridement following functional endoscopic sinus surgery, nasal and/or sinus cavity(s), unilateral or bilateral

◆ **S2344** Nasal/sinus endoscopy, surgical; with enlargement of sinus ostium opening using inflatable device (i.e., balloon sinuplasty)

◆ **S2348** Decompression procedure, percutaneous, of nucleus pulpous of intervertebral disc, using radiofrequency energy, single or multiple levels, lumbar

◆ **S2350** Diskectomy, anterior, with decompression of spinal cord and/or nerve root(s), including osteophytectomy; lumbar, single interspace

◆ **S2351** Diskectomy, anterior, with decompression of spinal cord and/or nerve root(s) including osteophytectomy; lumbar, each additional interspace (list separately in addition to code for primary procedure)

◆ **S2360** Percutaneous vertebroplasty, one vertebral body, unilateral or bilateral injection; cervical

◆ **S2361** Each additional cervical vertebral body (list separately in addition to code for primary procedure)

◆ **S2400** Repair, congenital diaphragmatic hernia in the fetus using temporary tracheal occlusion, procedure performed in utero

◆ **S2401** Repair, urinary tract obstruction in the fetus, procedure performed in utero

◆ **S2402** Repair, congenital cystic adenomatoid malformation in the fetus, procedure performed in utero

◆ **S2403** Repair, extralobar pulmonary sequestration in the fetus, procedure performed in utero

◆ **S2404** Repair, myelomeningocele in the fetus, procedure performed in utero

◆ **S2405** Repair of sacrococcygeal teratoma in the fetus, procedure performed in utero

◆ **S2409** Repair, congenital malformation of fetus, procedure performed in utero, not otherwise classified

◆ **S2411** Fetoscopic laser therapy for treatment of twin-to-twin transfusion syndrome

◆ **S2900** Surgical techniques requiring use of robotic surgical system (list separately in addition to code for primary procedure)

◆ **S3000** Diabetic indicator; retinal eye exam, dilated, bilateral

◆ **S3005** Performance measurement, evaluation of patient self assessment, depression

◆ **S3600** STAT laboratory request (situations other than S3601)

◆ **S3601** Emergency STAT laboratory charge for patient who is homebound or residing in a nursing facility

◆ **S3620** Newborn metabolic screening panel, includes test kit, postage and the laboratory tests specified by the state for inclusion in this panel (e.g. galactose; hemoglobin, electrophoresis; hydroxyprogesterone, 17-D; phenylalanine (PKU); and thyroxine, total)

◆ **S3625** Maternal serum triple marker screen including alpha-fetoprotein (AFP), estriol, and human chorionic gonadotropin (HCG)

◆ **S3626** Maternal serum quadruple marker screen including alpha-fetoprotein (AFP), estriol, human chorionic gonadotropin (HCG) and inhibin a

▶◆ **S3628** Placental alpha microglobulin-1 rapid immunoassay for detection of rupture of fetal membranes

◆ **S3630** Eosinophil count, blood, direct

◆ **S3645** HIV-1 antibody testing of oral mucosal transudate

◆ **S3650** Saliva test, hormone level; during menopause

◆ **S3652** Saliva test, hormone level; to assess preterm labor risk

◆ **S3655** Antisperm antibodies test (immunobead)

◆ **S3708** Gastrointestinal fat absorption study

▶◆ **S3711** Circulating tumor cell test

◆ **S3800** Genetic testing for amyotrophic lateral sclerosis (ALS)

◆ **S3818** Complete gene sequence analysis; BRCA1 gene

◀▶ New   ←→ Revised   ✔ Reinstated   ✖ Deleted

⊙ Special coverage instructions   ◆ Not covered or valid by Medicare   ✳ Carrier discretion   ▶ ASC payment group

◆ **S3819** Complete gene sequence analysis; BRCA2 gene

◆ **S3820** Complete BRCA1 and BRCA2 gene sequence analysis for susceptibility to breast and ovarian cancer

◆ **S3822** Single mutation analysis (in individual with a known BRCA1 or BRCA2 mutation in the family) for susceptibility to breast and ovarian cancer

◆ **S3823** Three-mutation BRCA1 and BRCA2 analysis for susceptibility to breast and ovarian cancer in Ashkenazi individuals

◆ **S3828** Complete gene sequence analysis; MLH1 gene

◆ **S3829** Complete gene sequence analysis; MLH2 gene

◆ **S3830** Complete MLH and MLH gene sequence analysis for hereditary nonpolyposis colorectal cancer (HNPCC) genetic testing

◆ **S3831** Single-mutation analysis (in individual with a known MLH and MLH mutation in the family) for hereditary nonpolyposis colorectal cancer (HNPCC) genetic testing

◆ **S3833** Complete APC gene sequence analysis for susceptibility to familial adenomatous polyposis (FAP) and attenuated FAP

◆ **S3834** Single-mutation analysis (in individual with a known APC mutation in the family) for susceptibility to familial adenomatous polyposis (FAP) and attenuated FAP

◆ **S3835** Complete gene sequence analysis for cystic fibrosis genetic testing

◆ **S3837** Complete gene sequence analysis for hemochromatosis genetic testing

◆ **S3840** DNA analysis for germline mutations of the RET proto-oncogene for susceptibility to multiple endocrine neoplasia type 2

◆ **S3841** Genetic testing for retinoblastoma

◆ **S3842** Genetic testing for von Hippel-Lindau disease

◆ **S3843** DNA analysis of the F5 gene for susceptibility to Factor V Leiden thrombophilia

◆ **S3844** DNA analysis of the connexin 26 gene (GJB2) for susceptibility to congenital, profound deafness

◆ **S3845** Genetic testing for alpha-thalassemia

◆ **S3846** Genetic testing for hemoglobin E beta-thalassemia

◆ **S3847** Genetic testing for Tay-Sachs disease

◆ **S3848** Genetic testing for Gaucher disease

◆ **S3849** Genetic testing for Niemann-Pick disease

◆ **S3850** Genetic testing for sickle cell anemia

◆ **S3851** Genetic testing for Canavan disease

◆ **S3852** DNA analysis for APOE epilson 4 allele for susceptibility to Alzheimer's disease

◆ **S3853** Genetic testing for myotonic muscular dystrophy

◆ **S3854** Gene expression profiling panel for use in the management of breast cancer treatment

◆ **S3855** Genetic testing for detection of mutations in the presenilin - 1 gene

▶ ◆ **S3860** Genetic testing, comprehensive cardiac ion channel analysis, for variants in 5 major cardiac ion channel genes for individuals with high index of suspicion for familial long QT syndrome (LQTS) or related syndromes

▶ ◆ **S3861** Genetic testing, sodium channel, voltage-gated, type V, alpha subunit (SCN5A) and variants for suspected Brugada syndrome

▶ ◆ **S3862** Genetic testing, family-specific ion channel analysis, for blood-relatives of individuals (index case) who have previously tested positive for a genetic variant of a cardiac ion channel syndrome using either one of the above test configurations or confirmed results from another laboratory

◆ **S3890** DNA analysis, fecal, for colorectal cancer screening

◆ **S3900** Surface electromyography (EMG)

◆ **S3902** Ballistrocardiogram

◆ **S3904** Masters two step

(Bill on paper. Requires a report.)

◆ **S3905** Non-invasive electrodiagnostic testing with automatic computerized hand-held device to stimulate and measure neuromuscular signals in diagnosing and evaluating systemic and entrapment neuropathies

◆ **S4005** Interim labor facility global (labor occurring but not resulting in delivery)

◆ **S4011** In vitro fertilization; including but not limited to identification and incubation of mature oocytes, fertilization with sperm, incubation of embryo(s), and subsequent visualization for determination of development

---

◀▶ New   ←→ Revised   ✔ Reinstated   ✖ Deleted

✿ Special coverage instructions   ◆ Not covered or valid by Medicare   ✳ Carrier discretion   ▶ ASC payment group

◆ **S4013** Complete cycle, gamete intrafallopian transfer (GIFT), case rate

◆ **S4014** Complete cycle, zygote intrafallopian transfer (ZIFT), case rate

◆ **S4015** Complete in vitro fertilization cycle, not otherwise specified, case rate

◆ **S4016** Frozen in vitro fertilization cycle, case rate

◆ **S4017** Incomplete cycle, treatment cancelled prior to stimulation, case rate

◆ **S4018** Frozen embryo transfer procedure cancelled before transfer, case rate

◆ **S4020** In vitro fertilization procedure cancelled before aspiration, case rate

◆ **S4021** In vitro fertilization procedure cancelled after aspiration, case rate

◆ **S4022** Assisted oocyte fertilization, case rate

◆ **S4023** Donor egg cycle, incomplete, case rate

◆ **S4025** Donor services for in vitro fertilization (sperm or embryo), case rate

◆ **S4026** Procurement of donor sperm from sperm bank

◆ **S4027** Storage of previously frozen embryos

◆ **S4028** Microsurgical epididymal sperm aspiration (MESA)

◆ **S4030** Sperm procurement and cryopreservation services; initial visit

◆ **S4031** Sperm procurement and cryopreservation services; subsequent visit

◆ **S4035** Stimulated intrauterine insemination (IUI), case rate

◆ **S4037** Cryopreserved embryo transfer, case rate

◆ **S4040** Monitoring and storage of cryopreserved embryos, per 30 days

◆ **S4042** Management of ovulation induction (interpretation of diagnostic tests and studies, non-face-to-face medical management of the patient), per cycle

◆ **S4981** Insertion of levonorgestrel-releasing intrauterine system

◆ **S4989** Contraceptive intrauterine device (e.g. Progestasert IUD), including implants and supplies

Other: Estring Vaginal Ring

◆ **S4990** Nicotine patches, legend

◆ **S4991** Nicotine patches, non-legend

◆ **S4993** Contraceptive pills for birth control

(May only be billed by Family Planning Clinics)

◆ **S4995** Smoking cessation gum

◆ **S5000** Prescription drug, generic

◆ **S5001** Prescription drug, brand name

◆ **S5010** 5% dextrose and 0.45% normal saline, 1000 ml

◆ **S5011** 5% dextrose in lactated Ringer's, 1000 ml

◆ **S5012** 5% dextrose with potassium chloride, 1000 ml

◆ **S5013** 5% dextrose/0.45% normal saline with potassium chloride and magnesium sulfate, 1000 ml

◆ **S5014** 5% dextrose/0.45% normal saline with potassium chloride and magnesium sulfate, 1500 ml

◆ **S5035** Home infusion therapy, routine service of infusion device (e.g. pump maintenance)

◆ **S5036** Home infusion therapy, repair of infusion device (e.g. pump repair)

◆ **S5100** Day care services, adult; per 15 minutes

◆ **S5101** Day care services, adult; per half day

◆ **S5102** Day care services, adult; per diem

◆ **S5105** Day care services, center-based; services not included in program fee, per diem

◆ **S5108** Home care training to home care client, per 15 minutes

◆ **S5109** Home care training to home care client, per session

◆ **S5110** Home care training, family; per 15 minutes

◆ **S5111** Home care training, family; per session

◆ **S5115** Home care training, non-family; per 15 minutes

◆ **S5116** Home care training, non-family; per session

◆ **S5120** Chore services; per 15 minutes

◆ **S5121** Chore services; per diem

◆ **S5125** Attendant care services; per 15 minutes

◆ **S5126** Attendant care services; per diem

◆ **S5130** Homemaker service, NOS; per 15 minutes

◆ **S5131** Homemaker service, NOS; per diem

◆ **S5135** Companion care, adult (e.g. IADL/ADL); per 15 minutes

◆ **S5136** Companion care, adult (e.g. IADL/ADL); per diem

◆ **S5140** Foster care, adult; per diem

◆ **S5141** Foster care, adult; per month

◀▶ New ←→ Revised ✔ Reinstated ✖ Deleted

○ Special coverage instructions ◆ Not covered or valid by Medicare ✳ Carrier discretion ▶ ASC payment group

◆ **S5145** Foster care, therapeutic, child; per diem

◆ **S5146** Foster care, therapeutic, child; per month

◆ **S5150** Unskilled respite care, not hospice; per 15 minutes

◆ **S5151** Unskilled respite care, not hospice; per diem

◆ **S5160** Emergency response system; installation and testing

◆ **S5161** Emergency response system; service fee, per month (excludes installation and testing)

◆ **S5162** Emergency response system; purchase only

◆ **S5165** Home modifications; per service

◆ **S5170** Home delivered meals, including preparation; per meal

◆ **S5175** Laundry service, external, professional; per order

◆ **S5180** Home health respiratory therapy, initial evaluation

◆ **S5181** Home health respiratory therapy, NOS, per diem

◆ **S5185** Medication reminder service, non-face-to-face; per month

◆ **S5190** Wellness assessment, performed by non-physician

◆ **S5199** Personal care item, NOS, each

◆ **S5497** Home infusion therapy, catheter care / maintenance, not otherwise classified; includes administrative services, professional pharmacy services, care coordination, and all necessary supplies and equipment (drugs and nursing visits coded separately), per diem

◆ **S5498** Home infusion therapy, catheter care / maintenance, simple (single lumen), includes administrative services, professional pharmacy services, care coordination and all necessary supplies and equipment, (drugs and nursing visits coded separately), per diem

◆ **S5501** Home infusion therapy, catheter care / maintenance, complex (more than one lumen), includes administrative services, professional pharmacy services, care coordination, and all necessary supplies and equipment (drugs and nursing visits coded separately), per diem

◆ **S5502** Home infusion therapy, catheter care / maintenance, implanted access device, includes administrative services, professional pharmacy services, care coordination, and all necessary supplies and equipment, (drugs and nursing visits coded separately), per diem (use this code for interim maintenance of vascular access not currently in use)

◆ **S5517** Home infusion therapy, all supplies necessary for restoration of catheter patency or declotting

◆ **S5518** Home infusion therapy, all supplies necessary for catheter repair

◆ **S5520** Home infusion therapy, all supplies (including catheter) necessary for a peripherally inserted central venous catheter (PICC) line insertion

(Bill on paper. Requires a report.)

◆ **S5521** Home infusion therapy, all supplies (including catheter) necessary for a midline catheter insertion

◆ **S5522** Home infusion therapy, insertion of peripherally inserted central venous catheter (PICC), nursing services only (no supplies or catheter included)

◆ **S5523** Home infusion therapy, insertion of midline central venous catheter, nursing services only (no supplies or catheter included)

◆ **S5550** Insulin, rapid onset, 5 units

◆ **S5551** Insulin, most rapid onset (Lispro or Aspart); 5 units

◆ **S5552** Insulin, intermediate acting (NPH or Lente); 5 units

◆ **S5553** Insulin, long acting; 5 units

◆ **S5560** Insulin delivery device, reusable pen; 1.5 ml size

◆ **S5561** Insulin delivery device, reusable pen; 3 ml size

◆ **S5565** Insulin cartridge for use in insulin delivery device other than pump; 150 units

◆ **S5566** Insulin cartridge for use in insulin delivery device other than pump; 300 units

◆ **S5570** Insulin delivery device, disposable pen (including insulin); 1.5 ml size

◆ **S5571** Insulin delivery device, disposable pen (including insulin); 3 ml size

◆ **S8030** Scleral application of tantalum ring(s) for localization of lesions for proton beam therapy

◆ **S8035** Magnetic source imaging

◀▶ New	←→ Revised	✔ Reinstated	✖ Deleted
⚙ Special coverage instructions	◆ Not covered or valid by Medicare	✳ Carrier discretion	▶ ASC payment group

◆ **S8037** Magnetic resonance cholangiopancreatography (MRCP)

◆ **S8040** Topographic brain mapping

◆ **S8042** Magnetic resonance imaging (MRI), low-field

◆ **S8049** Intraoperative radiation therapy (single administration)

◆ **S8055** Ultrasound guidance for multifetal pregnancy reduction(s), technical component (only to be used when the physician doing the reduction procedure does not perform the ultrasound, guidance is included in the CPT code for multifetal pregnancy reduction - 59866)

◆ **S8080** Scintimammography (radioimmunoscintigraphy of the breast), unilateral, including supply of radiopharmaceutical

◆ **S8085** Fluorine-18 fluorodeoxyglucose (F-18 FDG) imaging using dual-head coincidence detection system (non-dedicated PET scan)

◆ **S8092** Electron beam computed tomography (also known as ultrafast CT, cine CT)

◆ **S8096** Portable peak flow meter

◆ **S8097** Asthma kit (including but not limited to portable peak expiratory flow meter, instructional video, brochure, and/or spacer)

◆ **S8100** Holding chamber or spacer for use with an inhaler or nebulizer; without mask

◆ **S8101** Holding chamber or spacer for use with an inhaler or nebulizer; with mask

◆ **S8110** Peak expiratory flow rate (physician services)

◆ **S8120** Oxygen contents, gaseous, 1 unit equals 1 cubic foot

◆ **S8121** Oxygen contents, liquid, 1 unit equals 1 pound

◆ **S8185** Flutter device

◆ **S8186** Swivel adaptor

◆ **S8189** Tracheostomy supply, not otherwise classified

◆ **S8190** Electronic spirometer (or microspirometer)

◆ **S8210** Mucus trap

◆ **S8262** Mandibular orthopedic repositioning device, each

◆ **S8265** Haberman feeder for cleft lip/palate

◆ **S8270** Enuresis alarm, using auditory buzzer and/or vibration device

◆ **S8301** Infection control supplies, not otherwise specified

◆ **S8415** Supplies for home delivery of infant

◆ **S8420** Gradient pressure aid (sleeve and glove combination), custom made

◆ **S8421** Gradient pressure aid (sleeve and glove combination), ready made

◆ **S8422** Gradient pressure aid (sleeve), custom made, medium weight

◆ **S8423** Gradient pressure aid (sleeve), custom made, heavy weight

◆ **S8424** Gradient pressure aid (sleeve), ready made

◆ **S8425** Gradient pressure aid (glove), custom made, medium weight

◆ **S8426** Gradient pressure aid (glove), custom made, heavy weight

◆ **S8427** Gradient pressure aid (glove), ready made

◆ **S8428** Gradient pressure aid (gauntlet), ready made

◆ **S8429** Gradient pressure exterior wrap

◆ **S8430** Padding for compression bandage, roll

◆ **S8431** Compression bandage, roll

◆ **S8450** Splint, prefabricated, digit (specify digit by use of modifier)

◆ **S8451** Splint, prefabricated, wrist or ankle

◆ **S8452** Splint, prefabricated, elbow

◆ **S8460** Camisole, post-mastectomy

◆ **S8490** Insulin syringes (100 syringes, any size)

◆ **S8940** Equestrian/Hippotherapy, per session

◆ **S8948** Application of a modality (requiring constant provider attendance) to one or more areas; low-level laser; each 15 minutes

◆ **S8950** Complex lymphedema therapy, each 15 minutes

◆ **S8990** Physical or manipulative therapy performed for maintenance rather than restoration

◆ **S8999** Resuscitation bag (for use by patient on artificial respiration during power failure or other catastrophic event)

◆ **S9001** Home uterine monitor with or without associated nursing services

◆ **S9007** Ultrafiltration monitor

◆ **S9015** Automated EEG monitoring

◆ **S9024** Paranasal sinus ultrasound

◆ **S9025** Omnicardiogram/cardiointegram

◀▶ New   ←→ Revised   ✔ Reinstated   ✖ Deleted

⊘ Special coverage instructions   ◆ Not covered or valid by Medicare   ✳ Carrier discretion   ▶ ASC payment group

268

◆ **S9034** Extracorporeal shockwave lithotripsy for gall stones (if performed with ERCP, use 43265)

◆ **S9055** Procuren or other growth factor preparation to promote wound healing

◆ **S9056** Coma stimulation per diem

◆ **S9061** Home administration of aerosolized drug therapy (e.g., pentamidine); administrative services, professional pharmacy services, care coordination, all necessary supplies and equipment (drugs and nursing visits coded separately), per diem

◆ **S9075** Smoking cessation treatment

◆ **S9083** Global fee urgent care centers

◆ **S9088** Services provided in an urgent care center (list in addition to code for service)

◆ **S9090** Vertebral axial decompression, per session

~~**S9092** Canolith repositioning, per visit~~ ✖

◆ **S9097** Home visit for wound care

◆ **S9098** Home visit, phototherapy services (e.g. Bili-Lite), including equipment rental, nursing services, blood draw, supplies, and other services, per diem

◆ **S9109** Congestive heart failure telemonitoring, equipment rental, including telescale, computer system and software, telephone connections, and maintenance, per month

◆ **S9117** Back school, per visit

◆ **S9122** Home health aide or certified nurse assistant, providing care in the home; per hour

◆ **S9123** Nursing care, in the home; by registered nurse, per hour (use for general nursing care only, not to be used when CPT codes 99500-99602 can be used)

◆ **S9124** Nursing care, in the home; by licensed practical nurse, per hour

◆ **S9125** Respite care, in the home, per diem

◆ **S9126** Hospice care, in the home, per diem

◆ **S9127** Social work visit, in the home, per diem

◆ **S9128** Speech therapy, in the home, per diem

◆ **S9129** Occupational therapy, in the home, per diem

◆ **S9131** Physical therapy; in the home, per diem

◆ **S9140** Diabetic management program, follow-up visit to non-MD provider

◆ **S9141** Diabetic management program, follow-up visit to MD provider

◆ **S9145** Insulin pump initiation, instruction in initial use of pump (pump not included)

◆ **S9150** Evaluation by ocularist

◆ **S9152** Speech therapy, re-evaluation

◆ **S9208** Home management of preterm labor, including administrative services, professional pharmacy services, care coordination, and all necessary supplies or equipment (drugs and nursing visits coded separately), per diem (do not use this code with any home infusion per diem code)

◆ **S9209** Home management of preterm premature rupture of membranes (PPROM), including administrative services, professional pharmacy services, care coordination, and all necessary supplies or equipment (drugs and nursing visits coded separately), per diem (do not use this code with any home infusion per diem code)

◆ **S9211** Home management of gestational hypertension, includes administrative services, professional pharmacy services, care coordination, and all necessary supplies and equipment (drugs and nursing visits coded separately); per diem (do not use this code with any home infusion per diem code)

◆ **S9212** Home management of postpartum hypertension, includes administrative services, professional pharmacy services, care coordination, and all necessary supplies and equipment (drugs and nursing visits coded separately), per diem (do not use this code with any home infusion per diem code)

◆ **S9213** Home management of preeclampsia, includes administrative services, professional pharmacy services, care coordination, and all necessary supplies and equipment (drugs and nursing services coded separately); per diem (do not use this code with any home infusion per diem code)

◆ **S9214** Home management of gestational diabetes, includes administrative services, professional pharmacy services, care coordination, and all necessary supplies and equipment (drugs and nursing visits coded separately); per diem (do not use this code with any home infusion per diem code)

◀▶ New ← → Revised ✔ Reinstated ✖ Deleted

⊙ Special coverage instructions ◆ Not covered or valid by Medicare ✳ Carrier discretion ▶ ASC payment group

◆ **S9325**   Home infusion therapy, pain management infusion; administrative services, professional pharmacy services, care coordination, and all necessary supplies and equipment, (drugs and nursing visits coded separately), per diem (do not use this code with S9326, S9327 or S9328)

◆ **S9326**   Home infusion therapy, continuous (twenty-four hours or more) pain management infusion; administrative services, professional pharmacy services, care coordination, and all necessary supplies and equipment (drugs and nursing visits coded separately), per diem

◆ **S9327**   Home infusion therapy, intermittent (less than twenty-four hours) pain management infusion; administrative services, professional pharmacy services, care coordination, and all necessary supplies and equipment (drugs and nursing visits coded separately), per diem

◆ **S9328**   Home infusion therapy, implanted pump pain management infusion; administrative services, professional pharmacy services, care coordination, and all necessary supplies and equipment (drugs and nursing visits coded separately), per diem

◆ **S9329**   Home infusion therapy, chemotherapy infusion; administrative services, professional pharmacy services, care coordination, and all necessary supplies and equipment (drugs and nursing visits coded separately), per diem (do not use this code with S9330 or S9331)

◆ **S9330**   Home infusion therapy, continuous (twenty-four hours or more) chemotherapy infusion; administrative services, professional pharmacy services, care coordination, and all necessary supplies and equipment (drugs and nursing visits coded separately), per diem

◆ **S9331**   Home infusion therapy, intermittent (less than twenty-four hours) chemotherapy infusion; administrative services, professional pharmacy services, care coordination, and all necessary supplies and equipment (drugs and nursing visits coded separately), per diem

◆ **S9335**   Home therapy, hemodialysis; administrative services, professional pharmacy services, care coordination, and all necessary supplies and equipment (drugs and nursing services coded separately), per diem

◆ **S9336**   Home infusion therapy, continuous anticoagulant infusion therapy (e.g. heparin), administrative services, professional pharmacy services, care coordination, and all necessary supplies and equipment (drugs and nursing visits coded separately), per diem

◆ **S9338**   Home infusion therapy, immunotherapy, administrative services, professional pharmacy services, care coordination, and all necessary supplies and equipment (drug and nursing visits coded separately), per diem

◆ **S9339**   Home therapy; peritoneal dialysis, administrative services, professional pharmacy services, care coordination and all necessary supplies and equipment (drugs and nursing visits coded separately), per diem

◆ **S9340**   Home therapy; enteral nutrition; administrative services, professional pharmacy services, care coordination, and all necessary supplies and equipment (enteral formula and nursing visits coded separately), per diem

◆ **S9341**   Home therapy; enteral nutrition via gravity; administrative services, professional pharmacy services, care coordination, and all necessary supplies and equipment (enteral formula and nursing visits coded separately), per diem

◆ **S9342**   Home therapy; enteral nutrition via pump; administrative services, professional pharmacy services, care coordination, and all necessary supplies and equipment (enteral formula and nursing visits coded separately), per diem

◆ **S9343**   Home therapy; enteral nutrition via bolus; administrative services, professional pharmacy services, care coordination, and all necessary supplies and equipment (enteral formula and nursing visits coded separately), per diem

◆ **S9345**   Home infusion therapy, anti-hemophilic agent infusion therapy (e.g. Factor VIII); administrative services, professional pharmacy services, care coordination, and all necessary supplies and equipment (drugs and nursing visits coded separately), per diem

◄▶ New   ←→ Revised   ✔ Reinstated   ✖ Deleted
⊙ Special coverage instructions   ◆ Not covered or valid by Medicare   ✳ Carrier discretion   ▶ ASC payment group

◆ **S9346** Home infusion therapy, alpha-1-proteinase inhibitor (e.g., Prolastin); administrative services, professional pharmacy services, care coordination, and all necessary supplies and equipment (drugs and nursing visits coded separately), per diem

◆ **S9347** Home infusion therapy, uninterrupted, long-term, controlled rate intravenous or subcutaneous infusion therapy (e.g. Epoprostenol); administrative services, professional pharmacy services, care coordination, and all necessary supplies and equipment (drugs and nursing visits coded separately), per diem

◆ **S9348** Home infusion therapy, sympathomimetic/inotropic agent infusion therapy (e.g., Dobutamine); administrative services, professional pharmacy services, care coordination, all necessary supplies and equipment (drugs and nursing visits coded separately), per diem

◆ **S9349** Home infusion therapy, tocolytic infusion therapy; administrative services, professional pharmacy services, care coordination, and all necessary supplies and equipment (drugs and nursing visits coded separately), per diem

◆ **S9351** Home infusion therapy, continuous or intermittent anti-emetic infusion therapy; administrative services, professional pharmacy services, care coordination, and all necessary supplies and equipment (drugs and visits coded separately), per diem

◆ **S9353** Home infusion therapy, continuous insulin infusion therapy; administrative services, professional pharmacy services, care coordination, and all necessary supplies and equipment (drugs and nursing visits coded separately), per diem

◆ **S9355** Home infusion therapy, chelation therapy; administrative services, professional pharmacy services, care coordination, and all necessary supplies and equipment (drugs and nursing visits coded separately), per diem

◆ **S9357** Home infusion therapy, enzyme replacement intravenous therapy; (e.g. Imiglucerase); administrative services, professional pharmacy services, care coordination, and all necessary supplies and equipment (drugs and nursing visits coded separately), per diem

◆ **S9359** Home infusion therapy, anti-tumor necrosis factor intravenous therapy; (e.g. Infliximab); administrative services, professional pharmacy services, care coordination, and all necessary supplies and equipment (drugs and nursing visits coded separately), per diem

◆ **S9361** Home infusion therapy, diuretic intravenous therapy; administrative services, professional pharmacy services, care coordination, and all necessary supplies and equipment (drugs and nursing visits coded separately), per diem

◆ **S9363** Home infusion therapy, anti-spasmotic therapy; administrative services, professional pharmacy services, care coordination, and all necessary supplies and equipment (drugs and nursing visits coded separately), per diem

◆ **S9364** Home infusion therapy, total parenteral nutrition (TPN); administrative services, professional pharmacy services, care coordination, and all necessary supplies and equipment including standard TPN formula (lipids, specialty amino acid formulas, drugs other than in standard formula, and nursing visits coded separately) per diem (do not use with home infusion codes S9365-S9368 using daily volume scales)

◆ **S9365** Home infusion therapy, total parenteral nutrition (TPN); one liter per day, administrative services, professional pharmacy services, care coordination, and all necessary supplies and equipment including standard TPN formula (lipids, specialty amino acid formulas, drugs other than in standard formula and nursing visits coded separately), per diem

◆ **S9366** Home infusion therapy, total parenteral nutrition (TPN); more than one liter but no more than two liters per day, administrative services, professional pharmacy services, care coordination, and all necessary supplies and equipment including standard TPN formula; (lipids, specialty amino acid formulas, drugs other than in standard formula and nursing visits coded separately), per diem

---

◀ ▶ New   ← → Revised   ✔ Reinstated   ✖ Deleted

Ⓢ **Special coverage instructions**   ◆ **Not covered or valid by Medicare**   ✱ **Carrier discretion**   ▶ **ASC payment group**

◆ **S9367** Home infusion therapy, total parenteral nutrition (TPN); more than two liters but no more than three liters per day, administrative services, professional pharmacy services, care coordination, and all necessary supplies and equipment including standard TPN formula; (lipids, specialty amino acid formulas, drugs other than in standard formula and nursing visits coded separately), per diem

◆ **S9368** Home infusion therapy, total parenteral nutrition (TPN); more than three liters per day, administrative services, professional pharmacy services, care coordination, and all necessary supplies and equipment (including standard TPN formula; lipids, specialty amino acid formulas, drugs other than in standard formula and nursing visits coded separately), per diem

◆ **S9370** Home therapy, intermittent anti-emetic injection therapy; administrative services, professional pharmacy services, care coordination, and all necessary supplies and equipment (drugs and nursing visits coded separately), per diem

◆ **S9372** Home therapy; intermittent anticoagulant injection therapy (e.g., heparin); administrative services, professional pharmacy services, care coordination, and all necessary supplies and equipment (drugs and nursing visits coded separately), per diem (do not use this code for flushing of infusion devices with heparin to maintain patency)

◆ **S9373** Home infusion therapy, hydration therapy; administrative services, professional pharmacy services, care coordination, and all necessary supplies and equipment (drugs and nursing visits coded separately), per diem (do not use with hydration therapy codes S9374-S9377 using daily volume scales)

◆ **S9374** Home infusion therapy, hydration therapy; one liter per day, administrative services, professional pharmacy services, care coordination, and all necessary supplies and equipment (drugs and nursing visits coded separately), per diem

◆ **S9375** Home infusion therapy, hydration therapy; more than one liter but no more than two liters per day, administrative services, professional pharmacy services, care coordination, and all necessary supplies and equipment (drugs and nursing visits coded separately), per diem

◆ **S9376** Home infusion therapy, hydration therapy; more than two liters but no more than three liters per day, administrative services, professional pharmacy services, care coordination, and all necessary supplies and equipment (drugs and nursing visits coded separately), per diem

◆ **S9377** Home infusion therapy, hydration therapy; more than three liters per day, administrative services, professional pharmacy services, care coordination, and all necessary supplies (drugs and nursing visits coded separately), per diem

◆ **S9379** Home infusion therapy, infusion therapy, not otherwise classified; administrative services, professional pharmacy services, care coordination, and all necessary supplies and equipment (drugs and nursing visits coded separately), per diem

◆ **S9381** Delivery or service to high risk areas requiring escort or extra protection, per visit

◆ **S9401** Anticoagulation clinic, inclusive of all services except laboratory tests, per session

◆ **S9430** Pharmacy compounding and dispensing services

▶ ◆ **S9433** Medical food nutritionally complete, administered orally, providing 100% of nutritional intake

◆ **S9434** Modified solid food supplements for inborn errors of metabolism

◆ **S9435** Medical foods for inborn errors of metabolism

◆ **S9436** Childbirth preparation/Lamaze classes, non-physician provider, per session

◆ **S9437** Childbirth refresher classes, non-physician provider, per session

◆ **S9438** Cesarean birth classes, non-physician provider, per session

◆ **S9439** VBAC (vaginal birth after cesarean) classes, non-physician provider, per session

◆ **S9441** Asthma education, non-physician provider, per session

---

◀▶ New   ←→ Revised   ✔ Reinstated   ✖ Deleted

☺ Special coverage instructions   ◆ Not covered or valid by Medicare   ✳ Carrier discretion   ▶ ASC payment group

◆ **S9442**   Birthing classes, non-physician provider, per session

◆ **S9443**   Lactation classes, non-physician provider, per session

◆ **S9444**   Parenting classes, non-physician provider, per session

◆ **S9445**   Patient education, not otherwise classified, non-physician provider, individual, per session

◆ **S9446**   Patient education, not otherwise classified, non-physician provider, group, per session

◆ **S9447**   Infant safety (including CPR) classes, non-physician provider, per session

◆ **S9449**   Weight management classes, non-physician provider, per session

◆ **S9451**   Exercise classes, non-physician provider, per session

◆ **S9452**   Nutrition classes, non-physician provider, per session

◆ **S9453**   Smoking cessation classes, non-physician provider, per session

◆ **S9454**   Stress management classes, non-physician provider, per session

◆ **S9455**   Diabetic management program, group session

◆ **S9460**   Diabetic management program, nurse visit

◆ **S9465**   Diabetic management program, dietitian visit

◆ **S9470**   Nutritional counseling, dietitian visit

◆ **S9472**   Cardiac rehabilitation program, non-physician provider, per diem

◆ **S9473**   Pulmonary rehabilitation program, non-physician provider, per diem

◆ **S9474**   Enterostomal therapy by a registered nurse certified in enterostomal therapy, per diem

◆ **S9475**   Ambulatory setting substance abuse treatment or detoxification services, per diem

◆ **S9476**   Vestibular rehabilitation program, non-physician provider, per diem

◆ **S9480**   Intensive outpatient psychiatric services, per diem

◆ **S9482**   Family stabilization services, per 15 minutes

◆ **S9484**   Crisis intervention mental health services, per hour

◆ **S9485**   Crisis intervention mental health services, per diem

◆ **S9490**   Home infusion therapy, corticosteroid infusion; administrative services, professional pharmacy services, care coordination, and all necessary supplies and equipment (drugs and nursing visits coded separately), per diem

◆ **S9494**   Home infusion therapy, antibiotic, antiviral, or antifungal therapy; administrative services, professional pharmacy services, care coordination, and all necessary supplies and equipment (drugs and nursing visits coded separately, per diem), (do not use this code with home infusion codes for hourly dosing schedules S9497-S9504)

◆ **S9497**   Home infusion therapy, antibiotic, antiviral, or antifungal therapy; once every 3 hours; administrative services, professional pharmacy services, care coordination, and all necessary supplies and equipment (drugs and nursing visits coded separately), per diem

◆ **S9500**   Home infusion therapy, antibiotic, antiviral, or antifungal therapy; once every 24 hours; administrative services, professional pharmacy services, care coordination, and all necessary supplies and equipment (drugs and nursing visits coded separately), per diem

◆ **S9501**   Home infusion therapy, antibiotic, antiviral, or antifungal therapy; once every 12 hours; administrative services, professional pharmacy services, care coordination, and all necessary supplies and equipment (drugs and nursing visits coded separately), per diem

◆ **S9502**   Home infusion therapy, antibiotic, antiviral, or antifungal therapy; once every 8 hours, administrative services, professional pharmacy services, care coordination, and all necessary supplies and equipment (drugs and nursing visits coded separately), per diem

◆ **S9503**   Home infusion therapy, antibiotic, antiviral, or antifungal; once every 6 hours; administrative services, professional pharmacy services, care coordination, and all necessary supplies and equipment (drugs and nursing visits coded separately), per diem

◆ **S9504**   Home infusion therapy, antibiotic, antiviral, or antifungal; once every 4 hours; administrative services, professional pharmacy services, care coordination, and all necessary supplies and equipment (drugs and nursing visits coded separately), per diem

◀ ▶ **New**   ← → **Revised**   ✔ **Reinstated**   ✖ **Deleted**

♻ **Special coverage instructions**   ◆ **Not covered or valid by Medicare**   ✳ **Carrier discretion**   ▶ **ASC payment group**

◆ **S9529** Routine venipuncture for collection of specimen(s), single home bound, nursing home, or skilled nursing facility patient

◆ **S9537** Home therapy; hematopoietic hormone injection therapy (e.g. erythropoietin, G-CSF, GM-CSF); administrative services, professional pharmacy services, care coordination, and all necessary supplies and equipment (drugs and nursing visits coded separately), per diem

◆ **S9538** Home transfusion of blood product(s); administrative services, professional pharmacy services, care coordination, and all necessary supplies and equipment (blood products, drugs, and nursing visits coded separately), per diem

◆ **S9542** Home injectable therapy; not otherwise classified, including administrative services, professional pharmacy services, care coordination, and all necessary supplies and equipment (drugs and nursing visits coded separately), per diem

◆ **S9558** Home injectable therapy; growth hormone, including administrative services, professional pharmacy services, care coordination, and all necessary supplies and equipment (drugs and nursing visits coded separately), per diem

◆ **S9559** Home injectable therapy; interferon, including administrative services, professional pharmacy services, care coordination, and all necessary supplies and equipment (drugs and nursing visits coded separately), per diem

◆ **S9560** Home injectable therapy; hormonal therapy (e.g.; Leuprolide, Goserelin), including administrative services, professional pharmacy services, care coordination, and all necessary supplies and equipment (drugs and nursing visits coded separately), per diem

◆ **S9562** Home injectable therapy, palivizumab, including administrative services, professional pharmacy services, care coordination, and all necessary supplies and equipment (drugs and nursing visits coded separately), per diem

◆ **S9590** Home therapy, irrigation therapy (e.g. sterile irrigation of an organ or anatomical cavity); including administrative services, professional pharmacy services, care coordination, and all necessary supplies and equipment (drugs and nursing visits coded separately), per diem

◆ **S9810** Home therapy; professional pharmacy services for provision of infusion, specialty drug administration, and/or disease state management, not otherwise classified, per hour (do not use this code with any per diem code)

◆ **S9900** Services by authorized Christian Science Practitioner for the process of healing, per diem; not to be used for rest or study; excludes in-patient services

◆ **S9970** Health club membership, annual

◆ **S9975** Transplant related lodging, meals and transportation, per diem

◆ **S9976** Lodging, per diem, not otherwise classified

◆ **S9977** Meals, per diem, not otherwise specified

◆ **S9981** Medical records copying fee, administrative

◆ **S9982** Medical records copying fee, per page

◆ **S9986** Not medically necessary service (patient is aware that service not medically necessary)

◆ **S9988** Services provided as part of a Phase I clinical trial

◆ **S9989** Services provided outside of the United States of America (list in addition to code(s) for services(s))

◆ **S9990** Services provided as part of a Phase II clinical trial

◆ **S9991** Services provided as part of a Phase III clinical trial

◆ **S9992** Transportation costs to and from trial location and local transportation costs (e.g., fares for taxicab or bus) for clinical trial participant and one caregiver/companion

◆ **S9994** Lodging costs (e.g., hotel charges) for clinical trial participant and one caregiver/companion

◆ **S9996** Meals for clinical trial participant and one caregiver/companion

◆ **S9999** Sales tax

TEMPORARY NATIONAL CODES ESTABLISHED BY MEDICAID (T1000-T9999)

Not Valid For Medicare

- ◆ **T1000** Private duty/independent nursing service(s) - licensed, up to 15 minutes
- ◆ **T1001** Nursing assessment/evaluation
- ◆ **T1002** RN services, up to 15 minutes
- ◆ **T1003** LPN/LVN services, up to 15 minutes
- ◆ **T1004** Services of a qualified nursing aide, up to 15 minutes
- ◆ **T1005** Respite care services, up to 15 minutes
- ◆ **T1006** Alcohol and/or substance abuse services, family/couple counseling
- ◆ **T1007** Alcohol and/or substance abuse services, treatment plan development and/or modification
- ◆ **T1009** Child sitting services for children of the individual receiving alcohol and/or substance abuse services
- ◆ **T1010** Meals for individuals receiving alcohol and/or substance abuse services (when meals not included in the program)
- ◆ **T1012** Alcohol and/or substance abuse services, skills development
- ◆ **T1013** Sign language or oral interpretive services, per 15 minutes
- ◆ **T1014** Telehealth transmission, per minute, professional services bill separately
- ◆ **T1015** Clinic visit/encounter, all-inclusive
- ◆ **T1016** Case Management, each 15 minutes
- ◆ **T1017** Targeted Case Management, each 15 minutes
- ◆ **T1018** School-based individualized education program (IEP) services, bundled
- ◆ **T1019** Personal care services, per 15 minutes, not for an inpatient or resident of a hospital, nursing facility, ICF/MR or IMD, part of the individualized plan of treatment (code may not be used to identify services provided by home health aide or certified nurse assistant)
- ◆ **T1020** Personal care services, per diem, not for an inpatient or resident of a hospital, nursing facility, ICF/MR or IMD, part of the individualized plan of treatment (code may not be used to identify services provided by home health aide or certified nurse assistant)
- ◆ **T1021** Home health aide or certified nurse assistant, per visit
- ◆ **T1022** Contracted home health agency services, all services provided under contract, per day
- ◆ **T1023** Screening to determine the appropriateness of consideration of an individual for participation in a specified program, project or treatment protocol, per encounter
- ◆ **T1024** Evaluation and treatment by an integrated, specialty team contracted to provide coordinated care to multiple or severely handicapped children, per encounter
- ◆ **T1025** Intensive, extended multidisciplinary services provided in a clinic setting to children with complex medical, physical, mental and psychosocial impairments, per diem
- ◆ **T1026** Intensive, extended multidisciplinary services provided in a clinic setting to children with complex medical, physical, medical and psychosocial impairments, per hour
- ◆ **T1027** Family training and counseling for child development, per 15 minutes
- ◆ **T1028** Assessment of home, physical and family environment, to determine suitability to meet patient's medical needs
- ◆ **T1029** Comprehensive environmental lead investigation, not including laboratory analysis, per dwelling
- ◆ **T1030** Nursing care, in the home, by registered nurse, per diem
- ◆ **T1031** Nursing care, in the home, by licensed practical nurse, per diem
- ◆ **T1502** Administration of oral, intramuscular and/or subcutaneous medication by health care agency/professional, per visit
- ◆ **T1503** Administration of medication, other than oral and/or injectable, by a health care agency/professional, per visit
- ◆ **T1999** Miscellaneous therapeutic items and supplies, retail purchases, not otherwise classified; identify product in "remarks"
- ◆ **T2001** Non-emergency transportation; patient attendant/escort
- ◆ **T2002** Non-emergency transportation; per diem
- ◆ **T2003** Non-emergency transportation; encounter/trip
- ◆ **T2004** Non-emergency transport; commercial carrier, multi-pass

---

◄▶ New ←→ Revised ✔ Reinstated ✖ Deleted
 Special coverage instructions ◆ Not covered or valid by Medicare ✳ Carrier discretion ▶ ASC payment group

◆ **T2005**   Non-emergency transportation: stretcher van

◆ **T2007**   Transportation waiting time, air ambulance and non-emergency vehicle, one-half (1/2) hour increments

◆ **T2010**   Preadmission screening and resident review (PASRR) level I identification screening, per screen

◆ **T2011**   Preadmission screening and resident review (PASRR) level II evaluation, per evaluation

◆ **T2012**   Habilitation, educational; waiver, per diem

◆ **T2013**   Habilitation, educational, waiver; per hour

◆ **T2014**   Habilitation, prevocational, waiver; per diem

◆ **T2015**   Habilitation, prevocational, waiver; per hour

◆ **T2016**   Habilitation, residential, waiver; per diem

◆ **T2017**   Habilitation, residential, waiver; 15 minutes

◆ **T2018**   Habilitation, supported employment, waiver; per diem

◆ **T2019**   Habilitation, supported employment, waiver; per 15 minutes

◆ **T2020**   Day habilitation, waiver; per diem

◆ **T2021**   Day habilitation, waiver; per 15 minutes

◆ **T2022**   Case management, per month

◆ **T2023**   Targeted case management; per month

◆ **T2024**   Service assessment/plan of care development, waiver

◆ **T2025**   Waiver services; not otherwise specified (NOS)

◆ **T2026**   Specialized childcare, waiver; per diem

◆ **T2027**   Specialized childcare, waiver; per 15 minutes

◆ **T2028**   Specialized supply, not otherwise specified, waiver

◆ **T2029**   Specialized medical equipment, not otherwise specified, waiver

◆ **T2030**   Assisted living, waiver; per month

◆ **T2031**   Assisted living; waiver, per diem

◆ **T2032**   Residential care, not otherwise specified (NOS), waiver; per month

◆ **T2033**   Residential care, not otherwise specified (NOS), waiver; per diem

◆ **T2034**   Crisis intervention, waiver; per diem

◆ **T2035**   Utility services to support medical equipment and assistive technology/devices, waiver

◆ **T2036**   Therapeutic camping, overnight, waiver; each session

◆ **T2037**   Therapeutic camping, day, waiver; each session

◆ **T2038**   Community transition, waiver; per service

◆ **T2039**   Vehicle modifications, waiver; per service

◆ **T2040**   Financial management, self-directed, waiver; per 15 minutes

◆ **T2041**   Supports brokerage, self-directed, waiver; per 15 minutes

◆ **T2042**   Hospice routine home care; per diem

◆ **T2043**   Hospice continuous home care; per hour

◆ **T2044**   Hospice inpatient respite care; per diem

◆ **T2045**   Hospice general inpatient care; per diem

◆ **T2046**   Hospice long term care, room and board only; per diem

◆ **T2048**   Behavioral health; long-term care residential (non-acute care in a residential treatment program where stay is typically longer than 30 days), with room and board, per diem

◆ **T2049**   Non-emergency transportation; stretcher van, mileage; per mile

◆ **T2101**   Human breast milk processing, storage and distribution only

◆ **T4521**   Adult sized disposable incontinence product, brief/diaper, small, each

IOM: 100-03, 4, 280.1

◆ **T4522**   Adult sized disposable incontinence product, brief/diaper, medium, each

IOM: 100-03, 4, 280.1

◆ **T4523**   Adult sized disposable incontinence product, brief/diaper, large, each

IOM: 100-03, 4, 280.1

◆ **T4524**   Adult sized disposable incontinence product, brief/diaper, extra large, each

IOM: 100-03, 4, 280.1

◆ **T4525**   Adult sized disposable incontinence product, protective underwear/pull-on, small size, each

IOM: 100-03, 4, 280.1

◀▶ **New**   ←→ **Revised**   ✔ **Reinstated**   ✖ **Deleted**

⊙ **Special coverage instructions**   ◆ **Not covered or valid by Medicare**   ✳ **Carrier discretion**   ▶ **ASC payment group**

◆ **T4526** Adult sized disposable incontinence product, protective underwear/pull-on, medium size, each

IOM: 100-03, 4, 280.1

◆ **T4527** Adult sized disposable incontinence product, protective underwear/pull-on, large size, each

IOM: 100-03, 4, 280.1

◆ **T4528** Adult sized disposable incontinence product, protective underwear/pull-on, extra large size, each

IOM: 100-03, 4, 280.1

◆ **T4529** Pediatric sized disposable incontinence product, brief/diaper, small/medium size, each

IOM: 100-03, 4, 280.1

◆ **T4530** Pediatric sized disposable incontinence product, brief/diaper, large size, each

IOM: 100-03, 4, 280.1

◆ **T4531** Pediatric sized disposable incontinence product, protective underwear/pull-on, small/medium size, each

IOM: 100-03, 4, 280.1

◆ **T4532** Pediatric sized disposable incontinence product, protective underwear/pull-on, large size, each

IOM: 100-03, 4, 280.1

◆ **T4533** Youth sized disposable incontinence product, brief/diaper, each

IOM: 100-03, 4, 280.1

◆ **T4534** Youth sized disposable incontinence product, protective underwear/pull-on, each

IOM: 100-03, 4, 280.1

◆ **T4535** Disposable liner/shield/guard/pad/ undergarment, for incontinence, each

IOM: 100-03, 4, 280.1

◆ **T4536** Incontinence product, protective underwear/pull-on, reusable, any size, each

IOM: 100-03, 4, 280.1

◆ **T4537** Incontinence product, protective underpad, reusable, bed size, each

IOM: 100-03, 4, 280.1

◆ **T4538** Diaper service, reusable diaper, each diaper

IOM: 100-03, 4, 280.1

◆ **T4539** Incontinence product, diaper/brief, reusable, any size, each

IOM: 100-03, 4, 280.1

◆ **T4540** Incontinence product, protective underpad, reusable, chair size, each

IOM: 100-03, 4, 280.1

◆ **T4541** Incontinence product, disposable underpad, large, each

◆ **T4542** Incontinence product, disposable underpad, small size, each

◆ **T4543** Disposable incontinence product, brief/ diaper, bariatric, each

IOM: 100-03, 4, 280.1

◆ **T5001** Positioning seat for persons with special orthopedic needs, supply, not otherwise specified

◆ **T5999** Supply, not otherwise specified

◄ ▶ New   ← → Revised   ✔ Reinstated   ✖ Deleted

☺ **Special coverage instructions**   ◆ **Not covered or valid by Medicare**   ✳ **Carrier discretion**   ▶ **ASC payment group**

VISION SERVICES (V0000-V2999)

Frames

⊙ **V2020** Frames, purchases

(Includes cost of frame or replacement and dispensing fee. One unit of service represents one frame.)

IOM: 100-02, 15, 120

◆ **V2025** Deluxe frame

(Not a benefit, use V2020)

IOM: 100-04, 1, 30.3.5

Spectacle Lenses

NOTE: If a CPT procedure code for supply of spectacles or a permanent prosthesis is reported, recode with the specific lens type listed below. For aphakic temporary spectacle correction, see CPT.

Single Vision, Glass or Plastic

✴ **V2100** Sphere, single vision, plano to plus or minus 4.00, per lens

✴ **V2101** Sphere, single vision, plus or minus 4.12 to plus or minus 7.00d, per lens

✴ **V2102** Sphere, single vision, plus or minus 7.12 to plus or minus 20.00d, per lens

✴ **V2103** Spherocylinder, single vision, plano to plus or minus 4.00d sphere, .12 to 2.00d cylinder, per lens

✴ **V2104** Spherocylinder, single vision, plano to plus or minus 4.00d sphere, 2.12 to 4.00d cylinder, per lens

✴ **V2105** Spherocylinder, single vision, plano to plus or minus 4.00d sphere, 4.25 to 6.00d cylinder, per lens

✴ **V2106** Spherocylinder, single vision, plano to plus or minus 4.00d sphere, over 6.00d cylinder, per lens

✴ **V2107** Spherocylinder, single vision, plus or minus 4.25 to plus or minus 7.00 sphere, .12 to 2.00d cylinder, per lens

✴ **V2108** Spherocylinder, single vision, plus or minus 4.25d to plus or minus 7.00d sphere, 2.12 to 4.00d cylinder, per lens

✴ **V2109** Spherocylinder, single vision, plus or minus 4.25 to plus or minus 7.00d sphere, 4.25 to 6.00d cylinder, per lens

✴ **V2110** Sperocylinder, single vision, plus or minus 4.25 to 7.00d sphere, over 6.00d cylinder, per lens

✴ **V2111** Spherocylinder, single vision, plus or minus 7.25 to plus or minus 12.00d sphere, .25 to 2.25d cylinder, per lens

✴ **V2112** Spherocylinder, single vision, plus or minus 7.25 to plus or minus 12.00d sphere, 2.25d to 4.00d cylinder, per lens

✴ **V2113** Spherocylinder, single vision, plus or minus 7.25 to plus or minus 12.00d sphere, 4.25 to 6.00d cylinder, per lens

✴ **V2114** Spherocylinder, single vision, sphere over plus or minus 12.00d, per lens

✴ **V2115** Lenticular, (myodisc), per lens, single vision

✴ **V2118** Aniseikonic lens, single vision

⊙ **V2121** Lenticular lens, per lens, single

IOM: 100-02, 15, 120; 100-04, 3, 10.4

✴ **V2199** Not otherwise classified, single vision lens

(Bill on paper. Requires report of type of single vision lens and optical lab invoice.)

Bifocal, Glass or Plastic

✴ **V2200** Sphere, bifocal, plano to plus or minus 4.00d, per lens

✴ **V2201** Sphere, bifocal, plus or minus 4.12 to plus or minus 7.00d, per lens

✴ **V2202** Sphere, bifocal, plus or minus 7.12 to plus or minus 20.00d, per lens

✴ **V2203** Spherocylinder, bifocal, plano to plus or minus 4.00d sphere, .12 to 2.00d cylinder, per lens

✴ **V2204** Spherocylinder, bifocal, plano to plus or minus 4.00d sphere, 2.12 to 4.00d cylinder, per lens

✴ **V2205** Spherocylinder, bifocal, plano to plus or minus 4.00d sphere, 4.25 to 6.00d cylinder, per lens

✴ **V2206** Spherocylinder, bifocal, plano to plus or minus 4.00d sphere, over 6.00d cylinder, per lens

✴ **V2207** Spherocylinder, bifocal, plus or minus 4.25 to plus or minus 7.00d sphere, .12 to 2.00d cylinder, per lens

✴ **V2208** Spherocylinder, bifocal, plus or minus 4.25 to plus or minus 7.00d sphere, 2.12 to 4.00d cylinder, per lens

✴ **V2209** Spherocylinder, bifocal, plus or minus 4.25 to plus or minus 7.00d sphere, 4.25 to 6.00d cylinder, per lens

✴ **V2210** Spherocylinder, bifocal, plus or minus 4.25 to plus or minus 7.00d sphere, over 6.00d cylinder, per lens

---

◀▶ New   ←→ Revised   ✔ Reinstated   ✖ Deleted

⊙ **Special coverage instructions**   ◆ **Not covered or valid by Medicare**   ✴ **Carrier discretion**   ▶ **ASC payment group**

* **V2211** Spherocylinder, bifocal, plus or minus 7.25 to plus or minus 12.00d sphere, .25 to 2.25d cylinder, per lens

* **V2212** Spherocylinder, bifocal, plus or minus 7.25 to plus or minus 12.00d sphere, 2.25 to 4.00d cylinder, per lens

* **V2213** Spherocylinder, bifocal, plus or minus 7.25 to plus or minus 12.00d sphere, 4.25 to 6.00d cylinder, per lens

* **V2214** Spherocylinder, bifocal, sphere over plus or minus 12.00d, per lens

* **V2215** Lenticular (myodisc), per lens, bifocal

* **V2218** Aniseikonic, per lens, bifocal

* **V2219** Bifocal seg width over 28mm

* **V2220** Bifocal add over 3.25d

☺ **V2221** Lenticular lens, per lens, bifocal
IOM: 100-02, 15, 120; 100-04, 3, 10.4

* **V2299** Specialty bifocal (by report)
(Bill on paper. Requires report of type of specialty bifocal lens and optical lab invoice.)

Trifocal, Glass or Plastic

* **V2300** Sphere, trifocal, plano to plus or minus 4.00d, per lens

* **V2301** Sphere, trifocal, plus or minus 4.12 to plus or minus 7.00d per lens

* **V2302** Sphere, trifocal, plus or minus 7.12 to plus or minus 20.00, per lens

* **V2303** Spherocylinder, trifocal, plano to plus or minus 4.00d sphere, .12 to 2.00d cylinder, per lens

* **V2304** Spherocylinder, trifocal, plano to plus or minus 4.00d sphere, 2.25-4.00d cylinder, per lens

* **V2305** Spherocylinder, trifocal, plano to plus or minus 4.00d sphere, 4.25 to 6.00 cylinder, per lens

* **V2306** Spherocylinder, trifocal, plano to plus or minus 4.00d sphere, over 6.00d cylinder, per lens

* **V2307** Spherocylinder, trifocal, plus or minus 4.25 to plus or minus 7.00d sphere, .12 to 2.00d cylinder, per lens

* **V2308** Spherocylinder, trifocal, plus or minus 4.25 to plus or minus 7.00d sphere, 2.12 to 4.00d cylinder, per lens

* **V2309** Spherocylinder, trifocal, plus or minus 4.25 to plus or minus 7.00d sphere, 4.25 to 6.00d cylinder, per lens

* **V2310** Spherocylinder, trifocal, plus or minus 4.25 to plus or minus 7.00d sphere, over 6.00d cylinder, per lens

* **V2311** Spherocylinder, trifocal, plus or minus 7.25 to plus or minus 12.00d sphere, .25 to 2.25d cylinder, per lens

* **V2312** Spherocylinder, trifocal, plus or minus 7.25 to plus or minus 12.00d sphere, 2.25 to 4.00d cylinder, per lens

* **V2313** Spherocylinder, trifocal, plus or minus 7.25 to plus or minus 12.00d sphere, 4.25 to 6.00d cylinder, per lens

* **V2314** Spherocylinder, trifocal, sphere over plus or minus 12.00d, per lens

* **V2315** Lenticular, (myodisc), per lens, trifocal

* **V2318** Aniseikonic lens, trifocal

* **V2319** Trifocal seg width over 28 mm

* **V2320** Trifocal add over 3.25d

☺ **V2321** Lenticular lens, per lens, trifocal
IOM: 100-02, 15, 120; 100-04, 3, 10.4

* **V2399** Specialty trifocal (by report)
(Bill on paper. Requires report of type of trifocal lens and optical lab invoice.)

Variable Asphericity

* **V2410** Variable asphericity lens, single vision, full field, glass or plastic, per lens

* **V2430** Variable asphericity lens, bifocal, full field, glass or plastic, per lens

* **V2499** Variable sphericity lens, other type
(Bill on paper. Requires report of other type of lens and optical lab invoice.)

Contact Lenses

If a CPT procedure code for supply of contact lens is reported, recode with specific lens type listed below (per lens).

* **V2500** Contact lens, PMMA, spherical, per lens
(Requires prior authorization for patients under age 21.)

* **V2501** Contact lens, PMMA, toric or prism ballast, per lens
(Requires prior authorization for clients under age 21.)

* **V2502** Contact lens PMMA, bifocal, per lens
(Requires prior authorization for clients under age 21. Bill on paper. Requires optical lab invoice.)

◄► New   ←→ Revised   ✔ Reinstated   ✖ Deleted
☺ Special coverage instructions   ◆ Not covered or valid by Medicare   ✳ Carrier discretion   ▶ ASC payment group

* **V2503** Contact lens PMMA, color vision deficiency, per lens

   (Requires prior authorization for clients under age 21. Bill on paper. Requires optical lab invoice.)

* **V2510** Contact lens, gas permeable, spherical, per lens

   (Requires prior authorization for clients under age 21.)

* **V2511** Contact lens, gas permeable, toric, prism ballast, per lens

   (Requires prior authorization for clients under age 21.)

* **V2512** Contact lens, gas permeable, bifocal, per lens

   (Requires prior authorization for clients under age 21.)

* **V2513** Contact lens, gas permeable, extended wear, per lens

   (Requires prior authorization for clients under age 21.)

⊛ **V2520** Contact lens, hydrophilic, spherical, per lens

   (Requires prior authorization for clients under age 21.)

   IOM: 100-03, 1, 80.1; 100-03, 1, 80.4

⊛ **V2521** Contact lens, hydrophilic, toric, or prism ballast, per lens

   (Requires prior authorization for clients under age 21.)

   IOM: 100-03, 1, 80.1; 100-03, 1, 80.4

⊛ **V2522** Contact lens, hydrophilic, bifocal, per lens

   (Requires prior authorization for clients under age 21.)

   IOM: 100-03, 1, 80.1; 100-03, 1, 80.4

⊛ **V2523** Contact lens, hydrophilic, extended wear, per lens

   (Requires prior authorization for clients under age 21.)

   IOM: 100-03, 1, 80.1; 100-03, 1, 80.4

* **V2530** Contact lens, scleral, gas impermeable, per lens (for contact lens modification, see 92325)

   (Requires prior authorization for clients under age 21.)

⊛ **V2531** Contact lens, scleral, gas permeable, per lens (for contact lens modification, see 92325)

   (Requires prior authorization for clients under age 21. Bill on paper. Requires optical lab invoice.)

   IOM: 100-03, 1, 80.5

* **V2599** Contact lens, other type

   (Requires prior authorization for clients under age 21. Bill on paper. Requires report of other type of contact lens and optical invoice.)

Low Vision Aids

If a CPT procedure code for supply of low vision aid is reported, recode with specific systems listed below.

* **V2600** Hand held low vision aids and other nonspectacle mounted aids

   (Requires prior authorization.)

* **V2610** Single lens spectacle mounted low vision aids

   (Requires prior authorization.)

* **V2615** Telescopic and other compound lens system, including distance vision telescopic, near vision telescopes and compound microscopic lens system

   (Requires prior authorization. Bill on paper. Requires optical lab invoice.)

Prosthetic Eye

⊛ **V2623** Prosthetic eye, plastic, custom

   (Requires prior authorization. Bill on paper. Requires optical lab invoice.)

* **V2624** Polishing/resurfacing of ocular prosthesis

   (Requires prior authorization. Bill on paper. Requires optical lab invoice.)

* **V2625** Enlargement of ocular prosthesis

   (Requires prior authorization. Bill on paper. Requires optical lab invoice.)

* **V2626** Reduction of ocular prosthesis

   (Requires prior authorization. Bill on paper. Requires optical lab invoice.)

⊛ **V2627** Scleral cover shell

   (Requires prior authorization. Bill on paper. Requires optical lab invoice.)

   IOM: 100-03, 4, 280.2

◀▶ New	←→ Revised	✔ Reinstated	✖ Deleted
⊙ Special coverage instructions	◆ Not covered or valid by Medicare	⊛ Carrier discretion	▶ ASC payment group

* **V2628** Fabrication and fitting of ocular conformer

   (Requires prior authorization. Bill on paper. Requires optical lab invoice.)

* **V2629** Prosthetic eye, other type

   (Requires prior authorization. Bill on paper. Requires optical lab invoice.)

Intraocular Lenses

⊛ **V2630** Anterior chamber intraocular lens

   IOM: 100-02, 15, 120

⊛ **V2631** Iris supported intraocular lens

   IOM: 100-02, 15, 120

⊛ **V2632** Posterior chamber intraocular lens

   IOM: 100-02, 15, 120

Miscellaneous

* **V2700** Balance lens, per lens

◆ **V2702** Deluxe lens feature

   IOM: 100-02, 15, 120; 100-04, 3, 10.4

* **V2710** Slab off prism, glass or plastic, per lens

* **V2715** Prism, per lens

* **V2718** Press-on lens, Fresnel prism, per lens

* **V2730** Special base curve, glass or plastic, per lens

⊛ **V2744** Tint, photochromatic, per lens

   (Requires prior authorization.)

   IOM: 100-02, 15, 120; 100-04, 3, 10.4

⊛ **V2745** Addition to lens, tint, any color, solid, gradient or equal, excludes photochroatic, any lens material, per lens

   IOM: 100-02, 15, 120; 100-04, 3, 10.4

⊛ **V2750** Anti-reflective coating, per lens

   (Requires prior authorization.)

   IOM: 100-02, 15, 120; 100-04, 3, 10.4

⊛ **V2755** U-V lens, per lens

   IOM: 100-02, 15, 120; 100-04, 3, 10.4

* **V2756** Eye glass case

* **V2760** Scratch resistant coating, per lens

⊛ **V2761** Mirror coating, any type, solid, gradient or equal, any lens material, per lens

   IOM: 100-02, 15, 120; 100-04, 3, 10.4

⊛ **V2762** Polarization, any lens material, per lens

   IOM: 100-02, 15, 120; 100-04, 3, 10.4

* **V2770** Occluder lens, per lens

   (Requires prior authorization.)

* **V2780** Oversize lens, per lens

   (Requires prior authorization.)

* **V2781** Progressive lens, per lens

   (Requires prior authorization.)

⊛ **V2782** Lens, index 1.54 to 1.65 plastic or 1.60 to 1.79 glass, excludes polycarbonate, per lens

   IOM: 100-02, 15, 120; 100-04, 3, 10.4

⊛ **V2783** Lens, index greater than or equal to 1.66 plastic or greater than or equal to 1.80 glass, excludes polycarbonate, per lens

   IOM: 100-02, 15, 120; 100-04, 3, 10.4

⊛ **V2784** Lens, polycarbonate or equal, any index, per lens

   IOM: 100-02, 15, 120; 100-04, 3, 10.4

* **V2785▶** Processing, preserving and transporting corneal tissue

   (Bill on paper. Must attach eye bank invoice to claim.)

⊛ **V2786** Specialty occupational multifocal lens, per lens

   IOM: 100-02, 15, 120; 100-04, 3, 10.4

◆ **V2787** Astigmatism correcting function of intraocular lens

   Medicare Statute 1862(a)(7)

◆ **V2788** Presbyopia correcting function of intraocular lens

   Medicare Statute 1862a7

* **V2790** Amniotic membrane for surgical reconstruction, per procedure

* **V2797** Vision supply, accessory and/or service component of another HCPCS vision code

* **V2799** Vision service, miscellaneous

   (Bill on paper. Requires report of miscellaneous service and optical lab invoice.)

◀▶ **New**   ←→ **Revised**   ✔ **Reinstated**   ✖ **Deleted**

⊛ **Special coverage instructions**   ◆ **Not covered or valid by Medicare**   * **Carrier discretion**   ▶ **ASC payment group**

HEARING SERVICES (V5000-V5999)

NOTE: These codes are for non-physician services.

- ◆ **V5008** Hearing screening
  IOM: 100-02, 16, 90

- ◆ **V5010** Assessment for hearing aid
  Medicare Statute 1862a7

- ◆ **V5011** Fitting/orientation/checking of hearing aid
  Medicare Statute 1862a7

- ◆ **V5014** Repair/modification of a hearing aid
  Medicare Statute 1862a7

- ◆ **V5020** Conformity evaluation
  Medicare Statute 1862a7

- ◆ **V5030** Hearing aid, monaural, body worn, air conduction
  Medicare Statute 1862a7

- ◆ **V5040** Hearing aid, monaural, body worn, bone conduction
  Medicare Statute 1862a7

- ◆ **V5050** Hearing aid, monaural, in the ear
  Medicare Statute 1862a7

- ◆ **V5060** Hearing aid, monaural, behind the ear
  Medicare Statute 1862a7

- ◆ **V5070** Glasses, air conduction
  Medicare Statute 1862a7

- ◆ **V5080** Glasses, bone conduction
  Medicare Statute 1862a7

- ◆ **V5090** Dispensing fee, unspecified hearing aid
  Medicare Statute 1862a7

- ◆ **V5095** Semi-implantable middle ear hearing prosthesis
  Medicare Statute 1862a7

- ◆ **V5100** Hearing aid, bilateral, body worn
  Medicare Statute 1862a7

- ◆ **V5110** Dispensing fee, bilateral
  Medicare Statute 1862a7

- ◆ **V5120** Binaural, body
  Medicare Statute 1862a7

- ◆ **V5130** Binaural, in the ear
  Medicare Statute 1862a7

- ◆ **V5140** Binaural, behind the ear
  Medicare Statute 1862a7

- ◆ **V5150** Binaural, glasses
  Medicare Statute 1862a7

- ◆ **V5160** Dispensing fee, binaural
  Medicare Statute 1862a7

- ◆ **V5170** Hearing aid, CROS, in the ear
  Medicare Statute 1862a7

- ◆ **V5180** Hearing aid, CROS, behind the ear
  Medicare Statute 1862a7

- ◆ **V5190** Hearing aid, CROS, glasses
  Medicare Statute 1862a7

- ◆ **V5200** Dispensing fee, CROS
  Medicare Statute 1862a7

- ◆ **V5210** Hearing aid, BICROS, in the ear
  Medicare Statute 1862a7

- ◆ **V5220** Hearing aid, BICROS, behind the ear
  Medicare Statute 1862a7

- ◆ **V5230** Hearing aid, BICROS, glasses
  Medicare Statute 1862a7

- ◆ **V5240** Dispensing fee, BICROS
  Medicare Statute 1862a7

- ◆ **V5241** Dispensing fee, monaural hearing aid, any type
  Medicare Statute 1862a7

- ◆ **V5242** Hearing aid, analog, monaural, CIC (completely in the ear canal)
  Medicare Statute 1862a7

- ◆ **V5243** Hearing aid, analog, monaural, ITC (in the canal)
  Medicare Statute 1862a9

- ◆ **V5244** Hearing aid, digitally programmable analog, monaural, CIC
  Medicare Statute 1862a7

- ◆ **V5245** Hearing aid, digitally programmable, analog, monaural, ITC
  Medicare Statute 1862a7

- ◆ **V5246** Hearing aid, digitally programmable analog, monaural, ITE (in the ear)
  Medicare Statute 1862a7

- ◆ **V5247** Hearing aid, digitally programmable analog, monaural, BTE (behind the ear)
  Medicare Statute 1862a7

- ◆ **V5248** Hearing aid, analog, binaural, CIC
  Medicare Statute 1862a7

◀▶ New ←→ Revised ✔ Reinstated ✖ Deleted
⊙ Special coverage instructions ◆ Not covered or valid by Medicare ✳ Carrier discretion ▶ ASC payment group

◆ **V5249**   Hearing aid, analog, binaural, ITC

Medicare Statute 1862a7

◆ **V5250**   Hearing aid, digitally programmable analog, binaural, CIC

Medicare Statute 1862a7

◆ **V5251**   Hearing aid, digitally programmable analog, binaural, ITC

Medicare Statute 1862a7

◆ **V5252**   Hearing aid, digitally programmable, binaural, ITE

Medicare Statute 1862a7

◆ **V5253**   Hearing aid, digitally programmable, binaural, BTE

Medicare Statute 1862a7

◆ **V5254**   Hearing aid, digital, monaural, CIC

Medicare Statute 1862a7

◆ **V5255**   Hearing aid, digital, monaural, ITC

Medicare Statute 1862a7

◆ **V5256**   Hearing aid, digital, monaural, ITE

Medicare Statute 1862a7

◆ **V5257**   Hearing aid, digital, monaural, BTE

Medicare Statute 1862a7

◆ **V5258**   Hearing aid, digital, binaural, CIC

Medicare Statute 1862a7

◆ **V5259**   Hearing aid, digital, binaural, ITC

Medicare Statute 1862a7

◆ **V5260**   Hearing aid, digital, binaural, ITE

Medicare Statute 1862a7

◆ **V5261**   Hearing aid, digital, binaural, BTE

Medicare Statute 1862a7

◆ **V5262**   Hearing aid, disposable, any type, monaural

Medicare Statute 1862a7

◆ **V5263**   Hearing aid, disposable, any type, binaural

Medicare Statute 1862a7

◆ **V5264**   Ear mold/insert, not disposable, any type

Medicare Statute 1862a7

◆ **V5265**   Ear mold/insert, disposable, any type

Medicare Statute 1862a7

◆ **V5266**   Battery for use in hearing device

Medicare Statute 1862a7

◆ **V5267**   Hearing aid supplies/accessories

Medicare Statute 1862a7

◆ **V5268**   Assistive listening device, telephone amplifier, any type

Medicare Statute 1862a7

◆ **V5269**   Assistive listening device, alerting, any type

Medicare Statute 1862a7

◆ **V5270**   Assistive listening device, television amplifier, any type

Medicare Statute 1862a7

◆ **V5271**   Assistive listening device, television caption decoder

Medicare Statute 1862a7

◆ **V5272**   Assistive listening device, TDD

Medicare Statute 1862a7

◆ **V5273**   Assistive listening device, for use with cochlear implant

Medicare Statute 1862a7

◆ **V5274**   Assistive listening device, not otherwise specified

Medicare Statute 1862a7

◆ **V5275**   Ear impression, each

Medicare Statute 1862a7

◆ **V5298**   Hearing aid, not otherwise classified

Medicare Statute 1862a7

⊛ **V5299**   Hearing service, miscellaneous

IOM: 100-02, 16, 90

◀▶ **New**   ←→ **Revised**   ✔ **Reinstated**   ✖ **Deleted**

 Special coverage instructions   ◆ **Not covered or valid by Medicare**   ✳ **Carrier discretion**   ▶ **ASC payment group**

HEARING SERVICES

Speech-Language Pathology Services

NOTE: These codes are for non-physician services.

◆ **V5336** Repair/modification of augmentative communicative system or device (excludes adaptive hearing aid)

Medicare Statute 1862a7

◆ **V5362** Speech screening

Medicare Statute 1862a7

◆ **V5363** Language screening

Medicare Statute 1862a7

◆ **V5364** Dysphagia screening

Medicare Statute 1862a7

V5336 – V5364

◄ ► New   ← → Revised   ✔ Reinstated   ✖ Deleted

☺ Special coverage instructions   ◆ Not covered or valid by Medicare   ✳ Carrier discretion   ▶ ASC payment group

APPENDIX

APPENDIX A

Select Internet Only Manuals (IOM)

Updates available at http://www.cms.hhs.gov/Manuals/IOM/list.asp. IOM last accessed on October 22, 2008.

100-01 Chapter 3

20.5 - Blood Deductibles (Part A and Part B)

(Rev. 1, 09-11-02)

Program payment may not be made for the first 3 pints of whole blood or equivalent units of packed red cells received under Part A and Part B combined in a calendar year. However, blood processing (e.g., administration, storage) is not subject to the deductible.

The blood deductibles are in addition to any other applicable deductible and coinsurance amounts for which the patient is responsible.

The deductible applies only to the first 3 pints of blood furnished in a calendar year, even if more than one provider furnished blood.

20.5.1 - Part A Blood Deductible

(Rev. 1, 09-11-02)

Blood must be furnished on a Medicare covered day in a hospital or SNF to be counted under Part A. Blood furnished to an inpatient after benefits exhausted or before entitlement is not counted toward the combined deductible. Blood furnished during a lifetime extension election period is counted toward the combined A/B 3 pint total.

20.5.2 - Part B Blood Deductible

(Rev. 1, 09-11-02)

Blood is furnished on an outpatient basis or is subject to the Part B blood deductible and is counted toward the combined limit. It should be noted that payment for blood may be made to the hospital under Part B only for blood furnished in an outpatient setting. Blood is not covered for inpatient Part B services.

20.5.3 - Items Subject to Blood Deductibles

(Rev. 18, Issued: 03-04-05, Effective: 07-01-05, Implementation: 07-05-05)

The blood deductibles apply only to whole blood and packed red cells. The term whole blood means human blood from which none of the liquid or cellular components have been removed. Where packed red cells are furnished, a unit of packed red cells is considered equivalent to a pint of whole blood. Other components of blood such as platelets, fibrinogen, plasma, gamma globulin, and serum albumin are not subject to the blood deductible. However, these components of blood are covered as biologicals.

Refer to Pub. 100-04, Medicare Claims Processing Manual, Chapter 4, §231 regarding billing for blood and blood products under the Hospital Outpatient Prospective Payment System (OPPS).

20.5.4 - Obligations of the Beneficiary to Pay for or Replace Deductible Blood

(Rev. 1, 09-11-02)

A provider may charge the beneficiary or a third party its customary charge for whole blood or units of packed red cells which are subject to either the Part A or Part B blood deductible, unless the individual, another person, or a blood bank replaces the blood or arranges to have it replaced.

20.5.4.1 - Replacement of Blood

(Rev. 1, 09-11-02)

For replacement purposes, a pint of whole blood is considered equivalent to a unit of packed red cells. A deductible pint of whole blood or unit of packed red cells is considered replaced when a medically acceptable pint or unit is given or offered to the provider or, at the provider's request, to its blood supplier. Accordingly, where an individual or a blood bank offers blood as a replacement for a deductible pint or unit furnished a Medicare beneficiary, the provider may not charge the beneficiary for the blood, whether or not the provider or its blood supplier accepts the replacement offer. Thus a provider may not charge a beneficiary merely because it is the policy of the provider or its blood supplier not to accept blood from a particular source which has offered to replace blood on behalf of the beneficiary. However, a provider would not be barred from charging a beneficiary for deductible blood, if there is a reasonable basis for believing that replacement blood offered by or on behalf of the beneficiary would endanger the health of a recipient or that the prospective donor's health would be endangered by making a blood donation. Once a provider accepts a pint of replacement blood from a beneficiary or another individual acting on his/her behalf, the blood is deemed to have been replaced, and, the beneficiary may not be charged for the blood, even though the replacement blood is later found to be unfit and has to be discarded.

When a provider accepts blood donated in advance, in anticipation of need by a specific beneficiary, whether the beneficiary's own blood, that is, an autologous donation, or blood furnished by another individual or blood assurance group, such donations are considered replacement for pints or units subsequently furnished the beneficiary.

20.6 - Part B Premium

(Rev. 41, Issued: 10-27-06; Effective: 01-01-07; Implementation: 01-02-07)

The Centers for Medicare and Medicaid Services (CMS) updates the Part B premium each year. These adjustments are made according to formulas set by statute. By law, the monthly Part B premium must be sufficient to cover 25 percent of the program's costs, including the costs of maintaining a reserve against unexpected spending increases. The federal government pays the remaining 75 percent.

Below are the annual Part B premium amounts from Calendar Year (CY) 1996 to 2006. For these years, and years prior to 1996, the Part B premium is a single established rate for all beneficiaries.

Year	Part B Premium
1996	$42.50
1997	$43.80
1998	$43.80
1999	$45.50
2000	$45.50
2001	$50.00
2002	$54.00
2003	$58.70
2004	$66.60
2005	$78.20
2006	$88.50

Beginning on January 1, 2007, the Part B premium will be based on the income of the beneficiary. Below are the CY 2007 Part B premium amounts based on beneficiary income parameters.

Income Parameters for Determining Part B Premium

Premium/ month	Individual Income	Combined Income (Married)
$ 93.50	$ 80,000.00 or less	$160,000.00 or less
$105.80	$ 80,000.01 – $100,000.00	$160,000.01 – $200,000.00
$124.40	$100,000.01 – $150,000.00	$200,000.01 – $300,000.00
$142.90	$150,000.01 – $200,000.00	$300,000.01 – $400,000.00
$161.40	$200,000.01 or more	$400,000.01 or more

30 - Outpatient Mental Health Treatment Limitation

(Rev. 1, 09-11-02)

Regardless of the actual expenses a beneficiary incurs for treatment of mental, psychoneurotic, and personality disorders while the beneficiary is not an inpatient of a hospital at the time such expenses are incurred, the amount of those expenses that may be recognized for Part B deductible and payment purposes is limited to 62.5 percent of the Medicare allowed amount for these services. The limitation is called the outpatient mental health treatment limitation. Since Part B deductible also applies the program pays for about half of the allowed amount recognized for mental health therapy services.

Expenses for diagnostic services (e.g., psychiatric testing and evaluation to diagnose the patient's illness) are not subject to this limitation. This limitation applies only to therapeutic services and to services performed to evaluate the progress of a course of treatment for a diagnosed condition.

30.1 - Application of Mental Health Limitation - Status of Patient

(Rev. 1, 09-11-02)

The limitation is applicable to expenses incurred in connection with the treatment of an individual who is not an inpatient of a hospital. Thus, the limitation applies to mental health services furnished to a person in a physician's office, in the patient's home, in a skilled nursing facility, as an outpatient, and so forth. The term "hospital" in this context means an institution which is primarily engaged in providing to inpatients, by or under the supervision of a physician(s):

- Diagnostic and therapeutic services for medical diagnosis, and treatment, and care of injured, disabled, or sick persons:
- Rehabilitation services for injured, disabled, or sick persons; or
- Psychiatric services for the diagnosis and treatment of mentally ill patients.

30.2 - Disorders Subject to Mental Health Limitation

(Rev. 1, 09-11-02)

The term "mental, psychoneurotic, and personality disorders" is defined as the specific psychiatric conditions described in the American Psychiatric Association's Diagnostic and Statistical Manual of Mental Disorders, Third Edition - Revised (DSM-III-R).

If the treatment services rendered are for both a psychiatric condition and one or more nonpsychiatric conditions, the charges are separated to apply the limitation only to the mental health charge. Normally HCPCS code and diagnoses are used. Where HCPCS code is not available on the claim, revenue code is used.

If the service is primarily on the basis of a diagnosis of Alzheimer's Disease (coded 331.0 in the International Classification of Diseases, 9th Revision) or Alzheimer's or other disorders (coded 290.XX in DSM-III-R), treatment typically represents medical management of the patient's condition (rather than psychiatric treatment) and is not subject to the limitation.

30.3 - Diagnostic Services

(Rev. 1, 09-11-02)

The mental health limitation does not apply to tests and evaluations performed to establish or confirm the patient's diagnosis. Diagnostic services include psychiatric or psychological tests and interpretations, diagnostic consultations, and initial evaluations. However, testing services performed to evaluate a patient's progress during treatment are considered part of treatment and are subject to the limitation.

40 - Limitation on Physical Therapy, Occupational Therapy and Speech-Language Pathology Services

(Rev. 28; Issued: 08-12-05; Effective/Implementation: 09-12-05)

Coverage of outpatient physical therapy, occupational therapy, and speech-language pathology services under Part B has been limited in some years. For descriptions of these limitations see Pub 100-04, Chapter 5, §10.2.

Transmittals Issued for this Chapter

Rev #	Issue Date	Subject	Impl Date	CR#
R41GI	10/27/2006	Update to Medicare Deductible, Coinsurance and Premium Rates for 2007	01/02/2007	5345
R31GI	11/04/2005	Update to Medicare Deductible, Coinsurance and Premium Rates for 2006	01/03/2006	4132
R28GI	08/12/2005	Conforming Changes for Change Request 3648 to Pub. 100-01	09/12/2005	3912
R18GI	03/04/2005	Billing for Blood and Blood Products Under the Hospital Outpatient Prospective Payment System (OPPS)	07/05/2005	3681
R12GI	10/22/2004	New Policy and Refinements on Billing Noncovered Charges to Fiscal Intermediaries (FIs)	04/04/2005	3416
R11GI	10/22/2004	Manual Revision Regarding Waiver of Annual Deductible and Coinsurance for Both ASC Facility, and ASC/ Hospital Outpatient Department Physician Services	11/22/2004	3471
R10GI	09/10/2004	Update to Medicare Deductible, Coinsurance and Premium Rates for Calendar Year 2005	01/03/2005	3463
R09GI	09/03/2004	Update to Medicare Deductible, Coinsurance and Premium Rates for Calendar Year 2005	01/03/2005	3463
R03GI	03/12/2004	New Part B Annual Deductible	01/03/2005	3121
R01GI	09/11/2002	Initial Publication of Manual	NA	NA

100-01 Chapter 5

90.2—Laboratory Defined

(Rev. 1, 09-11-02)

Laboratory means a facility for the biological, microbiological, serological, chemical, immuno-hematological, hematological, biophysical, cytological, pathological, or other examination of materials derived from the human body for the purpose of providing information for the diagnosis, prevention, or treatment of any disease or impairment of, or the assessment of the health of, human beings. These examinations also include procedures to determine, measure, or otherwise describe the presence or absence of various substances or organisms in the body. Facilities only collecting or preparing specimens (or both) or only serving as a mailing service and not performing testing are not considered laboratories.

100-02 Chapter 1

10—Covered Inpatient Hospital Services Covered Under Part A

(Rev. 1, 10-01-03)

A3-3101, HO-210

Patients covered under hospital insurance are entitled to have payment made on their behalf for inpatient hospital services. (Inpatient hospital services do not include extended care services provided by hospitals pursuant to swing bed approvals. See Pub. 100-1, Chapter 8, §10.1, "Hospital Providers of Extended Care Services."). However, both inpatient hospital and inpatient SNF benefits are provided under Part A - Hospital Insurance Benefits for the Aged and Disabled, of Title XVIII).

Additional information concerning the following topics can be found in the following manual chapters:

- Benefit periods is found in Chapter 3, "Duration of Covered Inpatient Services";
- Copayment days is found in Chapter 2, "Duration of Covered Inpatient Services";
- Lifetime reserve days is found in Chapter 5, "Lifetime Reserve Days";

- Related payment information is housed in the Provider Reimbursement Manual.

Blood must be furnished on a day which counts as a day of inpatient hospital services to be covered as a Part A service and to count toward the blood deductible. Thus, blood is not covered under Part A and does not count toward the Part A blood deductible when furnished to an inpatient after the inpatient has exhausted all benefit days in a benefit period, or where the individual has elected not to use lifetime reserve days. However, where the patient is discharged on their first day of entitlement or on the hospital's first day of participation, the hospital is permitted to submit a billing form with no accommodation charge, but with ancillary charges including blood.

The records for all Medicare hospital inpatient discharges are maintained in CMS for statistical analysis and use in determining future PPS DRG classifications and rates.

Non-PPS hospitals do not pay for noncovered services generally excluded from coverage in the Medicare Program. This may result in denial of a part of the billed charges or in denial of the entire admission, depending upon circumstance. In PPS hospitals, the following are also possible:

1. In appropriately admitted cases where a noncovered procedure was performed, denied services may result in payment of a different DRG (i.e., one which excludes payment for the noncovered procedure); or
2. In appropriately admitted cases that become cost outlier cases, denied services may lead to denial of some or all of an outlier payment.

The following examples illustrate this principle. If care is noncovered because a patient does not need to be hospitalized, the intermediary denies the admission and makes no Part A (i.e., PPS) payment unless paid under limitation on liability. Under limitation on liability, Medicare payment may be made when the provider **and** the beneficiary were **not** aware the services were not necessary and could not reasonably be expected to know that he services were not necessary. For detailed instructions, see the Medicare Claims Processing Manual, Chapter 30, "Limitation on Liability." If a patient is appropriately hospitalized but receives (beyond routine services) only noncovered care, the admission is denied.

NOTE: The intermediary does not deny an admission that includes covered care, even if noncovered care was also rendered. Under PPS, Medicare assumes that it is paying for **only** the covered care rendered whenever covered services needed to treat and/or diagnose the illness were in fact provided.

If a noncovered procedure is provided along with covered nonroutine care, a DRG change rather than an admission denial might occur. If noncovered procedures are elevating costs into the cost outlier category, outlier payment is denied in whole or in part.

When the hospital is included in PPS, most of the subsequent discussion regarding coverage of inpatient hospital services is relevant only in the context of determining the appropriateness of admissions, which DRG, if any, to pay, and the appropriateness of payment for any outlier cases.

If a patient receives items or services in excess of, or more expensive than, those for which payment can be made, payment is made only for the covered items or services or for only the appropriate prospective payment amount. This provision applies not only to inpatient services, but also to all hospital services under Parts A and B of the program. If the items or services were requested by the patient, the hospital may charge him the difference between the amount customarily charged for the services requested and the amount customarily charged for covered services.

An **inpatient** is a person who has been admitted to a hospital for bed occupancy for purposes of receiving inpatient hospital services. Generally, a patient is considered an inpatient if formally admitted as inpatient with the expectation that he or she will remain at least overnight and occupy a bed even though it later develops that the patient can be discharged or transferred to another hospital and not actually use a hospital bed overnight.

The physician or other practitioner responsible for a patient's care at the hospital is also responsible for deciding whether the patient should be admitted as an inpatient. Physicians should use a 24-hour period as a benchmark, i.e., they should order admission for patients who are expected to need hospital care for 24 hours or more, and treat other patients on an outpatient basis. However, the decision to admit a patient is a complex medical judgment which can be made only after the physician has considered a number of factors, including the patient's medical history and current medical needs, the types of facilities available to inpatients and to outpatients, the hospital's by-laws and admissions policies, and the relative appropriateness of treatment in each setting. Factors to be considered when making the decision to admit include such things as:

- The severity of the signs and symptoms exhibited by the patient;
- The medical predictability of something adverse happening to the patient;
- The need for diagnostic studies that appropriately are outpatient services (i.e., their performance does not ordinarily require the patient to remain at the hospital for 24 hours or more) to assist in assessing whether the patient should be admitted; and

- The availability of diagnostic procedures at the time when and at the location where the patient presents.

Admissions of particular patients are not covered or noncovered solely on the basis of the length of time the patient actually spends in the hospital. In certain specific situations coverage of services on an inpatient or outpatient basis is determined by the following rules:

Minor Surgery or Other Treatment - When patients with known diagnoses enter a hospital for a specific minor surgical procedure or other treatment that is expected to keep them in the hospital for only a few hours (less than 24), they are considered **outpatients** for coverage purposes regardless of: the hour they came to the hospital, whether they used a bed, and whether they remained in the hospital past midnight.

Renal Dialysis - Renal dialysis treatments are usually covered only as outpatient services but may under certain circumstances be covered as inpatient services depending on the patient's condition. Patients staying at home, who are ambulatory, whose conditions are stable and who come to the hospital for routine chronic dialysis treatments, and not for a diagnostic workup or a change in therapy, are considered outpatients. On the other hand, patients undergoing short-term dialysis until their kidneys recover from an acute illness (acute dialysis), or persons with borderline renal failure who develop acute renal failure every time they have an illness and require dialysis (episodic dialysis) are usually inpatients. A patient may begin dialysis as an inpatient and then progress to an outpatient status.

Under original Medicare, the Quality Improvement Organization (QIO), for each hospital is responsible for deciding, during review of inpatient admissions on a case-by-case basis, whether the admission was medically necessary. Medicare law authorizes the QIO to make these judgments, and the judgments are binding for purposes of Medicare coverage. In making these judgments, however, QIOs consider only the medical evidence which was available to the physician at the time an admission decision had to be made. They do not take into account other information (e.g., test results) which became available only after admission, except in cases where considering the post-admission information would support a finding that an admission was medically necessary.

Refer to Parts 4 and 7 of the QIO Manual with regard to initial determinations for these services. The QIO will review the swing bed services in these PPS hospitals as well.

NOTE: When patients requiring extended care services are admitted to beds in a hospital, they are considered inpatients of the hospital. In such cases, the services furnished in the hospital will not be considered extended care services, and payment may not be made under the program for such services unless the services are extended care services furnished pursuant to a swing bed agreement granted to the hospital by the Secretary of Health and Human Services.

10.1—Bed and Board

(Rev. 1, 10-01-03)

A3-3101.1, HO-210.1

10.1.1—Accommodations - General

(Rev. 1, 10-01-03)

A3-3101.1.A, HO-210.1.A

The program will pay the same amount for routine accommodations services whether the patient has a private room not medically necessary, a private room medically necessary (Medicare does not pay for deluxe accommodations in any case), a semiprivate room (2-, 3-, or 4-bed accommodations), or ward accommodations, if its ward accommodations are consistent with program purposes (see §10.1.6 below).

A provider having both private and semiprivate accommodations may nevertheless charge the patient a differential for a private room if:

- The private room is not medically necessary; and
- The patient (or relative or other person acting on their behalf) has requested the private room, and the provider informs them of the amount of charge at the time of the request.

The private room differential may not exceed the difference between the customary charge for the accommodations furnished and the most prevalent semiprivate accommodation rate at the time of the patient's admission.

Where the provider bills for a private room as a covered service, i.e., shows the charge for the room as a covered charge on the Form CMS-1450, the intermediary will deem the private room to be medically necessary. Where the provider, on the other hand, shows a private differential as a noncovered charge, the intermediary will assume that the private room is not medically necessary.

If the beneficiary (or their representative) protests a charge for the private room on the grounds that the privacy was medically necessary, such protest will, if not in written form, be reduced to writing and forwarded to the intermediary. The intermediary will then develop the facts and make a specific determination regarding the medical necessity of the private room. (If an intermediary receives many protests of this kind, the provider may need guidance on what constitutes medical necessity for privacy). If the protest is received after the claim is processed, it will be treated as a request for reconsideration.

If at any time in the course of development (or thereafter within the period when the determination is not administratively final), the provider acknowledges that the private room was medically necessary; the intermediary will make an immediate finding to this effect.

Where it is necessary to develop the medical necessity of a private room, the guidelines in subsections §§10.1.2 and 10.1.3 below will apply.

10.1.2—Medical Necessity - Need for Isolation

(Rev. 1, 10-01-03)

A3-3101.1.B, HO-210.1.B

A private room is medically necessary where isolation of a beneficiary is required to avoid jeopardizing their health or recovery, or that of other patients who are likely to be alarmed or disturbed by the beneficiary's symptoms or treatment or subjected to infection by the beneficiary's communicable disease. For example, communicable diseases, heart attacks, cerebra-vascular accidents, and psychotic episodes may require isolation of the patient for certain periods. (See §10.1.3 below concerning medical necessity not based on need for isolation).

In establishing the medical necessity for isolation, the date of the physician's written statement is not controlling, nor is the presence of a written statement. The crucial question is whether a private room was ordered by the physician because it is necessary for the health of the patient himself or herself or of other patients. In the absence of such an order, a patient who requested the room with knowledge of the amount of the charge may be charged appropriately, even though a physician subsequently submits a statement that the room was medically necessary. There may be cases in which the physician's written statement of medical necessity, though dated after admission or even after discharge, merely confirms an order made informally at or before the time the beneficiary was admitted to the private room (e.g., the physician made arrangements by phone for the patient's admission, gave the diagnosis, and stated the beneficiary would need a private room). In such cases, assuming that the private room was medically necessary, the lack of a written statement by the physician, or the fact that the written statement was prepared after discharge, would not be controlling. The patient may not be charged.

10.1.3—Medical Necessity - Admission Required and Only Private Rooms Available

(Rev. 1, 10-01-03)

A3-3101.1.C, HO-210.1.C

A private room is considered to be medically necessary even though the beneficiary's condition does not require isolation if he/she needs immediate hospitalization (i.e., the beneficiary's medical condition is such that hospitalization cannot be deferred) and the hospital has no semiprivate or ward accommodations available at the time of admission.

It need not be considered whether semiprivate or ward accommodations were available in some other accessible hospital. Where medical necessity exists, the provider may not charge the beneficiary a private room differential until semiprivate or ward accommodations become available. Thereafter the provider may transfer the patient to the nonprivate accommodations, or allow them to continue occupancy of the private room, subject to an appropriate differential charge (described in §10.1.1 above) if they request the private room with knowledge of the amount of the charge.

If the admission could be deferred until semiprivate or ward accommodations become available, the beneficiary should be informed of the amount of the differential he/she must pay for a private room if he/she wishes to be admitted immediately. The beneficiary may be charged the specified differential if he/she has been admitted to the private room at their request (or at the request of their representative) with knowledge of the amount of the charge.

10.1.4—Charges for Deluxe Private Room

(Rev. 1, 10-01-03)

A3-3101.1.D, HO-210.1.D

Beneficiaries found to need a private room (either because they need isolation for medical reasons or because they need immediate admission when no other accommodations are available) may be assigned to any of the provider's private rooms. They do not have the right to insist on the private room of their choice, but their preferences should be given the same consideration as if they were paying all provider charges themselves. The program does not, under any circumstances, pay for personal comfort items. Thus, the program does not pay for deluxe accommodations and/or services. These would include a suite, or a room substantially more spacious than is required for treatment, or specially equipped or decorated, or serviced for the comfort and convenience of persons willing to pay a differential for such amenities. If the beneficiary (or representative) requests such deluxe accommodations, the provider should advise that there will be a charge, not covered by Medicare, of a specified amount per day (not exceeding the differential defined in the next sentence); and may charge the beneficiary that amount for each day he/she occupies the deluxe accommodations. The maximum amount the provider may charge the beneficiary for such accommodations is the differential between the most prevalent private room rate at the time of admission and the customary charge for the room occupied. Beneficiaries may not be charged this differential if they (or their representative) do not request the deluxe accommodations.

The beneficiary may not be charged such a differential in private room rates if that differential is based on factors other than personal comfort items. Such factors might include differences between older and newer wings, proximity to lounge, elevators or nursing stations, desirable view, etc. Such rooms are standard 1-bed units and not deluxe rooms for purposes of these instructions, even though the provider may call them deluxe and have a higher customary charge for them. No additional charge may be imposed upon the beneficiary who is assigned to a room that may be somewhat more desirable because of these factors.

10.1.5—All Private Room Providers

(Rev. 1, 10-01-03)

A3-3101.E, HO-210.1.E

If the patient is admitted to a provider which has only private accommodations, and no semiprivate or ward accommodations, medical necessity will be deemed to exist for the accommodations furnished. Beneficiaries may not be subjected to an extra charge for a private room in an all-private room provider.

10.1.6—Wards

(Rev. 1, 10-01-03)

A3-3101.1.F, HO-210.1.F

The law contemplates that Medicare patients should not be assigned to ward accommodations except at the patient's request or for a reason consistent with the purposes of the health insurance program.

When ward accommodations are furnished at the patient's request or for a reason determined to be consistent with the program's purposes, payment will be based on the average per diem cost of routine services (see §10.1.1 above). Where ward accommodations are assigned for other reasons, the law provides what may be a substantial penalty. (See §10.1.6.2 below).

Any request by the patient (or relative or other person responsible for his or her affairs) for ward accommodations must be obtained by the provider in writing and kept in its files.

10.1.6.1—Assignment Consistent With Program Purposes

(Rev. 1, 10-01-03)

A3-3101.1.F.1, HO-210.1.F.1

It is considered to be consistent with the program's purposes to assign the patient to ward accommodations if all semiprivate accommodations are occupied, or the facility has no semiprivate accommodations. However, the patient must be moved to semiprivate accommodations if they become available during the stay.

Some hospitals have a policy of placing in wards all patients who do not have private physicians. Such a practice may be consistent with the purposes of the program if the intermediary determines that the ward assignment inures to the benefit of the patient. In making this determination, the principal consideration is whether the assignment is likely to result in better medical treatment of the patient (e.g., it facilitates necessary medical and nursing supervision and treatment). The intermediary should ask a provider having this policy to submit a statement describing how the assignments are made, their purpose, and the effect on the care of patients so assigned.

If the intermediary makes a favorable determination on a practice affecting all ward assignments of Medicare patients in the institution, a reference should be made on the appropriate billing form for patients to whom the hospital assigned a ward pursuant to such practice.

10.1.6.2—Assignment Not Consistent With Program Purposes

(Rev. 1, 10-01-03)

A3-3101.1.F.2, HO-210.1.F.2

It is not consistent with the purposes of the law to assign a patient ward accommodation based on their social or economic status, their national origin, race, or religion, or their entitlement to benefits as a Medicare patient, or any other such discriminatory reason. It is also inconsistent with the purposes of the law to assign patients to ward accommodations merely for the convenience or financial advantage of the institution. Additionally, under DRGs, there no longer is a reduction to payment or an adjustment to the end of year settlement.

10.1.7—Charges

(Rev. 1, 10-01-03)

A3-3101.1.G, HO-210.1.G

Customary charges means amounts which the hospital or skilled nursing facility is uniformly charging patients currently for specific services and accommodations. The most prevalent rate or charge is the rate that applies to the greatest number of semiprivate or private beds in the institution.

100-02 Chapter 6

10—Medical and Other Health Services Furnished to Inpatients of Participating Hospitals

(Rev. 37, Issued: 08-12-05; Effective/Implementation: 09-12-05)

Payment may be made under **Part B** for physician services and for the nonphysician medical and other health services listed below when furnished by a participating hospital (either directly or under arrangements) to an inpatient of the hospital, but only if payment for these services cannot be made under Part A.

In PPS hospitals, this means that Part B payment could be made for these services if:

- No Part A prospective payment is made at all for the hospital stay because of patient exhaustion of benefit days before admission;
- The admission was disapproved as not reasonable and necessary (and waiver of liability payment was not made);
- The day or days of the otherwise covered stay during which the services were provided were not reasonable and necessary (and no payment was made under waiver of liability);
- The patient was not otherwise eligible for or entitled to coverage under Part A (See the Medicare Benefit Policy Manual, Chapter 1, §150, for services received as a result of noncovered services); or
- No Part A day outlier payment is made (for discharges before October 1997) for one or more outlier days due to patient exhaustion of benefit days after admission but before the case's arrival at outlier status, or because outlier days are otherwise not covered and waiver of liability payment is not made.

However, if only day outlier payment is denied under Part A (discharges before October 1997), Part B payment may be made for only the services covered under Part B and furnished on the denied outlier days.

In non-PPS hospitals, Part B payment may be made for services on **any** day for which Part A payment is denied (i.e., benefit days are exhausted; services are not at the hospital level of care; or patient is not otherwise eligible or entitled to payment under Part A).

Services payable are:

Diagnostic x-ray tests, diagnostic laboratory tests, and other diagnostic tests;

- X-ray, radium, and radioactive isotope therapy, including materials and services of technicians;
- Surgical dressings, and splints, casts, and other devices used for reduction of fractures and dislocations;
- Prosthetic devices (other than dental) which replace all or part of an internal body organ (including contiguous tissue), or all or part of the function of a permanently inoperative or malfunctioning internal body organ, including replacement or repairs of such devices;
- Leg, arm, back, and neck braces, trusses, and artificial legs, arms, and eyes including adjustments, repairs, and re-

placements required because of breakage, wear, loss, or a change in the patient's physical condition;
- Outpatient physical therapy, outpatient speech-language pathology services, and outpatient occupational therapy (see the Medicare Benefit Policy Manual, Chapter 15, "Covered Medical and Other Health Services," §§220 and 230);
- Screening mammography services;
- Screening pap smears;
- Influenza, pneumococcal pneumonia, and hepatitis B vaccines;
- Colorectal screening;
- Bone mass measurements;
- Diabetes self-management;
- Prostate screening;
- Ambulance services;
- Hemophilia clotting factors for hemophilia patients competent to use these factors without supervision;
- Immunosuppressive drugs;
- Oral anti-cancer drugs;
- Oral drug prescribed for use as an acute anti-emetic used as part of an anti-cancer chemotherapeutic regimen; and
- Epoetin Alfa (EPO).

Coverage rules for these services are described in the Medicare Benefit Policy Manual, Chapters: 11, "End Stage Renal Disease (ESRD);" 14, "Medical Devices;" or 15, "Medical and Other Health Services."

For services to be covered under Part A or Part B, a hospital **must** furnish nonphysician services to its inpatients directly or under arrangements. A nonphysician service is one which does not meet the criteria defining physicians' services specifically provided for in regulation at 42 CFR 415.102. Services "incident to" physicians' services (except for the services of nurse anesthetists employed by anesthesiologists) are nonphysician services for purposes of this provision. This provision is applicable to all hospitals participating in Medicare, including those paid under alternative arrangements such as State cost control systems, and to emergency hospital services furnished by nonparticipating hospitals.

In all hospitals, **every** service provided to a hospital inpatient other than those listed in the next paragraph must be treated as an inpatient hospital service to be paid for under Part A, if Part A coverage is available and the beneficiary is entitled to Part A. This is because every hospital must provide directly or arrange for any nonphysician service rendered to its inpatients, and a hospital can be paid under Part B for a service provided in this manner only if Part A coverage does not exist.

These services, when provided to a hospital inpatient, may be covered under Part B, even though the patient has Part A coverage for the hospital stay. This is because these services are covered under Part B and not covered under Part A. They are:

- Physicians' services (including the services of residents and interns in unapproved teaching programs);
- Influenza vaccine;
- Pneumoccocal vaccine and its administration;
- Hepatitis B vaccine and its administration;
- Screening mammography services;
- Screening pap smears and pelvic exams;
- Colorectal screening;
- Bone mass measurements;
- Diabetes self management training services; and
- Prostate screening.

However, note that in order to have any Medicare coverage at all (Part A or Part B), any nonphysician service rendered to a hospital inpatient must be provided directly or arranged for by the hospital.

100-02 Chapter 10

20—Coverage Guidelines for Ambulance Service Claims

(Rev. 1, 10-01-03)

B3-2125

Payment may be made for expenses incurred by a patient for ambulance service provided conditions l, 2, and 3 in the left-hand column have been met. The right-hand column indicates the documentation needed to establish that the condition has been met.

20.1—Mandatory Assignment Requirements

(Rev. 1, 10-01-03)

When an ambulance provider/supplier, or a third party under contract with the provider/supplier, furnishes a Medicare-covered ambulance service to a Medicare beneficiary and the service is not statutorily excluded under the particular circumstances, the provider/supplier must submit a claim to Medicare and accept assignment of the beneficiary's right to payment from Medicare.

20.1.1—Managed Care Providers/Suppliers

(Rev. 1, 10-01-03)

Mandatory assignment for ambulance services, in effect with the implementation of the ambulance fee schedule, applies to ambulance providers/suppliers under managed care as well as under fee-for-service. The ambulance fee schedule is effective for claims with a date of service on or after April 1, 2002.

Any provider or supplier without a contract establishing payment amounts for services provided to a beneficiary enrolled in a Medicare + Choice (M+C) coordinated care plan or M+C private fee-for-service plan must accept, as payment in full, the amounts that they could collect if the beneficiary were enrolled in original Medicare. The provider or supplier can collect from the M+C plan enrollee the cost-sharing amount required under the M+C plan, and collect the remainder from the M+C organization.

Conditions	Review Action

1. Patient was transported by an approved supplier of ambulance services.
2. The patient was suffering from an illness or injury, which contraindicated transportation by other means. (§10.2)
	1. Ambulance supplier is listed in the table of approved ambulance companies (§10.1.3)
	2. (a) The contractor presumes the requirement was met if the submitted documentation indicates that the patient:
	    • Was transported in an emergency situation, e.g., as a result of an accident, injury or acute illness, or
	    • Needed to be restrained to prevent injury to the beneficiary or others; or
	    • Was unconscious or in shock; or
	    • Required oxygen or other emergency treatment during transport to the nearest appropriate facility; or
	    • Exhibits signs and symptoms of acute respiratory distress or cardiac distress such as shortness of breath or chest pain; or
	    • Exhibits signs and symptoms that indicate the possibility of acute stroke; or
	    • Had to remain immobile because of a fracture that had not been set or the possibility of a fracture; or
	    • Was experiencing severe hemorrhage; or
	    • Could be moved only by stretcher; or
	    • Was bed-confined before and after the ambulance trip.
	(b) In the absence of any of the conditions listed in (a) above additional documentation should be obtained to establish medical need where the evidence indicates the existence of the circumstances listed below:
	    (i) Patient's condition would not ordinarily require movement by stretcher, or
	    (ii) The individual was not admitted as a hospital inpatient (except in accident cases), or
	    (iii) The ambulance was used solely because other means of transportation were unavailable, or
	    (iv) The individual merely needed assistance in getting from his room or home to a vehicle.
	(c) Where the information indicates a situation not listed in 2(a) or 2(b) above, refer the case to your supervisor.

3. The patient was transported from and to points listed below.
   (a) From patient's residence (or other place where need arose) to hospital or skilled nursing facility.

3. Claims should show the ZIP code of the point of pickup.
   (a)
       i. Condition met if trip began within the institution's service area as shown in the carrier's locality guide
       ii. Condition met where the trip began outside the institution's service area if the institution was the nearest one with appropriate facilities.

NOTE: A patient's residence is the place where he or she makes his/her home and dwells permanently, or for an extended period of time. A skilled nursing facility is one, which is listed in the Directory of Medical Facilities as a participating SNF or as an institution which meets §1861(j)(1) of the Act.

NOTE: A claim for ambulance service to a participating hospital or skilled nursing facility should not be denied on the grounds that there is a nearer nonparticipating institution having appropriate facilities.

(b) Skilled nursing facility to a hospital or hospital to a skilled nursing facility.

(b)
   (i) Condition met if the ZIP code of the pickup point is within the service area of the destination as shown in the carrier's locality guide.
   (ii) Condition met where the ZIP code of the pickup point is outside the service area of the destination if the destination institution was the nearest appropriate facility.

(c) Hospital to hospital or skilled nursing facility to skilled nursing facility.

(c) Condition met if the discharging institution was not an appropriate facility and the admitting institution was the nearest appropriate facility.

(d) From a hospital or skilled nursing facility to patient's residence.

(d)
   (i) Condition met if patient's residence is within the institution's service area as shown in the carrier's locality guide.
   (ii) Condition met where the patient's residence is outside the institution's service area if the institution was the nearest appropriate facility.

(e) Round trip for hospital or participating skilled nursing facility inpatients to the nearest hospital or nonhospital treatment facility.

(e) Condition met if the reasonable and necessary diagnostic or therapeutic service required by patient's condition is not available at the institution where the beneficiary is an inpatient.

NOTE: Ambulance service to a physician's office or a physician-directed clinic is not covered. See §10.3.7 above, where a stop is made at a physician's office en route to a hospital and §10.3.3 for additional exceptions.)

4. Ambulance services involving hospital admissions in Canada or Mexico are covered (Medicare Claims Processing Manual, Chapter 1, "General Billing Requirements, " §§10.1.3.) if the following conditions are met:

(a) The foreign hospitalization has been determined to be covered; and
(b) The ambulance service meets the coverage requirements set forth in §§10-10.3. If the foreign hospitalization has been determined to be covered on the basis of emergency services (See the Medicare Claims Processing Manual, Chapter 1, "General Billing Requirements," §10.1.3), the necessity requirement (§10.2) and the destination requirement (§10.3) are considered met.

5. The carrier will make partial payment for otherwise covered ambulance service, which exceeded limits defined in item 6. The carrier will base the payment on the amount payable had the patient been transported:

(a) From the pickup point to the nearest appropriate facility, or
(b) From the nearest appropriate facility to the beneficiary's residence where he or she is being returned home from a distant institution.

20.1.2—Beneficiary Signature Requirements

(Rev. 1, 10-01-03)

Medicare requires the signature of the beneficiary, or that of his or her representative, for both the purpose of accepting assignment and submitting a claim to Medicare. If the beneficiary is unable to sign because of a mental or physical condition, a representative payee, relative, friend, representative of the institution providing care, or a government agency providing assistance may sign on his/her behalf. A provider/supplier (or his/her employee) cannot request payment for services furnished except under circumstances fully docu-

mented to show that the beneficiary is unable to sign and that there is no other person who could sign.

Medicare does not require that the signature to authorize claim submission be obtained at the time of transport for the purpose of accepting assignment of Medicare payment for ambulance benefits. When a provider/supplier is unable to obtain the signature of the beneficiary, or that of his or her representative, at the time of transport, it may obtain this signature any time prior to submitting the claim to Medicare for payment. (Note: there is a 15 to 27 month period for filing a Medicare claim, depending upon the date of service.)

If the beneficiary/representative refuses to authorize the submission of a claim, including a refusal to furnish an authorizing signature, then the ambulance provider/supplier may not bill Medicare, but may bill the beneficiary (or his or her estate) for the full charge of the ambulance items and services furnished. If, after seeing this bill, the beneficiary/representative decides to have Medicare pay for these items and services, then a beneficiary/representative signature is required and the ambulance provider/supplier must afford the beneficiary/representative this option within the claims filing period.

100-02 Chapter 11

130—Inpatient Hospital Dialysis

(Rev. 1, 10-01-03)

A3-3173, A3-3173.1, A3-3173.2

Dialysis services provided by any participating Medicare hospital are covered if the inpatient stay is medically necessary and the primary reason for the admission is not maintenance dialysis. Reimbursement for the maintenance dialysis is included in the PPS reimbursement for the DRG that represents care for the actual reason for admission.

In many cases, ESRD patients who require inpatient care are experiencing complications that affect the nature of the dialysis services. Payment for medically necessary inpatient dialysis is not subject to the composite rate.

A hospital may decide not to provide dialysis services directly to an inpatient. In this situation, the hospital must make arrangements with a certified ESRD facility to provide the dialysis services.

Inpatient dialysis services are also covered if an ESRD emergency occurs. However, when the emergency is over, outpatient maintenance dialysis must be performed in an ESRD certified facility or coverage will be denied. The intermediary should examine all claims for inpatient dialysis services, from hospitals that are not certified under the ESRD conditions for coverage, to ensure that one or more of these special situations exist.

130.1—Inpatient Dialysis in Nonparticipating Hospitals

(Rev. 1, 10-01-03)

A3-3173.3

Emergency inpatient dialysis services provided by a nonparticipating U.S. hospital are covered if the requirements in §130 above are met.

130.2—Extended Intermittent Peritoneal Dialysis

(Rev. 1, 10-01-03)

A3-3173.4

Extended intermittent peritoneal dialysis (EIPD) is performed once a week, usually for 30 hours or more, and is provided in the hospital due to the duration of treatment. Although the services are provided in the hospital, they are billed as outpatient maintenance dialysis services and reimbursed under Part B as long as the patient is not admitted as an inpatient for another reason. EIPD is an acceptable, but not optimal

mode of treatment, appropriate only when the patient cannot attend a facility two or three times a week, for geographic or other reasons, and is not suited for home dialysis. (See §30.1.)

130.3—Services Provided Under an Agreement

(Rev. 1, 10-01-03)

A3-3173.5

An approved ESRD facility may make a written **agreement** with a second facility under which the second facility furnishes certain covered outpatient dialysis items or services to patients. When services are provided under an agreement, the first facility is discharged from professional responsibility for the services furnished. The second facility is responsible for obtaining reimbursement directly from the Medicare program and the beneficiary, but may not bill the beneficiary for amounts in excess of the normal coinsurance and any applicable deductible.

130.4—Services Provided Under an Arrangement

(Rev. 1, 10-01-03)

A3-3173.6

An approved ESRD facility may make written **arrangements** with a second facility to provide certain covered outpatient dialysis items or services to patients. When services are provided under an arrangement, the first facility retains professional responsibility for those services and also for obtaining reimbursement for them. The first facility may bill the patient any applicable coinsurance and deductible amounts. The second facility is permitted to seek payment only from the first facility, and may not bill the patient or the Medicare program.

130.5—Dialysis Services Provided Under Arrangements to Hospital Inpatients

(Rev. 1, 10-01-03)

A3-3173.7

Any nonphysician service provided to a hospital inpatient must either be provided directly by the hospital or be arranged for by the hospital. (See the Medicare Claims Processing Manual, Chapter 1, "General Billing Requirements.") Therefore, a hospital may not contract an agreement as described in §130.3 above, for care (except for physician's care) provided to its inpatients.

100-02 Chapter 15

20.1 - Physician Expense for Surgery, Childbirth, and Treatment for Infertility

(Rev. 1, 10-01-03)

B3-2005.L

A. Surgery and Childbirth

Skilled medical management is covered throughout the events of pregnancy, beginning with diagnosis, continuing through delivery and ending after the necessary postnatal care. Similarly, in the event of termination of pregnancy, regardless of whether terminated spontaneously or for therapeutic reasons (i.e., where the life of the mother would be endangered if the fetus were brought to term), the need for skilled medical management and/or medical services is equally important as in those cases carried to full term. After the infant is delivered and is a separate individual, items and services furnished to the infant are not covered on the basis of the mother's eligibility.

Most surgeons and obstetricians bill patients an all-inclusive package charge intended to cover all services associated with the surgical procedure or delivery of the child. All expenses for surgical and obstetrical care, including preoperative/prenatal examinations and tests and post-operative/postnatal services, are considered incurred on the date of surgery or delivery, as appropriate. This policy applies whether the physician bills on a package charge basis, or itemizes the bill separately for these items.

Occasionally, a physician's bill may include charges for additional services not directly related to the surgical procedure or the delivery. Such charges are considered incurred on the date the additional services are furnished.

The above policy applies only where the charges are imposed by one physician or by a clinic on behalf of a group of physicians. Where more than one physician imposes charges for surgical or obstetrical services, all preoperative/prenatal and post-operative/postnatal services performed by the physician who performed the surgery or delivery are considered incurred on the date of the surgery or delivery. Expenses for services rendered by other physicians are considered incurred on the date they were performed.

B. Treatment for Infertility

Reasonable and necessary services associated with treatment for infertility are covered under Medicare. Infertility is a condition sufficiently at variance with the usual state of health to make it appropriate for a person who normally is expected to be fertile to seek medical consultation and treatment.

50—Drugs and Biologicals

(Rev. 1, 10-01-03)

B3-2049, A3-3112.4.B, HO-230.4.B

The Medicare program provides limited benefits for outpatient drugs. The program covers drugs that are furnished "incident to" a physician's service provided that the drugs are not usually self-administered by the patients who take them.

Generally, drugs and biologicals are covered only if all of the following requirements are met:

- They meet the definition of drugs or biologicals (see §50.1);
- They are of the type that are not usually self-administered (see §50.2);
- They meet all the general requirements for coverage of items as incident to a physician's services (see §§50.1 and 50.3);
- They are reasonable and necessary for the diagnosis or treatment of the illness or injury for which they are administered according to accepted standards of medical practice (see §50.4);

- They are not excluded as noncovered immunizations (see §50.4.4.2); and
- They have not been determined by the FDA to be less than effective. (See §§50.4.4).

Medicare Part B does generally not cover drugs that can be self-administered, such as those in pill form, or are used for self-injection. However, the statute provides for the coverage of some self-administered drugs. Examples of self-administered drugs that are covered include blood-clotting factors, drugs used in immunosuppressive therapy, erythropoietin for dialysis patients, osteoporosis drugs for certain homebound patients, and certain oral cancer drugs. (See §110.3 for coverage of drugs, which are necessary to the effective use of Durable Medical Equipment (DME) or prosthetic devices.)

50.1—Definition of Drug or Biological

(Rev. 1, 10-01-03)

B3-2049.1

Drugs and biologicals must be determined to meet the statutory definition. Under the statute §1861(t)(1), payment may be made for a drug or biological only where it is included, or approved for inclusion, in the latest official edition of the United States Pharmacopoeia National Formulary (USP-NF), the United States Pharmacopoeia-Drug Information (USD-DI), or the American Dental Association (AOA) Guide to Dental Therapeutics, except for those drugs and biologicals unfavorably evaluated in the ADA Guide to Dental Therapeutics. The inclusion of an item in the USP DI does not necessarily mean that the item is a drug or biological. The USP DI is a database of drug information developed by the U.S. Pharmacopoeia but maintained by Micromedex, which contains medically accepted uses for generic and brand name drug products. Inclusion in such reference (or approval by a hospital committee) is a necessary condition for a product to be considered a drug or biological under the Medicare program, however, it is not enough. Rather, the product must also meet all other program requirements to be determined to be a drug or biological. Combination drugs are also included in the definition of drugs if the combination itself or all of the therapeutic ingredients of the combination are included, or approved for inclusion, in any of the above drug compendia.

Drugs and biologicals are considered approved for inclusion in a compendium if approved under the established procedure by the professional organization responsible for revision of the compendium.

50.2—Determining Self-Administration of Drug or Biological

(Rev. 1, 10-01-03)

AB-02-072, AB-02-139, B3-2049.2

The Medicare program provides limited benefits for outpatient prescription drugs. The program covers drugs that are furnished "incident to" a physician's service provided that the drugs are not usually self-administered by the patients who take them. Section 112 of the Benefits, Improvements & Protection Act of 2000 (BIPA) amended sections 1861(s)(2)(A) and 1861(s)(2)(B) of the Act to redefine this exclusion. The prior statutory language referred to those drugs "which cannot be self-administered." Implementation of the BIPA provision requires interpretation of the phrase "not usually self-administered by the patient".

A—Policy

Fiscal intermediaries and carriers are instructed to follow the instructions below when applying the exclusion for drugs that are usually self-administered by the patient. Each individual contractor must make its own individual determination on each drug. Contractors must continue to apply the policy that not only the drug is medically reasonable and necessary for any individual claim, but also that the route of administration is medically reasonable and necessary. That is, if a drug is available in both oral and injectable forms, the injectable form of the drug must be medically reasonable and necessary as compared to using the oral form.

For certain injectable drugs, it will be apparent due to the nature of the condition(s) for which they are administered or the usual course of treatment for those conditions, they are, or are not, usually self-administered. For example, an injectable drug used to treat migraine headaches is usually self-administered. On the other hand, an injectable drug, administered at the same time as chemotherapy, used to treat anemia secondary to chemotherapy is not usually self-administered.

B—Administered

The term "administered" refers only to the physical process by which the drug enters the patient's body. It does not refer to whether the process is supervised by a medical professional (for example, to observe proper technique or side-effects of the drug). Only injectable (including intravenous) drugs are eligible for inclusion under the "incident to" benefit. Other routes of administration including, but not limited to, oral drugs, suppositories, topical medications are all considered to be usually self-administered by the patient.

C—Usually

For the purposes of applying this exclusion, the term "usually" means more than 50 percent of the time for all Medicare beneficiaries who use the drug. Therefore, if a drug is self-administered by more than 50 percent of Medicare beneficiaries, the drug is excluded from coverage and the contractor may not make any Medicare payment for it. In arriving at a single determination as to whether a drug is usually self-administered, contractors should make a separate determination for each indication for a drug as to whether that drug is usually self-administered.

After determining whether a drug is usually self-administered for each indication, contractors should determine the relative contribution of each indication to total use of the drug (i.e., weighted average) in order to make an overall determination as to whether the drug is usually self-administered. For example, if a drug has three indications, is not self-administered for the first indication, but is self administered for the second and third indications, and the first indication makes up 40 percent of total usage, the second indication makes up 30 percent of total usage, and the third indication makes up 30 percent of total usage, then the drug would be considered usually self-administered.

Reliable statistical information on the extent of self-administration by the patient may not always be available. Consequently, CMS offers the following guidance for each contractor's consideration in making this determination in the absence of such data:

1. Absent evidence to the contrary, presume that drugs delivered intravenously are not usually self-administered by the patient.
2. Absent evidence to the contrary, presume that drugs delivered by intramuscular injection are not usually self-administered by the patient. (Avonex, for example, is delivered by intramuscular injection, not usually self-administered by the patient.) The contractor may consider the depth and nature of the particular intramuscular injection in applying this presumption. In applying this presumption, contractors should examine the use of the particular drug and consider the following factors:
3. Absent evidence to the contrary, presume that drugs delivered by subcutaneous injection are self-administered by the patient. However, contractors should examine the use of the particular drug and consider the following factors:
   A. **Acute Condition**—Is the condition for which the drug is used an acute condition? If so, it is less likely that a patient would self-administer the drug. If the condition were longer term, it would be more likely that the patient would self-administer the drug.
   B. **Frequency of Administration**—How often is the injection given? For example, if the drug is administered once per month, it is less likely to be self-administered by the patient. However, if it is administered once or more per week, it is likely that the drug is self-administered by the patient.

In some instances, carriers may have provided payment for one or perhaps several doses of a drug that would otherwise not be paid for because the drug is usually self-administered. Carriers may have exercised this discretion for limited coverage, for example, during a brief time when the patient is being trained under the supervision of a physician in the proper technique for self-administration. Medicare will no longer pay for such doses. In addition, contractors may no longer pay for any drug when it is administered on an outpatient emergency basis, if the drug is excluded because it is usually self-administered by the patient.

D—Definition of Acute Condition

For the purposes of determining whether a drug is usually self-administered, an acute condition means a condition that begins over a short time period, is likely to be of short duration and/or the expected course of treatment is for a short, finite interval. A course of treatment consisting of scheduled injections lasting less than two weeks, regardless of frequency or route of administration, is considered acute. Evidence to support this may include Food and Drug administration (FDA) approval language, package inserts, drug compendia, and other information.

E—By the Patient

The term "by the patient" means Medicare beneficiaries as a collective whole. The carrier includes only the patients themselves and not other individuals (that is, spouses, friends, or other care-givers are not considered the patient). The determination is based on whether the drug is self-administered by the patient a majority of the time that the drug is used on an outpatient basis by Medicare beneficiaries for medically necessary indications. The carrier ignores all instances when the drug is administered on an inpatient basis.

The carrier makes this determination on a drug-by-drug basis, not on a beneficiary-by-beneficiary basis. In evaluating whether beneficiaries as a collective whole self-administer, individual beneficiaries who do not have the capacity to self-administer any drug due to a condition other than the condition for which they are taking the drug in question are not considered. For example, an individual afflicted with paraplegia or advanced dementia would not have the capacity to self-administer any injectable drug, so such individuals would not be included in the population upon which the determination for self-administration by the patient was based. Note that some individuals afflicted with a less severe stage of an otherwise debilitating condition would be included in the population upon which the determination for "self-administered by the patient" was based; for example, an early onset of dementia.

F—Evidentiary Criteria

Contractors are only required to consider the following types of evidence: peer reviewed medical literature, standards of medical practice, evidence-based practice guidelines, FDA approved label, and package inserts. Contractors may also consider other evidence submitted by interested individuals or groups subject to their judgment.

Contractors should also use these evidentiary criteria when reviewing requests for making a determination as to whether a drug is usually self-administered, and requests for reconsideration of a pending or published determination.

Please note that prior to the August 1, 2002, one of the principal factors used to determine whether a drug was subject to the self-administered exclusion was whether the FDA label contained instructions for self-administration. However, CMS notes that under the new standard, the fact that the FDA label includes instructions for self-administration is not, by itself, a determining factor that a drug is subject to this exclusion.

G—Provider Notice of Noncovered Drugs

Contractors must describe on their Web site the process they will use to determine whether a drug is usually self-administered and thus does not meet the "incident to" benefit category. Contractors must publish a list of the injectable drugs that are subject to the self-administered exclusion on their Web site, including the data and rationale that led to the determination. Contractors will report the workload associated with developing new coverage statements in CAFM 21208.

Contractors must provide notice 45 days prior to the date that these drugs will not be covered. During the 45-day time period, contractors will maintain existing medical review and payment procedures. After the 45-day notice, contractors may deny payment for the drugs subject to the notice.

Contractors must not develop local medical review policies (LMRPs) for this purpose because further elaboration to describe drugs that do not meet the 'incident to' and the 'not usually self-administered' provisions of the statute are unnecessary. Current LMRPs based solely on these provisions must be withdrawn. LMRPs that address the self-administered exclusion and other information may be reissued absent the self-administered drug exclusion material. Contractors will report this workload in CAFM 21206. However, contractors may continue to use and write LMRPs to describe reasonable and necessary uses of drugs that are not usually self-administered.

H—Conferences Between Contractors

Contractors' Medical Directors may meet and discuss whether a drug is usually self-administered without reaching a formal consensus. Each contractor uses its discretion as to whether or not it will participate in such discussions. Each contractor must make its own individual determinations, except that fiscal intermediaries may, at their discretion, follow the determinations of the local carrier with respect to the self-administered exclusion.

I—Beneficiary Appeals

If a beneficiary's claim for a particular drug is denied because the drug is subject to the "self-administered drug" exclusion, the beneficiary may appeal the denial. Because it is a "benefit category" denial and not a denial based on medical necessity, an Advance Beneficiary Notice (ABN) is not required. A "benefit category" denial (i.e., a denial based on the fact that there is no benefit category under which the drug may be covered) does not trigger the financial liability protection provisions of Limitation On Liability (under §1879 of the Act). Therefore, physicians or providers may charge the beneficiary for an excluded drug.

J—Provider and Physician Appeals

A physician accepting assignment may appeal a denial under the provisions found in Chapter 29 of the Medicare Claims Processing Manual.

K—Reasonable and Necessary

Carriers and fiscal intermediaries will make the determination of reasonable and necessary with respect to the medical appropriateness of a drug to treat the patient's condition. Contractors will continue to make the determination of whether the intravenous or injection form of a drug is appropriate as opposed to the oral form. Contractors will also continue to make the determination as to whether a physician's office visit was reasonable and necessary. However, contractors should not make a determination of whether it was reasonable and necessary for the patient to choose to have his or her drug administered in the physician's office or outpatient hospital setting. That is, while a physician's office visit may not be reasonable and necessary in a specific situation, in such a case an injection service would be payable.

L—Reporting Requirements

Each carrier and intermediary must report to CMS, every September 1 and March 1, its complete list of injectable drugs that the contractor has determined are excluded when furnished incident to a physician's service on the basis that the drug is usually self-administered. The CMS anticipates that contractors will review injectable drugs on a rolling basis and publish their list of excluded drugs as it is developed. For example, contractors should not wait to publish this list until every drug has been reviewed. Contractors must send their exclusion list to the following e-mail address: drugdata@cms.hhs.gov a template that CMS will provide separately, consisting of the following data elements in order:

1. Carrier Name
2. State
3. Carrier ID#
4. HCPCS

5. Descriptor
6. Effective Date of Exclusion
7. End Date of Exclusion
8. Comments

Any exclusion list not provided in the CMS mandated format will be returned for correction.

To view the presently mandated CMS format for this report, open the file located at:

http://cms.hhs.gov/manuals/pm_trans/AB02_139a.zip

50.3—Incident-to Requirements

(Rev. 1, 10-01-03)

B3-2049.3

In order to meet all the general requirements for coverage under the incident-to provision, an FDA approved drug or biological must:

- Be of a form that is not usually self-administered;
- Must be furnished by a physician; and
- Must be administered by the physician, or by auxiliary personnel employed by the physician and under the physician's personal supervision.

The charge, if any, for the drug or biological must be included in the physician's bill, and the cost of the drug or biological must represent an expense to the physician. Drugs and biologicals furnished by other health professionals may also meet these requirements. (See §§170, 180, 190 and 200 for specific instructions.)

Whole blood is a biological, which cannot be self-administered and is covered when furnished incident to a physician's services. Payment may also be made for blood fractions if all coverage requirements are satisfied and the blood deductible has been met.

50.4—Reasonableness and Necessity

(Rev. 1, 10-01-03)

B3-2049.4

50.4.1—Approved Use of Drug

(Rev. 1, 10-01-03)

B3-2049.4

Use of the drug or biological must be safe and effective and otherwise reasonable and necessary. (See the Medicare Benefit Policy Manual, Chapter 16, "General Exclusions from Coverage," §20.) Drugs or biologicals approved for marketing by the Food and Drug Administration (FDA) are considered safe and effective for purposes of this requirement when used for indications specified on the labeling. Therefore, the program may pay for the use of an FDA approved drug or biological, if:

- It was injected on or after the date of the FDA's approval;
- It is reasonable and necessary for the individual patient; and
- All other applicable coverage requirements are met.

The carrier, DMERC, or intermediary will deny coverage for drugs and biologicals which have not received final marketing approval by the FDA unless it receives instructions from CMS to the contrary. For specific guidelines on coverage of Group C cancer drugs, see the Medicare National Coverage Determinations Manual.

If there is reason to question whether the FDA has approved a drug or biological for marketing, the carrier or intermediary must obtain satisfactory evidence of FDA's approval. Acceptable evidence includes:

- A copy of the FDA's letter to the drug's manufacturer approving the new drug application (NDA);
- A listing of the drug or biological in the FDA's "Approved Drug Products" or "FDA Drug and Device Product Approvals";
- A copy of the manufacturer's package insert, approved by the FDA as part of the labeling of the drug, containing its recommended uses and dosage, as well as possible adverse reactions and recommended precautions in using it; or
- Information from the FDA's Web site.

When necessary, the Regional Office (RO) may be able to help in obtaining information.

50.4.2—Unlabeled Use of Drug

(Rev. 1, 10-01-03)

B3-2049.3

An unlabeled use of a drug is a use that is not included as an indication on the drug's label as approved by the FDA. FDA approved drugs used for indications other than what is indicated on the official label may be covered under Medicare if the carrier determines the use to be medically accepted, taking into consideration the major drug compendia, authoritative medical literature and/or accepted standards of medical practice. In the case of drugs used in an anti-cancer chemotherapeutic regimen, unlabeled uses are covered for a medically accepted indication as defined in §50.5.

These decisions are made by the contractor on a case-by-case basis.

50.4.3—Examples of Not Reasonable and Necessary

(Rev. 1, 10-01-03)

B3-2049.4

Determinations as to whether medication is reasonable and necessary for an individual patient should be made on the same basis as all other such determinations (i.e., with the advice of medical consultants and with reference to accepted standards of medical practice and the medical circumstances of the individual case). The following guidelines identify three categories with specific examples of situations in which medications would not be reasonable and necessary according to accepted standards of medical practice:

1—Not for Particular Illness

Medications given for a purpose other than the treatment of a particular condition, illness, or injury are not covered (except for certain immunizations). Charges for medications, e.g., vitamins, given simply for the general good and welfare of the patient and not as accepted therapies for a particular illness are excluded from coverage.

2—Injection Method Not Indicated

Medication given by injection (parenterally) is not covered if standard medical practice indicates that the administration of the medication by mouth (orally) is effective and is an accepted or preferred method of administration. For example, the accepted standard of medical practice for the treatment of certain diseases is to initiate therapy with parenteral penicillin and to complete therapy with oral penicillin. Carriers exclude the entire charge for penicillin injections given after the initiation of therapy if oral penicillin is indicated unless there are special medical circumstances that justify additional injections.

3—Excessive Medications

Medications administered for treatment of a disease and which exceed the frequency or duration of injections indicated by accepted standards of medical practice are not covered. For example, the accepted standard of medical practice in the maintenance treatment of pernicious anemia is one vitamin B-12 injection per month. Carriers exclude the entire charge for injections given in excess of this frequency unless there are special medical circumstances that justify additional injections.

Carriers will supplement the guidelines as necessary with guidelines concerning appropriate use of specific injections in other situations. They will use the guidelines to screen out questionable cases for special review, further development, or denial when the injection billed for would not be reasonable and necessary. They will coordinate any type of drug treatment review with the Quality Improvement Organization (QIO).

If a medication is determined not to be reasonable and necessary for diagnosis or treatment of an illness or injury according to these guidelines, the carrier excludes the entire charge (i.e., for both the drug and its administration). Also, carriers exclude from payment any charges for other services (such as office visits) which were primarily for the purpose of administering a noncovered injection (i.e., an injection that is not reasonable and necessary for the diagnosis or treatment of an illness or injury).

50.4.4—Payment for Antigens and Immunizations

(Rev. 1, 10-01-03)

50.4.4.1—Antigens

(Rev. 1, 10-01-03)

B3-2049.4

Payment may be made for a reasonable supply of antigens that have been prepared for a particular patient if: (1) the antigens are prepared by a physician who is a doctor of medicine or osteopathy, and (2) the physician who prepared the antigens has examined the patient and has determined a plan of treatment and a dosage regimen.

Antigens must be administered in accordance with the plan of treatment and by a doctor of medicine or osteopathy or by a properly instructed person (who could be the patient) under the supervision of the doctor. The associations of allergists that CMS consulted advised that a reasonable supply of antigens is considered to be not more than a 12-month supply of antigens that has been prepared for a particular patient at any one time. The purpose of the reasonable supply limita-

tion is to assure that the antigens retain their potency and effectiveness over the period in which they are to be administered to the patient. (See §§20.2 and 50.2.)

50.4.4.2—Immunizations

(Rev. 1, 10-01-03)

A3-3157.A, B3-2049.4, HO-230.4.C

Vaccinations or inoculations are excluded as immunizations unless they are directly related to the treatment of an injury or direct exposure to a disease or condition, such as antirabies treatment, tetanus antitoxin or booster vaccine, botulin antitoxin, anti-venin sera, or immune globulin. In the absence of injury or direct exposure, preventive immunization (vaccination or inoculation) against such diseases as smallpox, polio, diphtheria, etc., is not covered. However, pneumococcal, hepatitis B, and influenza virus vaccines are exceptions to this rule. (See items A, B, and C below.) In cases where a vaccination or inoculation is excluded from coverage, related charges are also not covered.

A—Pneumococcal Pneumonia Vaccinations

Effective for services furnished on or after May 1, 1981, the Medicare Part B program covers pneumococcal pneumonia vaccine and its administration when furnished in compliance with any applicable State law by any provider of services or any entity or individual with a supplier number. This includes revaccination of patients at highest risk of pneumococcal infection. Typically, these vaccines are administered once in a lifetime except for persons at highest risk. Effective July 1, 2000, Medicare does not require for coverage purposes that a doctor of medicine or osteopathy order the vaccine. Therefore, the beneficiary may receive the vaccine upon request without a physician's order and without physician supervision.

An initial vaccine may be administered only to persons at high risk (see below) of pneumococcal disease. Revaccination may be administered only to persons at highest risk of serious pneumococcal infection and those likely to have a rapid decline in pneumococcal antibody levels, provided that at least five years have passed since the previous dose of pneumococcal vaccine.

Persons at high risk for whom an initial vaccine may be administered include all people age 65 and older; immunocompetent adults who are at increased risk of pneumococcal disease or its complications because of chronic illness (e.g., cardiovascular disease, pulmonary disease, diabetes mellitus, alcoholism, cirrhosis, or cerebrospinal fluid leaks); and individuals with compromised immune systems (e.g., splenic dysfunction or anatomic asplenia, Hodgkin's disease, lymphoma, multiple myeloma, chronic renal failure, HIV infection, nephrotic syndrome, sickle cell disease, or organ transplantation).

Persons at highest risk and those most likely to have rapid declines in antibody levels are those for whom revaccination may be appropriate. This group includes persons with functional or anatomic asplenia (e.g., sickle cell disease, splenectomy), HIV infection, leukemia, lymphoma, Hodgkin's disease, multiple myeloma, generalized malignancy, chronic renal failure, nephrotic syndrome, or other conditions associated with immunosuppression such as organ or bone marrow transplantation, and those receiving immunosuppressive chemotherapy. It is not appropriate for routine revaccination of people age 65 or older that are not at highest risk.

Those administering the vaccine should not require the patient to present an immunization record prior to administering the pneumococcal vaccine, nor should they feel compelled to review the patient's complete medical record if it is not available. Instead, provided that the patient is competent, it is acceptable to rely on the patient's verbal history to determine prior vaccination status. If the patient is uncertain about his or her vaccination history in the past five years, the vaccine should be given. However, if the patient is certain he/she was were vaccinated in the last five years, the vaccine should not be given. If the patient is certain that the vaccine was given more than five years ago, revaccination is covered only if the patient is at high risk.

B—Hepatitis B Vaccine

Effective for services furnished on or after September 1, 1984, P.L. 98-369 provides coverage under Part B for hepatitis B vaccine and its administration, furnished to a Medicare beneficiary who is at high or intermediate risk of contracting hepatitis B. This coverage is effective for services furnished on or after September 1, 1984. High-risk groups currently identified include (see exception below):

* ESRD patients;
* Hemophiliacs who receive Factor VIII or IX concentrates;
* Clients of institutions for the mentally retarded;
* Persons who live in the same household as an Hepatitis B Virus (HBV) carrier;
* Homosexual men; and
* Illicit injectable drug abusers.

Intermediate risk groups currently identified include:

* Staff in institutions for the mentally retarded; and
* Workers in health care professions who have frequent contact with blood or blood-derived body fluids during routine work.

EXCEPTION: Persons in both of the above-listed groups in paragraph B, would not be considered at high or intermediate risk of contracting hepatitis B, however, if there were laboratory evidence positive for antibodies to hepatitis B. (ESRD patients are routinely tested for hepatitis B antibodies as part of their continuing monitoring and therapy.)

For Medicare program purposes, the vaccine may be administered upon the order of a doctor of medicine or osteopathy, by a doctor of medicine or osteopathy, or by home health agencies, skilled nursing facilities, ESRD facilities, hospital outpatient departments, and persons recognized under the incident to physicians' services provision of law.

A charge separate from the ESRD composite rate will be recognized and paid for administration of the vaccine to ESRD patients.

C—Influenza Virus Vaccine

Effective for services furnished on or after May 1, 1993, the Medicare Part B program covers influenza virus vaccine and its administration when furnished in compliance with any applicable State law by any provider of services or any entity or individual with a supplier number. Typically, these vaccines are administered once a year in the fall or winter. Medicare does not require, for coverage purposes, that a doctor of medicine or osteopathy order the vaccine. Therefore, the beneficiary may receive the vaccine upon request without a physician's order and without physician supervision.

50.4.5—Unlabeled Use for Anti-Cancer Drugs

(Rev. 78, Issued: 09-21-07, Effective: 10-22-07, Implementation: 10-22-07)

Effective January 1, 1994, unlabeled uses of FDA approved drugs and biologicals used in an anti-cancer chemotherapeutic regimen for a medically accepted indication are evaluated under the conditions described in this paragraph. A regimen is a combination of anti-cancer agents which has been clinically recognized for the treatment of a specific type of cancer. An example of a drug regimen is: Cyclophosphamide + vincristine + prednisone (CVP) for non-Hodgkin's lymphoma.

In addition to listing the combination of drugs for a type of cancer, there may be a different regimen or combinations which are used at different times in the history of the cancer (induction, prophylaxis of CNS involvement, post remission, and relapsed or refractory disease). A protocol may specify the combination of drugs, doses, and schedules for administration of the drugs. For purposes of this provision, a cancer treatment regimen includes drugs used to treat toxicities or side effects of the cancer treatment regimen when the drug is administered incident to a chemotherapy treatment.

Do deny coverage based solely on the absence of FDA-approved labeling for the use, if the use is supported by one of the following and the use is **not** listed as "not indicated" in any of the three compendia. (See note at the end of this subsection.)

A—American Hospital Formulary Service Drug Information

Drug monographs are arranged in alphabetical order within therapeutic classifications. Within the text of the monograph, information concerning indications is provided; including both labeled and unlabeled uses. Unlabeled uses are identified with daggers. The text must be analyzed to make a determination whether a particular use is supported.

B—American Medical Association (AMA) Drug Evaluations

Drug evaluations are organized into sections and Chapters that are based on therapeutic classifications. The evaluation of a drug provides information concerning indications, including both labeled and unlabeled uses. Unlabeled uses are not specifically identified as such. The text must be analyzed to make a determination whether a particular use is supported. In making these determinations, also refer to the "AMA Drug Evaluations Subscription," Volume III, section 17 (Oncolytic Drugs), Chapter 1 (Principles of Cancer Chemotherapy), tables 1 and 2.

Table 1, Specific Agents Used In Cancer Chemotherapy, lists the antineoplastic agents which are currently available for use in various cancers. The indications presented in this table for a particular anticancer drug include labeled and unlabeled uses (although they are not identified as such). Any indication appearing in this table is considered to be a medically accepted use.

Table 2, Clinical Responses To Chemotherapy, lists some of the currently preferred regimens for various cancers. The table headings include (1) type of cancer, (2) drugs or regimens currently preferred, (3) alternative or secondary drugs or regimens, and (4) other drugs or regimens with reported activity.

A regimen appearing under the preferred or alternative/secondary headings is considered to be a medically ac cepted use.

A regimen appearing under the heading "Other Drugs or Regimens With Reported Activity" is considered to be for a medically accepted use provided:

- The preferred and alternative/secondary drugs or regimens are contraindicated;
- A preferred and/or alternative/secondary drug or regimen was used but was not tolerated or was ineffective; or
- There was tumor progression or recurrence after an initial response.

C—United States Pharmacopoeia Drug Information (USPDI)

Monographs are arranged in alphabetic order by generic or family name. Indications for use appear as accepted, unaccepted, or insufficient data. An indication is considered to be a medically accepted use only if the indication is listed as accepted. Unlabeled uses are identified with brackets. A separate indications index lists all indications included in USPDI along with the medically accepted drugs used in treatment or diagnosis.

D—A Use Supported by Clinical Research That Appears in Peer Reviewed Medical Literature

This applies only when an unlabeled use does not appear in any of the compendia or is listed as insufficient data or investigational. If an unlabeled use of a drug meets these criteria, the carrier will contact the compendia to see if a report regarding this use is forthcoming. If a report is forthcoming, the carrier uses this information as a basis for making decisions. The compendium process for making decisions concerning unlabeled uses is very thorough and continuously updated. Peer reviewed medical literature includes scientific, medical, and pharmaceutical publications in which original manuscripts are published, only after having been critically reviewed for scientific accuracy, validity, and reliability by unbiased independent experts. This does not include in-house publications of pharmaceutical manufacturing companies or abstracts (including meeting abstracts).

In determining whether there is supportive clinical evidence for a particular use of a drug, carrier medical staff (in consultation with local medical specialty groups) will evaluate the quality of the evidence in published peer reviewed medical literature. When evaluating this literature, they will consider (among other things) the following:

- The prevalence and life history of the disease when evaluating the adequacy of the number of subjects and the response rate. While a 20 percent response rate may be adequate for highly prevalent disease states, a lower rate may be adequate for rare diseases or highly unresponsive conditions.
- The effect on the patient's well-being and other responses to therapy that indicate effectiveness, e.g., a significant increase in survival rate or life expectancy or an objective and significant decrease in the size of the tumor or a reduction in symptoms related to the tumor. Stabilization is not considered a response to therapy.

- The appropriateness of the study design. The carrier will consider:
  1. Whether the experimental design in light of the drugs and conditions under investigation is appropriate to address the investigative question. (For example, in some clinical studies, it may be unnecessary or not feasible to use randomization, double blind trials, placebos, or crossover.);
  2. That nonrandomized clinical trials with a significant number of subjects may be a basis for supportive clinical evidence for determining accepted uses of drugs; and
  3. That case reports are generally considered uncontrolled and anecdotal information and do not provide adequate supportive clinical evidence for determining accepted uses of drugs.

The carrier will use peer-reviewed medical literature appearing in the regular editions of the following publications, not to include supplement editions privately funded by parties with a vested interest in the recommendations of the authors.

- American Journal of Medicine;
- Annals of Internal Medicine;
- Annals of Oncology;
- Annals of Surgical Oncology;
- Biology of Blood and Marrow Transplantation;
- Blood;
- Bone Marrow Transplantation;
- British Journal of Cancer;
- British Journal of Hematology;
- British Medical Journal;
- Cancer;
- Clinical Cancer Research;
- Drugs;
- European Journal of Cancer (formerly the European Journal of Cancer and Clinical Oncology);
- Gynecologic Oncology;
- International Journal of Radiation, Oncology, Biology, and Physics;
- The Journal of the American Medical Association;
- Journal of Clinical Oncology;
- Journal of the National Cancer Institute;
- Journal of the National Comprehensive Cancer Network (NCCN);
- Journal of Urology;
- Lancet;
- Lancet Oncology;
- Leukemia;
- The New England Journal of Medicine; or
- Radiation Oncology

The carrier is not required to maintain copies of these publications. If a claim raises a question about the use of a drug for a purpose not included in the FDA approved labeling or the compendia, the carrier will ask the physician to submit copies of relevant supporting literature.

Unlabeled uses may also be considered medically accepted if determined by the carrier to be medically accepted generally as safe and effective for the particular use.

NOTE: If a use is identified as not indicated by CMS or the FDA, or if a use is specifically identified as not indicated in one or more of the three compendia mentioned or if the carrier determines, based on peer reviewed medical literature, that a particular use of a drug is not safe and effective, the off-label usage is not supported and, therefore, the drug is not covered.

50.4.5.1 - Process for Amending the List of Compendia for Determination of Medically-Accepted Indications for Off-Label Uses of Drugs and Biologicals in an Anti-Cancer Chemotherapeutic Regimen

(Rev. 81; Issued: 02-07-08; Effective: 01-01-08; Implementation: 03-07-08)

A. Background

A compendium is defined as a comprehensive listing of FDA-approved drugs and biologicals or a comprehensive listing of a specific subset of drugs and biologicals in a specialty compendium, for example, a compendium of anti-cancer treatment. It includes a summary of the pharmacologic characteristics of each drug or biological and may include information on dosage, as well as recommended or endorsed uses in specific diseases; is indexed by drug or biological; and differs from a disease treatment guideline, which is indexed by disease. The list of compendia is located on the CMS Web site at http://www.cms.hhs.gov/CoverageGenInfo/02_compendia.asp.

B. Desirable Characteristics of Compendia

Following are desirable characteristics of compendia to determine medically-accepted indications of drugs and biologicals in anti-cancer therapy:

- Extensive breadth of listings.
- Quick processing from application for inclusion to listing.
- Detailed description of the evidence reviewed for every individual listing.
- Use of pre-specified published criteria for weighing evidence.
- Use of prescribed published process for making recommendations.
- Publicly transparent process for evaluating therapies.
- Explicit "Not recommended" listing when validated evidence is appropriate.
- Explicit listing and recommendations regarding therapies, including sequential use or combination in relation to other therapies.
- Explicit "Equivocal" listing when validated evidence is equivocal.
- Process for public identification and notification of potential conflicts of interest of the compendia's parent and sibling organizations, reviewers, and committee members, with an established procedure to manage recognized conflicts.

C. Process for Changing List of Compendia

CMS will provide an annual 30-day open request period starting January 15th for the public to submit requests for additions or deletions to the compendia list contained on the CMS Web site at http://www.cms.hhs.gov/CoverageGenInfo/02_compendia.asp. Complete requests as defined in section 50.4.5.1.D will be posted to the Web site by March 15th for public notice and comment. The request will identify the requestor and the requested action to the list. Public comments will be accepted for a 30-day period beginning on the day the request is posted on the Web site.

In addition to the annual process, CMS may generate a request for changes to the list at any time an urgent action is needed to protect the interests of the Medicare program and its beneficiaries.

D. Content of Requests

For a request to be considered complete and therefore accepted for review, it must include the following information:

- The full name and contact information (including the mailing address, e-mail address, and telephone number) of the requestor. If the requestor is not an individual person, the information shall identify the officer or other representative who is authorized to act for the requestor on all matters related to the request.
- Full identification of the compendium that is the subject of the request, including name, publisher, edition if applicable, date of publication, and any other information needed for the accurate and precise identification of the specific compendium.
- A complete written copy of the compendium that is the subject of the request. If the complete compendium is available electronically, it may be submitted electronically in place of hard copy. If the compendium is available online, the requestor may provide CMS with electronic access by furnishing at no cost to the Federal government sufficient accounts for the purposes and duration of the review of the application in place of hard copy.
- The specific action that the requestor wishes CMS to take, for example to add or delete a specific compendium.
- Detailed, specific documentation that the compendium that is the subject of the request does or does not comply with the conditions of this rule. Broad, nonspecific claims without supporting documentation cannot be efficiently reviewed; therefore, they will not be accepted.

A request may have only a single compendium as its subject. This will provide greater clarity on the scope of the agency's review of a given request. A requestor may submit multiple requests, each requesting a different action.

E. Submission of Requests

Requests must be in writing and submitted in one of the following two ways (no duplicates please):

- Electronic requests are encouraged to facilitate administrative efficiency. Each solicitation will include the electronic address for submissions.
- Hard copy requests can be sent to:

> Centers for Medicare & Medicaid Services
> Coverage and Analysis Group
> Mailstop C1–09–06
> 7500 Security Boulevard
> Baltimore, MD, 21244

Allow sufficient time for hard copies to be received prior to the close of the open request period.

F. Review of Requests

CMS will consider a compendium's attainment of the desirable characteristics of compendia specified in 50.4.5.1.B when reviewing requests. CMS may consider additional reasonable factors in making a determination. (For example, CMS may consider factors that are likely to impact the compendium's suitability for this use, such as a change in ownership or affiliation, the standards applicable to the evidence considered by the compendium, and any relevant conflicts of interest. CMS may consider that broad accessibility by the general public to the information contained in the compendium may assist beneficiaries, their treating physicians or both in choosing among treatment options.) CMS will also consider a compendium's grading of evidence used in making recommendations regarding off-label uses and the process by which the compendium grades the evidence. CMS may, at its discretion, combine and consider multiple requests that refer to the same compendium, even if those requests are for different actions. This facilitates administrative efficiency in the review of requests.

G. Publishing Review Results

CMS will publish decisions on the CMS Web site within 90 days after the close of the public comment period.

50.4.6—Less Than Effective Drug

(Rev. 1, 10-01-03)

B3-2049.4.C.5

This is a drug that has been determined by the Food and Drug Administration (FDA) to lack substantial evidence of effectiveness for all labeled indications. Also, a drug that has been the subject of a Notice of an Opportunity for a Hearing (NOOH) published in the "Federal Register" before being withdrawn from the market, and for which the Secretary has not determined there is a compelling justification for its medical need, is considered less than effective. This includes any other drug product that is identical, similar, or related. Payment may not be made for a less than effective drug.

Because the FDA has not yet completed its identification of drug products that are still on the market, existing FDA efficacy decisions must be applied to all similar products once they are identified.

50.4.7—Denial of Medicare Payment for Compounded Drugs Produced in Violation of Federal Food, Drug, and Cosmetic Act

(Rev. 1, 10-01-03)

B3-2049.4.C.6

The Food and Drug Administration (FDA) has found that, from time to time, firms established as retail pharmacies engage in mass production of compounded drugs, beyond the normal scope of pharmaceutical practice, in violation of the Federal Food, Drug, and Cosmetic Act (FFDCA). By compounding drugs on a large scale, a company may be operating as a drug manufacturer within the meaning of the FFDCA, without complying with requirements of that law. Such companies may be manufacturing drugs which are subject to the new drug application (NDA) requirements of the FFDCA, but for which FDA has not approved an NDA or which are misbranded or adulterated. If the FDA has not approved the manufacturing and processing procedures used by these facilities, the FDA has no assurance that the drugs these companies are producing are safe and effective. The safety and effectiveness issues pertain to such factors as chemical stability, purity, strength, bioequivalency, and biovailability.

Section 1862(a)(1)(A) of the Act requires that drugs must be reasonable and necessary in order to by covered under Medicare. This means, in the case of drugs, the FDA must approve them for marketing. Section 50.4.1 instructs carriers and intermediaries to deny coverage for drugs that have not received final marketing approval by the FDA, unless instructed otherwise by CMS. The Medicare Benefit Policy Manual, Chapter 16, "General Exclusions from Coverage," §180, instructs carriers to deny coverage of services related to the use of noncovered drugs as well. Hence, if DME or a prosthetic device is used to administer a noncovered drug, coverage is denied for both the nonapproved drug and the DME or prosthetic device.

In those cases in which the FDA has determined that a company is producing compounded drugs in violation of the FFDCA, Medicare does not pay for the drugs because they do not meet the FDA approval requirements of the Medicare program. In addition, Medicare does not pay for the DME or prosthetic device used to administer such a drug if FDA determines that a required NDA has not been approved or that the drug is misbranded or adulterated.

The CMS will notify the carrier when the FDA has determined that compounded drugs are being produced in violation of the FFDCA. The carrier does not stop Medicare payment for such a drug unless it is notified that it is appropriate to do so through a subsequent instruction. In addition, if the carrier or Regional Offices (ROs) become aware that other companies are possibly operating in violation of the FFDCA, the carrier or RO notifies:

Centers for Medicare & Medicaid Services
Center for Medicare Management
7500 Security Blvd.
Baltimore, MD 21244-1850

50.4.8—Process for Amending the List of Compendia for Determination of Medically-Accepted Indications for Off-Label Uses of Drugs and Biologicals in an Anti-Cancer Chemotherapeutic Regimen

50.5—Self-Administered Drugs and Biologicals

(Rev. 1, 10-01-03)

B3-2049.5

Medicare Part B does not cover drugs that are usually self-administered by the patient unless the statute provides for such coverage. The statute explicitly provides coverage, for blood clotting factors, drugs used in immunosuppressive therapy, erythropoietin for dialysis patients, certain oral anti-cancer drugs and anti-emetics used in certain situations.

50.5.1—Immunosuppressive Drugs

(Rev. 1, 10-01-03)

A3-3112.4.B.3, HO-230.4.B.3, AB-01-10

Until January 1, 1995, immunosuppressive drugs were covered under Part B for a period of one year following discharge from a hospital for a Medicare covered organ transplant. The CMS interpreted the 1-year period after the date of the transplant procedure to mean 365 days from the day on which an inpatient is discharged from the hospital. Beneficiaries are eligible to receive additional Part B coverage **within** 18 months after the discharge date for drugs furnished in 1995; **within** 24 months for drugs furnished in 1996; **within** 30 months for drugs furnished in 1997; and **within** 36 months for drugs furnished after 1997.

For immunosuppressive drugs furnished on or after December 21, 2000, this time limit for coverage is eliminated.

Covered drugs include those immunosuppressive drugs that have been specifically labeled as such and approved for marketing by the FDA. (This is an exception to the standing drug policy which permits coverage of FDA approved drugs for **nonlabeled** uses, where such uses are found to be reasonable and necessary in an individual case.)

Covered drugs also include those prescription drugs, such as prednisone, that are used in conjunction with immunosuppressive drugs as part of a therapeutic regimen reflected in FDA approved labeling for immunosuppressive drugs. Therefore, antibiotics, hypertensives, and other drugs that are not directly related to rejection are not covered.

The FDA has identified and approved for marketing the following specifically labeled immunosuppressive drugs. They are:

Sandimmune (cyclosporine), Sandoz Pharmaceutical;
Imuran (azathioprine), Burroughs Wellcome;
Atgam (antithymocyte globulin), Upjohn;
Orthoclone OKT3 (Muromonab-CD3), Ortho Pharmaceutical;
Prograf (tacrolimus), Fujisawa USA, Inc;
Celicept (mycophenolate mefetil), Roche Laboratories;
Daclizumab (Zenapax);
Cyclophosphamide (Cytoxan);
Prednisone; and
Prednosolone.

The CMS expects contractors to keep informed of FDA additions to the list of the **immunosuppressive drugs.**

50.5.2—Erythropoietin (EPO)

(Rev. 1, 10-01-03)

A3-3112.4.B.4, HO-230.4.B.4

The statute provides that EPO is covered for the treatment of anemia for patients with chronic renal failure who are on dialysis. Coverage is available regardless of whether the drug is administered by the patient or the patient's caregiver. EPO is a biologically engineered protein which stimulates the bone marrow to make new red blood cells.

NOTE: Non-ESRD patients who are receiving EPO to treat anemia induced by other conditions such as chemotherapy or the drug zidovudine (commonly called AZT) must meet the coverage requirements in §50.

EPO is covered for the treatment of anemia for patients with chronic renal failure who are on dialysis when:

- It is administered in the renal dialysis facility; or
- It is self-administered in the home by any dialysis patient (or patient caregiver) who is determined competent to use the drug and meets the other conditions detailed below.

NOTE: Payment may not be made for EPO under the incident to provision when EPO is administered in the renal dialysis facility.

Also, in the office setting, reimbursement will be made for the administration charge only for non-ESRD patients receiving EPO.

50.5.2.1—Requirements for Medicare Coverage for EPO

(Rev. 1, 10-01-03)

B3-2049.5

Medicare covers EPO and items related to its administration for dialysis patients who use EPO in the home when the following conditions are met:

A—Patient Care Plan

A dialysis patient who uses EPO in the home must have a current care plan (a copy of which must be maintained by the designated backup facility for Method II patients) for monitoring home use of EPO that includes the following:

1. Review of diet and fluid intake for aberrations as indicated by hyperkalemia and elevated blood pressure secondary to volume overload;
2. Review of medications to ensure adequate provision of supplemental iron;
3. Ongoing evaluations of hematocrit and iron stores;
4. Reevaluation of the dialysis prescription taking into account the patient's increased appetite and red blood cell volume;
5. Method for physician and facility (including backup facility for Method II patients) follow-up on blood tests and a mechanism (such as a patient log) for keeping the physician informed of the results;
6. Training of the patient to identify the signs and symptoms of hypotension and hypertension; and
7. The decrease or discontinuance of EPO if hypertension is uncontrollable.

B—Patient Selection

The dialysis facility, or the physician responsible for all dialysis-related services furnished to the patient, must make a comprehensive assessment that includes the following:

1. **Preselection Monitoring**—The patient's hematocrit (or hemoglobin), serum iron, transferrin saturation, serum ferritin, and blood pressure must be measured.
2. **Conditions the Patient Must Meet**—The assessment must find that the patient meets the following conditions:
   a. Is a dialysis patient;
   b. Has a hematocrit (or comparable hemoglobin level) that is as follows:

   - For a patient who is initiating EPO treatment, no higher than 30 percent unless there is medical documentation showing the need for EPO despite a hematocrit (or comparable hemoglobin level) higher than 30 percent. Patients with severe angina, severe pulmonary distress, or severe hypotension may require EPO to prevent adverse symptoms even if they have higher hematocrit or hemoglobin levels.
   - For a patient who has been receiving EPO from the facility or the physician, between 30 and 36 percent.
   c. Is under the care of:
   - A physician who is responsible for all dialysis-related services and who prescribes the EPO and

follows the drug labeling instructions when monitoring the EPO home therapy; and

- A renal dialysis facility that establishes the plan of care and monitors the progress of the home EPO therapy.

3. **The assessment must find that the patient or a caregiver meets the following conditions:**
   - Is trained by the facility to inject EPO and is capable of carrying out the procedure;
   - Is capable of reading and understanding the drug labeling; and
   - Is trained in, and capable of observing, aseptic techniques.

4. **Care and Storage of Drug**—The assessment must find that EPO can be stored in the patient's residence under refrigeration and that the patient is aware of the potential hazard of a child's having access to the drug and syringes.

C—Responsibilities of Physician or Dialysis Facility

The patient's physician or dialysis facility must:

- Develop a protocol that follows the drug label instructions;
- Make the protocol available to the patient to ensure safe and effective home use of EPO;
- Through the amounts prescribed, ensure that the drug on hand at any time does not exceed a 2-month supply;
- Maintain adequate records to allow quality assurance for review by the Network and State Survey Agencies. For Method II patients, current records must be provided to and maintained by the designated backup facility; and
- The dialysis facility must submit claims for EPO, if the facility provides it.

See the Medicare Claims Processing Manual, Chapter 11, "End Stage Renal Disease," for instructions for billing and processing claims for EPO under Method 1 and Method 2. Note that hematocrit readings are required on claims. It is expected that the ESRD facility or hospital outpatient department will maintain the following information in each patient's medical record to permit the review of the medical necessity of EPO.

1. Diagnostic coding;
2. Most recent creatinine prior to initiation of EPO therapy;
3. Date of most recent creatinine prior to initiation of EPO therapy;
4. Most recent hematocrit (HCT) prior to initiation of EPO therapy;
5. Date of most recent hematocrit (HCT) prior to initiation of EPO therapy;
6. Dosage in units/kg;
7. Weight in kgs; and
8. Number of units administered.

50.5.2.2—Medicare Coverage of Epoetin Alfa (Procrit) for Preoperative Use

(Rev. 1, 10-01-03)

PM-AB-99-59, DATED 8/1/99

This instruction pertains exclusively to the preoperative surgical indication of the drug Procrit, in which it is administered to specific patients prior to surgery to reduce risk of transfusion. It does not affect Medicare policies related to

other Food and Drug Administration (FDA) approved uses of Procrit. **It is not a national coverage decision.**

Procrit as Preventive Service

The carrier may determine that Procrit is covered for individuals who:

1. Are undergoing hip or knee surgery
2. Have an anemia with a hemoglobin between 10 and 13 mg/dL;
3. Are not a candidate for autologous blood transfusion;
4. Are expected to lose more than 2 units of blood; and
5. Have had a workup so that their anemia appears to be that of chronic disease.

The preoperative use of Procrit may be afforded to these individuals when carriers, exercising their discretion, determine that this treatment is reasonable and necessary. In other cases, Procrit is considered a preventive service and therefore not covered.

50.5.3—Oral Anti-Cancer Drugs

(Rev. 1, 10-01-03)

A3-3112.4.B.5, HO-230.4.B.5

Effective January 1, 1994, Medicare Part B coverage is extended to include oral anti-cancer drugs that are prescribed as anti-cancer chemotherapeutic agents providing they have the same active ingredients and are used for the same indications as anti-cancer chemotherapeutic agents which would be covered if they were not self-administered and they were furnished incident to a physician's service as drugs and biologicals.

For an oral anti-cancer drug to be covered under Part B, it must:

- Be prescribed by a physician or other practitioner licensed under State law to prescribe such drugs as anti-cancer chemotherapeutic agents;
- Be a drug or biological that has been approved by the Food and Drug Administration (FDA);
- Have the same active ingredients as a non-self-administrable anti-cancer chemotherapeutic drug or biological that is covered when furnished incident to a physician's service. The oral anti-cancer drug and the non-self-administrable drug must have the same chemical/generic name as indicated by the FDA's "Approved Drug Products" (Orange Book), "Physician's Desk Reference" (PDR), or an authoritative drug compendium;
- Be used for the same indications, including unlabeled uses, as the non-self-administrable version of the drug; and
- Be reasonable and necessary for the individual patient.

50.5.4—Oral Anti-Nausea (Anti-Emetic) Drugs

(Rev. 1, 10-01-03)

PM AB-97-26

Effective January 1, 1998, Medicare also covers self-administered anti-emetics which are necessary for the administration and absorption of the anti-neoplastic chemotherapeutic agents when a high likelihood of vomiting exists. The anti-emetic drug is covered as a necessary means for administration of the antineoplastic chemotherapeutic agents. Oral drugs prescribed for use with the primary drug, which enhance the anti-neoplastic effect of the primary drug or permit the patient to tolerate the primary anti-neoplastic drug in higher doses for longer periods are not covered. Self-administered anti-emetics to reduce the side effects of nausea and vomiting brought on by the primary drug are not included beyond the administration necessary to achieve drug absorption.

Section 1861(s)(2) of the Act extends coverage to oral anti-emetic drugs that are used as full replacement for intravenous dosage forms of a cancer regimen under the following conditions:

- Coverage is provided only for oral drugs approved by the Food and Drug Administration (FDA) for use as anti-emetics;
- The oral anti-emetic must either be administered by the treating physician or in accordance with a written order from the physician as part of a cancer chemotherapy regimen;
- Oral anti-emetic drugs administered with a particular chemotherapy treatment must be initiated within two hours of the administration of the chemotherapeutic agent and may be continued for a period not to exceed 48 hours from that time;
- The oral anti-emetic drugs provided must be used as a full therapeutic replacement for the intravenous anti-emetic drugs that would have otherwise been administered at the time of the chemotherapy treatment.

Only drugs pursuant to a physician's order at the time of the chemotherapy treatment qualify for this benefit. The dispensed number of dosage units may not exceed a loading dose administered within two hours of the treatment, plus a supply of additional dosage units not to exceed 48 hours of therapy.

Oral drugs that are not approved by the FDA for use as anti-emetics and which are used by treating physicians adjunctively in a manner incidental to cancer chemotherapy are not covered by this benefit and are not reimbursable within the scope of this benefit.

It is recognized that a limited number of patients will fail on oral anti-emetic drugs. Intravenous anti-emetics may be covered (subject to the rules of medical necessity) when furnished to patients who fail on oral anti-emetic therapy.

More than one oral anti emetic drug may be prescribed and may be covered for concurrent use if needed to fully replace the intravenous drugs that otherwise would be given.

50.5.5—Hemophilia Clotting Factors

(Rev. 1, 10-01-03)

A3-3112.4.B.2, HO-230.4.B.2

Section 1861(s)(2)(I) of the Act provides Medicare coverage of blood clotting factors for hemophilia patients competent to use such factors to control bleeding without medical supervision, and items related to the administration of such factors. Hemophilia, a blood disorder characterized by prolonged coagulation time, is caused by deficiency of a factor in plasma necessary for blood to clot. For purposes of Medicare

Part B coverage, hemophilia encompasses the following conditions:

- Factor VIII deficiency (classic hemophilia);
- Factor IX deficiency (also termed plasma thromboplastin component (PTC) or Christmas factor deficiency); and
- Von Willebrand's disease.

Claims for blood clotting factors for hemophilia patients with these diagnoses may be covered if the patient is competent to use such factors without medical supervision.

The amount of clotting factors determined to be necessary to have on hand and thus covered under this provision is based on the historical utilization pattern or profile developed by the contractor for each patient. It is expected that the treating source, e.g., a family physician or comprehensive hemophilia diagnostic and treatment center, have such information. From this data, the contractor is able to anticipate and make reasonable projections concerning the quantity of clotting factors the patient will need over a specific period of time. Unanticipated occurrences involving extraordinary events, such as automobile accidents or inpatient hospital stays, will change this base line data and should be appropriately considered. In addition, changes in a patient's medical needs over a period of time require adjustments in the profile.

50.6 – Coverage of Intravenous Immune Globulin for Treatment of Primary Immune Deficiency Diseases in the Home

(Rev. 6, 01-23-04)

Beginning for dates of service on or after January 1, 2004, The Medicare Prescription Drug, Improvement, and Modernization Act of 2003 provides coverage of intravenous immune globulin (IVIG) for the treatment of primary immune deficiency diseases (ICD-9 diagnosis codes 279.04, 279.05, 279.06, 279.12, and 279.2) in the home. The corresponding HCPCS codes are J1563 and J1564. The Act defines "intravenous immune globulin" as an approved pooled plasma derivative for the treatment of primary immune deficiency disease. It is covered under this benefit when the patient has a diagnosed primary immune deficiency disease, it is administered in the home of a patient with a diagnosed primary immune deficiency disease, and the physician determines that administration of the derivative in the patient's home is medically appropriate. The benefit does not include coverage for items or services related to the administration of the derivative. For coverage of IVIG under this benefit, it is not necessary for the derivative to be administered through a piece of durable medical equipment.

80—Requirements for Diagnostic X-Ray, Diagnostic Laboratory, and Other Diagnostic Tests

(Rev. 51, Issued: 06-23-06, Effective: 01-01-05, Implemented: 09-21-06)

B3-2070

This section describes the levels of physician supervision required for furnishing the technical component of diagnostic tests for a Medicare beneficiary who is not a hospital inpatient or outpatient. Section 410.32(b) of the Code of Federal Regulations (CFR) requires that diagnostic tests covered under §1861(s)(3) of the Act (the Act) and payable under the physician fee schedule, with certain exceptions listed in the regulation, have to be performed under the supervision of an individual meeting the definition of a physician (§1861(r) of the Act) to be considered reasonable and necessary and, therefore, covered under Medicare. The regulation defines these levels of physician supervision for diagnostic tests as follows:

General Supervision—means the procedure is furnished under the physician's overall direction and control, but the physician's presence is not required during the performance of the procedure. Under general supervision, the training of the nonphysician personnel who actually performs the diagnostic procedure and the maintenance of the necessary equipment and supplies are the continuing responsibility of the physician.

Direct Supervision—in the office setting means the physician must be present in the office suite and immediately available to furnish assistance and direction throughout the performance of the procedure. It does not mean that the physician must be present in the room when the procedure is performed.

Personal Supervision—means a physician must be in attendance in the room during the performance of the procedure.

One of the following numerical levels is assigned to each CPT or HCPCS code in the Medicare Physician Fee Schedule Database:

0   Procedure is not a diagnostic test or procedure is a diagnostic test which is not subject to the physician supervision policy.

1   Procedure must be performed under the general supervision of a physician.

2   Procedure must be performed under the direct supervision of a physician.

3   Procedure must be performed under the personal supervision of a physician.

4   Physician supervision policy does not apply when procedure is furnished by a qualified, independent psychologist or a clinical psychologist or furnished under the general supervision of a clinical psychologist; otherwise must be performed under the general supervision of a physician.

5   Physician supervision policy does not apply when procedure is furnished by a qualified audiologist; otherwise must be performed under the general supervision of a physician.

6   Procedure must be performed by a physician or by a physical therapist (PT) who is certified by the American Board of Physical Therapy Specialties (ABPTS) as a qualified electrophysiologic clinical specialist and is permitted to provide the procedure under State law.

6a Supervision standards for level 66 apply; in addition, the PT with ABPTS certification may supervise another PT but only the PT with ABPTS certification may bill.

7a Supervision standards for level 77 apply; in addition, the PT with ABPTS certification may supervise another PT but only the PT with ABPTS certification may bill.

9   Concept does not apply.

21 Procedure must be performed by a technician with certification under general supervision of a physician; otherwise must be performed under direct supervision of a physician.

22 Procedure may be performed by a technician with on-line real-time contact with physician.

66 Procedure must be performed by a physician or by a PT with ABPTS certification and certification in this specific procedure.

77 Procedure must be performed by a PT with ABPTS certification or by a PT without certification under direct supervision of a physician, or by a technician with certification under general supervision of a physician.

Nurse practitioners, clinical nurse specialists, and physician assistants are not defined as physicians under §1861(r) of the Act. Therefore, they may not function as supervisory physicians under the diagnostic tests benefit (§1861(s)(3) of the Act). However, when these practitioners personally perform diagnostic tests as provided under §1861(s)(2)(K) of the Act, §1861(s)(3) does not apply and they may perform diagnostic tests pursuant to State scope of practice laws and under the applicable State requirements for physician supervision or collaboration.

Because the diagnostic tests benefit set forth in §1861(s)(3) of the Act is separate and distinct from the incident to benefit set forth in §1861(s)(2) of the Act, diagnostic tests need not meet the incident to requirements. Diagnostic tests may be furnished under situations that meet the incident to requirements but this is not required. However, carriers must not scrutinize claims for diagnostic tests utilizing the incident to requirements.

80.1—Clinical Laboratory Services

(Rev. 79; Issued: 10-19-07; Effective: 01-01-03; Implementation: 11-19-07)

Section 1833 and 1861 of the Act provides for payment of clinical laboratory services under Medicare Part B. Clinical laboratory services involve the biological, microbiological, serological, chemical, immunohematological, hematological, biophysical, cytological, pathological, or other examination of materials derived from the human body for the diagnosis, prevention, or treatment of a disease or assessment of a medical condition. Laboratory services must meet all applicable requirements of the Clinical Laboratory Improvement Amendments of 1988 (CLIA), as set forth at 42 CFR part 493. Section 1862(a)(1)(A) of the Act provides that Medicare payment may not be made for services that are not reasonable and necessary. Clinical laboratory services must be ordered and used promptly by the physician who is treating the beneficiary as described in 42CFR410.32(a), or by a qualified nonphysician practitioner, as described in 42CFR410.32(a)(3).

See section 80.6 of this manual for related physician ordering instructions.

See the Medicare Claims Processing Manual Chapter 16 for related claims processing instructions.

80.1.1—Certification Changes

(Rev. 1, 10-01-03)

B3-2070.1.E

Each page of the lists of approved specialties also includes a column "Certification Changed" in which the following codes are used:

"C" indicates a change in the laboratory's approved certification since the preceding listing.

"A" discloses an accretion.

"TERM"—Laboratory not approved for payment after the indicated date which follows the code. The reason for termination also is given in the following codes:

1. Involuntary termination—no longer meets requirements
2. Voluntary withdrawal
3. Laboratory closed, merged with other interests, or organizational change
4. Ownership change with new ownership participating under different name
5. Ownership change with new owner not participating
6. Change in ownership—new provider number assigned
7. Involuntary termination—failure to abide by agreement
8. Former "emergency" hospital now fully participating

80.1.2—Carrier Contacts With Independent Clinical Laboratories

(Rev. 1, 10-01-03)

B3-2070.1.F

An important role of the carrier is as a communicant of necessary information to independent clinical laboratories. Experience has shown that the failure to inform laboratories of Medicare regulations and claims processing procedures may have an adverse effect on prosecution of laboratories suspected of fraudulent activities with respect to tests performed by, or billed on behalf of, independent laboratories. United States Attorneys often have to prosecute under a handicap or may simply refuse to prosecute cases where there is no evidence that a laboratory has been specifically informed of Medicare regulations and claims processing procedures.

Carriers must follow the Provider Education and Training (PET) guidelines to assure that laboratories are aware of Medicare regulations and the carrier's policy when any changes are made in coverage policy or claims processing procedures. The PET guidelines require carriers to use various methods of communication (such as print, Internet, face-to-face instruction). Newsletters/bulletins that contain program and billing information must be produced at least quarterly and posted on the carrier Web site where duplicate copies may be obtained.

Some items which should be communicated to laboratories and responsibilities that laboratories are required to perform are:

- The requirements to have the same fee schedule for Medicare and private patients;
- To specify whether the tests are manual or automated;
- To document fully the medical necessity for pickup of specimens from a skilled nursing facility or a beneficiary's home, and
- In cases when a laboratory service is referred from one independent laboratory to another independent laboratory, to identify the laboratory actually performing the test.

Additionally, when carrier professional relations representatives make personal contacts with particular laboratories, the representative should prepare and retain reports of contact indicating dates, persons present, and issues discussed. Fi-

nally, carriers should inform independent laboratories that the Medicare National Coverage Determinations Manual as well as other guidelines contained in the manual for determining medical necessity are on the Web site. Carriers should also publish local guidelines on its Web site; the carrier should not duplicate national instructions here. Timely paper or electronic communications concerning the Internet publications to independent laboratories new to the carrier's service area are essential.

80.1.3—Independent Laboratory Service to a Patient in the Patient's Home or an Institution

(Rev. 1, 10-01-03)

B3-2070.1.G

Where it is medically necessary for an independent laboratory to visit a patient to obtain a specimen, the service would be covered in the following circumstances:

1—Patient Confined to Home

If a patient is confined to the home or other place of residence used as his or her home (see §60.4.1 for the definition of a "homebound patient"), medical necessity would exist (e.g., where a laboratory technician draws a blood specimen). However, where the specimen is a type which would require only the services of a messenger and would not require the skills of a laboratory technician, e.g., urine or sputum, a specimen pickup service would not be considered medically necessary.

2—Place of Residence is an Institution

Medical necessity could also exist where the patient's place of residence is an institution, including a skilled nursing facility that does not perform venipunctures. This would apply even though the institution meets the basic definition of a skilled nursing facility and would not ordinarily be considered a beneficiary's home. (This policy is intended for independent laboratories only and does not expand the range of coverage of services to homebound patients under the incident to provision.) A trip by an independent laboratory technician to a facility (other than a hospital) for the purpose of performing a venipuncture is considered medically necessary only if:

a. The patient was confined to the facility; and
b. The facility did not have on duty personnel qualified to perform this service.

When facility personnel actually obtained and prepared the specimens for the independent laboratory to pick them up, the laboratory provides this pickup service as a service to the facility in the same manner as it does for physicians.

80.2—Psychological Tests and Neuropsychological Tests

(Rev. 55, Issued: 09-29-06, Effective: 01-01-06, Implementation: 12-28-06)

Medicare Part B coverage of psychological tests and neuropsychological tests is authorized under section 1861(s)(2)(C) of the Social Security Act. Payment for psychological and neuropsychological tests is authorized under section 1842(b)(2)(A) of the Social Security Act. The payment amounts for the new psychological and neuropsychological tests (CPT codes 96102, 96103, 96119 and 96120) that are effective January 1, 2006, and are billed for tests administered by a technician or a computer reflect a site of service payment differential for the facility and non-facility settings. Additionally, there is no authorization for payment for diagnostic tests when performed on an "incident to" basis.

Under the diagnostic tests provision, all diagnostic tests are assigned a certain level of supervision. Generally, regulations governing the diagnostic tests provision require that only physicians can provide the assigned level of supervision for diagnostic tests. However, there is a regulatory exception to the supervision requirement for diagnostic psychological and neuropsychological tests in terms of who can provide the supervision. That is, regulations allow a clinical psychologist (CP) or a physician to perform the general supervision assigned to diagnostic psychological and neuropsychological tests.

In addition, nonphysician practitioners such as nurse practitioners (NPs), clinical nurse specialists (CNSs) and physician assistants (PAs) who personally perform diagnostic psychological and neuropsychological tests are excluded from having to perform these tests under the general supervision of a physician or a CP. Rather, NPs and CNSs must perform such tests under the requirements of their respective benefit instead of the requirements for diagnostic psychological and neuropsychological tests. Accordingly, NPs and CNSs must perform tests in collaboration (as defined under Medicare law at section 1861(aa)(6) of the Act) with a physician. PAs perform tests under the general supervision of a physician as required for services furnished under the PA benefit.

Furthermore, physical therapists (PTs), occupational therapists (OTs) and speech language pathologists (SLPs) are authorized to bill three test codes as "sometimes therapy" codes. Specifically, CPT codes 96105, 96110 and 96111 may be performed by these therapists. However, when PTs, OTs and SLPs perform these three tests, they must be performed under the general supervision of a physician or a CP.

Who May Bill for Diagnostic Psychological and Neuropsychological Tests

- CPs – see qualifications under chapter 15, section 160 of the Benefits Policy Manual, Pub. 100-02.
- NPs –to the extent authorized under State scope of practice. See qualifications under chapter 15, section 200 of the Benefits Policy Manual, Pub. 100-02.
- CNSs –to the extent authorized under State scope of practice. See qualifications under chapter 15, section 210 of the Benefits Policy Manual, Pub. 100-02.
- PAs – to the extent authorized under State scope of practice. See qualifications under chapter 15, section 190 of the Benefits Policy Manual, Pub. 100-02.
- Independently Practicing Psychologists (IPPs)
- PTs, OTs and SLPs – see qualifications under chapter 15, sections 220-230.6 of the Benefits Policy Manual, Pub. 100-02.

Psychological and neuropsychological tests performed by a psychologist (who is not a CP) practicing independently of an institution, agency, or physician's office are covered when a physician orders such tests. An IPP is any psychologist who is licensed or certified to practice psychology in the State or jurisdiction where furnishing services or, if the jurisdiction does not issue licenses, if provided by any practicing psychologist. (It is CMS' understanding that all States, the District of Columbia, and Puerto Rico license psychologists, but that some trust territories do not. Examples of psychologists, other than CPs, whose psychological and neuropsychological

tests are covered under the diagnostic tests provision include, but are not limited to, educational psychologists and counseling psychologists.)

The carrier must secure from the appropriate State agency a current listing of psychologists holding the required credentials to determine whether the tests of a particular IPP are covered under Part B in States that have statutory licensure or certification. In States or territories that lack statutory licensing or certification, the carrier checks individual qualifications before provider numbers are issued. Possible reference sources are the national directory of membership of the American Psychological Association, which provides data about the educational background of individuals and indicates which members are board-certified, the records and directories of the State or territorial psychological association, and the National Register of Health Service Providers. If qualification is dependent on a doctoral degree from a currently accredited program, the carrier verifies the date of accreditation of the school involved, since such accreditation is not retroactive. If the listed reference sources do not provide enough information (e.g., the psychologist is not a member of one of these sources), the carrier contacts the psychologist personally for the required information. Generally, carriers maintain a continuing list of psychologists whose qualifications have been verified.

NOTE: When diagnostic psychological tests are performed by a psychologist who is not practicing independently, but is on the staff of an institution, agency, or clinic, that entity bills for the psychological tests.

The carrier considers psychologists as practicing independently when:

- They render services on their own responsibility, free of the administrative and professional control of an employer such as a physician, institution or agency;
- The persons they treat are their own patients; and
- They have the right to bill directly, collect and retain the fee for their services.

A psychologist practicing in an office located in an institution may be considered an independently practicing psychologist when both of the following conditions exist:

- The office is confined to a separately-identified part of the facility which is used solely as the psychologist's office and cannot be construed as extending throughout the entire institution; and
- The psychologist conducts a private practice, i.e., services are rendered to patients from outside the institution as well as to institutional patients.

Payment for Diagnostic Psychological and Neuropsychological Tests

Expenses for diagnostic psychological and neuropsychological tests are not subject to the outpatient mental health treatment limitation, that is, the payment limitation on treatment services for mental, psychoneurotic and personality disorders as authorized under Section 1833(c) of the Act. The payment amount for the new psychological and neuropsychological tests (CPT codes 96102, 96103, 96119 and 96120) that are billed for tests performed by a technician or a computer reflect a site of service payment differential for the facility and non-facility settings. CPs, NPs, CNSs and PAs are required by law to accept assigned payment for psychological and neuropsychological tests. However, while IPPs are not required by law to accept assigned payment for these tests, they must report the name and address of the physician who ordered the test on the claim form when billing for tests.

CPT Codes for Diagnostic Psychological and Neuropsychological Tests

The range of CPT codes used to report psychological and neuropsychological tests is 96101-96120. CPT codes 96101, 96102, 96103, 96105, 96110, and 96111 are appropriate for use when billing for psychological tests. CPT codes 96116, 96118, 96119 and 96120 are appropriate for use when billing for neuropsychological tests.

All of the tests under this CPT code range 96101-96120 are indicated as active codes under the physician fee schedule database and are covered if medically necessary.

Payment and Billing Guidelines for Psychological and Neuropsychological Tests

The technician and computer CPT codes for psychological and neuropsychological tests include practice expense, malpractice expense and professional work relative value units. Accordingly, CPT psychological test code 96101 should not be paid when billed for the same tests or services performed under psychological test codes 96102 or 96103. CPT neuropsychological test code 96118 should not be paid when billed for the same tests or services performed under neuropsychological test codes 96119 or 96120. However, CPT codes 96101 and 96118 can be paid separately on the rare occasion when billed on the same date of service for different and separate tests from 96102, 96103, 96119 and 96120.

Under the physician fee schedule, there is no payment for services performed by students or trainees. Accordingly, Medicare does not pay for services represented by CPT codes 96102 and 96119 when performed by a student or a trainee. However, the presence of a student or a trainee while the test is being administered does not prevent a physician, CP, IPP, NP, CNS or PA from performing and being paid for the psychological test under 96102 or the neuropsychological test under 96119.

80.3 - Audiological Diagnostic Testing

(Rev. 84; Issued: 02-29-08; Effective: 04-01-08; Implementation: 04-07-08)

References.

> 1861(ll)(3)(B) of the Social Security Act for qualifications of audiologists.
> Pub. 100-04, chapter 12, section 30.3 for coding and billing information related to audiological services and aural rehabilitation.
> Pub. 100-02, chapter 15, sections 220 and 230 for the physical therapy and speech-language pathology policies relative to aural rehabilitation and balance, section 60 for services incident to a physician, and section 80.5 for policies relevant to ordering for diagnostic tests.
> Pub. 100-02, chapter 16, section 100 for hearing aid policies.

Benefit. Audiological diagnostic testing refers to tests of the audiological and vestibular systems, e.g., hearing, balance, auditory processing, tinnitus and diagnostic programming of certain prosthetic devices, performed by qualified audiologists. Audiological testing is covered as "other diagnostic tests" under §1861(s)(3) of the Act when a physician orders such testing for the purpose of obtaining information necessary for the physician's diagnostic medical evaluation or to determine the appro-

priate medical or surgical treatment of a hearing deficit or related medical problem. For the purposes of ordering audiological diagnostic tests, a nonphysician practitioner may perform the same service as a physician when the nonphysician practitioner orders diagnostic tests within their scope of practice, State and local laws and any policies applicable to the setting. See subsections of section 80 of this chapter for policies relative to ordering diagnostic tests.

Audiological diagnostic tests are not covered under the benefit for incident to a physician (described in Pub. 100-02, chapter 15, section 60), because they have their own benefit as "other diagnostic tests". See Pub. 100-04, chapter 13 for diagnostic test policies.

Orders

If a beneficiary undergoes diagnostic testing performed by an audiologist without a physician order, the tests are not covered even if the audiologist discovers a pathologic condition. See the policies on ordering diagnostic tests in section 80.6 of this chapter.

When a qualified physician or qualified nonphysician practitioner orders a specific audiological test using the CPT descriptor for the test, only that test may be provided on that order. Further orders are necessary if the ordered test indicates that other tests are necessary to evaluate, for example, the type or cause of the condition. Orders for specific tests are required for technicians.

When the qualified physician or qualified nonphysician practitioner orders diagnostic audiological tests by an audiologist without naming specific tests, the audiologist may select the appropriate battery of tests.

Coverage and Payment for Audiological Services. Diagnostic services performed by a qualified audiologist and meeting the requirements at §1861(ll)(3)(B) are payable as "other diagnostic tests." Audiological diagnostic tests are not covered as services incident to physician's services or as services incident to audiologist's services.

The payment for audiological diagnostic tests is determined by the reason the tests were performed, rather than by the diagnosis or the patient's condition.

Payment for audiological diagnostic tests is not allowed by virtue of §1862(a)(7) when:

- The type and severity of the current hearing, tinnitus or balance status needed to determine the appropriate medical or surgical treatment is known to the physician before the test; or
- The test was ordered for the specific purpose of fitting or modifying a hearing aid.

Payment of audiological diagnostic tests is allowed for other reasons (see Documentation subsection below) and is not limited, for example, by:

- Any information resulting from the test including, for example:
  - Confirmation of a prior diagnosis;
  - Post-evaluation diagnoses; or
  - Treatment provided after diagnosis, including hearing aids, or
- The type of evaluation or treatment the physician anticipates before the diagnostic test; or

- Timing of re-evaluation. Re-evaluation is appropriate at a schedule dictated by the ordering physician when the information provided by the diagnostic test is required, for example, to determine changes in hearing, to evaluate the appropriate medical or surgical treatment or evaluate the results of treatment. For example, re-evaluation may be appropriate, even when the evaluation was recent, in cases where the hearing loss, balance or tinnitus may be progressive or fluctuating, the patient or caregiver complains of new symptoms, or treatment (such as medication or surgery) may have changed the patient's audiological condition with or without awareness by the patient.

Payment for these services is based on the physician fee schedule amount except for audiology services furnished in a hospital outpatient department, which are paid under the Outpatient Prospective Payment System.

Computer-administered hearing tests are screening tests, do not require the skilled services of an audiologist and are not covered or payable using codes for diagnostic audiological testing. Examples include, but are not limited to "otograms" and pure tone or immitance screening devices that do not require the skills of an audiologist.

Diagnostic analysis of cochlear or brainstem implant and programming are audiology diagnostic services covered under the "other diagnostic test" benefit. Audiological diagnostic tests before and periodically after implantation of auditory prosthetic devices are covered services.

For descriptions of hearing aids and auditory prosthetic devices including osseointegrated devices, see Pub. 100-02, chapter16, section 100.

If a physician refers a beneficiary to an audiologist for testing related to signs or symptoms associated with hearing loss, balance disorder, tinnitus, ear disease, or ear injury, the audiologist's diagnostic testing services should be covered even if the only outcome is the prescription of a hearing aid.

Individuals Who Provide Audiological Tests. Some diagnostic audiological tests require, for both the technical and professional components, the skills of an audiologist to perform the test and interpret not only the data output, but also the manner of the patient's response to the test. These tests must be personally furnished by an audiologist or a physician. The skills of an audiologist required when furnishing the ordered diagnostic tests involve skilled judgment or assessment including but not limited to:

- Interpretation, comparison or consideration of the anatomical or physiological implications of test results or patient responsiveness to stimuli during the test;
- Modification of the stimulus based on responses obtained during the test;
- Choices for subsequent presentations of stimuli, or tests in a battery of tests;
- Tests related to implantation of auditory prosthetic devices, central auditory processing, contralateral masking; and/or
- Tests designed to identify central auditory processing disorders, tinnitus, or nonorganic hearing loss.

The technical components of certain audiological diagnostic tests i.e., tympanometry (92567) and vestibular function tests (e.g., 92541) that do not require the skills of an audiologist

may be performed by a qualified technician or by an audiologist, physician or nonphysician practitioner acting within their scope of practice. If performed by a technician, the service must be provided under the direct supervision [42 CFR §410.32(3)] of a physician or qualified nonphysician practitioner who is responsible for all clinical judgment and for the appropriate provision of the service. The physician or qualified nonphysician practitioner bills the directly supervised service as a diagnostic test.

Documenting for Audiological Tests. The "other diagnostic tests" benefit requires an order from a physician, or, where allowed by State and local law, by a non-physician practitioner. See section 80.6 of this chapter for policies concerning orders for diagnostic tests.

The reason for the test should be documented either on the order, on the audiological evaluation report, or in the patient's medical record. (See subsection of this section titled "Benefit".) Examples of appropriate reasons include but are not limited to:

- Evaluation of suspected change in hearing, tinnitus, or balance;
- Evaluation of the cause of disorders of hearing, tinnitus, or balance.
- Determination of the effect of medication, surgery or other treatment;

Reevaluation to follow-up changes in hearing, tinnitus or balance that may be caused for example, but not limited to otosclerosis, atelectatic tympanic membrane, tymposclerosis, cholesteatoma, resolving middle ear infection, Meniere's disease, sudden idiopathic sensorineural hearing loss, autoimmune inner ear disease, acoustic neuroma, demyelinating diseases, ototoxicity secondary to medications, genetic, vascular and viral conditions. Screening tests are not payable, but failure of a screening test may be an appropriate reason for diagnostic audiological tests.

The medical record shall identify the name and professional identity of the person who ordered and the person who actually performed the service. When the medical record is subject to medical review, it is necessary that the contractor determine that the service qualifies as an audiological diagnostic test that requires the skills of an audiologist. A technician must meet qualifications determined by the Medicare contractor to whom the claim is billed. At a minimum, the qualifications must include the requirements of any applicable State or local laws, and successful completion of a curriculum including both classroom training and supervised clinical experience in administration of the audiological service.

If a technician performs the technical component of a service that does not require the skills of an audiologist, the physician supervisor shall provide and document the physician's professional component of the service including, e.g., clinical decision making, and other active participation in the delivery of the service. This participation may not also be billed as evaluation and management or as part of other billed services.

Audiological Treatment. There is no provision in the law for Medicare to pay audiologists for therapeutic services. For example, vestibular treatment, auditory rehabilitation and auditory processing treatment, while they are within the scope of practice of audiologists, are not diagnostic tests, and therefore, shall not be billed by audiologists to Medicare. Services related to hearing aid evaluation and fitting are not covered regardless of how they are billed. Services identified as "always" therapy in Pub. 100-04 chapter 5, section 20 may not be billed when provided by audiologists. (See also Pub 100-04, chapter 12, section 30.3.)

Services that are not diagnostic tests and are also not "always" therapy (according to the list and the policy in Pub.100-04, chapter 5, section 20) and are provided by qualified personnel (who may be audiologists), may be billed "incident to" when all other appropriate requirements are met. (See policies in Pub. 100-02, chapter 15, sections 60, 200, and 230.)

Treatment related to hearing may be covered under the speech-language pathology benefit when the services are provided by speech-language pathologists. Treatment related to balance (e.g., using "always therapy" codes 97001-97004, 97110, 97112, 97116, and 97750) may be covered under the physical therapy or occupational therapy benefit when the services are provided by physical or occupational therapists or their assistants, where appropriate. Covered therapy services incident to a physician's service must conform to policies in chapter 15, sections 60, 220 and 230. Audiological treatment provided under the benefit for physical therapy and speech-language pathology services may be personally provided and billed by physicians and nonphysician practitioners when the services are within their scope of practice and consistent with State and local laws.

For example, aural rehabilitation and signed communication training may be payable according to the benefit for speech-language pathology services or as speech-language pathology services incident to a physician's or nonphysician practitioner's service. Treatment for balance disorders may be payable according to the benefit for physical therapy services or as a physical therapy service incident to the services of a physician or nonphysician practitioner. See the policies in Pub 100-02, chapter 15, section 220 and 230 for details.

Assignment. Nonhospital entities billing for the audiologist's services may accept assignment under the usual procedure or, if not accepting assignment, may charge the patient and submit a nonassigned claim on their behalf.

80.3.1 - Definition of Qualified Audiologist

(Rev. 84; Issued: 02-29-08; Effective: 04-01-08; Implementation: 04-07-08)

Audiological tests require the skills of an audiologist and shall be furnished by qualified audiologists, or, in States where it is allowed by State and local laws, by a physician or non-physician practitioner. Medicare is not authorized to pay for these services when performed by audiological aides, assistants, technicians, or others who do not meet the qualifications below. In cases where it is not clear, the Medicare contractor shall determine whether a service is an audiological service that requires the skills of an audiologist and whether the qualifications for an audiologist have been met.

Section 1861(ll)(3) of the Act, provides that a qualified audiologist is an individual with a master's or doctoral degree in audiology. Therefore, a Doctor of Audiology (AuD) 4th year student with a provisional license from a State does not qualify unless he or she also holds a master's or doctoral degree in audiology. In addition, a qualified audiologist is an individual who:

- Is licensed as an audiologist by the State in which the individual furnishes such services, or

- In the case of an individual who furnishes services in a State which does not license audiologists has:
  - Successfully completed 350 clock hours of supervised clinical practicum (or is in the process of accumulating such supervised clinical experience), and
  - Performed not less than 9 months of supervised full-time audiology services after obtaining a master's or doctoral degree in audiology or a related field, and
  - Successfully completed a national examination in audiology approved by the Secretary.

If it is necessary to determine whether a particular audiologist is qualified under the above definition, the carrier should check references. Carriers in States that have statutory licensure or certification should secure from the appropriate State agency a current listing of audiologists holding the required credentials. Additional references for determining an audiologist's professional qualifications are the national directory published annually by the American Speech-Language-Hearing Association and records and directories, which may be available from the State Licensing Authority.

80.4—Coverage of Portable X-Ray Services Not Under the Direct Supervision of a Physician

(Rev. 1, 10-01-03)

B3-2070.4

80.4.1—Diagnostic X-Ray Tests

(Rev. 1, 10-01-03)

B3-2070.4.A

Diagnostic x-ray services furnished by a portable x-ray supplier are covered under Part B when furnished in a place or residence used as the patient's home and in nonparticipating institutions. These services must be performed under the general supervision of a physician, the supplier must meet FDA certification requirements, and certain conditions relating to health and safety (as prescribed by the Secretary) must be met.

Diagnostic portable x-ray services are also covered under Part B when provided in participating SNFs and hospitals, under circumstances in which they cannot be covered under hospital insurance, i.e., the services are not furnished by the participating institution either directly or under arrangements that provide for the institution to bill for the services. (See §250 for Part B services furnished to inpatients of participating and nonparticipating institutions.)

80.4.2—Applicability of Health and Safety Standards

(Rev. 1, 10-01-03)

B3-2070.4.B

The health and safety standards apply to all suppliers of portable x-ray services, except physicians who provide immediate personal supervision during the administration of diagnostic x-ray services. Payment is made only for services of approved suppliers who have been found to meet the standards. Notice of the coverage dates for services of approved suppliers are given to carriers by the RO.

When the services of a supplier of portable x-ray services no longer meet the conditions of coverage, physicians having an interest in the supplier's certification status must be notified. The notification action regarding suppliers of portable x-ray equipment is the same as required for decertification of independent laboratories, and the procedures explained in §80.1.3 are followed.

80.4.3—Scope of Portable X-Ray Benefit

(Rev. 71, Issued: 05-25-07, Effective: N/A; Implementation: July 2, 2007)

In order to avoid payment for services, which are inadequate or hazardous to the patient, the scope of the covered portable x-ray benefit is defined as:

- Skeletal films involving the extremities, pelvis, vertebral column, or skull;
- Chest films which do not involve the use of contrast media (except routine screening procedures and tests in connection with routine physical examinations);
- Abdominal films which do not involve the use of contrast media; and
- Diagnostic mammograms if the approved portable x-ray supplier, as defined in 42 CFR part 486, subpart C, meets the certification requirements of section 354 of the Public Health Services Act, as implemented by 21 CFR part 900, subpart B.

80.4.4—Exclusions From Coverage as Portable X-Ray Services

(Rev. 1, 10-01-03)

B3-2070.4.D

Procedures and examinations which are not covered under the portable x-ray provision include the following:

- Procedures involving fluoroscopy;
- Procedures involving the use of contrast media;
- Procedures requiring the administration of a substance to the patient or injection of a substance into the patient and/or special manipulation of the patient;
- Procedures which require special medical skill or knowledge possessed by a doctor of medicine or doctor of osteopathy or which require that medical judgment be exercised;
- Procedures requiring special technical competency and/or special equipment or materials;
- Routine screening procedures; and
- Procedures which are not of a diagnostic nature.

80.4.5—Electrocardiograms

(Rev. 1, 10-01-03)

B3-2070.4.F

The taking of an electrocardiogram tracing by an approved supplier of portable x-ray services may be covered as an "other diagnostic test." The health and safety standards referred to in §80.4.2 are applicable to such diagnostic EKG services, e.g., the technician must meet the personnel qualification requirements in the conditions for coverage of portable x-ray services.

80.5—Bone Mass Measurements (BMMs)

(Rev.70, Issued: 05-11-07, Effective: 01-01-07, Implementation: 07-02-07)

80.5.1—Background

(Rev. 70, Issued: 05-11-07, Effective: 01-01-07, Implementation: 07-02-07)

On June 24, 1998, CMS published an Interim Final Rule with Comment Period (IFC) in the **Federal Register** entitled "Medicare Coverage of and Payment for Bone Mass Measurements." This IFC implemented section 4106 of the Balanced Budget Act of 1997 by establishing conditions for coverage and frequency standards thereby providing uniform coverage under Medicare Part B. It was effective July 1, 1998.

On December 1, 2006, CMS published the CY 2007 Physician Fee Schedule final rule. This rule implemented several changes effective January 1, 2007, which are reflected below.

80.5.2—Authority

(Rev. 70, Issued: 05-11-07, Effective: 01-01-07, Implementation: 07-02-07)

Definitions can be found in sections 1861(s)(15) and (rr)(1) of the Social Security Act (the Act). Conditions for coverage and frequency standards can be found in 42 CFR 410.31. Denials as not reasonable and necessary can be found at §1862(a)(1)(A) of the Act, 42 CFR 410.31(e), and 42 CFR 411.15(k).

80.5.3—Definition

(Rev. 70, Issued: 05-11-07, Effective: 01-01-07, Implementation: 07-02-07)

BMM means a radiologic, radioisotopic, or other procedure that meets all of the following conditions:

- Is performed to identify bone mass, detect bone loss, or determine bone quality.
- Is performed with either a bone densitometer (other than single-photon or dual-photon absorptiometry) or a bone sonometer system that has been cleared for marketing for BMM by the Food and Drug Administration (FDA) under 21 CFR part 807, or approved for marketing under 21 CFR part 814.
- Includes a physician's interpretation of the results.

80.5.4—Conditions for Coverage

(Rev. 70, Issued: 05-11-07, Effective: 01-01-07, Implementation: 07-02-07)

Medicare covers BMM under the following conditions:

1. Is ordered by the physician or qualified nonphysician practitioner who is treating the beneficiary following an evaluation of the need for a BMM and determination of the appropriate BMM to be used.

A physician or qualified nonphysician practitioner treating the beneficiary for purposes of this provision is one who furnishes a consultation or treats a beneficiary for a specific medical problem, and who uses the results in the management of the patient. For the purposes of the BMM benefit, qualified nonphysician practitioners include physician assistants, nurse practitioners, clinical nurse specialists, and certified nurse midwives.

2. Is performed under the appropriate level of physician supervision as defined in 42 CFR 410.32(b).

3. Is reasonable and necessary for diagnosing and treating

the condition of a beneficiary who meets the conditions described in §80.5.6.

4. In the case of an individual being monitored to assess the response to or efficacy of an FDA-approved osteoporosis drug therapy, is performed with a dual-energy x-ray absorptiometry system (axial skeleton).

5. In the case of any individual who meets the conditions of 80.5.6 and who has a confirmatory BMM, is performed by a dual-energy x-ray absorptiometry system (axial skeleton) if the initial BMM was not performed by a dual-energy x-ray absorptiometry system (axial skeleton). A confirmatory baseline BMM is not covered if the initial BMM was performed by a dual-energy x-ray absorptiometry system (axial skeleton).

80.5.5—Frequency Standards

(Rev. 70, Issued: 05-11-07, Effective: 01-01-07, Implementation: 07-02-07)

Medicare pays for a screening BMM once every 2 years (at least 23 months have passed since the month the last covered BMM was performed).

When medically necessary, Medicare may pay for more frequent BMMs. Examples include, but are not limited to, the following medical circumstances:

• Monitoring beneficiaries on long-term glucocorticoid (steroid) therapy of more than 3 months.
• Confirming baseline BMMs to permit monitoring of beneficiaries in the future.

80.5.6—Beneficiaries Who May be Covered

(Rev. 70, Issued: 05-11-07, Effective: 01-01-07, Implementation: 07-02-07)

To be covered, a beneficiary must meet at least one of the five conditions listed below:

1. A woman who has been determined by the physician or qualified nonphysician practitioner treating her to be estrogen-deficient and at clinical risk for osteoporosis, based on her medical history and other findings.

NOTE: Since not every woman who has been prescribed estrogen replacement therapy (ERT) may be receiving an "adequate" dose of the therapy, the fact that a woman is receiving ERT should not preclude her treating physician or other qualified treating nonphysician practitioner from ordering a bone mass measurement for her. If a BMM is ordered for a woman following a careful evaluation of her medical need, however, it is expected that the ordering treating physician (or other qualified treating nonphysician practitioner) will document in her medical record why he or she believes that the woman is estrogen-deficient and at clinical risk for osteoporosis.

2. An individual with vertebral abnormalities as demonstrated by an x-ray to be indicative of osteoporosis, osteopenia, or vertebral fracture.

3. An individual receiving (or expecting to receive) glucocorticoid (steroid) therapy equivalent to an average of 5.0 mg of prednisone, or greater, per day, for more than 3 months.

4. An individual with primary hyperparathyroidism.

5. An individual being monitored to assess the response to or efficacy of an FDA-approved osteoporosis drug therapy.

80.5.7—Noncovered BMMs

(Rev. 70, Issued: 05-11-07, Effective: 01-01-07, Implementation: 07-02-07)

The following BMMs are noncovered under Medicare because they are not considered reasonable and necessary under section 1862(a)(1)(A) of the Act.

• Single photon absorptiometry (effective January 1, 2007).
• Dual photon absorptiometry (established in 1983).

80.5.8—Claims Processing

(Rev. 70, Issued: 05-11-07, Effective: 01-01-07, Implementation: 07-02-07)

For instructions concerning payment methodology, HCPCS coding, and Medicare summary notice and remittance advice messages, see chapter 13, section 140 of Pub. 100-04, Medicare Claims Processing Manual.

80.5.9—National Coverage Determinations (NCDs)

(Rev. 70, Issued: 05-11-07, Effective: 01-01-07, Implementation: 07-02-07)

In addition to these conditions for coverage, CMS may determine through the NCD process that additional BMM systems are reasonable and necessary under section 1862(a)(1) of the Act for monitoring and confirming baseline BMMs.

80.6—Requirements for Ordering and Following Orders for Diagnostic Tests

(Rev. 94, Issued: 08-29-08, Effective: 01-01-03, Implementation: 09-30-08)

The following sections provide instructions about ordering diagnostic tests and for complying with such orders for Medicare payment.

NOTE: Unless specified, these sections are not applicable in a hospital setting.

80.6.1—Definitions

(Rev. 94, Issued: 08-29-08, Effective: 01-01-03, Implementation: 09-30-08)

Diagnostic Test

A "diagnostic test" includes all diagnostic x-ray tests, all diagnostic laboratory tests, and other diagnostic tests furnished to a beneficiary.

Treating Physician

A "treating physician" is a physician, as defined in §1861(r) of the Social Security Act (the Act), who furnishes a consultation or treats a beneficiary for a specific medical problem, and who uses the results of a diagnostic test in the management of the beneficiary's specific medical problem.

A radiologist performing a therapeutic interventional procedure is considered a treating physician. A radiologist performing a diagnostic interventional or diagnostic procedure is not considered a treating physician.

Treating Practitioner

A "treating practitioner" is a nurse practitioner, clinical nurse specialist, or physician assistant, as defined in §1861(s)(2)(K) of the Act, who furnishes, pursuant to State law, a consultation or treats a beneficiary for a specific medical problem, and who uses the result of a diagnostic test in the management of the beneficiary's specific medical problem.

Testing Facility

A "testing facility" is a Medicare provider or supplier that furnishes diagnostic tests. A testing facility may include a physician or a group of physicians (e.g., radiologist, pathologist), a laboratory, or an independent diagnostic testing facility (IDTF).

Order

An "order" is a communication from the treating physician/practitioner requesting that a diagnostic test be performed for a beneficiary. The order may conditionally request an additional diagnostic test for a particular beneficiary if the result of the initial diagnostic test ordered yields to a certain value determined by the treating physician/practitioner (e.g., if test X is negative, then perform test Y). An order may be delivered via the following forms of communication:

- A written document signed by the treating physician/practitioner, which is hand-delivered, mailed, or faxed to the testing facility; NOTE: No signature is required on orders for clinical diagnostic tests paid on the basis of the clinical laboratory fee schedule, the physician fee schedule, or for physician pathology services;
- A telephone call by the treating physician/practitioner or his/her office to the testing facility; and
- An electronic mail by the treating physician/practitioner or his/her office to the testing facility.

If the order is communicated via telephone, both the treating physician/practitioner or his/her office, and the testing facility must document the telephone call in their respective copies of the beneficiary's medical records. While a physician order is not required to be signed, the physician must clearly document, in the medical record, his or her intent that the test be performed.

80.6.2—Interpreting Physician Determines a Different Diagnostic Test is Appropriate

(Rev. 80; Issued: 01-11-08; Effective: 01-01-03; Implementation: 11-19-07)

When an interpreting physician, e.g., radiologist, cardiologist, family practitioner, general internist, neurologist, obstetrician, gynecologist, ophthalmologist, thoracic surgeon, vascular surgeon, at a testing facility determines that an ordered diagnostic radiology test is clinically inappropriate or suboptimal, and that a different diagnostic test should be performed (e.g., an MRI should be performed instead of a CT scan because of the clinical indication), the interpreting physician/testing facility may not perform the unordered test until a new order from the treating physician/practitioner has been received. Similarly, if the result of an ordered diagnostic test is normal and the interpreting physician believes that another diagnostic test should be performed (e.g., a renal sonogram was normal and based on the clinical indication, the interpreting physician believes an MRI will reveal the

diagnosis), an order from the treating physician must be received prior to performing the unordered diagnostic test.

80.6.3—Rules for Testing Facility to Furnish Additional Tests

(Rev. 80; Issued: 01-11-08; Effective: 01-01-03; Implementation: 11-19-07)

If the testing facility cannot reach the treating physician/practitioner to change the order or obtain a new order and documents this in the medical record, then the testing facility may furnish the additional diagnostic test if all of the following criteria apply:

- The testing center performs the diagnostic test ordered by the treating physician/practitioner;
- The interpreting physician at the testing facility determines and documents that, because of the abnormal result of the diagnostic test performed, an additional diagnostic test is medically necessary;
- Delaying the performance of the additional diagnostic test would have an adverse effect on the care of the beneficiary;
- The result of the test is communicated to and is used by the treating physician/practitioner in the treatment of the beneficiary; and
- The interpreting physician at the testing facility documents in his/her report why additional testing was done.

EXAMPLE:

The last cut of an abdominal CT scan with contrast shows a mass requiring a pelvic CT scan to further delineate the mass; (b) a bone scan reveals a lesion on the femur requiring plain films to make a diagnosis.

80.6.4—Rules for Testing Facility Interpreting Physician to Furnish Different or Additional Tests

(Rev. 80; Issued: 01-11-08; Effective: 01-01-03; Implementation: 11-19-07)

The following applies to an interpreting physician of a testing facility who furnishes a diagnostic test to a beneficiary who is not a hospital inpatient or outpatient. The interpreting physician must document accordingly in his/her report to the treating physician/practitioner.

Test Design

Unless specified in the order, the interpreting physician may determine, without notifying the treating physician/practitioner, the parameters of the diagnostic test (e.g., number of radiographic views obtained, thickness of tomographic sections acquired, use or non-use of contrast media).

Clear Error

The interpreting physician may modify, without notifying the treating physician/practitioner, an order with clear and obvious errors that would be apparent to a reasonable layperson, such as the patient receiving the test (e.g., x-ray of wrong foot ordered).

Patient Condition

The interpreting physician may cancel, without notifying the treating physician/practitioner, an order because the beneficiary's physical condition at the time of diagnostic testing will not permit performance of the test (e.g., a barium enema cannot be performed because of residual stool in colon on scout KUB; 170.5PA/LAT of the chest cannot be performed because the patient is unable to stand). When an ordered diagnostic test is cancelled, any medically necessary preliminary or scout testing performed is payable.

80.6.5—Surgical/Cytopathology Exception

(Rev. 80; Issued: 01-11-08; Effective: 01-01-03; Implementation: 11-19-07)

This exception applies to an independent laboratory's pathologist or a hospital pathologist who furnishes a pathology service to a beneficiary who is not a hospital inpatient or outpatient, and where the treating physician/practitioner does not specifically request additional tests the pathologist may need to perform. When a surgical or cytopathology specimen is sent to the pathology laboratory, it typically comes in a labeled container with a requisition form that reveals the patient demographics, the name of the physician/practitioner, and a clinical impression and/or brief history. There is no specific order from the surgeon or the treating physician/practitioner for a certain type of pathology service. While the pathologist will generally perform some type of examination or interpretation on the cells or tissue, there may be additional tests, such as special stains, that the pathologist may need to perform, even though they have not been specifically requested by the treating physician/practitioner. The pathologist may perform such additional tests under the following circumstances:

- These services are medically necessary so that a complete and accurate diagnosis can be reported to the treating physician/practitioner;
- The results of the tests are communicated to and are used by the treating physician/practitioner in the treatment of the beneficiary; and
- The pathologist documents in his/her report why additional testing was done.

EXAMPLE:

A lung biopsy is sent by the surgeon to the pathology department, and the pathologist finds a granuloma which is suspicious for tuberculosis. The pathologist cultures the granuloma, sends it to bacteriology, and requests smears for acid fast bacilli (tuberculosis). The pathologist is expected to determine the need for these studies so that the surgical pathology examination and interpretation can be completed and the definitive diagnosis reported to the treating physician for use in treating the beneficiary.

100—Surgical Dressings, Splints, Casts, and Other Devices Used for Reductions of Fractures and Dislocations

(Rev. 1, 10-01-03)

B3-2079, A3-3110.3, HO-228.3

Surgical dressings are limited to primary and secondary dressings required for the treatment of a wound caused by, or treated by, a surgical procedure that has been performed by a physician or other health care professional to the extent permissible under State law. In addition, surgical dressings re-

quired after debridement of a wound are also covered, irrespective of the type of debridement, as long as the debridement was reasonable and necessary and was performed by a health care professional acting within the scope of his/her legal authority when performing this function. Surgical dressings are covered for as long as they are medically necessary.

Primary dressings are therapeutic or protective coverings applied directly to wounds or lesions either on the skin or caused by an opening to the skin. Secondary dressing materials that serve a therapeutic or protective function and that are needed to secure a primary dressing are also covered. Items such as adhesive tape, roll gauze, bandages, and disposable compression material are examples of secondary dressings. Elastic stockings, support hose, foot coverings, leotards, knee supports, surgical leggings, gauntlets, and pressure garments for the arms and hands are examples of items that are not ordinarily covered as surgical dressings. Some items, such as transparent film, may be used as a primary or secondary dressing.

If a physician, certified nurse midwife, physician assistant, nurse practitioner, or clinical nurse specialist applies surgical dressings as part of a professional service that is billed to Medicare, the surgical dressings are considered incident to the professional services of the health care practitioner. (See §§60.1, 180, 190, 200, and 210.) When surgical dressings are not covered incident to the services of a health care practitioner and are obtained by the patient from a supplier (e.g., a drugstore, physician, or other health care practitioner that qualifies as a supplier) on an order from a physician or other health care professional authorized under State law or regulation to make such an order, the surgical dressings are covered separately under Part B.

Splints and casts, and other devices used for reductions of fractures and dislocations are covered under Part B of Medicare. This includes dental splints.

110—Durable Medical Equipment—General

(Rev. 1, 10-01-03)

B3-2100, A3-3113, HO-235, HHA-220

Expenses incurred by a beneficiary for the rental or purchases of durable medical equipment (DME) are reimbursable if the following three requirements are met:

- The equipment meets the definition of DME (§110.1);
- The equipment is necessary and reasonable for the treatment of the patient's illness or injury or to improve the functioning of his or her malformed body member (§110.1); and
- The equipment is used in the patient's home.

The decision whether to rent or purchase an item of equipment generally resides with the beneficiary, but the decision on how to pay rests with CMS. For some DME, program payment policy calls for lump sum payments and in others for periodic payment. Where covered DME is furnished to a beneficiary by a supplier of services other than a provider of services, the DMERC makes the reimbursement. If a provider of services furnishes the equipment, the intermediary makes the reimbursement. The payment method is identified in the annual fee schedule update furnished by CMS.

The CMS issues quarterly updates to a fee schedule file that contains rates by HCPCS code and also identifies the classification of the HCPCS code within the following categories.

Category Code	Definition
IN	Inexpensive and Other Routinely Purchased Items
FS	Frequently Serviced Items
CR	Capped Rental Items
OX	Oxygen and Oxygen Equipment
OS	Ostomy, Tracheostomy & Urological Items
SD	Surgical Dressings
PO	Prosthetics & Orthotics
SU	Supplies
TE	Transcutaneous Electrical Nerve Stimulators

The DMERCs, carriers, and intermediaries, where appropriate, use the CMS files to determine payment rules. See the Medicare Claims Processing Manual, Chapter 20, "Durable Medical Equipment, Surgical Dressings and Casts, Orthotics and Artificial Limbs, and Prosthetic Devices," for a detailed description of payment rules for each classification.

Payment may also be made for repairs, maintenance, and delivery of equipment and for expendable and nonreusable items essential to the effective use of the equipment subject to the conditions in §110.2.

See the Medicare Benefit Policy Manual, Chapter 11, "End Stage Renal Disease," for hemodialysis equipment and supplies.

110.1—Definition of Durable Medical Equipment

(Rev. 1, 10-01-03)

B3-2100.1, A3-3113.1, HO-235.1, HHA-220.1, B3-2100.2, A3-3113.2, HO-235.2, HHA-220.2

Durable medical equipment is equipment which:

- Can withstand repeated use;
- Is primarily and customarily used to serve a medical purpose;
- Generally is not useful to a person in the absence of an illness or injury; and
- Is appropriate for use in the home.

All requirements of the definition must be met before an item can be considered to be durable medical equipment.

The following describes the underlying policies for determining whether an item meets the definition of DME and may be covered.

A—Durability

An item is considered durable if it can withstand repeated use, i.e., the type of item that could normally be rented. Medical supplies of an expendable nature, such as incontinent pads, lambs wool pads, catheters, ace bandages, elastic stockings, surgical facemasks, irrigating kits, sheets, and bags are not considered "durable" within the meaning of the definition. There are other items that, although durable in nature, may fall into other coverage categories such as supplies, braces, prosthetic devices, artificial arms, legs, and eyes.

B—Medical Equipment

Medical equipment is equipment primarily and customarily used for medical purposes and is not generally useful in the absence of illness or injury. In most instances, no development will be needed to determine whether a specific item of equipment is medical in nature. However, some cases will require development to determine whether the item constitutes medical equipment. This development would include the advice of local medical organizations (hospitals, medical schools, medical societies) and specialists in the field of physical medicine and rehabilitation. If the equipment is new on the market, it may be necessary, prior to seeking professional advice, to obtain information from the supplier or manufacturer explaining the design, purpose, effectiveness and method of using the equipment in the home as well as the results of any tests or clinical studies that have been conducted.

1. **Equipment Presumptively Medical**—Items such as hospital beds, wheelchairs, hemodialysis equipment, iron lungs, respirators, intermittent positive pressure breathing machines, medical regulators, oxygen tents, crutches, canes, trapeze bars, walkers, inhalators, nebulizers, commodes, suction machines, and traction equipment presumptively constitute medical equipment. (Although hemodialysis equipment is covered as a prosthetic device (§120), it also meets the definition of DME, and reimbursement for the rental or purchase of such equipment for use in the beneficiary's home will be made only under the provisions for payment applicable to DME. See the Medicare Benefit Policy Manual, Chapter 11, "End Stage Renal Disease," §30.1, for coverage of home use of hemodialysis.) **NOTE:** There is a wide variety in types of respirators and suction machines. The DMERC's medical staff should determine whether the apparatus specified in the claim is appropriate for home use.

2. **Equipment Presumptively Nonmedical**—Equipment which is primarily and customarily used for a nonmedical purpose may not be considered "medical" equipment for which payment can be made under the medical insurance program. This is true even though the item has some remote medically related use. For example, in the case of a cardiac patient, an air conditioner might possibly be used to lower room temperature to reduce fluid loss in the patient and to restore an environment conducive to maintenance of the proper fluid balance. Nevertheless, because the primary and customary use of an air conditioner is a nonmedical one, the air conditioner cannot be deemed to be medical equipment for which payment can be made.

Other devices and equipment used for environmental control or to enhance the environmental setting in which the beneficiary is placed are not considered covered DME. These include, for example, room heaters, humidifiers, dehumidifiers, and electric air cleaners. Equipment which basically serves comfort or convenience functions or is primarily for the convenience of a person caring for the patient, such as elevators, stairway elevators, and posture chairs, do not constitute medical equipment. Similarly, physical fitness equipment (such as an exercycle), first-aid or precautionary-type equipment (such as preset portable oxygen units), self-help devices (such as safety grab bars), and training equipment (such as Braille training texts) are considered nonmedical in nature.

3. **Special Exception Items**—Specified items of equipment may be covered under certain conditions even though they do not meet the definition of DME because they are not primarily and customarily used to serve a medical purpose and/or are generally useful in the absence of illness or injury. These items would be covered when it is clearly established that they serve a therapeutic purpose in an individual case and would include:

a. Gel pads and pressure and water mattresses (which generally serve a preventive purpose) when prescribed for a patient who had bed sores or there is medical evidence indicating that they are highly susceptible to such ulceration; and

b. Heat lamps for a medical rather than a soothing or cosmetic purpose, e.g., where the need for heat therapy has been established.

In establishing medical necessity for the above items, the evidence must show that the item is included in the physician's course of treatment and a physician is supervising its use.

NOTE: The above items represent special exceptions and no extension of coverage to other items should be inferred

C—Necessary and Reasonable

Although an item may be classified as DME, it may not be covered in every instance. Coverage in a particular case is subject to the requirement that the equipment be necessary and reasonable for treatment of an illness or injury, or to improve the functioning of a malformed body member. These considerations will bar payment for equipment which cannot reasonably be expected to perform a therapeutic function in an individual case or will permit only partial therapeutic function in an individual case or will permit only partial payment when the type of equipment furnished substantially exceeds that required for the treatment of the illness or injury involved.

See the Medicare Claims Processing Manual, Chapter 1, "General Billing Requirements;" §60, regarding the rules for providing advance beneficiary notices (ABNs) that advise beneficiaries, before items or services actually are furnished, when Medicare is likely to deny payment for them. ABNs allow beneficiaries to make an informed consumer decision about receiving items or services for which they may have to pay out-of-pocket and to be more active participants in their own health care treatment decisions.

1. **Necessity for the Equipment**—Equipment is necessary when it can be expected to make a meaningful contribution to the treatment of the patient's illness or injury or to the improvement of his or her malformed body member. In most cases the physician's prescription for the equipment and other medical information available to the DMERC will be sufficient to establish that the equipment serves this purpose.

2. **Reasonableness of the Equipment**—Even though an item of DME may serve a useful medical purpose, the DMERC or intermediary must also consider to what extent, if any, it would be reasonable for the Medicare program to pay for the item prescribed. The following considerations should enter into the determination of reasonableness:

1. Would the expense of the item to the program be clearly disproportionate to the therapeutic benefits which could ordinarily be derived from use of the equipment?

2. Is the item substantially more costly than a medically appropriate and realistically feasible alternative pattern of care?

3. Does the item serve essentially the same purpose as equipment already available to the beneficiary?

3. **Payment Consistent With What is Necessary and Reasonable**—Where a claim is filed for equipment containing features of an aesthetic nature or features of a medical nature which are not required by the patient's condition or where there exists a reasonably feasible and medically appropriate alternative pattern of care which is less costly than the equipment furnished, the amount payable is based on the rate for the equipment or alternative treatment which meets the patient's medical needs.

The acceptance of an assignment binds the supplier-assignee to accept the payment for the medically required equipment or service as the full charge and the supplier-assignee cannot charge the beneficiary the differential attributable to the equipment actually furnished.

4. **Establishing the Period of Medical Necessity**—Generally, the period of time an item of durable medical equipment will be considered to be medically necessary is based on the physician's estimate of the time that his or her patient will need the equipment. See the Medicare Program Integrity Manual, Chapters 5 and 6, for medical review guidelines.

D—Definition of a Beneficiary's Home

For purposes of rental and purchase of DME a beneficiary's home may be his/her own dwelling, an apartment, a relative's home, a home for the aged, or some other type of institution. However, an institution may not be considered a beneficiary's home if it:

• Meets at least the basic requirement in the definition of a hospital, i.e., it is primarily engaged in providing by or under the supervision of physicians, to inpatients, diagnostic and therapeutic services for medical diagnosis, treatment, and care of injured, disabled, and sick persons, or rehabilitation services for the rehabilitation of injured, disabled, or sick persons; or

• Meets at least the basic requirement in the definition of a skilled nursing facility, i.e., it is primarily engaged in providing to inpatients skilled nursing care and related services for patients who require medical or nursing care, or rehabilitation services for the rehabilitation of injured, disabled, or sick persons.

Thus, if an individual is a patient in an institution or distinct part of an institution which provides the services described in the bullets above, the individual is not entitled to have separate Part B payment made for rental or purchase of DME. This is because such an institution may not be considered the individual's home. The same concept applies even if the patient resides in a bed or portion of the institution not certified for Medicare.

If the patient is at home for part of a month and, for part of the same month is in an institution that cannot qualify as his or her home, or is outside the U.S., monthly payments may be made for the entire month. Similarly, if DME is returned to the provider before the end of a payment month because the beneficiary died in that month or because the equipment became unnecessary in that month, payment may be made for the entire month.

110.2—Repairs, Maintenance, Replacement, and Delivery

(Rev. 30, Issued: 02-18-05, Effective/Implementation: Not Applicable)

Under the circumstances specified below, payment may be made for repair, maintenance, and replacement of medically required DME, including equipment which had been in use before the user enrolled in Part B of the program. However, do not pay for repair, maintenance, or replacement of equipment in the frequent and substantial servicing or oxygen equipment payment categories. In addition, payments for repair and maintenance may not include payment for parts and labor covered under a manufacturer's or supplier's warranty.

A—Repairs

To repair means to fix or mend and to put the equipment back in good condition after damage or wear. Repairs to equipment which a beneficiary owns are covered when necessary to make the equipment serviceable. However, do not pay for repair of previously denied equipment or equipment in the frequent and substantial servicing or oxygen equipment payment categories. If the expense for repairs exceeds the estimated expense of purchasing or renting another item of equipment for the remaining period of medical need, no payment can be made for the amount of the excess. (See subsection C where claims for repairs suggest malicious damage or culpable neglect.)

Since renters of equipment recover from the rental charge the expenses they incur in maintaining in working order the equipment they rent out, separately itemized charges for repair of rented equipment are not covered. This includes items in the frequent and substantial servicing, oxygen equipment, capped rental, and inexpensive or routinely purchased payment categories which are being rented.

A new Certificate of Medical Necessity (CMN) and/or physician's order is not needed for repairs.

For replacement items, see Subsection C below.

B—Maintenance

Routine periodic servicing, such as testing, cleaning, regulating, and checking of the beneficiary's equipment, is not covered. The owner is expected to perform such routine maintenance rather than a retailer or some other person who charges the beneficiary. Normally, purchasers of DME are given operating manuals which describe the type of servicing an owner may perform to properly maintain the equipment. It is reasonable to expect that beneficiaries will perform this maintenance. Thus, hiring a third party to do such work is for the convenience of the beneficiary and is not covered. However, more extensive maintenance which, based on the manufacturers' recommendations, is to be performed by authorized technicians, is covered as repairs for medically necessary equipment which a beneficiary owns. This might include, for example, breaking down sealed components and

performing tests which require specialized testing equipment not available to the beneficiary. Do not pay for maintenance of purchased items that require frequent and substantial servicing or oxygen equipment.

Since renters of equipment recover from the rental charge the expenses they incur in maintaining in working order the equipment they rent out, separately itemized charges for maintenance of rented equipment are generally not covered. Payment may not be made for maintenance of rented equipment other than the maintenance and servicing fee established for capped rental items. For capped rental items which have reached the 15-month rental cap, contractors pay claims for maintenance and servicing fees after 6 months have passed from the end of the final paid rental month or from the end of the period the item is no longer covered under the supplier's or manufacturer's warranty, whichever is later. See the Medicare Claims Processing Manual, Chapter 20, "Durable Medical Equipment, Prosthetics and Orthotics, and Supplies (DMEPOS)," for additional instruction and an example.

A new CMN and/or physician's order is not needed for covered maintenance.

C—Replacement

Replacement refers to the provision of an identical or nearly identical item. Situations involving the provision of a different item because of a change in medical condition are not addressed in this section.

Equipment which the beneficiary owns or is a capped rental item may be replaced in cases of loss or irreparable damage. Irreparable damage refers to a specific accident or to a natural disaster (e.g., fire, flood). A physician's order and/or new Certificate of Medical Necessity (CMN), when required, is needed to reaffirm the medical necessity of the item.

Irreparable wear refers to deterioration sustained from day-to-day usage over time and a specific event cannot be identified. Replacement of equipment due to irreparable wear takes into consideration the reasonable useful lifetime of the equipment. If the item of equipment has been in continuous use by the patient on either a rental or purchase basis for the equipment's useful lifetime, the beneficiary may elect to obtain a new piece of equipment. Replacement may be reimbursed when a new physician order and/or new CMN, when required, is needed to reaffirm the medical necessity of the item.

The reasonable useful lifetime of durable medical equipment is determined through program instructions. In the absence of program instructions, carriers may determine the reasonable useful lifetime of equipment, but in no case can it be less than 5 years. Computation of the useful lifetime is based on when the equipment is delivered to the beneficiary, not the age of the equipment. Replacement due to wear is not covered during the reasonable useful lifetime of the equipment. During the reasonable useful lifetime, Medicare does cover repair up to the cost of replacement (but not actual replacement) for medically necessary equipment owned by the beneficiary. (See subsection A.)

Charges for the replacement of oxygen equipment, items that require frequent and substantial servicing or inexpensive or routinely purchased items which are being rented are not covered.

Cases suggesting malicious damage, culpable neglect, or wrongful disposition of equipment should be investigated and denied where the DMERC determines that it is unreasonable to make program payment under the circumstances. DMERCs refer such cases to the program integrity specialist in the RO.

D—Delivery

Payment for delivery of DME whether rented or purchased is generally included in the fee schedule allowance for the item. See Pub. 100-04, Medicare Claims Processing Manual, Chapter 20, "Durable Medical Equipment, Prosthetics and Orthotics, and Supplies (DMEPOS)," for the rules that apply to making reimbursement for exceptional cases.

110.3—Coverage of Supplies and Accessories

(Rev. 1, 10-01-03)

B3-2100.5, A3-3113.4, HO-235.4, HHA-220.5

Payment may be made for supplies, e.g., oxygen, that are necessary for the effective use of durable medical equipment. Such supplies include those drugs and biologicals which must be put directly into the equipment in order to achieve the therapeutic benefit of the durable medical equipment or to assure the proper functioning of the equipment, e.g., tumor chemotherapy agents used with an infusion pump or heparin used with a home dialysis system. However, the coverage of such drugs or biologicals does not preclude the need for a determination that the drug or biological itself is reasonable and necessary for treatment of the illness or injury or to improve the functioning of a malformed body member.

In the case of prescription drugs, other than oxygen, used in conjunction with durable medical equipment, prosthetic, orthotics, and supplies (DMEPOS) or prosthetic devices, the entity that dispenses the drug must furnish it directly to the patient for whom a prescription is written. The entity that dispenses the drugs must have a Medicare supplier number, must possess a current license to dispense prescription drugs in the State in which the drug is dispensed, and must bill and receive payment in its own name. A supplier that is not the entity that dispenses the drugs cannot purchase the drugs used in conjunction with DME for resale to the beneficiary. Reimbursement may be made for replacement of essential accessories such as hoses, tubes, mouthpieces, etc., for necessary DME, only if the beneficiary owns or is purchasing the equipment.

110.4—Miscellaneous Issues Included in the Coverage of Equipment

(Rev. 1, 10-01-03)

B3-2100.6, A3-3113.5, HO-235.5, HHA-220.6

Payment can be made for the purchase of DME even though rental payments may have been made for prior months. This could occur where, because of a change in his/her condition, the beneficiary feels that it would be to his/her advantage to purchase the equipment rather than to continue to rent it.

A beneficiary may sell or otherwise dispose of equipment for which they have no further use, for example, because of recovery from the illness or injury that gave rise to the need for the equipment. (There is no authority for the program to re-possess the equipment.) If after such disposal there is again medical need for similar equipment, payment can be made for the rental or purchase of that equipment.

However, where an arrangement is motivated solely by a desire to create artificial expenses to be met by the program and to realize a profit thereby, such expenses would not be covered under the program. The resolution of questions involving the disposition and subsequent acquisition of durable medical equipment must be made on a case-by-case basis.

Cases where it appears that there has been an attempt to create an artificial expense and realize a profit thereby should be developed and when appropriate denied. After adjudication the DMERC would refer such cases to the program integrity specialist in the RO.

When payments stop because the beneficiary's condition has changed and the equipment is no longer medically necessary, the beneficiary is responsible for the remaining noncovered charges. Similarly, when payments stop because the beneficiary dies, the beneficiary's estate is responsible for the remaining noncovered charges.

Contractors do not get involved in issues relating to ownership or title of property.

110.5—Incurred Expense Dates for Durable Medical Equipment

(Rev. 1, 10-01-03)

A3-3113.7.B, HO-235.7.B, B3-3011

The date of service on the claim must be the date that the beneficiary or authorized representative received the DME-POS item. If the date of delivery is not specified on the bill, the contractor should assume, in the absence of evidence to the contrary, that the date of purchase was the date of delivery.

For mail order DMEPOS items, the date of service on the claim must be the shipping date.

The date of service on the claim must be the date that the DME-POS item(s) was received by the nursing facility if the supplier delivered it or the shipping date if the supplier utilized a delivery/shipping service.

An exception to the preceding statements concerning the date of service on the claim occurs when items are provided in anticipation of discharge from a hospital or nursing facility. If a DMEPOS item is delivered to a patient in a hospital up to two days prior to discharge to home and it is for the benefit of the patient for purposes of fitting or training of the patient on its use, the supplier should bill the date of service on the claim as the date of discharge to home and should use POS = 12.

See the Medicare Program Integrity Manual, Chapter 5, "Items and Services Having Special DMERC Review Considerations," for additional information pertaining to the date of service on the claim. Also see the Medicare Claims Processing Manual, Chapter 20, "Durable Medical Equipment, Surgical dressings and Casts, Orthotics and Artificial Limbs, and Prosthetic Devices," for additional DME billing and claims processing information.

110.6—Determining Months for Which Periodic Payments May Be Made for Equipment Used in an Institution

(Rev. 1, 10-01-03)

A3-3113.7.D, HO-235.7.C

If a patient uses equipment subject to the monthly payment rule in an institution, which does not qualify as his or her home, the used months during which the beneficiary was institutionalized are not covered.

110.7—No Payment for Purchased Equipment Delivered Outside the United States or Before Beneficiary's Coverage Began

(Rev. 1, 10-01-03)

A3-3113.7.C

In the case of equipment subject to the lump sum payment rules, the beneficiary must have been in the United States and must have had Medicare coverage at the time the item was delivered. Therefore, where an item of durable medical equipment paid for as a lump sum was delivered to an individual outside the United States or before his or her coverage period began, the entire expense of the item would be excluded from coverage. Payment cannot be made in such cases even though the individual later uses the item inside the United States or after his or her coverage begins.

If the individual is outside the U.S. for more than 30 days and then returns to the U.S., the DMERC determines medical necessity as in an initial case before resuming payments.

120—Prosthetic Devices

(Rev. 1, 10-01-03)

B3-2130, A3-3110.4, HO-228.4, A3-3111, HO-229

A—General

Prosthetic devices (other than dental) which replace all or part of an internal body organ (including contiguous tissue), or replace all or part of the function of a permanently inoperative or malfunctioning internal body organ are covered when furnished on a physician's order. This does not require a determination that there is no possibility that the patient's condition may improve sometime in the future. If the medical record, including the judgment of the attending physician, indicates the condition is of long and indefinite duration, the test of permanence is considered met. (Such a device may also be covered under §60.l as a supply when furnished incident to a physician's service.)

Examples of prosthetic devices include artificial limbs, parenteral and enteral (PEN) nutrition, cardiac pacemakers, prosthetic lenses (see subsection B), breast prostheses (including a surgical brassiere) for postmastectomy patients, maxillofacial devices, and devices which replace all or part of the ear or nose. A urinary collection and retention system with or without a tube is a prosthetic device replacing bladder function in case of permanent urinary incontinence. The Foley catheter is also considered a prosthetic device when ordered for a patient with permanent urinary incontinence. However, chucks, diapers, rubber sheets, etc., are supplies that are not covered under this provision. Although hemodialysis equipment is a prosthetic device, payment for the rental or purchase of such equipment in the home is made only for use under the provisions for payment applicable to durable medical equipment.

An exception is that if payment cannot be made on an inpatient's behalf under Part A, hemodialysis equipment, supplies, and services required by such patient could be covered under Part B as a prosthetic device, which replaces the function of a kidney. See the Medicare Benefit Policy Manual, Chapter 11, "End Stage Renal Disease," for payment for hemodialysis equipment used in the home. See the Medicare Benefit Policy Manual, Chapter 1, "Inpatient Hospital Services," §10, for additional instructions on hospitalization for renal dialysis.

NOTE: Medicare does not cover a prosthetic device dispensed to a patient prior to the time at which the patient undergoes the procedure that makes necessary the use of the device. For example, the carrier does not make a separate Part B payment for an intraocular lens (IOL) or pacemaker that a physician, during an office visit prior to the actual surgery, dispenses to the patient for his or her use. Dispensing a prosthetic device in this manner raises health and safety issues. Moreover, the need for the device cannot be clearly established until the procedure that makes its use possible is successfully performed. Therefore, dispensing a prosthetic device in this manner is not considered reasonable and necessary for the treatment of the patient's condition.

Colostomy (and other ostomy) bags and necessary accouterments required for attachment are covered as prosthetic devices. This coverage also includes irrigation and flushing equipment and other items and supplies directly related to ostomy care, whether the attachment of a bag is required.

Accessories and/or supplies which are used directly with an enteral or parenteral device to achieve the therapeutic benefit of the prosthesis or to assure the proper functioning of the device may also be covered under the prosthetic device benefit subject to the additional guidelines in the Medicare National Coverage Determinations Manual.

Covered items include catheters, filters, extension tubing, infusion bottles, pumps (either food or infusion), intravenous (I.V.) pole, needles, syringes, dressings, tape, Heparin Sodium (parenteral only), volumetric monitors (parenteral only), and parenteral and enteral nutrient solutions. Baby food and other regular grocery products that can be blenderized and used with the enteral system are not covered. Note that some of these items, e.g., a food pump and an I.V. pole, qualify as DME. Although coverage of the enteral and parenteral nutritional therapy systems is provided on the basis of the prosthetic device benefit, the payment rules relating to lump sum or monthly payment for DME apply to such items.

The coverage of prosthetic devices includes replacement of and repairs to such devices as explained in subsection D.

Finally, the Benefits Improvement and Protection Act of 2000 amended §1834(h)(1) of the Act by adding a provision (1834 (h)(1)(G)(i)) that requires Medicare payment to be made for the replacement of prosthetic devices which are artificial limbs, or for the replacement of any part of such devices, without regard to continuous use or useful lifetime restrictions if an ordering physician determines that the replacement device, or replacement part of such a device, is necessary.

Payment may be made for the replacement of a prosthetic device that is an artificial limb, or replacement part of a device if the ordering physician determines that the replacement device or part is necessary because of any of the following:

1. A change in the physiological condition of the patient;
2. An irreparable change in the condition of the device, or in a part of the device; or
3. The condition of the device, or the part of the device, requires repairs and the cost of such repairs would be more than 60 percent of the cost of a replacement device, or, as the case may be, of the part being replaced.

This provision is effective for items replaced on or after April 1, 2001. It supersedes any rule that that provided a 5-year or other replacement rule with regard to prosthetic devices.

B—Prosthetic Lenses

The term "internal body organ" includes the lens of an eye. Prostheses replacing the lens of an eye include post-surgical lenses customarily used during convalescence from eye surgery in which the lens of the eye was removed. In addition, permanent lenses are also covered when required by an individual lacking the organic lens of the eye because of surgical removal or congenital absence. Prosthetic lenses obtained on or after the beneficiary's date of entitlement to supplementary medical insurance benefits may be covered even though the surgical removal of the crystalline lens occurred before entitlement.

1. **Prosthetic Cataract Lenses**—One of the following prosthetic lenses or combinations of prosthetic lenses furnished by a physician (see §30.4 for coverage of prosthetic lenses prescribed by a doctor of optometry) may be covered when determined to be reasonable and necessary to restore essentially the vision provided by the crystalline lens of the eye:
   • Prosthetic bifocal lenses in frames;
   • Prosthetic lenses in frames for far vision, and prosthetic lenses in frames for near vision; or
   • When a prosthetic contact lens(es) for far vision is pre scribed (including cases of binocular and monocular aphakia), make payment for the contact lens(es) and prosthetic lenses in frames for near vision to be worn at the same time as the contact lens(es), and prosthetic lenses in frames to be worn when the contacts have been removed.

Lenses which have ultraviolet absorbing or reflecting properties may be covered, in lieu of payment for regular (untinted) lenses, if it has been determined that such lenses are medically reasonable and necessary for the individual patient.

Medicare does not cover cataract sunglasses obtained in addition to the regular (untinted) prosthetic lenses since the sunglasses duplicate the restoration of vision function performed by the regular prosthetic lenses.

2. **Payment for Intraocular Lenses (IOLs) Furnished in Ambulatory Surgical Centers (ASCs)**—Effective for services furnished on or after March 12, 1990, payment for intraocular lenses (IOLs) inserted during or subsequent to cataract surgery in a Medicare certified ASC is included with the payment for facility services that are furnished in connection with the covered surgery.

Refer to the Medicare Claims Processing Manual, Chapter 14, "Ambulatory Surgical Centers," for more information.

3. **Limitation on Coverage of Conventional Lenses**—One pair of conventional eyeglasses or conventional contact lenses furnished after each cataract surgery with insertion of an IOL is covered.

C—Dentures

Dentures are excluded from coverage. However, when a denture or a portion of the denture is an integral part (built-in) of a covered prosthesis (e.g., an obturator to fill an opening in the palate), it is covered as part of that prosthesis.

D—Supplies, Repairs, Adjustments, and Replacement

Supplies are covered that are necessary for the effective use of a prosthetic device (e.g., the batteries needed to operate an artificial larynx). Adjustment of prosthetic devices required by wear or by a change in the patient's condition is covered when ordered by a physician. General provisions relating to the repair and replacement of durable medical equipment in §110.2 for the repair and replacement of prosthetic devices are applicable. (See the Medicare Benefit Policy Manual, Chapter 16, "General Exclusions from Coverage," §40.4, for payment for devices replaced under a warranty.) Replacement of conventional eyeglasses or contact lenses furnished in accordance with §120.B.3 is not covered.

Necessary supplies, adjustments, repairs, and replacements are covered even when the device had been in use before the user enrolled in Part B of the program, so long as the device continues to be medically required.

130—Leg, Arm, Back, and Neck Braces, Trusses, and Artificial Legs, Arms, and Eyes

(Rev. 1, 10-01-03)

B3-2133, A3-3110.5, HO-228.5, AB-01-06 DATED 1/18/01

These appliances are covered under Part B when furnished incident to physicians' services or on a physician's order. A brace includes rigid and semi-rigid devices which are used for the purpose of supporting a weak or deformed body member or restricting or eliminating motion in a diseased or injured part of the body. Elastic stockings, garter belts, and similar devices do not come within the scope of the definition of a brace. Back braces include, but are not limited to, special corsets, e.g., sacroiliac, sacrolumbar, dorsolumbar corsets, and belts. A terminal device (e.g., hand or hook) is covered under this provision whether an artificial limb is required by the patient. Stump stockings and harnesses (including replacements) are also covered when these appliances are essential to the effective use of the artificial limb.

Adjustments to an artificial limb or other appliance required by wear or by a change in the patient's condition are covered when ordered by a physician.

Adjustments, repairs and replacements are covered even when the item had been in use before the user enrolled in Part B of the program so long as the device continues to be medically required.

140—Therapeutic Shoes for Individuals with Diabetes

(Rev. 1, 10-01-03)

B3-2134

Coverage of therapeutic shoes (depth or custom-molded) along with inserts for individuals with diabetes is available as of May 1, 1993. These diabetic shoes are covered if the requirements as specified in this section concerning certification and prescription are fulfilled. In addition, this benefit provides for a pair of diabetic shoes even if only one foot suffers from diabetic foot disease. Each shoe is equally equipped so that the affected limb, as well as the remaining limb, is protected. Claims for therapeutic shoes for diabetics are processed by the Durable Medical Equipment Regional Carriers (DMERCs).

Therapeutic shoes for diabetics are not DME and are not considered DME nor orthotics, but a separate category of coverage under Medicare Part B. (See §1861(s)(12) and §1833(o) of the Act.)

A. Definitions

The following items may be covered under the diabetic shoe benefit:

1. Custom-Molded Shoes

Custom-molded shoes are shoes that:

- Are constructed over a positive model of the patient's foot;
- Are made from leather or other suitable material of equal quality;
- Have removable inserts that can be altered or replaced as the patient's condition warrants; and
- Have some form of shoe closure.

2. Depth Shoes

Depth shoes are shoes that:

- Have a full length, heel-to-toe filler that, when removed, provides a minimum of 3/16 inch of additional depth used to accommodate custom-molded or customized inserts;
- Are made from leather or other suitable material of equal quality;
- Have some form of shoe closure; and
- Are available in full and half sizes with a minimum of three widths so that the sole is graded to the size and width of the upper portions of the shoes according to the American standard last sizing schedule or its equivalent. (The American standard last sizing schedule is the numerical shoe sizing system used for shoes sold in the United States.)

3. Inserts

Inserts are total contact, multiple density, removable inlays that are directly molded to the patient's foot or a model of the patient's foot and that are made of a suitable material with regard to the patient's condition.

B. Coverage

1. Limitations

For each individual, coverage of the footwear and inserts is limited to one of the following within one calendar year:

- No more than one pair of custom-molded shoes (including inserts provided with such shoes) and two additional pairs of inserts; or
- No more than one pair of depth shoes and three pairs of inserts (not including the noncustomized removable inserts provided with such shoes).

2. Coverage of Diabetic Shoes and Brace

Orthopedic shoes, as stated in the Medicare Claims Processing Manual, Chapter 20, "Durable Medical Equipment, Surgical Dressings and Casts, Orthotics and Artificial Limbs, and Prosthetic Devices," generally are not covered. This exclusion does not apply to orthopedic shoes that are an integral part of a leg brace. In situations in which an individual qualifies for both diabetic shoes and a leg brace, these items are covered separately. Thus, the diabetic shoes may be covered if the requirements for this section are met, while the brace may be covered if the requirements of §130 are met.

3. Substitution of Modifications for Inserts

An individual may substitute modification(s) of custom-molded or depth shoes instead of obtaining a pair(s) of inserts in any combination. Payment for the modification(s) may not exceed the limit set for the inserts for which the individual is entitled. The following is a list of the most common shoe modifications available, but it is not meant as an exhaustive list of the modifications available for diabetic shoes:

- **Rigid Rocker Bottoms** - These are exterior elevations with apex positions for 51 percent to 75 percent distance measured from the back end of the heel. The apex is a narrowed or pointed end of an anatomical structure. The apex must be positioned behind the metatarsal heads and tapered off sharply to the front tip of the sole. Apex height helps to eliminate pressure at the metatarsal heads. Rigidity is ensured by the steel in the shoe. The heel of the shoe tapers off in the back in order to cause the heel to strike in the middle of the heel;
- **Roller Bottoms (Sole or Bar)** - These are the same as rocker bottoms, but the heel is tapered from the apex to the front tip of the sole;
- **Metatarsal Bars** - An exterior bar is placed behind the metatarsal heads in order to remove pressure from the metatarsal heads. The bars are of various shapes, heights, and construction depending on the exact purpose;
- **Wedges (Posting)** - Wedges are either of hind foot, fore foot, or both and may be in the middle or to the side. The function is to shift or transfer weight bearing upon standing or during ambulation to the opposite side for added support, stabilization, equalized weight distribution, or balance; and
- **Offset Heels** - This is a heel flanged at its base either in the middle, to the side, or a combination, that is then extended upward to the shoe in order to stabilize extreme positions of the hind foot. Other modifications to diabetic shoes include, but are not limited to flared heels, Velcro closures, and inserts for missing toes.

4. Separate Inserts

Inserts may be covered and dispensed independently of diabetic shoes if the supplier of the shoes verifies in writing that the patient has appropriate footwear into which the insert can be placed. This footwear must meet the definitions found above for depth shoes and custom-molded shoes.

C. Certification

The need for diabetic shoes must be certified by a physician who is a doctor of medicine or a doctor of osteopathy and who is responsible for diagnosing and treating the patient's diabetic systemic condition through a comprehensive plan of care. This managing physician must:

- Document in the patient's medical record that the patient has diabetes;
- Certify that the patient is being treated under a comprehensive plan of care for diabetes, and that the patient needs diabetic shoes; and
- Document in the patient's record that the patient has one or more of the following conditions:
  - Peripheral neuropathy with evidence of callus formation;
  - History of pre-ulcerative calluses;
  - History of previous ulceration;
  - Foot deformity;
  - Previous amputation of the foot or part of the foot; or
  - Poor circulation.

D. Prescription

Following certification by the physician managing the patient's systemic diabetic condition, a podiatrist or other qualified physician who is knowledgeable in the fitting of diabetic shoes and inserts may prescribe the particular type of footwear necessary.

E. Furnishing Footwear

The footwear must be fitted and furnished by a podiatrist or other qualified individual such as a pedorthist, an orthotist, or a prosthetist. The certifying physician may not furnish the diabetic shoes unless the certifying physician is the only qualified individual in the area. It is left to the discretion of each carrier to determine the meaning of "in the area."

150—Dental Services

(Rev. 1, 10-01-03)

B3-2136

As indicated under the general exclusions from coverage, items and services in connection with the care, treatment, filling, removal, or replacement of teeth or structures directly supporting the teeth are not covered. "Structures directly supporting the teeth" means the periodontium, which includes the gingivae, dentogingival junction, periodontal membrane, cementum of the teeth, and alveolar process.

In addition to the following, see Pub 100-01, the Medicare General Information, Eligibility, and Entitlement Manual, Chapter 5, Definitions and Pub 3, the Medicare National Coverage Determinations Manual for specific services which may be covered when furnished by a dentist. If an otherwise non-covered procedure or service is performed by a dentist as incident to and as an integral part of a covered procedure or service performed by the dentist, the total service performed by the dentist on such an occasion is covered.

EXAMPLE 1:

The reconstruction of a ridge performed primarily to prepare the mouth for dentures is a noncovered procedure. However, when the reconstruction of a ridge is performed as a result of and at the same time as the surgical removal of a tumor (for other than dental purposes), the totality of surgical procedures is a covered service.

EXAMPLE 2:

Medicare makes payment for the wiring of teeth when this is done in connection with the reduction of a jaw fracture.

The extraction of teeth to prepare the jaw for radiation treatment of neoplastic disease is also covered. This is an exception to the requirement that to be covered, a noncovered procedure or service performed by a dentist must be an incident to and an integral part of a covered procedure or service performed by the dentist. Ordinarily, the dentist extracts the patient's teeth, but another physician, e.g., a radiologist, administers the radiation treatments.

When an excluded service is the primary procedure involved, it is not covered, regardless of its complexity or difficulty. For example, the extraction of an impacted tooth is not covered. Similarly, an alveoplasty (the surgical improvement of the shape and condition of the alveolar process) and a frenectomy are excluded from coverage when either of these procedures is performed in connection with an excluded service, e.g., the preparation of the mouth for dentures. In a like manner, the removal of a torus palatinus (a bony protuberance of the hard palate) may be a covered service. However, with rare exception, this surgery is performed in connection with an excluded service, i.e., the preparation of the mouth for dentures. Under such circumstances, Medicare does not pay for this procedure.

Dental splints used to treat a dental condition are excluded from coverage under 1862(a)(12) of the Act. On the other hand, if the treatment is determined to be a covered medical condition (i.e., dislocated upper/lower jaw joints), then the splint can be covered. Whether such services as the administration of anesthesia, diagnostic x-rays, and other related procedures are covered depends upon whether the primary procedure being performed by the dentist is itself covered. Thus, an x-ray taken in connection with the reduction of a fracture of the jaw or facial bone is covered. However, a single x-ray or xray survey taken in connection with the care or treatment of teeth or the periodontium is not covered.

Medicare makes payment for a covered dental procedure no matter where the service is performed. The hospitalization or nonhospitalization of a patient has no direct bearing on the coverage or exclusion of a given dental procedure.

Payment may also be made for services and supplies furnished incident to covered dental services. For example, the services of a dental technician or nurse who is under the direct supervision of the dentist or physician are covered if the services are included in the dentist's or physician's bill.

150.1—Treatment of Temporomandibular Joint (TMJ) Syndrome

(Rev. 1, 10-01-03)

PASS MEMO READ.014

There are a wide variety of conditions that can be characterized as TMJ, and an equally wide variety of methods for treating these conditions. Many of the procedures fall within the Medicare program's statutory exclusion that prohibits payment for items and services that have not been demonstrated to be reasonable and necessary for the diagnosis and treatment of illness or injury (§1862(a)(1) of the Act). Other services and appliances used to treat TMJ fall within the Medicare program's statutory exclusion at 1862(a)(12), which prohibits payment "for services in connection with the care, treatment, filling, removal, or replacement of teeth or structures directly supporting teeth...." For these reasons, a diagnosis of TMJ on a claim is insufficient. The actual condition or symptom must be determined.

200—Nurse Practitioner (NP) Services

(Rev. 75, Issued: 08-17-07, Effective: 11-19-07, Implementation: 11-19-07)

Effective for services rendered after January 1, 1998, any individual who is participating under the Medicare program as a nurse practitioner (NP) for the first time ever, may have his or her professional services covered if he or she meets the qualifications listed below, and he or she is legally authorized to furnish NP services in the State where the services are performed. NPs who were issued billing provider numbers prior to January 1, 1998, may continue to furnish services under the NP benefit.

Payment for NP services is effective on the date of service, that is, on or after January 1, 1998, and payment is made on an assignment-related basis only.

A. Qualifications for NPs

In order to furnish covered NP services, an NP must meet the conditions as follows:

- Be a registered professional nurse who is authorized by the State in which the services are furnished to practice as a nurse practitioner in accordance with State law; and be certified as a nurse practitioner by a recognized national certifying body that has established standards for nurse practitioners; or
- Be a registered professional nurse who is authorized by the State in which the services are furnished to practice as a nurse practitioner by December 31, 2000.

The following organizations are recognized national certifying bodies for NPs at the advanced practice level:

- American Academy of Nurse Practitioners;
- American Nurses Credentialing Center;
- National Certification Corporation for Obstetric, Gynecologic and Neonatal Nursing Specialties;
- Pediatric Nursing Certification Board (previously named the National Certification Board of Pediatric Nurse Practitioners and Nurses);
- Oncology Nurses Certification Corporation;
- AACN Certification Corporation; and
- National Board on Certification of Hospice and Palliative Nurses.

The NPs applying for a Medicare billing number for the first time on or after January 1, 2001, must meet the requirements as follows:

- Be a registered professional nurse who is authorized by the State in which the services are furnished to practice as a nurse practitioner in accordance with State law; and

- Be certified as a nurse practitioner by a recognized national certifying body that has established standards for nurse practitioners.

The NPs applying for a Medicare billing number for the first time on or after January 1, 2003, must meet the requirements as follows:

- Be a registered professional nurse who is authorized by the State in which the services are furnished to practice as a nurse practitioner in accordance with State law;
- Be certified as a nurse practitioner by a recognized national certifying body that has established standards for nurse practitioners; and
- Possess a master's degree in nursing.

B. Covered Services

Coverage is limited to the services an NP is legally authorized to perform in accordance with State law (or State regulatory mechanism established by State law).

1. General

The services of an NP may be covered under Part B if all of the following conditions are met:

- They are the type that are considered physician's services if furnished by a doctor of medicine or osteopathy (MD/DO);
- They are performed by a person who meets the definition of an NP (see subsection A);
- The NP is legally authorized to perform the services in the State in which they are performed;
- They are performed in collaboration with an MD/DO (see subsection D); and
- They are not otherwise precluded from coverage because of one of the statutory exclusions. (See subsection C.2.)

2. Incident To

If covered NP services are furnished, services and supplies furnished incident to the services of the NP may also be covered if they would have been covered when furnished incident to the services of an MD/DO as described in §60.

C. Application of Coverage Rules

1. Types of NP Services That May Be Covered

State law or regulation governing an NP's scope of practice in the State in which the services are performed applies. Consider developing a list of covered services based on the State scope of practice. Examples of the types of services that NP's may furnish include services that traditionally have been reserved to physicians, such as physical examinations, minor surgery, setting casts for simple fractures, interpreting x-rays, and other activities that involve an independent evaluation or treatment of the patient's condition. Also, if authorized under the scope of their State license, NPs may furnish services billed under all levels of evaluation and management codes and diagnostic tests if furnished in collaboration with a physician.

See §60.2 for coverage of services performed by NPs incident to the services of physicians.

2. Services Otherwise Excluded From Coverage

The NP services may not be covered if they are otherwise excluded from coverage even though an NP may be authorized by State law to perform them. For example, the Medicare law excludes from coverage routine foot care, routine physical checkups, and services that are not reasonable and necessary for the diagnosis or treatment of an illness or injury or to improve the functioning of a malformed body member. Therefore, these services are precluded from coverage even though they may be within an NP's scope of practice under State law.

D. Collaboration

Collaboration is a process in which an NP works with one or more physicians (MD/DO) to deliver health care services, with medical direction and appropriate supervision as required by the law of the State in which the services are furnished. In the absence of State law governing collaboration, collaboration is to be evidenced by NPs documenting their scope of practice and indicating the relationships that they have with physicians to deal with issues outside their scope of practice.

The collaborating physician does not need to be present with the NP when the services are furnished or to make an independent evaluation of each patient who is seen by the NP.

E. Direct Billing and Payment

Direct billing and payment for NP services may be made to the NP.

F. Assignment

Assignment is mandatory.

230—Practice of Physical Therapy, Occupational Therapy, and Speech-Language Pathology

(Rev. 63, Issued: 12-29-06, Effective: 01-01-07, Implementation: on or before 01-29-07)

A. Group Therapy Services. Contractors pay for outpatient physical therapy services (which includes outpatient speech-language pathology services) and outpatient occupational therapy services provided simultaneously to two or more individuals by a practitioner as group therapy services (97150). The individuals can be, but need not be performing the same activity. The physician or therapist involved in group therapy services must be in constant attendance, but one-on-one patient contact is not required.

B. Therapy Students

1. General

Only the services of the therapist can be billed and paid under Medicare Part B. The services performed by a student are not reimbursed even if provided under "line of sight" supervision of the therapist; however, the presence of the student "in the room" does not make the service unbillable. Pay for the direct (one-to-one) patient contact services of the physician or therapist provided to Medicare Part B patients. Group therapy services performed by a therapist or physician may be billed when a student is also present "in the room".

EXAMPLES:

Therapists may bill and be paid for the provision of services in the following scenarios:

- The qualified practitioner is present and in the room for the entire session. The student participates in the delivery of services when the qualified practitioner is directing the service, making the skilled judgment, and is responsible for the assessment and treatment.
- The qualified practitioner is present in the room guiding the student in service delivery when the therapy student and the therapy assistant student are participating in the provision of services, and the practitioner is not engaged in treating another patient or doing other tasks at the same time.
- The qualified practitioner is responsible for the services and as such, signs all documentation. (A student may, of course, also sign but it is not necessary since the Part B payment is for the clinician's service, not for the student's services).

2. Therapy Assistants as Clinical Instructors

Physical therapist assistants and occupational therapy assistants are not precluded from serving as clinical instructors for therapy students, while providing services within their scope of work and performed under the direction and supervision of a licensed physical or occupational therapist to a Medicare beneficiary.

3. Services Provided Under Part A and Part B

The payment methodologies for Part A and B therapy services rendered by a student are different. Under the MPFS (Medicare Part B), Medicare pays for services provided by physicians and practitioners that are specifically authorized by statute. Students do not meet the definition of practitioners under Medicare Part B. Under SNF PPS, payments are based upon the case mix or Resource Utilization Group (RUG) category that describes the patient. In the rehabilitation groups, the number of therapy minutes delivered to the patient determines the RUG category. Payment levels for each category are based upon the costs of caring for patients in each group rather than providing specific payment for each therapy service as is done in Medicare Part B.

230.1—Practice of Physical Therapy

(Rev. 88, Issued: 05-07-08, Effective: 01-01-08, Implementation: 06-09-08)

A—General

Physical therapy services are those services provided within the scope of practice of physical therapists and necessary for the diagnosis and treatment of impairments, functional limitations, disabilities or changes in physical function and health status. (See Pub. 100-03, the Medicare National Coverage Determinations Manual, for specific conditions or services.) For descriptions of aquatic therapy in a community center pool see section 220C of this chapter.

B—Qualified Physical Therapist Defined

Reference: 42CFR484.4

The new personnel qualifications for physical therapists were discussed in the 2008 Physician Fee Schedule. See the Federal Register of November 27, 2007, for the full text. See also the correction notice for this rule, published in the Federal Register on January 15, 2008.

The regulation provides that a qualified physical therapist (PT) is a person who is licensed, if applicable, as a PT by the state in which he or she is practicing unless licensure does not apply, has graduated from an accredited PT education program and passed a national examination approved by the state in which PT services are provided. The phrase, "by the state in which practicing" includes any authorization to practice provided by the same state in which the service is provided, including temporary licensure, regardless of the location of the entity billing the services. The curriculum accreditation is provided by the Commission on Accreditation in Physical Therapy Education (CAPTE) or, for those who graduated before CAPTE, curriculum approval was provided by the American Physical Therapy Association (APTA). For internationally educated PTs, curricula are approved by a credentials evaluation organization either approved by the APTA or identified in 8 CFR 212.15(e) as it relates to PTs. For example, in 2007, 8 CFR 212.15(e) approved the credentials evaluation provided by the Federation of State Boards of Physical Therapy (FSBPT) and the Foreign Credentialing Commission on Physical Therapy (FCCPT). The requirements above apply to all PTs effective January 1, 2010, if they have not met any of the following requirements prior to January 1, 2010.

Physical therapists whose current license was obtained on or prior to December 31, 2009, qualify to provide PT services to Medicare beneficiaries if they:

- graduated from a CAPTE approved program in PT on or before December 31, 2009 (examination is not required); or,
- graduated on or before December 31, 2009, from a PT program outside the U.S. that is determined to be substantially equivalent to a U.S. program by a credentials evaluating organization approved by either the APTA or identified in 8 CFR 212.15(e) and also passed an examination for PTs approved by the state in which practicing.

Or, PTs whose current license was obtained before January 1, 2008, may meet the requirements in place on that date (i.e., graduation from a curriculum approved by either the APTA, the Committee on Allied Health Education and Accreditation of the American Medical Association, or both).

Or, PTs meet the requirements who are currently licensed and were licensed or qualified as a PT on or before December 31, 1977, and had 2 years appropriate experience as a PT, and passed a proficiency examination conducted, approved, or sponsored by the U.S. Public Health Service.

Or, PTs meet the requirements if they are currently licensed and before January 1, 1966, they were:

- admitted to membership by the APTA; or
- admitted to registration by the American Registry of Physical Therapists; or
- graduated from a 4-year PT curriculum approved by a State Department of Education; or
- licensed or registered and prior to January 1, 1970, they had 15 years of fulltime experience in PT under the order

and direction of attending and referring doctors of medicine or osteopathy.

Or, PTs meet requirements if they are currently licensed and they were trained outside the U.S. before January 1, 2008, and after 1928 graduated from a PT curriculum approved in the country in which the curriculum was located, if that country had an organization that was a member of the World Confederation for Physical Therapy, and that PT qualified as a member of the organization.

For outpatient PT services that are provided incident to the services of physicians/NPPs, the requirement for PT licensure does not apply; all other personnel qualifications do apply. The qualified personnel providing PT services incident to the services of a physician/NPP must be trained in an accredited PT curriculum. For example, a person who, on or before December 31, 2009, graduated from a PT curriculum accredited by CAPTE, but who has not passed the national examination or obtained a license, could provide Medicare outpatient PT therapy services incident to the services of a physician/NPP if the physician assumes responsibility for the services according to the incident to policies. On or after January 1, 2010, although licensure does not apply, both education and examination requirements that are effective January 1, 2010, apply to qualified personnel who provide PT services incident to the services of a physician/NPP.

C—Services of Physical Therapy Support Personnel

Reference: 42CFR 484.4

Personnel Qualifications. The new personnel qualifications for physical therapist assistants (PTA) were discussed in the 2008 Physician Fee Schedule. See the Federal Register of November 27, 2007, for the full text. See also the correction notice for this rule, published in the Federal Register on January 15, 2008.

The regulation provides that a qualified PTA is a person who is licensed as a PTA unless licensure does not apply, is registered or certified, if applicable, as a PTA by the state in which practicing, and graduated from an approved curriculum for PTAs, and passed a national examination for PTAs. The phrase, "by the state in which practicing" includes any authorization to practice provided by the same state in which the service is provided, including temporary licensure, regardless of the location or the entity billing for the services. Approval for the curriculum is provided by CAPTE or, if internationally or military trained PTAs apply, approval will be through a credentialing body for the curriculum for PTAs identified by either the American Physical Therapy Association or identified in 8 CFR 212.15(e). A national examination for PTAs is, for example the one furnished by the Federation of State Boards of Physical Therapy. These requirements above apply to all PTAs effective January 1, 2010, if they have not met any of the following requirements prior to January 1, 2010.

Those PTAs also qualify who, on or before December 31, 2009, are licensed, registeredor certified as a PTA and met one of the two following requirements:

1. Is licensed or otherwise regulated in the state in which practicing; or
2. In states that have no licensure or other regulations, or where licensure does not apply, PTAs have:

- graduated on or before December 31, 2009, from a 2-year college-level program approved by the APTA or CAPTE; and
- effective January 1, 2010, those PTAs must have both graduated from a CAPTE approved curriculum and passed a national examination for PTAs; or

PTAs may also qualify if they are licensed, registered or certified as a PTA, if applicable and meet requirements in effect before January 1, 2008, that is,

- they have graduated before January 1, 2008, from a 2 year college level program approved by the APTA; or
- on or before December 31, 1977, they were licensed or qualified as a PTA and passed a proficiency examination conducted, approved, or sponsored by the U.S. Public Health Service.

Services. The services of PTAs used when providing covered therapy benefits are included as part of the covered service. These services are billed by the supervising physical therapist. PTAs may not provide evaluation services, make clinical judgments or decisions or take responsibility for the service. They act at the direction and under the supervision of the treating physical therapist and in accordance with state laws.

A physical therapist must supervise PTAs. The level and frequency of supervision differs by setting (and by state or local law). General supervision is required for PTAs in all settings except private practice (which requires direct supervision) unless state practice requirements are more stringent, in which case state or local requirements must be followed. See specific settings for details. For example, in clinics, rehabilitation agencies, and public health agencies, 42CFR485.713 indicates that when a PTA provides services, either on or off the organization's premises, those services are supervised by a qualified physical therapist who makes an onsite supervisory visit at least once every 30 days or more frequently if required by state or local laws or regulation.

The services of a PTA shall not be billed as services incident to a physician/NPP's service, because they do not meet the qualifications of a therapist.

The cost of supplies (e.g., theraband, hand putty, electrodes) used in furnishing covered therapy care is included in the payment for the HCPCS codes billed by the physical therapist, and are, therefore, not separately billable. Separate coverage and billing provisions apply to items that meet the definition of brace in §130.

Services provided by aides, even if under the supervision of a therapist, are not therapy services in the outpatient setting and are not covered by Medicare. Although an aide may help the therapist by providing unskilled services, those services that are unskilled are not covered by Medicare and shall be denied as not reasonable and necessary if they are billed as therapy services.

D—Application of Medicare Guidelines to PT Services

This subsection will be used in the future to illustrate the application of the above guidelines to some of the physical therapy modalities and procedures utilized in the treatment of patients.

230.2—Practice of Occupational Therapy

(Rev. 88, Issued: 05-07-08, Effective: 01-01-08, Implementation: 06-09-08)

A—General

Occupational therapy services are those services provided within the scope of practice of occupational therapists and necessary for the diagnosis and treatment of impairments, functional disabilities or changes in physical function and health status. (See Pub. 100-03, the Medicare National Coverage Determinations Manual, for specific conditions or services.)

Occupational therapy is medically prescribed treatment concerned with improving or restoring functions which have been impaired by illness or injury or, where function has been permanently lost or reduced by illness or injury, to improve the individual's ability to perform those tasks required for independent functioning. Such therapy may involve:

The evaluation, and reevaluation as required, of a patient's level of function by administering diagnostic and prognostic tests;

The selection and teaching of task-oriented therapeutic activities designed to restore physical function; e.g., use of woodworking activities on an inclined table to restore shoulder, elbow, and wrist range of motion lost as a result of burns;

The planning, implementing, and supervising of individualized therapeutic activity programs as part of an overall "active treatment" program for a patient with a diagnosed psychiatric illness; e.g., the use of sewing activities which require following a pattern to reduce confusion and restore reality orientation in a schizophrenic patient;

The planning and implementing of therapeutic tasks and activities to restore sensory-integrative function; e.g., providing motor and tactile activities to increase sensory input and improve response for a stroke patient with functional loss resulting in a distorted body image;

The teaching of compensatory technique to improve the level of independence in the activities of daily living, for example:

- Teaching a patient who has lost the use of an arm how to pare potatoes and chop vegetables with one hand;
- Teaching an upper extremity amputee how to functionally utilize a prosthesis;
- Teaching a stroke patient new techniques to enable the patient to perform feeding, dressing, and other activities as independently as possible; or
- Teaching a patient with a hip fracture/hip replacement techniques of standing tolerance and balance to enable the patient to perform such functional activities as dressing and homemaking tasks.

The designing, fabricating, and fitting of orthotics and self-help devices; e.g., making a hand splint for a patient with rheumatoid arthritis to maintain the hand in a functional position or constructing a device which would enable an individual to hold a utensil and feed independently; or

Vocational and prevocational assessment and training, subject to the limitations specified in item B below.

Only a qualified occupational therapist has the knowledge, training, and experience required to evaluate and, as necessary, reevaluate a patient's level of function, determine whether an occupational therapy program could reasonably be expected to improve, restore, or compensate for lost function and, where appropriate, recommend to the physician/ NPP a plan of treatment.

B—Qualified Occupational Therapist Defined

Reference: 42CFR484.4

The new personnel qualifications for occupational therapists (OT) were discussed in the 2008 Physician Fee Schedule. See the Federal Register of November 27, 2007, for the full text. See also the correction notice for this rule, published in the Federal Register on January 15, 2008.

The regulation provides that a qualified OT is an individual who is licensed, if licensure applies, or otherwise regulated, if applicable, as an OT by the state in which practicing, and graduated from an accredited education program for OTs, and is eligible to take or has passed the examination for OTs administered by the National Board for Certification in Occupational Therapy, Inc. (NBCOT). The phrase, "by the state in which practicing" includes any authorization to practice provided by the same state in which the service is provided, including temporary licensure, regardless of the location of the entity billing the services. The education program for U.S. trained OTs is accredited by the Accreditation Council for Occupational Therapy Education (ACOTE). The requirements above apply to all OTs effective January 1, 2010, if they have not met any of the following requirements prior to January 1, 2010.

The OTs may also qualify if on or before December 31, 2009:

- they are licensed or otherwise regulated as an OT in the state in which practicing (regardless of the qualifications they met to obtain that licensure or regulation); or
- when licensure or other regulation does not apply, OTs have graduated from an OT education program accredited by ACOTE and are eligible to take, or have successfully completed the NBCOT examination for OTs.

Also, those OTs who met the Medicare requirements for OTs that were in 42CFR484.4 prior to January 1, 2008, qualify to provide OT services for Medicare beneficiaries if:

- on or before January 1, 2008, they graduated an OT program approved jointly by the American Medical Association and the AOTA, or
- they are eligible for the National Registration Examination of AOTA or the National Board for Certification in OT.

Also, they qualify who on or before December 31, 1977, had 2 years of appropriate experience as an occupational therapist, and had achieved a satisfactory grade on a proficiency examination conducted, approved, or sponsored by the U.S. Public Health Service.

Those educated outside the U.S. may meet the same qualifications for domestic trained OTs. For example, they qualify if they were licensed or otherwise regulated by the state in which practicing on or before December 31, 2009. Or they are qualified if they:

- graduated from an OT education program accredited as substantially equivalent to a U.S. OT education program by ACOTE, the World Federation of Occupational Therapists, or a credentialing body approved by AOTA; and
- passed the NBCOT examination for OT; and

- Effective January 1, 2010, are licensed or otherwise regulated, if applicable as an OT by the state in which practicing.

For outpatient OT services that are provided incident to the services of physicians/NPPs, the requirement for OT licensure does not apply; all other personnel qualifications do apply. The qualified personnel providing OT services incident to the services of a physician/NPP must be trained in an accredited OT curriculum. For example, a person who, on or before December 31, 2009, graduated from an OT curriculum accredited by ACOTE and is eligible to take or has successfully completed the entry-level certification examination for OTs developed and administered by NBCOT, could provide Medicare outpatient OT services incident to the services of a physician/NPP if the physician assumes responsibility for the services according to the incident to policies. On or after January 1, 2010, although licensure does not apply, both education and examination requirements that are effective January 1, 2010, apply to qualified personnel who provide OT services incident to the services of a physician/NPP.

C—Services of Occupational Therapy Support Personnel

Reference: 42CFR 484.4

The new personnel qualifications for occupational therapy assistants were discussed in the 2008 Physician Fee Schedule. See the Federal Register of November 27, 2007, for the full text. See also the correction notice for this rule, published in the Federal Register on January 15, 2008.

The regulation provides that an occupational therapy assistant is a person who is licensed, unless licensure does not apply, or otherwise regulated, if applicable, as an OTA by the state in which practicing, and graduated from an OTA education program accredited by ACOTE and is eligible to take or has successfully completed the NBCOT examination for OTAs. The phrase, "by the state in which practicing" includes any authorization to practice provided by the same state in which the service is provided, including temporary licensure, regardless of the location of the entity billing the services.

If the requirements above are not met, an OTA may qualify if, on or before December 31, 2009, the OTA is licensed or otherwise regulated as an OTA, if applicable, by the state in which practicing, or meets any qualifications defined by the state in which practicing.

Or, where licensure or other state regulation does not apply, OTAs may qualify if they have, on or before December 31, 2009:

- completed certification requirements to practice as an OTA established by a credentialing organization approved by AOTA; and
- after January 1, 2010, they have also completed an education program accredited by ACOTE and passed the NBCOT examination for OTAs.

OTAs who qualified under the policies in effect prior to January 1, 2008, continue to qualify to provide OT directed and supervised OTA services to Medicare beneficiaries. Therefore, OTAs qualify who after December 31, 1977, and on or before December 31, 2007:

- completed certification requirements to practice as an OTA established by a credentialing organization approved by AOTA; or

- completed the requirements to practice as an OTA applicable in the state in which practicing.

Those OTAs who were educated outside the U.S. may meet the same requirements as domestically trained OTAs. Or, if educated outside the U.S. on or after January 1, 2008, they must have graduated from an OTA program accredited as substantially equivalent to OTA entry level education in the U.S. by ACOTE, its successor organization, or the World Federation of Occupational Therapists or a credentialing body approved by AOTA. In addition, they must have passed an exam for OTAs administered by NBCOT.

Services. The services of OTAs used when providing covered therapy benefits are included as part of the covered service. These services are billed by the supervising occupational therapist. OTAs may not provide evaluation services, make clinical judgments or decisions or take responsibility for the service. They act at the direction and under the supervision of the treating occupational therapist and in accordance with state laws.

An occupational therapist must supervise OTAs. The level and frequency of supervision differs by setting (and by state or local law). General supervision is required for OTAs in all settings except private practice (which requires direct supervision) unless state practice requirements are more stringent, in which case state or local requirements must be followed. See specific settings for details. For example, in clinics, rehabilitation agencies, and public health agencies, 42CFR485.713 indicates that when an OTA provides services, either on or off the organization's premises, those services are supervised by a qualified occupational therapist who makes an onsite supervisory visit at least once every 30 days or more frequently if required by state or local laws or regulation.

The services of an OTA shall not be billed as services incident to a physician/NPP's service, because they do not meet the qualifications of a therapist.

The cost of supplies (e.g., looms, ceramic tiles, or leather) used in furnishing covered therapy care is included in the payment for the HCPCS codes billed by the occupational therapist and are, therefore, not separately billable. Separate coverage and billing provisions apply to items that meet the definition of brace in §130 of this manual.

Services provided by aides, even if under the supervision of a therapist, are not therapy services in the outpatient setting and are not covered by Medicare. Although an aide may help the therapist by providing unskilled services, those services that are unskilled are not covered by Medicare and shall be denied as not reasonable and necessary if they are billed as therapy services.

D—Application of Medicare Guidelines to Occupational Therapy Services

Occupational therapy may be required for a patient with a specific diagnosed psychiatric illness. If such services are required, they are covered assuming the coverage criteria are met. However, where an individual's motivational needs are not related to a specific diagnosed psychiatric illness, the meeting of such needs does not usually require an individualized therapeutic program. Such needs can be met through general activity programs or the efforts of other professional personnel involved in the care of the patient. Patient motivation is an appropriate and inherent function of all health disciplines, which is interwoven with other functions performed by such personnel for the patient. Accordingly, since the special skills of an occupational therapist are not required, an occupational therapy program for individuals who do not have a specific diagnosed psychiatric illness is not to be considered reasonable and necessary for the treatment of an illness or injury. Services furnished under such a program are not covered.

Occupational therapy may include vocational and prevocational assessment and training. When services provided by an occupational therapist are related solely to specific employment opportunities, work skills, or work settings, they are not reasonable or necessary for the diagnosis or treatment of an illness or injury and are not covered. However, carriers and intermediaries exercise care in applying this exclusion, because the assessment of level of function and the teaching of compensatory techniques to improve the level of function, especially in activities of daily living, are services which occupational therapists provide for both vocational and nonvocational purposes. For example, an assessment of sitting and standing tolerance might be nonvocational for a mother of young children or a retired individual living alone, but could also be a vocational test for a sales clerk. Training an amputee in the use of prosthesis for telephoning is necessary for everyday activities as well as for employment purposes. Major changes in life style may be mandatory for an individual with a substantial disability. The techniques of adjustment cannot be considered exclusively vocational or nonvocational.

230.3—Practice of Speech-Language Pathology

(Rev. 88, Issued: 05-07-08, Effective: 01-01-08, Implementation: 06-09-08)

A—GENERAL

Speech-language pathology services are those services provided within the scope of practice of speech-language pathologists and necessary for the diagnosis and treatment of speech and language disorders, which result in communication disabilities and for the diagnosis and treatment of swallowing disorders (dysphagia), regardless of the presence of a communication disability. (See Pub. 100-03, chapter 1, §170.3)

B—Qualified Speech-Language Pathologist Defined

A qualified speech-language pathologist for program coverage purposes meets one of the following requirements:

- The education and experience requirements for a Certificate of Clinical Competence in (speech-language pathology or audiology) granted by the American Speech-Language Hearing Association; or
- Meets the educational requirements for certification and is in the process of accumulating the supervised experience required for certification.

For outpatient speech-language pathology services that are provided incident to the services of physicians/NPPs, the requirement for speech-language pathology licensure does not apply; all other personnel qualifications do apply. Therefore, qualified personnel providing speech-language pathology services incident to the services of a physician/NPP must meet the above qualifications.

C—Services of Speech-Language Pathology Support Personnel

Services of speech-language pathology assistants are not recognized for Medicare coverage. Services provided by speech-language pathology assistants, even if they are licensed to provide services in their states, will be considered unskilled services and denied as not reasonable and necessary if they are billed as therapy services.

Services provided by aides, even if under the supervision of a therapist, are not therapy services and are not covered by Medicare. Although an aide may help the therapist by providing unskilled services, those services are not covered by Medicare and shall be denied as not reasonable and necessary if they are billed as therapy services.

D—Application of Medicare Guidelines to Speech-Language Pathology Services

1—Evaluation Services

Speech-language pathology evaluation services are covered if they are reasonable and necessary and not excluded as routine screening by §1862(a)(7) of the Act. The speech-language pathologist employs a variety of formal and informal speech, language, and dysphagia assessment tests to ascertain the type, causal factor(s), and severity of the speech and language or swallowing disorders. Reevaluation of patients for whom speech, language, and swallowing were previously contraindicated is covered only if the patient exhibits a change in medical condition. However, monthly reevaluations; e.g., a Western Aphasia Battery, for a patient undergoing a rehabilitative speech-language pathology program, are considered a part of the treatment session and shall not be covered as a separate evaluation for billing purposes. Although hearing screening by the speech-language pathologist may be part of an evaluation, it is not billable as a separate service.

2—Therapeutic Services

The following are examples of common medical disorders and resulting communication deficits, which may necessitate active rehabilitative therapy. This list is not all-inclusive:

Cerebrovascular disease such as cerebral vascular accidents presenting with dysphagia, aphasia/dysphasia, apraxia, and dysarthria;

Neurological disease such as Parkinsonism or Multiple Sclerosis with dysarthria, dysphagia, inadequate respiratory volume/control, or voice disorder; or

Laryngeal carcinoma requiring laryngectomy resulting in aphonia.

3—Impairments of the Auditory System

The terms, aural rehabilitation, auditory rehabilitation, auditory processing, lipreading and speech reading are among the terms used to describe covered services related to perception and comprehension of sound through the auditory system. See Pub. 100-04, chapter 12, section 30.3 for billing instructions. For example:

- Auditory processing evaluation and treatment may be covered and medically necessary. Examples include but are not limited to services for certain neurological impairments or the absence of natural auditory stimulation that results in impaired ability to process sound. Certain auditory processing disorders require diagnostic audiological tests in addition to speech-language pathology evaluation and treatment.

- Evaluation and treatment for disorders of the auditory system may be covered and medically necessary, for example, when it has been determined by a speech-language pathologist in collaboration with an audiologist that the hearing impaired beneficiary's current amplification options (hearing aid, other amplification device or cochlear implant) will not sufficiently meet the patient's functional communication needs. Audiologists and speech-language pathologists both evaluate beneficiaries for disorders of the auditory system using different skills and techniques, but only speech-language pathologists may provide treatment.

Assessment for the need for rehabilitation of the auditory system (but not the vestibular system) may be done by a speech language pathologist. Examples include but are not limited to: evaluation of comprehension and production of language in oral, signed or written modalities, speech and voice production, listening skills, speech reading, communications strategies, and the impact of the hearing loss on the patient/client and family.

Examples of rehabilitation include but are not limited to treatment that focuses on comprehension, and production of language in oral, signed or written modalities; speech and voice production, auditory training, speech reading, multimodal (e.g., visual, auditory-visual, and tactile) training, communication strategies, education and counseling. In determining the necessity for treatment, the beneficiary's performance in both clinical and natural environment should be considered.

4—Dysphagia

Dysphagia, or difficulty in swallowing, can cause food to enter the airway, resulting in coughing, choking, pulmonary problems, aspiration, or inadequate nutrition and hydration with resultant weight loss, failure to thrive, pneumonia, and death. It is most often due to complex neurological and/or structural impairments including head and neck trauma, cerebrovascular accident, neuromuscular degenerative diseases, head and neck cancer, dementias, and encephalopathies. For these reasons, it is important that only qualified professionals with specific training and experience in this disorder provide evaluation and treatment.

The speech-language pathologist performs clinical and instrumental assessments and analyzes and integrates the diagnostic information to determine candidacy for intervention as well as appropriate compensations and rehabilitative therapy techniques. The equipment that is used in the examination may be fixed, mobile, or portable. Professional guidelines recommend that the service be provided in a team setting with a physician/NPP who provides supervision of the radiological examination and interpretation of medical conditions revealed in it.

Swallowing assessment and rehabilitation are highly specialized services. The professional rendering care must have education, experience, and demonstrated competencies. Competencies include but are not limited to: identifying abnormal upper aero-digestive tract structure and function; conducting an oral, pharyngeal, laryngeal and respiratory function examination as it relates to the functional assessment of swallowing; recommending methods of oral intake and risk precautions; and developing a treatment plan employing appropriate compensations and therapy techniques.

230.4—Services Furnished by a Physical or Occupational Therapist in Private Practice

(Rev. 88, Issued: 05-07-08, Effective: 01-01-08, Implementation: 06-09-08)

A—GENERAL

In order to qualify to bill Medicare directly as a therapist, each individual must be enrolled as a private practitioner and employed in one of the following practice types: an unincorporated solo practice, unincorporated partnership, unincorporated group practice, physician/NPP group or groups that are not professional corporations, if allowed by state and local law. Physician/NPP group practices may employ physical therapists in private practice (PTPP) and/or occupational therapists in private practice (OTPP) if state and local law permits this employee relationship.

For purposes of this provision, a physician/NPP group practice is defined as one or more physicians/NPPs enrolled with Medicare who may bill as one entity. For further details on issues concerning enrollment, see the provider enrollment Web site at www.cms.hhs.gov/providers/enrollment.

Private practice also includes therapists who are practicing therapy as employees of another supplier, of a professional corporation or other incorporated therapy practice. Private practice does not include individuals when they are working as employees of an institutional provider.

Services should be furnished in the therapist's or group's office or in the patient's home. The office is defined as the location(s) where the practice is operated, in the state(s) where the therapist (and practice, if applicable) is legally authorized to furnish services, during the hours that the therapist engages in the practice at that location. If services are furnished in a private practice office space, that space shall be owned, leased, or rented by the practice and used for the exclusive purpose of operating the practice. For descriptions of aquatic therapy in a community center pool see section 220C of this chapter.

Therapists in private practice must be approved as meeting certain requirements, but do not execute a formal provider agreement with the Secretary.

If therapists who have their own Medicare Personal Identification number (PIN) or National Provider Identifier (NPI) are employed by therapist groups, physician/NPP groups, or groups that are not professional organizations, the requirement that therapy space be owned, leased, or rented may be satisfied by the group that employs the therapist. Each physical or occupational therapist employed by a group should enroll as a PT or OT in private practice.

When therapists with a Medicare PIN/NPI provide services in the physician's/NPP's office in which they are employed, and bill using their PIN/NPI for each therapy service, then the direct supervision requirement for PTAs and OTAs apply.

When the PT or OT who has a Medicare PIN/NPI is employed in a physician's/NPP's office the services are ordinarily billed as services of the PT or OT, with the PT or OT identified on the claim as the supplier of services. However, services of the PT or OT who has a Medicare PIN/NPI may also be billed by the physician/NPP as services incident to the physician's/NPP's service. (See §230.5 for rules related to PTA and OTA services incident to a physician.) In that case, the physician/NPP is the supplier of service, the Unique Provider Identification Number (UPIN) or NPI of the physician/NPP (ordering or supervising, as indicated) is reported on the claim with the service and all the rules for incident to services (§230.5) must be followed.

B—Private Practice Defined

Reference: **Federal Register** November, 1998, pages 58863-58869; 42CFR 410.38(b)

The carrier considers a therapist to be in private practice if the therapist maintains office space at his or her own expense and furnishes services only in that space or the patient's home. Or, a therapist is employed by another supplier and furnishes services in facilities provided at the expense of that supplier.

The therapist need not be in full-time private practice but must be engaged in private practice on a regular basis; i.e., the therapist is recognized as a private practitioner and for that purpose has access to the necessary equipment to provide an adequate program of therapy.

The physical or occupational therapy services must be provided either by or under the direct supervision of the therapist in private practice. Each physical or occupational therapist in a practice should be enrolled as a Medicare provider. If a physical or occupational therapist is not enrolled, the services of that therapist must be directly supervised by an enrolled physical or occupational therapist. Direct supervision requires that the supervising private practice therapist be present in the office suite at the time the service is performed. These direct supervision requirements apply only in the private practice setting and only for physical therapists and occupational therapists and their assistants. In other outpatient settings, supervision rules differ. The services of support personnel must be included in the therapist's bill. The supporting personnel, including other therapists, must be W-2 or 1099 employees of the therapist in private practice or other qualified employer.

Coverage of outpatient physical therapy and occupational therapy under Part B includes the services of a qualified therapist in private practice when furnished in the therapist's office or the beneficiary's home. For this purpose, "home" includes an institution that is used as a home, but not a hospital, CAH or SNF, (**Federal Register** Nov. 2, 1998, pg 58869). Place of Service (POS) includes:

- 03/School, only if residential,
- 04/Homeless Shelter,
- 12/Home, other than a facility that is a private residence,
- 14/Group Home,
- 33/Custodial Care Facility.

C—Assignment

Reference: Nov. 2, 1998 **Federal Register,** pg. 58863
          See also Pub. 100-04 chapter 1, 30.2.

When physicians, NPPs, PTPPs or OTPPs obtain provider numbers, they have the option of accepting assignment (participating) or not accepting assignment (nonparticipating). In contrast, providers, such as outpatient hospitals, SNFs, rehabilitation agencies, and CORFs, do not have the option. For these providers, assignment is mandatory.

If physicians/NPPs, PTPPs or OTPPs accept assignment (are participating), they must accept the Medicare Physician Fee Schedule amount as payment. Medicare pays 80% and the patient is responsible for 20%. In contrast, if they do not accept assignment, Medicare will only pay 95% of the fee schedule amount. However, when these services are not furnished on an assignment-related basis, the limiting charge applies. (See §1848(g)(2)(c) of the Act.)

NOTE: Services furnished by a therapist in the therapist's office under arrangements with hospitals in rural communities and public health agencies (or services provided in the beneficiary's home under arrangements with a provider of outpatient physical or occupational therapy services) are not covered under this provision. See section 230.6.

230.5—Physical Therapy, Occupational Therapy and Speech-Language Pathology Services Provided Incident to the Services of Physicians and Non-Physician Practitioners (NPP)

(Rev. 36, Issued: 06-24-05, Effective: 06-06-05, Implementation: 06-06-05)

References: §1861(s)(2)(A) of the Act
42 CFR 410.10(b)
42 CFR 410.26
Pub. 100-02, ch. 15, § 60.

The Benefit. Therapy services have their own benefit under §1861 of the Social Security Act and shall be covered when provided according to the standards and conditions of the benefit described in Medicare manuals. The statute 1862(a)(20) requires that payment be made for a therapy service billed by a physician/NPP only if the service meets the standards and conditions—other than licensing—that would apply to a therapist. (For example, see coverage requirements in Pub. 100-08, Chapter 13, §13.5.1(C), Pub. 100-04, Chapter 5, and also the requirements of this manual, §220 and §230.)

Incident to a Therapist. There is no coverage for services provided incident to the services of a therapist. Although PTAs and OTAs work under the supervision of a therapist and their services may be billed by the therapist, their services are covered under the benefit for therapy services and not by the benefit for services incident to a physician/NPP. The services furnished by PTAs and OTAs are not incident to the therapist's service.

Qualifications of Auxiliary Personnel. Therapy services appropriately billed incident to a physician's/NPP's service shall be subject to the same requirements as therapy services that would be furnished by a physical therapist, occupational therapist or speech-language pathologist in any other outpatient setting with one exception. When therapy services are performed incident to a physician's/NPP's service, the qualified personnel who perform the service do not need to have a license to practice therapy, unless it is required by state law. The qualified personnel must meet all the other requirements except licensure. Qualifications for therapists are found in 42CFR484.4 and in section 230.1, 230.2, and 230.3 of this manual. In effect, these rules require that the person who furnishes the service to the patient must, at least, be a graduate of a program of training for one of the therapy services as described above. Regardless of any state licensing that allows other health professionals to provide therapy services, Medicare is authorized to pay only for services provided by those trained specifically in physical therapy, occupational therapy or speech-language pathology. That means that the services of athletic trainers, massage therapists, recreation therapists, kinesiotherapists, low vision specialists or any other profession may not be billed as therapy services.

The services of PTAs and OTAs also may not be billed incident to a physician's/NPP's service. However, if a PT and PTA (or an OT and OTA) are both employed in a physician's office, the services of the PTA, when directly supervised by the PT or the services of the OTA, when directly supervised by the OT may be billed by the physician group as PT or OT services using the PIN/NPI of the enrolled PT (or OT). (See Section 230.4 for private practice rules on billing services performed in a physician's office.) If the PT or OT is not enrolled, Medicare shall not pay for the services of a PTA or OTA billed incident to the physician's service, because they do not meet the qualification standards in 42CFR484.4.

Therapy services provided and billed incident to the services of a physician/NPP also must meet all incident-to requirements in this manual in Chapter 15, §60. Where the policies have different requirements, the more stringent requirement shall be met.

For example, when therapy services are billed as incident to a physician/NPP services, the requirement for direct supervision by the physician/NPP and other incident to requirements must be met, even though the service is provided by a licensed therapist who may perform the services unsupervised in other settings.

The mandatory assignment provision does not apply to therapy services furnished by a physician/NPP or "incident to" a physician's/NPP's service. However, when these services are not furnished on an assignment-related basis; the limiting charge applies.

For emphasis, following are some of the standards that apply to therapy services billed incident-to the services of a physician/NPP in the physician's/NPP's office or the beneficiary's residence.

A. Therapy services provided to the beneficiary must be covered and payable outpatient rehabilitation services as described, for example, in this section as well as Pub. 100-08, Chapter 13, §13.5.1.

B. Therapy services must be provided by, or under the direct supervision of a physician (a doctor of medicine or osteopathy) or NPP who is legally authorized to practice therapy services by the state in which he or she performs such function or action. Direct supervision requirements are the same as in 42CFR410.32(b)(3). The supervisor must be present in the office suite and immediately available to furnish assistance and direction throughout the performance of the procedure. It does not mean that the physician/NPP must be present in the same room in the office where the service is performed.

C. The services must be of a level of complexity that require that they be performed by a therapist or under the direct supervision of the therapist, physician/NPP who is licensed to perform them. Services that do not require the performance or supervision of the therapist, physician/NPP, are not considered reasonable or necessary therapy services even if they are performed or supervised by a physician/NPP or other qualified professional.

D. Services must be furnished under a plan of treatment as in §220.1.2 of this chapter. The services provided must relate directly to the physician/NPP service to which it is incident.

230.6—Therapy Services Furnished Under Arrangements With Providers and Clinics

(Rev. 36, Issued: 06-24-05, Effective: 06-06-05, Implementation: 06-06-05)

References: See also Pub. 100-01, chapter 5, §10.3.

A—General

For rules regarding services provided under arrangement, see Pub. 100-01, chapter 5, §10.3.

A provider may have others furnish outpatient therapy (physical therapy, occupational therapy, or speech-language pathology) services through arrangements under which receipt of payment by the provider for the services discharges the liability of the beneficiary or any other person to pay for the service.

However, it is not intended that the provider merely serve as a billing mechanism for the other party. For such services to be covered the provider must assume professional responsibility for the services.

The provider's professional supervision over the services requires application of many of the same controls that are applied to services furnished by salaried employees. The provider must:

- Accept the patient for treatment in accordance with its admission policies;
- Maintain a complete and timely clinical record on the patient which includes diagnosis, medical history, orders, and progress notes relating to all services received;
- Maintain liaison with the attending physician/NPP with regard to the progress of the patient and to assure that the required plan of treatment is periodically reviewed by the physician/NPP;
- Secure from the physician/NPP the required certifications and recertifications; and
- Ensure that the medical necessity of such service is reviewed on a sample basis by the agency's staff or an outside review group.

In addition, when a provider provides outpatient services under an arrangement with others, such services must be furnished in accordance with the terms of a written contract, which provides for retention by the provider of responsibility for and control and supervision of such services. The terms of the contract should include at least the following:

- Provide that the therapy services are to be furnished in accordance with the plan of care established according to Medicare policies for therapy plans of care in Section 220.1.2 of this chapter;
- Specify the geographical areas in which the services are to be furnished;
- Provide that contracted personnel and services meet the same requirements as those which would be applicable if the personnel and services were furnished directly by the provider;

- Provide that the therapist will participate in conferences required to coordinate the care of an individual patient;
- Provide for the preparation of treatment records, with progress notes and observations, and for the prompt incorporation of such into the clinical records of the clinic;
- Specify the financial arrangements. The contracting organization or individual may not bill the patient or the health insurance program; and
- Specify the period of time the contract is to be in effect and the manner of termination or renewal.

B—Special Rules for Hospitals

- A hospital may bill Medicare for outpatient therapy (physical therapy, occupational therapy, or speech-language pathology) services that it furnishes to its outpatients either directly or under arrangements in the hospital's outpatient department. If a hospital furnishes medically necessary therapy services in its outpatient department to individuals who are registered as its outpatients, those services must be billed directly by the hospital using bill type 13X or 85X for critical access hospitals. Note that services provided to residents of a Medicare-certified SNF may not be billed by the hospital as services to its outpatients.
- When a hospital sends its therapists to the home of an individual who is registered as an outpatient of the hospital but who is unable, for medical reasons, to come to the hospital to receive medically necessary therapy services, the services must meet the requirements applicable to outpatient hospital therapy services, as set forth in the regulations and applicable Medicare manuals. The hospital may bill for those services directly using bill type 13X or 85X for critical access hospitals.
- If a hospital sends its therapists to provide therapy services to individuals who are registered as its outpatients and who are residing in the non-certified part of a SNF, or in another residential setting (e.g., a group home, assisted living facility or domiciliary care home), the hospital may bill for the services as hospital outpatient services if the services meet the requirements applicable to outpatient hospital therapy services, as set forth in the regulations and applicable Medicare manuals.
- A hospital may make an arrangement with another entity such as an Outpatient Rehab Facility (Rehabilitation Agency) or a private practice, to provide therapy services to individuals who are registered as outpatients of the hospital. These services must meet the requirements applicable to services furnished under arrangements and the requirements applicable to the outpatient hospital therapy services as set forth in the regulations and applicable Medicare manuals. The hospital uses bill type 13X or 85X for critical access hospitals to bill for the services that another entity furnishes under arrangement to its outpatients.
- Where the provider is a public health agency or a hospital in a rural community, it may enter into arrangements to have outpatient physical therapy services furnished in the private office of a qualified physical therapist if the agency or hospital does not have the capacity to provide on its premises all of the modalities of treatment, tests, and measurements that are included in an adequate outpatient physical therapy program and the services and modalities which the public health agency or hospital cannot provide on its premises are not available on an outpatient basis in another accessible certified facility.

- In certain settings and under certain circumstances, hospitals may not bill Medicare for therapy services as services of the hospital:
  - If a hospital sends its therapists to provide therapy services to patients of another hospital, including a patient at an inpatient rehabilitation facility or a long term care facility, the services must be furnished under arrangements made with the hospital sending the therapists by the hospital having the patients and billed as hospital services by the facility whose patients are treated. These services would be subject to existing hospital bundling rules and would be paid under the payment method applicable to the hospital at which the individuals are patients.
  - A hospital may not send its therapists to provide therapy services to individuals who are receiving services from an HHA under a home health plan of care and bill for the therapy services as hospital outpatient services. For patients under a home health plan of care, payment for therapy services (unless provided by physicians/NPPs) is included or bundled into Medicare's episodic payment to the HHA, and those services must be billed by the HHA under the HHA consolidated billing rules. For patients receiving HHA services under an HHA plan of care, therapy services must be furnished directly or under arrangements made by the HHA, and only the HHA may bill for those services.
  - If a hospital sends its therapists to provide services under arrangements made by a SNF to residents of the Medicare-certified part of a SNF, SNF consolidated billing rules apply. For arrangements specific to SNF Part A, see Pub. 100-04, chapter 6, §10.4. This means that therapy services furnished to SNF residents in the Medicare-certified part of a SNF cannot be billed by any entity other than the SNF. Therefore, a hospital may not bill Medicare for PT/OT/SLP services furnished to residents of a Medicare-certified part of a SNF by its therapists as services of the hospital.

NOTE: If the SNF resident is in a covered Part A stay, the therapy services would be included in the SNF's global PPS per diem payment for the covered Part A stay itself. If the resident is in a noncovered stay (Part A benefits exhausted, no prior qualifying hospital stay, etc.), but remains in the Medicare-certified part of a SNF, the SNF would submit the Part B therapy bill to its fiscal intermediary.

SNF Setting	Applicable Rules	
Medicare Part A or B	Consolidated Billing Rules Apply?	Hospital May Bill For Outpatient Services?
Part A (Medicare Covered/PPS) Resident in Medicare-certified part of a SNF	Yes	No
Medicare Part B Resident in Medicare-certified part of a SNF	Yes	No
Medicare Part B Not a Resident in Medicare-certified part of a SNF	No	Yes

- A hospital may not send therapy staff to provide therapy services in non-residential health care settings and bill for the services as if they were provided at the hospital, even if the hospital owns the other facility or entity. Examples of such non-residential settings include CORFs, rehabilitation agencies, ORFs and offices of physicians/NPPs or other practitioners, such as physical therapists. For example, services furnished to patients of a CORF must be billed as CORF services and not as outpatient hospital services. Even if a CORF contracts with a hospital to furnish services to CORF patients, the hospital may not bill Medicare for the services as hospital outpatient services. However, the CORF could have the hospital furnish services to its patients under arrangements, in which case the CORF would bill for the services.

Psychiatric hospitals are treated the same as other hospitals for the purpose of therapy billing.

290—Foot Care

(Rev. 1, 10-01-03)

A3-3158, B3-2323, HO-260.9, B3-4120.1

A—Treatment of Subluxation of Foot

Subluxations of the foot are defined as partial dislocations or displacements of joint surfaces, tendons ligaments, or muscles of the foot. Surgical or nonsurgical treatments undertaken for the sole purpose of correcting a subluxated structure in the foot as an isolated entity are not covered.

However, medical or surgical treatment of subluxation of the ankle joint (talo-crural joint) is covered. In addition, reasonable and necessary medical or surgical services, diagnosis, or treatment for medical conditions that have resulted from or are associated with partial displacement of structures is covered. For example, if a patient has osteoarthritis that has resulted in a partial displacement of joints in the foot, and the primary treatment is for the osteoarthritis, coverage is provided.

B—Exclusions from Coverage

The following foot care services are generally excluded from coverage under both Part A and Part B. (See §290.F and §290. G for instructions on applying foot care exclusions.)

1. **Treatment of Flat Foot**—The term "flat foot" is defined as a condition in which one or more arches of the foot have flattened out. Services or devices directed toward the care or correction of such conditions, including the prescription of supportive devices, are not covered.
2. **Routine Foot Care**—Except as provided above, routine foot care is excluded from coverage. Services that normally are considered routine and not covered by Medicare include the following:

   - The cutting or removal of corns and calluses;
   - The trimming, cutting, clipping, or debriding of nails; and
   - Other hygienic and preventive maintenance care, such as cleaning and soaking the feet, the use of skin creams to maintain skin tone of either ambulatory or bedfast patients, and any other service performed in the absence of localized illness, injury, or symptoms involving the foot.

3. **Supportive Devices for Feet**—Orthopedic shoes and other supportive devices for the feet generally are not covered. However, this exclusion does not apply to such a shoe if it is an integral part of a leg brace, and its expense is included as part of the cost of the brace. Also, this exclusion does not apply to therapeutic shoes furnished to diabetics.

C—Exceptions to Routine Foot Care Exclusion

1. **Necessary and Integral Part of Otherwise Covered Services**—In certain circumstances, services ordinarily considered to be routine may be covered if they are performed as a necessary and integral part of otherwise covered services, such as diagnosis and treatment of ulcers, wounds, or infections.
2. **Treatment of Warts on Foot**—The treatment of warts (including plantar warts) on the foot is covered to the same extent as services provided for the treatment of warts located elsewhere on the body.
3. **Presence of Systemic Condition**—The presence of a systemic condition such as metabolic, neurologic, or peripheral vascular disease may require scrupulous foot care by a professional that in the absence of such condition(s) would be considered routine (and, therefore, excluded from coverage). Accordingly, foot care that would otherwise be considered routine may be covered when systemic condition(s) result in severe circulatory embarrassment or areas of diminished sensation in the individual's legs or feet. (See subsection A.)

In these instances, certain foot care procedures that otherwise are considered routine (e.g., cutting or removing corns and calluses, or trimming, cutting, clipping, or debriding nails) may pose a hazard when performed by a nonprofessional person on patients with such systemic conditions. (See §290.G for procedural instructions.)

4. **Mycotic Nails**—In the absence of a systemic condition, treatment of mycotic nails may be covered.

The treatment of mycotic nails for an ambulatory patient is covered only when the physician attending the patient's mycotic condition documents that (1) there is clinical evidence of mycosis of the toenail, and (2) the patient has marked limitation of ambulation, pain, or secondary infection resulting from the thickening and dystrophy of the infected toenail plate.

The treatment of mycotic nails for a nonambulatory patient is covered only when the physician attending the patient's mycotic condition documents that (1) there is clinical evidence of mycosis of the toenail, and (2) the patient suffers from pain or secondary infection resulting from the thickening and dystrophy of the infected toenail plate.

For the purpose of these requirements, documentation means any written information that is required by the carrier in order for services to be covered. Thus, the information submitted with claims must be substantiated by information found in the patient's medical record. Any information, including that contained in a form letter, used for documentation purposes is subject to carrier verification in order to ensure that the information adequately justifies coverage of the treatment of mycotic nails.

D—Systemic Conditions That Might Justify Coverage

Although not intended as a comprehensive list, the following metabolic, neurologic, and peripheral vascular diseases (with synonyms in parentheses) most commonly represent the underlying conditions that might justify coverage for routine foot care.

- Diabetes mellitus*
- Arteriosclerosis obliterans (A.S.O., arteriosclerosis of the extremities, occlusive peripheral arteriosclerosis)
- Buerger's disease (thromboangiitis obliterans)
- Chronic thrombophlebitis*
- Peripheral neuropathies involving the feet—
  - Associated with malnutrition and vitamin deficiency*
    - Malnutrition (general, pellagra)
    - Alcoholism
    - Malabsorption (celiac disease, tropical sprue)
    - Pernicious anemia
  - Associated with carcinoma*
  - Associated with diabetes mellitus*
  - Associated with drugs and toxins*
  - Associated with multiple sclerosis*
  - Associated with uremia (chronic renal disease)*
  - Associated with traumatic injury
  - Associated with leprosy or neurosyphilis
  - Associated with hereditary disorders
    - Hereditary sensory radicular neuropathy
    - Angiokeratoma corporis diffusum (Fabry's)
    - Amyloid neuropathy

When the patient's condition is one of those designated by an asterisk (*), routine procedures are covered only if the patient is under the active care of a doctor of medicine or osteopathy who documents the condition.

E—Supportive Devices for Feet

Orthopedic shoes and other supportive devices for the feet generally are not covered. However, this exclusion does not apply to such a shoe if it is an integral part of a leg brace, and its expense is included as part of the cost of the brace. Also, this exclusion does not apply to therapeutic shoes furnished to diabetics.

F—Presumption of Coverage

In evaluating whether the routine services can be reimbursed, a presumption of coverage may be made where the evidence available discloses certain physical and/or clinical findings consistent with the diagnosis and indicative of severe peripheral involvement. For purposes of applying this presumption the following findings are pertinent:

Class A Findings

- Nontraumatic amputation of foot or integral skeletal portion thereof.

Class B Findings

- Absent posterior tibial pulse;
- Advanced trophic changes as: hair growth (decrease or absence) nail changes (thickening) pigmentary changes (discoloration) skin texture (thin, shiny) skin color (rubor or redness) (Three required); and
- Absent dorsalis pedis pulse.

Class C Findings

- Claudication;
- Temperature changes (e.g., cold feet);
- Edema;
- Paresthesias (abnormal spontaneous sensations in the feet); and
- Burning.

The presumption of coverage may be applied when the physician rendering the routine foot care has identified:

1. A Class A finding;
2. Two of the Class B findings; or
3. One Class B and two Class C findings.

Cases evidencing findings falling short of these alternatives may involve podiatric treatment that may constitute covered care and should be reviewed by the intermediary's medical staff and developed as necessary.

For purposes of applying the coverage presumption where the routine services have been rendered by a podiatrist, the contractor may deem the active care requirement met if the claim or other evidence available discloses that the patient has seen an M.D. or D.O. for treatment and/or evaluation of the complicating disease process during the 6-month period prior to the rendition of the routine-type services. The intermediary may also accept the podiatrist's statement that the diagnosing and treating M.D. or D.O. also concurs with the podiatrist's findings as to the severity of the peripheral involvement indicated.

Services ordinarily considered routine might also be covered if they are performed as a necessary and integral part of otherwise covered services, such as diagnosis and treatment of diabetic ulcers, wounds, and infections.

G—Application of Foot Care Exclusions to Physician's Services

The exclusion of foot care is determined by the nature of the service. Thus, payment for an excluded service should be denied whether performed by a podiatrist, osteopath, or a doctor of medicine, and without regard to the difficulty or complexity of the procedure.

When an itemized bill shows both covered services and non-covered services not integrally related to the covered service, the portion of charges attributable to the noncovered services should be denied. (For example, if an itemized bill shows surgery for an ingrown toenail and also removal of calluses not necessary for the performance of toe surgery, any additional charge attributable to removal of the calluses should be denied.)

In reviewing claims involving foot care, the carrier should be alert to the following exceptional situations:

1. Payment may be made for incidental noncovered services performed as a necessary and integral part of, and secondary to, a covered procedure. For example, if trimming of toenails is required for application of a cast to a fractured foot, the carrier need not allocate and deny a portion of the charge for the trimming of the nails. However, a separately itemized charge for such excluded service should be disallowed. When the primary procedure is covered the administration of anesthesia necessary for the performance of such procedure is also covered.

2. Payment may be made for **initial** diagnostic services performed in connection with a specific symptom or complaint if it seems likely that its treatment would be covered even though the resulting diagnosis may be one requiring only noncovered care.

The name of the M.D. or D.O. who diagnosed the complicating condition must be submitted with the claim. In those cases, where active care is required, the approximate date the beneficiary was last seen by such physician must also be indicated.

NOTE: Section 939 of P.L. 96-499 removed "warts" from the routine foot care exclusion effective July 1, 1981.

Relatively few claims for routine-type care are anticipated considering the severity of conditions contemplated as the basis for this exception. Claims for this type of foot care should not be paid in the absence of convincing evidence that nonprofessional performance of the service would have been hazardous for the beneficiary because of an underlying systemic disease. The mere statement of a diagnosis such as those mentioned in §D above does not of itself indicate the severity of the condition. Where development is indicated to verify diagnosis and/or severity the carrier should follow existing claims processing practices which may include review of carrier's history and medical consultation as well as physician contacts.

The rules in §290.F concerning presumption of coverage also apply.

Codes and policies for routine foot care and supportive devices for the feet are not exclusively for the use of podiatrists. These codes must be used to report foot care services regardless of the specialty of the physician who furnishes the services. Carriers must instruct physicians to use the most appropriate code available when billing for routine foot care.

100-02 Chapter 16

10—General Exclusions From Coverage

(Rev. 1, 10-01-03)

A3-3150, HO-260, HHA-232, B3-2300

No payment can be made under either the hospital insurance or supplementary medical insurance program for certain items and services, when the following conditions exist:

- Not reasonable and necessary (§20);
- No legal obligation to pay for or provide (§40);
- Paid for by a governmental entity (§50);
- Not provided within United States (§60);
- Resulting from war (§70);
- Personal comfort (§80);
- Routine services and appliances (§90);
- Custodial care (§110);
- Cosmetic surgery (§120);
- Charges by immediate relatives or members of household (§130);
- Dental services (§140);
- Paid or expected to be paid under workers' compensation (§150);

- Nonphysician services provided to a hospital inpatient that were not provided directly or arranged for by the hospital (§170);
- Services Related to and Required as a Result of Services Which are not Covered Under Medicare (§180);
- Excluded foot care services and supportive devices for feet (§30); or
- Excluded investigational devices (See Chapter 14, §30).

20—Services Not Reasonable and Necessary

(Rev. 1, 10-01-03)

A3-3151, HO-260.1, B3-2303, AB-00-52 - 6/00

Items and services which are not reasonable and necessary for the diagnosis or treatment of illness or injury or to improve the functioning of a malformed body member are not covered, e.g., payment cannot be made for the rental of a special hospital bed to be used by the patient in their home unless it was a reasonable and necessary part of the patient's treatment. See also §80.

A health care item or service for the purpose of causing, or assisting to cause, the death of any individual (assisted suicide) is not covered. This prohibition does not apply to the provision of an item or service for the purpose of alleviating pain or discomfort, even if such use may increase the risk of death, so long as the item or service is not furnished for the specific purpose of causing death.

90—Routine Services and Appliances

(Rev. 1, 10-01-03)

A3-3157, HO-260.7, B3-2320, R-1797A3 - 5/00

Routine physical checkups; eyeglasses, contact lenses, and eye examinations for the purpose of prescribing, fitting, or changing eyeglasses; eye refractions by whatever practitioner and for whatever purpose performed; hearing aids and examinations for hearing aids; and immunizations are not covered.

The routine physical checkup exclusion applies to (a) examinations performed without relationship to treatment or diagnosis for a specific illness, symptom, complaint, or injury; and (b) examinations required by third parties such as insurance companies, business establishments, or Government agencies.

If the claim is for a diagnostic test or examination performed solely for the purpose of establishing a claim under title IV of Public Law 91-173, "Black Lung Benefits," the service is not covered under Medicare and the claimant should be advised to contact their Social Security office regarding the filing of a claim for reimbursement under the "Black Lung" program.

The exclusions apply to eyeglasses or contact lenses, and eye examinations for the purpose of prescribing, fitting, or changing eyeglasses or contact lenses for refractive errors. The exclusions do not apply to physicians' services (and services incident to a physicians' service) performed in conjunction with an eye disease, as for example, glaucoma or cataracts, or to post-surgical prosthetic lenses which are customarily used during convalescence from eye surgery in which the lens of the eye was removed, or to permanent prosthetic lenses required by an individual lacking the organic lens of the eye, whether by surgical removal or con-

genital disease. Such prosthetic lens is a replacement for an internal body organ - the lens of the eye. (See the Medicare Benefit Policy Manual, Chapter 15, "Covered Medical and Other Health Services," §120).

Expenses for all refractive procedures, whether performed by an ophthalmologist (or any other physician) or an optometrist and without regard to the reason for performance of the refraction, are excluded from coverage.

A. Immunizations

Vaccinations or inoculations are excluded as immunizations unless they are either

- Directly related to the treatment of an injury or direct exposure to a disease or condition, such as antirabies treatment, tetanus antitoxin or booster vaccine, botulin antitoxin, antivenin sera, or immune globulin.(In the absence of injury or direct exposure, preventive immunization (vaccination or inoculation) against such diseases as smallpox, polio, diphtheria, etc., is not covered.); or
- Specifically covered by statute, as described in the Medicare Benefit Policy Manual, Chapter 15, "Covered Medical and Other Health Services," §50.

B. Antigens

Prior to the Omnibus Reconciliation Act of 1980, a physician who prepared an antigen for a patient could not be reimbursed for that service unless the physician also administered the antigen to the patient. Effective January 1, 1981, payment may be made for a reasonable supply of antigens that have been prepared for a particular patient even though they have not been administered to the patient by the same physician who prepared them if:

- The antigens are prepared by a physician who is a doctor of medicine or osteopathy, and
- The physician who prepared the antigens has examined the patient and has determined a plan of treatment and a dosage regimen.

A reasonable supply of antigens is considered to be not more than a 12-week supply of antigens that has been prepared for a particular patient at any one time. The purpose of the reasonable supply limitation is to assure that the antigens retain their potency and effectiveness over the period in which they are to be administered to the patient. (See the Medicare Benefit Policy Manual, Chapter 15, "Covered Medical and Other Health Services," §50.4.4.2)

100 - Hearing Aids and Auditory Implants

(Rev. 39; Issued: 11-10-05; Effective: 11-10-05; Implementation: 12-12-05)

Section 1862(a)(7) of the Social Security Act states that no payment may be made under part A or part B for any expenses incurred for items or services "where such expenses are for . . . hearing aids or examinations therefore. . . ." This policy is further reiterated at 42 CFR 411.15(d) which specifically states that "hearing aids or examination for the purpose of prescribing, fitting, or changing hearing aids" are excluded from coverage.

Hearing aids are amplifying devices that compensate for impaired hearing. Hearing aids include air conduction devices that provide acoustic energy to the cochlea via stimulation of the tympanic membrane with amplified sound. They also include bone conduction devices that provide mechanical energy to the cochlea via stimulation of the scalp with amplified mechanical vibration or by direct contact with the tympanic membrane or middle ear ossicles.

Certain devices that produce perception of sound by replacing the function of the middle ear, cochlea or auditory nerve are payable by Medicare as prosthetic devices. These devices are indicated only when hearing aids are medically inappropriate or cannot be utilized due to congenital malformations, chronic disease, severe sensorineural hearing loss or surgery.

The following are prosthetic devices:

- Cochlear implants and auditory brainstem implants, i.e., devices that replace the function of cochlear structures or auditory nerve and provide electrical energy to auditory nerve fibers and other neural tissue via implanted electrode arrays.
- Osseointegrated implants, i.e., devices implanted in the skull that replace the function of the middle ear and provide mechanical energy to the cochlea via a mechanical transducer.

Medicare contractors deny payment for an item of service that is associated with any hearing aid as defined above. See §180 for policy for the medically necessary treatment of complications of implantable hearing aids, such as medically necessary removals of implantable hearing aids due to infection.

110 - Custodial Care

(Rev. 1, 10-01-03)

A3-3159, HO-260.10, HO-261, B3-2326

Custodial care is excluded from coverage. Custodial care serves to assist an individual in the activities of daily living, such as assistance in walking, getting in and out of bed, bathing, dressing, feeding, and using the toilet, preparation of special diets, and supervision of medication that usually can be self-administered. Custodial care essentially is personal care that does not require the continuing attention of trained medical or paramedical personnel. In determining whether a person is receiving custodial care, the intermediary or carrier considers the level of care and medical supervision required and furnished. It does not base the decision on diagnosis, type of condition, degree of functional limitation, or rehabilitation potential.

Institutional care that is below the level of care covered in a SNF is custodial care. (See the Medicare Benefit Policy Manual, Chapter 8, "Coverage of Extended Care (SNF) Services Under Hospital Insurance," §30). Some examples of custodial care in hospitals and SNFs are:

- A stroke patient who is ambulatory, has no bladder or bowel involvement, no serious associated or secondary illnesses and does not require medical or paramedical care but requires only the assistance of an aide in feeding, dressing, and bathing;
- A cardiac patient who is stable and compensated and has reasonable cardiac reserve and no associated illnesses, but who because of advanced age has difficulty in managing alone in the home, and requires assistance in meeting the activities of daily living; and

- A senile patient who has diabetes which remains stabilized as long as someone sees to it that the patient takes oral medication and sticks to a prescribed diet.

Even if a patient's stay in a hospital or SNF is determined to be custodial, some individual services may still be covered under Part B if they are reasonable and necessary. For example, periodic visits by a physician to their patient are covered under Part B if such services are reasonable and necessary to the treatment of the patient's illness or injury even though a finding has been made that the care being furnished the patient in the hospital of SNF is custodial care and, therefore, not covered. Similarly, such a finding of custodial care does not preclude payment for a Part B claim for ancillary services which are medically necessary (see the Medicare Benefit Policy Manual, Chapter 15, "Covered Medical and Other Health Services," §250). (See the Medicare Benefit Policy Manual, Chapter 6, "Hospital Services Covered Under Part B," §10, and Chapter 8, §80.)

110.1 - Custodial Care Under a Hospice Program

(Rev. 1, 10-01-03)

A3-3159.1

Care furnished to an individual who has elected the hospice care option is custodial only if it is not reasonable and necessary for the palliation or management of the terminal illness or related conditions. (See the Medicare Benefit Policy Manual, Chapter 9, "Coverage of Hospice Services Under Hospital Insurance," §40.)

100-02 Chapter 16

140—Dental Services Exclusion

(Rev. 1, 10-01-03)

A3-3162, HO-260.13, B3-2336

Items and services in connection with the care, treatment, filling, removal, or replacement of teeth, or structures directly supporting the teeth are not covered. Structures directly supporting the teeth mean the periodontium, which includes the gingivae, dentogingival junction, periodontal membrane, cementum, and alveolar process. However, payment may be made for certain other services of a dentist. (See the Medicare Benefit Policy Manual, Chapter 15, "Covered Medical and Other Health Services," §150.)

The hospitalization or nonhospitalization of a patient has no direct bearing on the coverage or exclusion of a given dental procedure.

When an excluded service is the primary procedure involved, it is not covered regardless of its complexity or difficulty. For example, the extraction of an impacted tooth is not covered. Similarly, an alveoplasty (the surgical improvement of the shape and condition of the alveolar process) and a frenectomy are excluded from coverage when either of these procedures is performed in connection with an excluded service, e.g., the preparation of the mouth for dentures. In like manner, the removal of the torus palatinus (a bony protuberance of the hard palate) could be a covered service. However, with rare exception, this surgery is performed in connection with an excluded service, i.e., the preparation of the mouth for dentures. Under such circumstances, reimbursement is not made for this purpose.

The extraction of teeth to prepare the jaw for radiation treatments of neoplastic disease is also covered. This is an exception to the requirement that to be covered, a noncovered procedure or service performed by a dentist must be an incident to and an integral part of a covered procedure or service performed by the dentist. Ordinarily, the dentist extracts the patient's teeth, but another physician, e.g., a radiologist, administers the radiation treatments.

Whether such services as the administration of anesthesia, diagnostic x-rays, and other related procedures are covered depends upon whether the primary procedure being performed by the dentist is covered. Thus, an x-ray taken in connection with the reduction of a fracture of the jaw or facial bone is covered. However, a single x-ray or x-ray survey taken in connection with the care or treatment of teeth or the periodontium is not covered.

See also the Medicare Benefit Policy Manual, Chapter 1, "Inpatient Hospital Services," §70, and Chapter 15, "Covered Medical and Other Health Services," §150 for additional information on dental services.

100-03 Part 1

20.8—Cardiac Pacemakers (Effective April 30, 2004)

(Rev. 16, 06-25-04)

Cardiac pacemakers are self-contained, battery-operated units that send electrical stimulation to the heart. They are generally implanted to alleviate symptoms of decreased cardiac output related to abnormal heart rate and/or rhythm. Pacemakers are generally used for persistent, symptomatic second- or third-degree atrioventricular (AV) block and symptomatic sinus bradycardia.

Cardiac pacemakers are covered as prosthetic devices under the Medicare program, subject to the following conditions and limitations. While cardiac pacemakers have been covered under Medicare for many years, there were no specific guidelines for their use other than the general Medicare requirement that covered services be reasonable and necessary for the treatment of the condition. Services rendered for cardiac pacing on or after the effective dates of this instruction are subject to these guidelines, which are based on certain assumptions regarding the clinical goals of cardiac pacing. While some uses of pacemakers are relatively certain or unambiguous, many other uses require considerable expertise and judgment.

Consequently, the medical necessity for permanent cardiac pacing must be viewed in the context of overall patient management. The appropriateness of such pacing may be conditional on other diagnostic or therapeutic modalities having been undertaken. Although significant complications and adverse side effects of pacemaker use are relatively rare, they cannot be ignored when considering the use of pacemakers for dubious medical conditions, or marginal clinical benefit.

These guidelines represent current concepts regarding medical circumstances in which permanent cardiac pacing may be appropriate or necessary. As with other areas of medicine, advances in knowledge and techniques in cardiology are ex-

pected. Consequently, judgments about the medical necessity and acceptability of new uses for cardiac pacing in new classes of patients may change as more conclusive evidence becomes available. This instruction applies only to permanent cardiac pacemakers, and does not address the use of temporary, non-implanted pacemakers.

The two groups of conditions outlined below deal with the necessity for cardiac pacing for patients in general. These are intended as guidelines in assessing the medical necessity for pacing therapies, taking into account the particular circumstances in each case. However, as a general rule, the two groups of current medical concepts may be viewed as representing:

Group I: Single-Chamber Cardiac Pacemakers – a) conditions under which single chamber pacemaker claims may be considered covered without further claims development; and b) conditions under which single-chamber pacemaker claims would be denied unless further claims development shows that they fall into the covered category, or special medical circumstances exist of the sufficiency to convince the contractor that the claim should be paid.

Group II: Dual-Chamber Cardiac Pacemakers - a) conditions under which dual-chamber pacemaker claims may be considered covered without further claims development, and b) conditions under which dual-chamber pacemaker claims would be denied unless further claims development shows that they fall into the covered categories for single- and dual-chamber pacemakers, or special medical circumstances exist sufficient to convince the contractor that the claim should be paid.

The CMS opened the NCD on Cardiac Pacemakers to afford the public an opportunity to comment on the proposal to revise the language contained in the instruction. The revisions transfer the focus of the NCD from the actual pacemaker implantation procedure itself to the reasonable and necessary medical indications that justify cardiac pacing. This is consistent with our findings that pacemaker implantation is no longer considered routinely harmful or an experimental procedure.

Group I: Single-Chamber Cardiac Pacemakers (Effective March 16, 1983)

A. Nationally Covered Indications

Conditions under which cardiac pacing is generally considered acceptable or necessary, provided that the conditions are chronic or recurrent and not due to transient causes such as acute myocardial infarction, drug toxicity, or electrolyte imbalance. (In cases where there is a rhythm disturbance, if the rhythm disturbance is chronic or recurrent, a single episode of a symptom such as syncope or seizure is adequate to establish medical necessity.)

1. Acquired complete (also referred to as third-degree) AV heart block.
2. Congenital complete heart block with severe bradycardia (in relation to age), or significant physiological deficits or significant symptoms due to the bradycardia.
3. Second-degree AV heart block of Type II (i.e., no progressive prolongation of P-R interval prior to each blocked beat. P-R interval indicates the time taken for an impulse to travel from the atria to the ventricles on an electrocardiogram).

4. Second-degree AV heart block of Type I (i.e., progressive prolongation of P-R interval prior to each blocked beat) with significant symptoms due to hemodynamic instability associated with the heart block.

5. Sinus bradycardia associated with major symptoms (e.g., syncope, seizures, congestive heart failure); or substantial sinus bradycardia (heart rate less than 50) associated with dizziness or confusion. The correlation between symptoms and bradycardia must be documented, or the symptoms must be clearly attributable to the bradycardia rather than to some other cause.

6. In selected and few patients, sinus bradycardia of lesser severity (heart rate 50-59) with dizziness or confusion. The correlation between symptoms and bradycardia must be documented, or the symptoms must be clearly attributable to the bradycardia rather than to some other cause.

7. Sinus bradycardia is the consequence of long-term necessary drug treatment for which there is no acceptable alternative when accompanied by significant symptoms (e.g., syncope, seizures, congestive heart failure, dizziness or confusion). The correlation between symptoms and bradycardia must be documented, or the symptoms must be clearly attributable to the bradycardia rather than to some other cause.

8. Sinus node dysfunction with or without tachyarrhythmias or AV conduction block (i.e., the bradycardia-tachycardia syndrome, sino-atrial block, sinus arrest) when accompanied by significant symptoms (e.g., syncope, seizures, congestive heart failure, dizziness or confusion).

9. Sinus node dysfunction with or without symptoms when there are potentially life-threatening ventricular arrhythmias or tachycardia secondary to the bradycardia (e.g., numerous premature ventricular contractions, couplets, runs of premature ventricular contractions, or ventricular tachycardia).

10. Bradycardia associated with supraventricular tachycardia (e.g., atrial fibrillation, atrial flutter, or paroxysmal atrial tachycardia) with high-degree AV block which is unresponsive to appropriate pharmacological management and when the bradycardia is associated with significant symptoms (e.g., syncope, seizures, congestive heart failure, dizziness or confusion).

11. The occasional patient with hypersensitive carotid sinus syndrome with syncope due to bradycardia and unresponsive to prophylactic medical measures.

12. Bifascicular or trifascicular block accompanied by syncope which is attributed to transient complete heart block after other plausible causes of syncope have been reasonably excluded.

13. Prophylactic pacemaker use following recovery from acute myocardial infarction during which there was temporary complete (third-degree) and/or Mobitz Type II second-degree AV block in association with bundle branch block.

14. In patients with recurrent and refractory ventricular tachycardia, "overdrive pacing" (pacing above the basal rate) to prevent ventricular tachycardia.

(Effective May 9, 1985)

15. Second-degree AV heart block of Type I with the QRS complexes prolonged.

B. Nationally Noncovered Indications

Conditions which, although used by some physicians as a basis for permanent cardiac pacing, are considered unsupported by adequate evidence of benefit and therefore should not generally be considered appropriate uses for single-chamber pacemakers in the absence of the above indications. Contractors should review claims for pacemakers with these indications to determine the need for further claims development prior to denying the claim, since additional claims development may be required. The object of such further development is to establish whether the particular claim actually meets the conditions in a) above. In claims where this is not the case or where such an event appears unlikely, the contractor may deny the claim

1. Syncope of undetermined cause.
2. Sinus bradycardia without significant symptoms.
3. Sino-atrial block or sinus arrest without significant symptoms.
4. Prolonged P-R intervals with atrial fibrillation (without third-degree AV block) or with other causes of transient ventricular pause.
5. Bradycardia during sleep.
6. Right bundle branch block with left axis deviation (and other forms of fascicular or bundle branch block) without syncope or other symptoms of intermittent AV block).
7. Asymptomatic second-degree AV block of Type I unless the QRS complexes are prolonged or electrophysiological studies have demonstrated that the block is at or beyond the level of the His bundle (a component of the electrical conduction system of the heart).

Effective October 1, 2001

8. Asymptomatic bradycardia in post-mycardial infarction patients about to initiate long-term beta-blocker drug therapy.

C. Other

All other indications for single-chamber cardiac pacing for which CMS has not specifically indicated coverage remain nationally noncovered, except for Category B Investigational Device Exemption (IDE) clinical trials, or as routine costs of single-chamber cardiac pacing associated with clinical trials, in accordance with section 310.1 of the NCD Manual.

Group II: Dual-Chamber Cardiac Pacemakers – (Effective May 9, 1985)

A. Nationally Covered Indications

Conditions under dual-chamber cardiac pacing are considered acceptable or necessary in the general medical community unless conditions 1 and 2 under Group II. B., are present:

1. Patients in who single-chamber (ventricular pacing) at the time of pacemaker insertion elicits a definite drop in blood pressure, retrograde conduction, or discomfort.
2. Patients in whom the pacemaker syndrome (atrial ventricular asynchrony), with significant symptoms, has already been experienced with a pacemaker that is being replaced.
3. Patients in whom even a relatively small increase in cardiac efficiency will importantly improve the quality of life, e.g., patients with congestive heart failure despite adequate other medical measures.

4. Patients in whom the pacemaker syndrome can be anticipated, e.g., in young and active people, etc.

Dual-chamber pacemakers may also be covered for the conditions, as listed in Group I. A., if the medical necessity is sufficiently justified through adequate claims development. Expert physicians differ in their judgments about what constitutes appropriate criteria for dual-chamber pacemaker use. The judgment that such a pacemaker is warranted in the patient meeting accepted criteria must be based upon the individual needs and characteristics of that patient, weighing the magnitude and likelihood of anticipated benefits against the magnitude and likelihood of disadvantages to the patient.

B. Nationally Noncovered Indications

Whenever the following conditions (which represent overriding contraindications) are present, dual-chamber pacemakers are not covered:

1. Ineffective atrial contractions (e.g., chronic atrial fibrillation or flutter, or giant left atrium).
2. Frequent or persistent supraventricular tachycardias, except where the pacemaker is specifically for the control of the tachycardia.
3. A clinical condition in which pacing takes place only intermittently and briefly, and which is not associated with a reasonable likelihood that pacing needs will become prolonged, e.g., the occasional patient with hypersensitive carotid sinus syndrome with syncope due to bradycardia and unresponsive to prophylactic medical measures.
4. Prophylactic pacemaker use following recovery from acute myocardial infarction during which there was temporary complete (third-degree) and/or Type II second-degree AV block in association with bundle branch block.

C. Other

All other indications for dual-chamber cardiac pacing for which CMS has not specifically indicated coverage remain nationally noncovered, except for Category B IDE clinical trials, or as routine costs of dual-chamber cardiac pacing associated with clinical trials, in accordance with section 310.1 of the NCD Manual.

(This NCD last reviewed June 2004.)

20.8.1—Cardiac Pacemaker Evaluation Services

(Rev. 1, 10-03-03)

CIM 50-1

Medicare covers a variety of services for the post-implant followup and evaluation of implanted cardiac pacemakers. The following guidelines are designed to assist contractors in identifying and processing claims for such services.

NOTE: These new guidelines are limited to lithium battery-powered pacemakers, because mercury-zinc battery-powered pacemakers are no longer being manufactured and virtually all have been replaced by lithium units. Contractors still receiving claims for monitoring such units should continue to apply the guidelines published in 1980 to those units until they are replaced.

There are two general types of pacemakers in current use—single-chamber pacemakers which sense and pace the ventricles of the heart, and dual-chamber pacemakers which sense and pace both the atria and the ventricles. These differences require different monitoring patterns over the expected life of the units involved. One fact of which contractors should be aware is that many dual-chamber units may be programmed to pace only the ventricles; this may be done either at the time the pacemaker is implanted or at some time afterward. In such cases, a dual-chamber unit, when programmed or reprogrammed for ventricular pacing, should be treated as a single-chamber pacemaker in applying screening guidelines.

The decision as to how often any patient's pacemaker should be monitored is the responsibility of the patient's physician who is best able to take into account the condition and circumstances of the individual patient. These may vary over time, requiring modifications of the frequency with which the patient should be monitored. In cases where monitoring is done by some entity other than the patient's physician, such as a commercial monitoring service or hospital outpatient department, the physician's prescription for monitoring is required and should be periodically renewed (at least annually) to assure that the frequency of monitoring is proper for the patient. Where a patient is monitored both during clinic visits and transtelephonically, the contractor should be sure to include frequency data on both types of monitoring in evaluating the reasonableness of the frequency of monitoring services received by the patient. Since there are over 200 pacemaker models in service at any given point, and a variety of patient conditions that give rise to the need for pacemakers, the question of the appropriate frequency of monitoring is a complex one. Nevertheless, it is possible to develop guidelines within which the vast majority of pacemaker monitoring will fall and contractors should do this, using their own data and experience, as well as the frequency guidelines which follow, in order to limit extensive claims development to those cases requiring special attention.

20.8.1.1—Transtelephonic Monitoring of Cardiac Pacemakers

(Rev. 1, 10-03-03)

CIM 50-1

A—General

Transtelephonic monitoring of pacemakers is furnished by commercial suppliers, hospital outpatient departments and physicians' offices.

Telephone monitoring of cardiac pacemakers as described below is medically efficacious in identifying early signs of possible pacemaker failure, thus reducing the number of sudden pacemaker failures requiring emergency replacement. All systems that monitor the pacemaker rate (bpm) in both the free-running and/or magnetic mode are effective in detecting subclinical pacemaker failure due to battery depletion. More sophisticated systems are also capable of detecting internal electronic problems within the pulse generator itself and other potential problems. In the case of dual chamber pacemakers in particular, such monitoring may detect failure of synchronization of the atria and ventricles, and the need for adjustment and reprogramming of the device.

NOTE: The transmitting device furnished to the patient is simply one component of the diagnostic system, and is not covered as durable medical equipment. Those engaged in transtelephonic pacemaker monitoring should reflect the costs of the transmitters in setting their charges for monitoring.

B—Definition of Transtelephonic Monitoring

In order for transtelephonic monitoring services to be covered, the services must consist of the following elements:

- A minimum 30-second readable strip of the pacemaker in the free-running mode;
- Unless contraindicated, a minimum 30-second readable strip of the pacemaker in the magnetic mode; and
- A minimum 30 seconds of readable ECG strip.

C—Frequency Guidelines for Transtelephonic Monitoring

The guidelines below constitute a system which contractors should use, in conjunction with their knowledge of local medical practices, to screen claims for transtelephonic monitoring prior to payment. It is important to note that they are not recommendations with respect to a minimum frequency for such monitorings, but rather a maximum frequency (within which payment may be made without further claims development). As with previous guidelines, more frequent monitorings may be covered in cases where contractors are satisfied that such monitorings are medically necessary; e.g., based on the condition of the patient, or with respect to pacemakers exhibiting unexpected defects or premature failure. Contractors should seek written justification for more frequent monitorings from the patient's physician and/or any monitoring service involved.

These guidelines are divided into two broad categories—Guideline I which will apply to the majority of pacemakers now in use, and Guideline II which will apply only to pacemaker systems (pacemaker and leads) for which sufficient long-term clinical information exists to assure that they meet the standards of the Inter-Society Commission for Heart Disease Resources (ICHD) for longevity and end-of-life decay. (The ICHD standards are: (l) 90 percent cumulative survival at 5 years following implant; and (2) an end-of-life decay of less than a 50 percent drop of output voltage and less than 20 percent deviation of magnet rate, or a drop of 5 beats per minute or less, over a period of 3 months or more.) Contractors should consult with their medical advisers and other appropriate individuals and organizations (such as the North American Society of Pacing and Electrophysiology which publishes product reliability information) should questions arise over whether a pacemaker system meets the ICHD standards.

The two groups of guidelines are then further broken down into two general categories—single chamber and dual-chamber pacemakers. Contractors should be aware that the frequency with which a patient is monitored may be changed from time to time for a number of reasons, such as a change in the patient's overall condition, a reprogramming of the patient's pacemaker, the development of better information on the pacemaker's longevity or failure mode, etc. Consequently, changes in the proper set of guidelines may be required. Contractors should inform physicians and monitoring services to alert contractors to any changes in the patient's monitoring prescription that might necessitate changes in the screening guidelines applied to that patient. (Of particular importance is the reprogramming of a dual-chamber pacemaker to a single-chamber mode of operation. Such reprogramming would shift the patient from the appropriate dual-chamber guideline to the appropriate single-chamber guideline.)

Guideline I

1. Single-chamber pacemakers
   1st month—every 2 weeks.
   2nd through 36th month—every 8 weeks.
   37th month to failure—every 4 weeks.

2. Dual-chamber pacemaker
   1st month—every 2 weeks.
   2nd through 6th month—every 4 weeks.
   7th through 36th month—every 8 weeks.
   37th month to failure—every 4 weeks.

Guideline II

1. Single-chamber pacemakers
   1st month—every 2 weeks.
   2nd through 48th month—every 12 weeks.
   49th through 72nd month—every 8 weeks.
   Thereafter—every 4 weeks.

2. Dual-chamber pacemaker
   1st month—every 2 weeks.
   2nd through 30th month—every 12 weeks.
   31st through 48th month—every 8 weeks.
   Thereafter—every 4 weeks.

D—Pacemaker Clinic Services

1. General

Pacemaker monitoring is also covered when done by pacemaker clinics. Clinic visits may be done in conjunction with transtelephonic monitoring or as a separate service; however, the services rendered by a pacemaker clinic are more extensive than those currently possible by telephone. They include, for example, physical examination of patients and reprogramming of pacemakers. Thus, the use of one of these types of monitoring does not preclude concurrent use of the other.

2. Frequency Guidelines

As with transtelephonic pacemaker monitoring, the frequency of clinic visits is the decision of the patient's physician, taking into account, among other things, the medical condition of the patient. However, contractors can develop monitoring guidelines that will prove useful in screening claims. The following are recommendations for monitoring guidelines on lithium-battery pacemakers:

- For single-chamber pacemakers—twice in the first 6 months following implant, then once every 12 months.
- For dual-chamber pacemakers—twice in the first 6 months, then once every 6 months.

20.8.2—Self-Contained Pacemaker Monitors

(Rev. 1, 10-03-03)

CIM 60-7

Self-contained pacemaker monitors are accepted devices for monitoring cardiac pacemakers. Accordingly, program payment may be made for the rental or purchase of either of the following pacemaker monitors when a physician for a patient prescribes it with a cardiac pacemaker:

A—Digital Electronic Pacemaker Monitor

This device provides the patient with an instantaneous digital readout of his pacemaker pulse rate. Use of this device does not involve professional services until there has been a change of five pulses (or more) per minute above or below the initial rate of the pacemaker; when such change occurs, the patient contacts his physician.

B—Audible/Visible Signal Pacemaker Monitor

This device produces an audible and visible signal which indicates the pacemaker rate. Use of this device does not involve professional services until a change occurs in these signals; at such time, the patient contacts his physician.

NOTE: The design of the self-contained pacemaker monitor makes it possible for the patient to monitor his pacemaker periodically and minimizes the need for regular visits to the outpatient department of the provider.

Therefore, documentation of the medical necessity for pacemaker evaluation in the outpatient department of the provider should be obtained where such evaluation is employed in addition to the self-contained pacemaker monitor used by the patient in his home.

Cross-reference: §20.8.1

100-03 Part 1

20.9—Artificial Hearts And Related Devices (Effective March 27, 2007)

(Rev. 68, Issued: 04-13-07, Effective: 03-27-07, Implementation: 05-14-07)

A. General

A ventricular assist device (VAD) or left ventricular assist device (LVAD) is used to assist a damaged or weakened heart in pumping blood. These devices are used for support of blood circulation post-cardiotomy, as a bridge to a heart transplant, or as destination therapy.

B. Nationally Covered Indications

1. Postcardiotomy (effective for services performed on or after October 18, 1993)

Post-cardiotomy is the period following open-heart surgery. VADs used for support of blood circulation post-cardiotomy are covered only if they have received approval from the Food and Drug Administration (FDA) for that purpose, and the VADs are used according to the FDA- approved labeling instructions.

2. Bridge-to-Transplant (effective for services performed on or after January 22, 1996)

The VADs used for bridge-to-transplant are covered only if they have received approval from the FDA for that purpose, and the VADs are used according to the FDA-approved labeling instructions. All of the following criteria must be fulfilled in order for Medicare coverage to be provided for a VAD used as a bridge-to-transplant:

a. The patient is approved and listed as a candidate for heart transplantation by a Medicare-approved heart transplant center; and
b. The implanting site, if different than the Medicare-approved transplant center, must receive written permission from the Medicare-approved heart transplant center under which the patient is listed prior to implantation of the VAD.

The Medicare-approved heart transplant center should make every reasonable effort to transplant patients on such devices as soon as medically reasonable. Ideally, the Medicare-approved heart transplant centers should determine patient-specific timetables for transplantation, and should not maintain such patients on VADs if suitable hearts become available.

3. Destination Therapy (effective for services performed on or after October 1, 2003 with facility criteria updated March 27, 2007)

Destination therapy is for patients that require permanent mechanical cardiac support. The VADs used for destination therapy are covered only if they have received approval from the FDA for that purpose, and the device is used according to the FDA-approved labeling instructions.

Patient Selection

The VADs are covered for patients who have chronic end-stage heart failure (New York Heart Association Class IV end-stage left ventricular failure for at least 90 days with a life expectancy of less than 2 years), are not candidates for heart transplantation, and meet all of the following conditions:

a. The patient's Class IV heart failure symptoms have failed to respond to optimal medical management, including dietary salt restriction, diuretics, digitalis, beta-blockers, and ACE inhibitors (if tolerated) for at least 60 of the last 90 days;
b. The patient has a left ventricular ejection fraction (LVEF) < 25%;
c. The patient has demonstrated functional limitation with a peak oxygen consumption of < 12 ml/kg/min; or the patient has a continued need for intravenous inotropic therapy owing to symptomatic hypotension, decreasing renal function, or worsening pulmonary congestion; and,
d. The patient has the appropriate body size ($\geq$ 1.5 m²) to support the VAD implantation.

Facility Criteria

a. Facilities must have at least one member of the team with experience implanting at least 10 VADs (as bridge to transplant or destination therapy) or artificial hearts over the course of the previous 36 months;
b. Facilities must be a member of the Interagency Registry for Mechanically Assisted Circulatory Support (INTERMACS); and
c. By March 27, 2009, all facilities must meet the above facility criteria and be credential by the Joint Commission under the Disease Specific Certification Program for Ventricular Assist Devices (standard February 2007).

The Web site

http://www.cms.hhs.gov/MedicareApprovedFacilitie/VAD/list.asp#TopOfPage will be updated continuously to list all approved facilities. Facilities gaining Joint Commission certification (including prior to March 27, 2009) will be added to the Web site when certification is obtained. Hospitals also must have in place staff and procedures that ensure that prospective VAD recipients receive all information necessary to assist them in giving appropriate informed consent for the procedure so that they and their families are fully aware of the aftercare requirements and potential limitations, as well as benefits, following VAD implantation.

C. Nationally Non-Covered Indications (effective for services performed on or after May 19, 1986)

1. Artificial Heart

Since there is no authoritative evidence substantiating the safety and effectiveness of a VAD used as a replacement for the human heart, Medicare does not cover this device when used as an artificial heart.

All other indications for the use of VADs not otherwise listed remain noncovered, except in the context of Category B IDE clinical trials (42 CFR 405) or as a routine cost in clinical trials defined under section 310.1 of the NCD manual (old CIM 30-1).

(This NCD last reviewed March 2007.)

20.15—Electrocardiographic Services

(Rev. 26, Issued: 12-10-04, Effective: 08-26-04, Implementation: 12-10-04)

A—General

1. An electrocardiogram (EKG) is a graphic representation of electrical activity within the heart. Electrodes placed on the body in predetermined locations sense this electrical activity, which is then recorded by various means for review and interpretation. EKG recordings are used to diagnose a wide range of heart disease and other conditions that manifest themselves by abnormal cardiac electrical activity.

    KG services are covered diagnostic tests when there are documented signs and symptoms or other clinical indications for providing the service. Coverage includes the review interpretation of EKGs only by a physician. There is no age for EKG services when rendered as a screening test or part of a routine examination unless performed as part one-time, "Welcome to Medicare" preventive physical exa ion under section 611 of the Medicare Prescription Dru rovement, and Modernization Act of 2003.

2. An ry electrocardiography (AECG) refers to services tim n an outpatient setting over a specified period of ties, ally while a patient is engaged in daily activi- vide ing sleep. AECG devices are intended to pro- mia, ician with documented episodes of arrhyth- EKG. ay not be detected using a standard 12-lead that ma most typically used to evaluate symptoms and/or nte with intermittent cardiac arrhythmias cope, diz ischemia. Such symptoms include syn- hest pain, palpitations, or shortness of

breath. Additionally, AECG is used to evaluate patient response to initiation, revision, or discontinuation of arrhythmic drug therapy.

3. The Centers for Medicare & Medicaid Services (CMS), through the national coverage determination (NCD) process, may create new ambulatory EKG monitoring device categories if published, peer-reviewed clinical studies demonstrate evidence of improved clinical utility, or equal utility with additional advantage to the patient, as indicated by improved patient management and/or improved health outcomes in the Medicare population (such as superior ability to detect serious or life-threatening arrhythmias) as compared to devices or services in the currently described categories below.

Descriptions of Ambulatory EKG Monitoring Technologies

1. Dynamic electrocardiography devices that continuously record a real-time EKG, commonly known as Holter™ monitors, typically record over a 24-hour period. The recording is captured either on a magnetic tape or other digital medium. The data are then computer-analyzed at a later time, and a physician interprets the computer-generated report. A 24-hour recording is generally adequate to detect most transient arrhythmias. Documentation of medical necessity is required for monitoring longer than 24 hours. The recording device itself is not covered as durable medical equipment (DME) separate from the total diagnostic service.

2. An event monitor, or event recorder, is a patient-activated or event-activated EKG device that intermittently records cardiac arrhythmic events as they occur. The EKG is recorded on magnetic tape or other digital medium.

Cardiac event monitor technology varies among different devices. For patient-activated event monitors, the patient initiates recording when symptoms appear or when instructed to do so by a physician (e.g., following exercise). For self-sensing, automatically triggered monitors, an EKG is automatically recorded when the device detects an arrhythmia, without patient intervention. Some devices permit a patient to transmit EKG data trans-telephonically (i. e., via telephone) to a receiving center where the data are reviewed. A technician may be available at these centers to review transmitted data 24-hours per day. In some instances, when the EKG is determined to be outside certain pre-set criteria by a technician or other non-physician, a physician is available 24-hours per day to review the transmitted data and to make clinical decisions regarding the patient. These services are known as "24-hour attended monitoring". In other instances, transmitted EKG data are reviewed at a later time and are, therefore, considered "non-attended."

Cardiac event monitors without trans-telephonic capability must be removed from the patient and taken to a location for review of the stored EKG data. Some devices also permit a "time sampling" mode of operation. The "time sampling" mode is not covered under ambulatory EKG monitoring technology. Some cardiac event monitoring devices with trans-telephonic capabilities require the patient to dial the phone number of a central EKG data reception center and initiate transmission of EKG data. Other devices use Internet-based in-home computers to capture and store EKG data. When such devices detect pre-programmed arrhythmias, data is automatically sent via modem and standard telephone lines to a central receiving center, or independent diagnostic testing facility (IDTF), where the data are reviewed. Internet-based in-home computer systems may also provide the receiving center with a daily computer-generated report that summarizes 24 hours of EKG data.

Certain cardiac event monitors capture electrical activity with a single electrode attached to the skin. Other devices may employ multiple electrodes in order to record more complex EKG tracings. Additionally, devices may be individually programmed to detect patient-specific factors, electrode malfunction, or other factors. Cardiac event monitors can be further categorized as either "pre-event" or "post-event" recorders, based on their memory capabilities:

a. Pre-symptom Memory Loop Recorder (MLR)

Upon detecting symptoms, the wearer presses a button, which activates the recorder to save (i.e., memorize) an interval of pre-symptom EKG data along with data during and subsequent to the symptomatic event. Self-sensing recorders (also known as event-activated or automatic trigger) do not require patient input to capture these data. Single or multiple events may be recorded. The device is worn at all times, usually for up to 30 days.

• Implantable (or Insertable Loop) Recorder (ILR)

Another type of pre-symptom MLR, it is implanted subcutaneously in a patient's upper left chest and may remain implanted for many months. An ILR is used when syncope is thought to be cardiac-related, but is too infrequent to be detected by either a Holter™ monitor or a traditional pre-symptom MLR.

b. Post-symptom Recorder

The patient temporarily places this device against the chest when symptoms occur and activates it by pressing a button. These recorders represent old technology, as they do not include a memory loop. The device transmits EKG data telephonically in real-time and is usually used for up to 30 days.

B—Nationally Covered Indications

The following indications are covered nationally unless otherwise indicated:

1. Computer analysis of EKGs when furnished in a setting and under the circumstances required for coverage of other EKG services.
2. EKG services rendered by an independent diagnostic testing facility (IDTF), including physician review and interpretation. Separate physician services are not covered unless he/she is the patient's attending or consulting physician.
3. Emergency EKGs (i.e., when the patient is or may be experiencing a life-threatening event) performed as a laboratory or diagnostic service by a portable x-ray supplier only when a physician is in attendance at the time the service is performed or immediately thereafter.
4. Home EKG services with documentation of medical necessity.
5. Trans-telephonic EKG transmissions (effective March 1, 1980) as a diagnostic service for the indications described below, when performed with equipment meeting the stan-

dards described below, subject to the limitations and conditions specified below. Coverage is further limited to the amounts payable with respect to the physician's service in interpreting the results of such transmissions, including charges for rental of the equipment. The device used by the beneficiary is part of a total diagnostic system and is not considered DME separately. Covered uses are to:

a. Detect, characterize, and document symptomatic transient arrhythmias;
b. Initiate, revise, or discontinue arrhythmic drug therapy; or,
c. Carry out early post-hospital monitoring of patients discharged after myocardial infarction (MI); (only if 24-hour coverage is provided, see C.5. below).

Certain uses other than those specified above may be covered if, in the judgment of the local contractor, such use is medically necessary.

Additionally, the transmitting devices must meet at least the following criteria:

a. They must be capable of transmitting EKG Leads, I, II, or III; and,
b. The tracing must be sufficiently comparable to a conventional EKG.

24-hour attended coverage used as early post-hospital monitoring of patients discharged after MI is only covered if provision is made for such 24-hour attended coverage in the manner described below:

24-hour attended coverage means there must be, at a monitoring site or central data center, an EKG technician or other non-physician, receiving calls and/or EKG data; tape recording devices do not meet this requirement. Further, such technicians should have immediate, 24-hour access to a physician to review transmitted data and make clinical decisions regarding the patient. The technician should also be instructed as to when and how to contact available facilities to assist the patient in case of emergencies.

C—Nationally Non-covered Indications

The following indications are non-covered nationally unless otherwise specified below:

1. The time-sampling mode of operation of ambulatory EKG cardiac event monitoring/recording.
2. Separate physician services other than those rendered an IDTF unless rendered by the patient's attending or consulting physician.
3. Home EKG services without documentation of medical necessity.
4. Emergency EKG services by a portable x-ray supplier without a physician in attendance at the time of service or immediately thereafter.
5. 24-hour attended coverage used as early post-hospital monitoring of patients discharged after MI unless provision is made for such 24-hour attended coverage in the manner described in section B.5. above.
6. Any marketed Food and Drug Administration (FDA)-approved ambulatory cardiac monitoring or service that cannot be categorized according to the framework below.

D—Other

Ambulatory cardiac monitoring performed with a marketed, FDA-approved device, is eligible for coverage if it can be categorized according to the framework below. Unless there is a specific NCD for that device or service, determination as to whether a device or service that fits into the framework is reasonable and necessary is according to local contractor discretion.

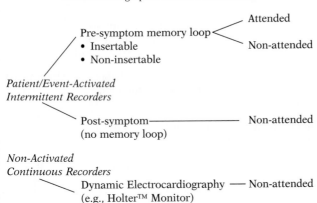

Electrocardiographic Services Framework

Pre-symptom memory loop
- Insertable
- Non-insertable

Attended

Non-attended

Patient/Event-Activated Intermittent Recorders

Post-symptom —————— Non-attended
(no memory loop)

Non-Activated Continuous Recorders

Dynamic Electrocardiography —— Non-attended
(e.g., Holter™ Monitor)

(This NCD last reviewed December 2004.)

20.19—Ambulatory Blood Pressure Monitoring

(Rev. 1, 10-03-03)

CIM 50-42

Ambulatory blood pressure monitoring (ABPM) involves the use of a noninvasive device which is used to measure blood pressure in 24-hour cycles. These 24-hour measurements are stored in the device and are later interpreted by the physician. ABPM must be performed for at least 24 hours to meet coverage criteria.

The ABPM is only covered for those patients with suspected white coat hypertension. Suspected white coat hypertension is defined as

Office blood pressure > 140/90 mm Hg on at least three separate clinic/office visits with two separate measurements made at each visit;
least two documented blood pressure measurements en outside the office which are < 140/90 mm Hg; and evidence of end-organ damage.

Th
determination obtained by ABPM is necessary in order to
is n the appropriate management of the patient. ABPM
that red for any other uses. In the rare circumstance
tient, needs to be performed more than once in a pa-
each s lifying criteria described above must be met for
ABPM ant ABPM test. For those patients that undergo
with no e an ambulatory blood pressure of < 135/85
cardiovas of end-organ damage, it is likely that their
should be sk is similar to that of normotensives. They
onstrates al over time. Patients for which ABPM dem-
cardiovascu ressure of > 135/85 may be at increased
antihyperten and a physician may wish to consider
apy.

20.20—External Counterpulsation (ECP) Therapy for Severe Angina (Effective March 20, 2006)

(Rev. 50, Issued: 03-31-06; Effective: 03-20-06; Implementation: 04-03-06)

CIM 35-74

A. General

External counterpulsation (ECP), commonly referred to as enhanced external counterpulsation, is a noninvasive outpatient treatment for coronary artery disease refractory to medical and/or surgical therapy. Although ECP devices are cleared by the Food and Drug Administration (FDA) for use in treating a variety of cardiac conditions, including stable or unstable angina pectoris, acute myocardial infarction and cardiogenic shock, the use of this device to treat cardiac conditions other than stable angina pectoris is not covered, since only that use has developed sufficient evidence to demonstrate its medical effectiveness. Noncoverage of hydraulic versions of these types of devices remains in force.

B. Nationally Covered Indications

Effective for services performed on or after July 1, 1999, coverage is provided for the use of ECP for patients who have been diagnosed with disabling angina (Class III or Class IV, Canadian Cardiovascular Society Classification or equivalent classification) who, in the opinion of a cardiologist or cardiothoracic surgeon, are not readily amenable to surgical intervention, such as PTCA or cardiac bypass because:

1. Their condition is inoperable, or at high risk of operative complications or post-operative failure;
2. Their coronary anatomy is not readily amenable to such procedures; or
3. They have co-morbid states that create excessive risk.

A full course of therapy usually consists of 35 one-hour treatments which may be offered once or twice daily, usually five days per week. The patient is placed on a treatment table where their lower trunk and lower extremities are wrapped in a series of three compressive air cuffs which inflate and deflate in synchronization with the patient's cardiac cycle.

During diastole, the three sets of air cuffs are inflated sequentially (distal to proximal) compressing the vascular beds within the muscles of the calves, lower thighs and upper thighs. This action results in an increase in diastolic pressure, generation of retrograde arterial blood flow and an increase in venous return. The cuffs are deflated simultaneously just prior to systole which produces a rapid drop in vascular impedance, a decrease in ventricular workload and an increase in cardiac output.

The augmented diastolic pressure and retrograde aortic flow appear to improve myocardial perfusion, while systolic unloading appears to reduce cardiac workload and oxygen requirements. The increased venous return coupled with enhanced systolic flow appears to increase cardiac output. As a result of this treatment, most patients experience increased time until onset of ischemia, increased exercise tolerance, and a reduction in the number and severity of anginal episodes. Evidence was presented that this effect lasted well beyond the immediate post-treatment phase, with patients symptom-free for several months to two years.

This procedure must be done under direct supervision of a physician.

C. Nationally Non-Covered Indications

All other cardiac conditions not otherwise specified as nationally covered for the use of ECP remain nationally non-covered.

(This NCD last reviewed March 2006.)

20.21—Chelation Therapy for Treatment of Atherosclerosis

(Rev. 1, 10-03-03)

CIM 35-64

Chelation therapy is the application of chelation techniques for the therapeutic or preventive effects of removing unwanted metal ions from the body. The application of chelation therapy using ethylenediamine-tetra-acetic acid (EDTA) for the treatment and prevention of atherosclerosis is controversial. There is no widely accepted rationale to explain the beneficial effects attributed to this therapy. Its safety is questioned and its clinical effectiveness has never been established by well-designed, controlled clinical trials. It is not widely accepted and practiced by American physicians. EDTA chelation therapy for atherosclerosis is considered experimental. For these reasons, EDTA chelation therapy for the treatment or prevention of atherosclerosis is not covered. Some practitioners refer to this therapy as chemoendarterectomy and may also show a diagnosis other than atherosclerosis, such as arteriosclerosis or calcinosis. Claims employing such variant terms should also be denied under this section.

Cross-reference: §20.22.

20.22—Ethylenediamine-Tetra-Acetic (EDTA) Chelation Therapy for Treatment of Atherosclerosis

(Rev. 1, 10-03-03)

CIM 45-20

The use of EDTA as a chelating agent to treat atherosclerosis, arteriosclerosis, calcinosis, or similar generalized condition not listed by the FDA as an approved use is not covered. Any such use of EDTA is considered experimental. See §20.21 for an explanation of this conclusion.

20.24—Displacement Cardiography

(Rev. 1, 10-03-03)

CIM 50-50

Displacement cardiography, including cardiokymography and photokymography, is a noninvasive diagnostic test used in evaluating coronary artery disease.

A—Cardiokymography

Cardiokymography is covered for services rendered on or after October 12, 1988.

Cardiokymography is a covered service only when it is used as an adjunct to electrocardiographic stress testing in evaluating coronary artery disease and only when the following clinical indications are present:

- For male patients, atypical angina pectoris or nonischemic chest pain; or
- For female patients, angina, either typical or atypical.

B—Photokymography—Not Covered

Photokymography remains excluded from coverage.

20.29—Hyperbaric Oxygen Therapy

(Rev. 48, Issued: 03-17-06; Effective/Implementation Dates: 06-19-06)

CIM 35-10

For purposes of coverage under Medicare, hyperbaric oxygen (HBO) therapy is a modality in which the entire body is exposed to oxygen under increased atmospheric pressure.

A—Covered Conditions

Program reimbursement for HBO therapy will be limited to that which is administered in a chamber (including the one man unit) and is limited to the following conditions:

1. Acute carbon monoxide intoxication.
2. Decompression illness.
3. Gas embolism.
4. Gas gangrene.
5. Acute traumatic peripheral ischemia. HBO therapy is a valuable adjunctive treatment to be used in combination with accepted standard therapeutic measures when loss of function, limb, or life is threatened.
6. Crush injuries and suturing of severed limbs. As in the previous conditions, HBO therapy would be an adjunctive treatment when loss of function, limb, or life is threatened.
7. Progressive necrotizing infections (necrotizing fasciitis).
8. Acute peripheral arterial insufficiency.
9. Preparation and preservation of compromised skin grafts (not for primary management of wounds).
10. Chronic refractory osteomyelitis, unresponsive to conventional medical and surgical management.
11. Osteoradionecrosis as an adjunct to conventional treatment.
12. Soft tissue radionecrosis as an adjunct to conventional treatment.
13. Cyanide poisoning.
14. Actinomycosis, only as an adjunct to conventional therapy when the disease process is refractory to antibiotics and surgical treatment.
15. Diabetic wounds of the lower extremities in patients who meet the following three criteria:
    a. Patient has type I or type II diabetes and has a lower extremity wound that is due to diabetes;
    b. Patient has a wound classified as Wagner grade III or higher; and
    c. Patient has failed an adequate course of standard wound therapy.

The use of HBO therapy is covered as adjunctive therapy only after there are no measurable signs of healing for at least 30 days of treatment with standard wound therapy and must be used in addition to standard wound care. Standard wound care in patients with diabetic wounds includes: assessment of a patient's vascular status and correction of any vascular problems in the affected limb if possible, optimization of nutritional status, optimization of glucose control, debridement by any means to remove devitalized tissue, maintenance of a clean, moist bed of granulation tissue with appropriate moist dressings, appropriate off-loading, and necessary treatment to resolve any infection that might be present. Failure to respond to standard wound care occurs when there are no measurable signs of healing for at least 30 consecutive days. Wounds must be evaluated at least every 30 days during administration of HBO therapy. Continued treatment with HBO therapy is not covered if measurable signs of healing have not been demonstrated within any 30-day period of treatment.

B—Noncovered Conditions

All other indications not specified under §270.4(A) are not covered under the Medicare program. No program payment may be made for any conditions other than those listed in §270.4(A).

No program payment may be made for HBO in the treatment of the following conditions:

1. Cutaneous, decubitus, and stasis ulcers
2. Chronic peripheral vascular insufficiency
3. Anaerobic septicemia and infection other than clostridial
4. Skin burns (thermal).
5. Senility.
6. Myocardial infarction.
7. Cardiogenic shock.
8. Sickle cell anemia.
9. Acute thermal and chemical pulmonary damage, i.e., smoke inhalation with pulmonary insufficiency
10. Acute or chronic cerebral vascular insufficiency.
11. Hepatic necrosis.
12. Aerobic septicemia.
13. Nonvascular causes of chronic brain syndrome (Pick's disease, Alzheimer's disease, Korsakoff's disease)
14. Tetanus.
15. Systemic aerobic infection.
16. Organ transplantation.
17. Organ storage.
18. Pulmonary emphysema.
19. Exceptional blood loss anemia.
    Multiple Sclerosis.
    Arthritic Diseases.
    Acute cerebral edema.

C—Topical Application of Oxygen

This definition of administering oxygen does not meet the efficacy HBO therapy as stated above. Also, its clinical reimbur not been established. Therefore, no Medicare oxygen. t may be made for the topical application of

Cross refe
§270.5 of this manual.

30.8—Cellular Therapy

(Rev. 1, 10-03-03)

CIM 35-5

Not Covered

Cellular therapy involves the practice of injecting humans with foreign proteins like the placenta or lungs of unborn lambs. Cellular therapy is without scientific or statistical evidence to document its therapeutic efficacy and, in fact, is considered a potentially dangerous practice. Accordingly, cellular therapy is not considered reasonable and necessary within the meaning of §1862(a)(1) of the Act.

40.2—Home Blood Glucose Monitors

(Rev. 48, Issued: 03-17-06; Effective/Implementation Dates: 06-19-06)

CIM 60-11

There are several different types of blood glucose monitors that use reflectance meters to determine blood glucose levels. Medicare coverage of these devices varies, with respect to both the type of device and the medical condition of the patient for whom the device is prescribed.

Reflectance colorimeter devices used for measuring blood glucose levels in clinical settings are not covered as durable medical equipment for use in the home because their need for frequent professional recalibration makes them unsuitable for home use. However, some types of blood glucose monitors which use a reflectance meter specifically designed for home use by diabetic patients may be covered as durable medical equipment, subject to the conditions and limitations described below.

Blood glucose monitors are meter devices that read color changes produced on specially treated reagent strips by glucose concentrations in the patient's blood. The patient, using a disposable sterile lancet, draws a drop of blood, places it on a reagent strip and, following instructions which may vary with the device used, inserts it into the device to obtain a reading. Lancets, reagent strips, and other supplies necessary for the proper functioning of the device are also covered for patients for whom the device is indicated. Home blood glucose monitors enable certain patients to better control their blood glucose levels by frequently checking and appropriately contacting their attending physician for advice and treatment. Studies indicate that the patient's ability to carefully follow proper procedures is critical to obtaining satisfactory results with these devices. In addition, the cost of the devices, with their supplies, limits economical use to patients who must make frequent checks of their blood glucose levels. Accordingly, coverage of home blood glucose monitors is limited to patients meeting the following conditions:

1. The patient has been diagnosed as having diabetes;
2. The patient's physician states that the patient is capable of being trained to use the particular device prescribed in an appropriate manner. In some cases, the patient may not be able to perform this function, but a responsible individual can be trained to use the equipment and monitor the patient to assure that the intended effect is achieved. This is permissible if the record is properly documented by the patient's physician; and
3. The device is designed for home rather than clinical use.

There is also a blood glucose monitoring system designed especially for use by those with visual impairments. The monitors used in such systems are identical in terms of reliability and sensitivity to the standard blood glucose monitors described above. They differ by having such features as voice synthesizers, automatic timers, and specially designed arrangements of supplies and materials to enable the visually impaired to use the equipment without assistance.

These special blood glucose monitoring systems are covered under Medicare if the following conditions are met:

- The patient and device meet the three conditions listed above for coverage of standard home blood glucose monitors; and
- The patient's physician certifies that he or she has a visual impairment severe enough to require use of this special monitoring system.

The additional features and equipment of these special systems justify a higher reimbursement amount than allowed for standard blood glucose monitors. Separately identify claims for such devices and establish a separate reimbursement amount for them.

50—Ear, Nose and Throat (ENT)

(Rev. 1, 10-03-03)

50.1—Speech Generating Devices

(Rev. 1, 10-03-03)

CIM 60-23

Effective January 1, 2001, augmentative and alternative communication devices or communicators which are hereafter referred to as "speech generating devices" are now considered to fall within the DME benefit category established by §1861(n) of the Social Security Act. They may be covered if the contractor's medical staff determines that the patient suffers from a severe speech impairment and that the medical condition warrants the use of a device based on the following definitions.

Definition of Speech Generating Devices

Speech generating devices are defined as speech aids that provide an individual who has a severe speech impairment with the ability to meet his functional speaking needs. Speech generating are characterized by:

- Being a dedicated speech device, used solely by the individual who has a severe speech impairment;
- May have digitized speech output, using prerecorded messages, less than or equal to 8 minutes recording time;
- May have digitized speech output, using prerecorded messages, greater than 8 minutes recording time;
- May have synthesized speech output which requires message formulation by spelling and device access by physical contact with the device-direct selection techniques;
- May have synthesized speech output which permits multiple methods of message formulation and multiple methods of device access; or
- May be software that allows a laptop computer, desktop computer or personal digital assistant (PDA) to function as a speech generating device.

Devices that would not meet the definition of speech generating devices and therefore, do not fall within the scope of §1861(n) of the Act are characterized by:

- Devices that are not dedicated speech devices, but are devices that are capable of running software for purposes other than for speech generation, e.g., devices that can also run a word processing package, an accounting program, or perform other than non-medical function.
- Laptop computers, desktop computers, or PDAs which may be programmed to perform the same function as a speech generating device, are noncovered since they are not primarily medical in nature and do not meet the definition of DME. For this reason, they cannot be considered speech-generating devices for Medicare coverage purposes.
- A device that is useful to someone without severe speech impairment is not considered a speech-generating device for Medicare coverage purposes.

50.2—Electronic Speech Aids

(Rev. 1, 10-03-03)

CIM 65-5

Electronic speech aids are covered under Part B as prosthetic devices when the patient has had a laryngectomy or his larynx is permanently inoperative. There are two types of speech aids. One operates by placing a vibrating head against the throat; the other amplifies sound waves through a tube which is inserted into the user's mouth. A patient who has had radical neck surgery and/or extensive radiation to the anterior part of the neck would generally be able to use only the "oral tube" model or one of the more sensitive and more expensive "throat contact" devices.

Cross-reference:

The Medicare Benefit Policy Manual, Chapter 15, "Covered Medical and Other Health Services," §120.

50.3—Cochlear Implantation (Effective April 4, 2005)

(Rev. 42, Issued: 06/24/05; Effective: 04-04-05; Implementation: 07-25-05)

A. General

A cochlear implant device is an electronic instrument, part of which is implanted surgically to stimulate auditory nerve fibers, and part of which is worn or carried by the individual to capture, analyze and code sound. Cochlear implant devices are available in single channel and multi-channel models. The purpose of implanting the device is to provide an awareness and identification of sounds and to facilitate communication for persons who are profoundly hearing impaired.

B. Nationally Covered Indications

1. Effective for services performed on or after April 4, 2005, cochlear implantation may be covered for treatment of bilateral pre- or post-linguistic, sensorineural, moderate-to-profound hearing loss in individuals who demonstrate limited benefit from amplification. Limited benefit from amplification is defined by test scores of less than or equal to 40% correct in the best-aided listening condition on tape-recorded tests of open-set sentence cognition. Medicare coverage is provided only for those patients who meet all of the following selection guidelines.

- Diagnosis of bilateral severe-to-profound sensorineural hearing impairment with limited benefit from appropriate hearing (or vibrotactile) aids;
- Cognitive ability to use auditory clues and a willingness to undergo an extended program of rehabilitation;
- Freedom from middle ear infection, an accessible cochlear lumen that is structurally suited to implantation, and freedom from lesions in the auditory nerve and acoustic areas of the central nervous system;
- No contraindications to surgery; and
- The device must be used in accordance with the FDA-approved labeling.

2. Effective for services performed on or after April 4, 2005, cochlear implantation may be covered for individuals meeting the selection guidelines above and with hearing test scores of greater than 40% and less than or equal to 60% only when the provider is participating in, and patients are enrolled in, either an FDA-approved category B investigational device exemption clinical trial as defined at 42 CFR 405.201, a trial under the Centers for Medicare & Medicaid (CMS) Clinical Trial Policy as defined at section 310.1 of the National Coverage Determinations Manual, or a prospective, controlled comparative trial approved by CMS as consistent with the evidentiary requirements for National Coverage Analyses and meeting specific quality standards.

C. Nationally Noncovered Indications

Medicare beneficiaries not meeting all of the coverage criteria for cochlear implantation listed are deemed not eligible for Medicare coverage under section 1862(a)(1)(A) of the Social Security Act.

D. Other

All other indications for cochlear implantation not otherwise indicated as nationally covered or non-covered above remain at local contractor discretion.

(This NCD last reviewed May 2005.)

70.2.1—Services Provided for the Diagnosis and Treatment of Diabetic Sensory Neuropathy with Loss of Protective Sensation (aka Diabetic Peripheral Neuropathy)

(Rev. 1, 10-03-03)

CIM 50-8.1

Presently, peripheral neuropathy, or diabetic sensory neuropathy, is the most common factor leading to amputation in people with diabetes. In diabetes, sensory neuropathy is an anatomically diffuse process primarily affecting sensory and autonomic fibers; however, distal motor findings may be present in advanced cases. Long nerves are affected first, with symptoms typically beginning insidiously in the toes and then advancing proximally. This leads to loss of protective sensation (LOPS), whereby a person is unable to feel minor trauma from mechanical, thermal, or chemical sources. When foot lesions are present, the reduction in autonomic nerve functions may also inhibit wound healing.

Diabetic sensory neuropathy with LOPS is a localized illness of the feet and falls within the regulation's exception to the general exclusionary rule (see 42 CFR 411.15(l)(1)(i)). Foot exams for people with diabetic sensory neuropathy with LOPS are reasonable and necessary to allow for early inter-vention in serious complications that typically afflict diabetics with the disease.

Effective for services furnished on or after July 1, 2002, Medicare covers, as a physician service, an evaluation (examination and treatment) of the feet no more often than every six months for individuals with a documented diagnosis of diabetic sensory neuropathy and LOPS, as long as the beneficiary has not seen a foot care specialist for some other reason in the interim. LOPS shall be diagnosed through sensory testing with the 5.07 monofilament using established guidelines, such as those developed by the National Institute of Diabetes and Digestive and Kidney Diseases guidelines. Five sites should be tested on the plantar surface of each foot, according to the National Institute of Diabetes and Digestive and Kidney Diseases guidelines. The areas must be tested randomly since the loss of protective sensation may be patchy in distribution, and the patient may get clues if the test is done rhythmically. Heavily callused areas should be avoided. As suggested by the American Podiatric Medicine Association, an absence of sensation at two or more sites out of 5 tested on either foot when tested with the 5.07 Semmes-Weinstein monofilament must be present and documented to diagnose peripheral neuropathy with loss of protective sensation.

The examination includes:

1. A patient history, and
2. A physical examination that must consist of at least the following elements:
   - Visual inspection of forefoot and hindfoot (including toe web spaces);
   - Evaluation of protective sensation;
   - Evaluation of foot structure and biomechanics;
   - Evaluation of vascular status and skin integrity;
   - Evaluation of the need for special footwear; and
3. Patient education.

A. Treatment includes, but is not limited to:

- Local care of superficial wounds;
- Debridement of corns and calluses; and
- Trimming and debridement of nails.

The diagnosis of diabetic sensory neuropathy with LOPS should be established and documented prior to coverage of foot care. Other causes of peripheral neuropathy should be considered and investigated by the primary care physician prior to initiating or referring for foot care for persons with LOPS.

80—Eye

(Rev. 1, 10-03-03)

80.1—Hydrophilic Contact Lens for Corneal Bandage

(Rev. 1, 10-03-03)

CIM 45-7

Some hydrophilic contact lenses are used as moist corneal bandages for the treatment of acute or chronic corneal pathology, such as bulbous keratopathy, dry eyes, corneal ulcers and erosion, keratitis, corneal edema, descemetocele, corneal ectasis, Mooren's ulcer, anterior corneal dystrophy, neurotrophic keratoconjunctivitis, and for other therapeutic reasons.

Payment may be made under §1861(s)(2) of the Act for a hydrophilic contact lens approved by the Food and Drug Administration (FDA) and used as a supply incident to a physician's service. Payment for the lens is included in the payment for the physician's service to which the lens is incident. Contractors are authorized to accept an FDA letter of approval or other FDA published material as evidence of FDA approval. (See §80.4 for coverage of a hydrophilic contact lens as a prosthetic device.) See the Medicare Benefit Policy Manual, Chapter 15, "Covered Medical and Other Health Services," and the Medicare Benefit Policy Manual, Chapter 6, "Hospital Services Covered Under Part B," §20.4.

80.2—Photodynamic Therapy

(Rev. 1, 10-03-03)

CIM 35-100

Photodynamic therapy is a medical procedure which involves the infusion of a photosensitive (light-activated) drug with a very specific absorption peak. This drug is chemically designed to have a unique affinity for the diseased tissue intended for treatment. Once introduced to the body, the drug accumulates and is retained in diseased tissue to a greater degree than in normal tissue. Infusion is followed by the targeted irradiation of this tissue with a non-thermal laser, calibrated to emit light at a wavelength that corresponds to the drug's absorption peak. The drug then becomes active and locally treats the diseased tissue.

Ocular photodynamic therapy (OPT)

The OPT is used in the treatment of ophthalmologic diseases. OPT is only covered when used in conjunction with verteporfin (see §80.3, "Photosensitive Drugs").

- Classic Subfoveal Choroidal Neovascular (CNV) Lesions - OPT is covered with a diagnosis of neovascular age-related macular degeneration (AMD) with predominately classic subfoveal choroidal neovascular (CNV) lesions (where the area of classic CNV occupies ≥ 50 percent of the area of the entire lesion) at the initial visit as determined by a fluorescein angiogram. Subsequent follow-up visits will require a fluorescein angiogram prior to treatment. There are no requirements regarding visual acuity, lesion size, and number of re-treatments.
- Occult Subfoveal Choroidal Neovascular (CNV) Lesions - OPT is noncovered for patients with a diagnosis of age-related macular degeneration (AMD) with occult and no classic CNV lesions.
- Other Conditions - Use of OPT with verteporfin for other types of AMD (e.g., patients with minimally classic CNV lesions, atrophic, or dry AMD) is noncovered. OPT with verteporfin for other ocular indications such as pathologic myopia or presumed ocular histoplasmosis syndrome, is eligible for coverage through individual contractor discretion.

80.2.1—Ocular Photodynamic Therapy (OPT) - Effective April 1, 2004 (see also 80.3 Photosensitive Drugs)

(Rev. 9, 04-01-04)

General

The OPT is used in the treatment of ophthalmologic diseases; specifically, for age-related macular degeneration (AMD), a common eye disease among the elderly. OPT involves the infusion of an intravenous photosensitizing drug called verte-

porfin followed by exposure to a laser. OPT is only covered when used in conjunction with verteporfin. Effective July 1, 2001, OPT with verteporfin was approved for a diagnosis of neovascular AMD with predominately classic subfoveal choroidal neovascularization (CNV) lesions (where the area of classic CNV occupies ≥ 50% of the area of the entire lesion) at the initial visit as determined by a fluorescein angiogram.

On October 17, 2001, CMS announced its "intent to cover" OPT with verteporfin for AMD patients with occult and no classic subfoveal CNV as determined by a fluorescein angiogram. The October 17, 2001, decision was never implemented.

On March 28, 2002, after thorough review and reconsideration of the October 17, 2001, intent to cover policy, CMS determined that the current noncoverage policy for OPT for verteporfin for AMD patients with occult and no classic subfoveal CNV as determined by a fluorescein angiogram should remain in effect.

Effective August 20, 2002, CMS issued a noncovered instruction for OPT with verteporfin for AMD patients with occult and no classic subfoveal CNV as determined by a fluorescein angiogram.

Covered Indications

Effective April 1, 2004, OPT with verteporfin continues to be approved for a diagnosis of neovascular AMD with predominately classic subfoveal CNV lesions (where the area of classic CNV occupies ≥ 50% of the area of the entire lesion) at the initial visit as determined by a fluorescein angiogram. (CNV lesions are comprised of classic and/or occult components.) Subsequent follow-up visits require a fluorescein angiogram prior to treatment. There are no requirements regarding visual acuity, lesion size, and number of re-treatments when treating predominantly classic lesions.

In addition, after thorough review and reconsideration of the August 20, 2002, noncoverage policy, CMS determines that the evidence is adequate to conclude that OPT with verteporfin is reasonable and necessary for treating:

1. Subfoveal occult with no classic CNV associated with AMD; and
2. Subfoveal minimally classic CNV (where the area of classic CNV occupies <50% of the area of the entire lesion) associated with AMD.

The above 2 indications are considered reasonable and necessary only when:

1. The lesions are small (4 disk areas or less in size) at the time of initial treatment or within the 3 months prior to initial treatment; and
2. The lesions have shown evidence of progression within the 3 months prior to initial treatment. Evidence of progression must be documented by deterioration of visual acuity (at least 5 letters on a standard eye examination chart), lesion growth (an increase in at least 1 disk area), or the appearance of blood associated with the lesion.

Noncovered Indications

Other uses of OPT with verteporfin to treat AMD not already addressed by CMS will continue to be noncovered. These include, but are not limited to, the following AMD indications:

- Juxtafoveal or extrafoveal CNV lesions (lesions outside the fovea),
- Inability to obtain a fluorescein angiogram,
- Atrophic or "dry" AMD.

Other

The OPT with verteporfin for other ocular indications, such as pathologic myopia or presumed ocular histoplasmosis syndrome, continue to be eligible for local coverage determinations through individual contractor discretion.

(This NCD last reviewed March 2004.)

80.3—Photosensitive Drugs

(Rev. 1, 10-03-03)

CIM 45-30

Photosensitive drugs are the light-sensitive agents used in photodynamic therapy. Once introduced into the body, these drugs selectively identify and adhere to diseased tissue. The drugs remain inactive until they are exposed to a specific wavelength of light, by means of a laser, that corresponds to their absorption peak. The activation of a photosensitive drug results in a photochemical reaction which treats the diseased tissue without affecting surrounding normal tissue.

Verteporfin

Verteporfin, a benzoporphyrin derivative, is an intravenous lipophilic photosensitive drug with an absorption peak of 690 nm. This drug was first approved by the Food and Drug Administration (FDA) on April 12, 2000, and subsequently, approved for inclusion in the United States Pharmacopoeia on July 18, 2000, meeting Medicare's definition of a drug when used in conjunction with ocular photodynamic therapy (see §80.2, "Photodynamic Therapy") when furnished intravenously incident to a physician's service. For patients with age-related macular degeneration, Verteporfin is only covered with a diagnosis of neovascular age-related macular degeneration (ICD-9-CM 362.52) with predominately classic subfoveal choroidal neovascular (CNV) lesions (where the area of classic CNV occupies ≥ 50 percent of the area of the entire lesion) at the initial visit as determined by a fluorescein angiogram (CPT code 92235). Subsequent follow-up visits will require a fluorescein angiogram prior to treatment. OPT with verteporfin is covered for the above indication and will remain noncovered for all other indications related to AMD (see §80.2). OPT with Verteporfin for use in non-AMD conditions is eligible for coverage through individual contractor discretion.

80.3.1- Verteporfin - Effective April 1, 2004 (see also 80.2.1 Ocular Photodynamic Therapy (OPT))

(Rev 9, 04-01-04)

General

Verteporfin, a benzoporphyrin derivative, is an intravenous lipophilic photosensitive drug with an absorption peak of 690 nm. Verteporfin was first approved by the Food and Drug Administration on April 12, 2000, and subsequently approved for inclusion in the United States Pharmacopoeia on July 18, 2000, meeting Medicare's definition of a drug as defined under §1861(t)(1) of the Social Security Act. Verteporfin is only covered when used in conjunction with ocular photodynamic therapy OPT) when furnished intravenously incident to a physician's service.

Covered Indications

Effective April 1, 2004, OPT with verteporfin is covered for patients with a diagnosis of neovascular age-related macular degeneration (AMD) with:

- Predominately classic subfoveal choroidal neovascularization (CNV) lesions (where the area of classic CNV occupies ≥ 50% of the area of the entire lesion) at the initial visit as determined by a fluorescein angiogram. (CNV lesions are comprised of classic and/or occult components.) Subsequent follow-up visits require a fluorescein angiogram prior to treatment. There are no requirements regarding visual acuity, lesion size, and number of retreatments when treating predominantly classic lesions.
- Subfoveal occult with no classic associated with AMD.
- Subfoveal minimally classic CNV CNV (where the area of classic CNV occupies < 50% of the area of the entire lesion) associated with AMD.
- The above 2 indications are considered reasonable and necessary only when:

1. The lesions are small (4 disk areas or less in size) at the time of initial treatment or within the 3 months prior to initial treatment; and,
2. The lesions have shown evidence of progression within the 3 months prior to initial treatment. Evidence of progression must be documented by deterioration of visual acuity (at least 5 letters on a standard eye examination chart), lesion growth (an increase in at least 1 disk area), or the appearance of blood associated with the lesion.

Noncovered Indications

Other uses of OPT with verteporfin to treat AMD not already addressed by CMS will continue to be noncovered. These include, but are not limited to, the following AMD indications: juxtafoveal or extrafoveal CNV lesions (lesions outside the fovea), inability to obtain a fluorescein angiogram, or atrophic or "dry" AMD.

Other

The OPT with verteporfin for other ocular indications, such as pathologic myopia or presumed ocular histoplasmosis syndrome, continue to be eligible for local coverage determinations through individual contractor discretion.

(This NCD last reviewed March 2004.)

80.4—Hydrophilic Contact Lenses

(Rev. 1, 10-03-03)

CIM 65-1

Hydrophilic contact lenses are eyeglasses within the meaning of the exclusion in §1862(a)(7) of the Act and are not covered when used in the treatment of nondiseased eyes with spherical ametrophia, refractive astigmatism, and/or corneal astigmatism. Payment may be made under the prosthetic device benefit, however, for hydrophilic contact lenses when prescribed for an aphakic patient.

Contractors are authorized to accept an FDA letter of approval or other FDA published material as evidence of FDA approval. (See §80.1 for coverage of a hydrophilic lens as a corneal bandage.)

Cross-references:

The Medicare Benefit Policy Manual, Chapter 15, "Covered Medical and Other Health Services," §100 and §120.

The Medicare Benefit Policy Manual, Chapter 16, "General Exclusions from Coverage," §20 and §90.

100-03 Part 2

110.2—Certain Drugs Distributed by the National Cancer Institute

(Rev. 1, 10-03-03)

CIM 45-16

Under its Cancer Therapy Evaluation, the Division of Cancer Treatment of the National Cancer Institute (NCI), in cooperation with the Food and Drug Administration, approves and distributes certain drugs for use in treating terminally ill cancer patients. One group of these drugs, designated as Group C drugs, unlike other drugs distributed by the NCI, are not limited to use in clinical trials for the purpose of testing their efficacy. Drugs are classified as Group C drugs only if there is sufficient evidence demonstrating their efficacy within a tumor type and that they can be safely administered.

A physician is eligible to receive Group C drugs from the Division of Cancer Treatment only if the following requirements are met:

- A physician must be registered with the NCI as an investigator by having completed an FD-Form 1573;
- A written request for the drug, indicating the disease to be treated, must be submitted to the NCI;
- The use of the drug must be limited to indications outlined in the NCIs guidelines; and
- All adverse reactions must be reported to the Investigational Drug Branch of the Division of Cancer Treatment.

In view of these NCI controls on distribution and use of Group C drugs, intermediaries may assume, in the absence of evidence to the contrary, that a Group C drug and the related hospital stay are covered if all other applicable coverage requirements are satisfied.

If there is reason to question coverage in a particular case, the matter should be resolved with the assistance of the Quality Improvement Organization (QIO), or if there is none, the assistance of the contractor's medical consultants. Information regarding those drugs which are classified as Group C drugs may be obtained from:

Office of the Chief, Investigational Drug Branch
Division of Cancer Treatment, CTEP, Landow Building
Room 4C09, National Cancer Institute
Bethesda, Maryland 20205

110.3—Anti-Inhibitor Coagulant Complex (AICC)

(Rev. 1, 10-03-03)

CIM 45-24

Anti-inhibitor coagulant complex, AICC, is a drug used to treat hemophilia in patients with factor VIII inhibitor anti-bodies. AICC has been shown to be safe and effective and has Medicare coverage when furnished to patients with hemophilia A and inhibitor antibodies to factor VIII who have major bleeding episodes and who fail to respond to other, less expensive therapies.

140.2—Breast Reconstruction Following Mastectomy

(Rev. 1, 10-03-03)

CIM 35-47

During recent years, there has been a considerable change in the treatment of diseases of the breast such as fibrocystic disease and cancer. While extirpation of the disease remains of primary importance, the quality of life following initial treatment is increasingly recognized as of great concern. The increased use of breast reconstruction procedures is due to several factors:

- A change in epidemiology of breast cancer, including an apparent increase in incidence;
- Improved surgical skills and techniques;
- The continuing development of better prostheses; and
- Increasing awareness by physicians of the importance of postsurgical psychological adjustment.

Reconstruction of the affected and the contralateral unaffected breast following a medically necessary mastectomy is considered a relatively safe and effective noncosmetic procedure. Accordingly, program payment may be made for breast reconstruction surgery following removal of a breast for any medical reason.

Program payment may not be made for breast reconstruction for cosmetic reasons. (Cosmetic surgery is excluded from coverage under §1862(a)(10) of the Act.)

150.2—Osteogenic Stimulator (Various Effective Dates Below)

(Rev.41, Issued: 06-24-05, Effective: 04-27-05, Implementation: 08-01-05)

CIM 35-48
Electrical Osteogenic Stimulators

A. General

Electrical stimulation to augment bone repair can be attained either invasively or noninvasively. Invasive devices provide electrical stimulation directly at the fracture site either through percutaneously placed cathodes or by implantation of a coiled cathode wire into the fracture site. The power pack for the latter device is implanted into soft tissue near the fracture site and subcutaneously connected to the cathode, creating a self-contained system with no external components. The power supply for the former device is externally placed and the leads connected to the inserted cathodes. With the noninvasive device, opposing pads, wired to an external power supply, are placed over the cast. An electromagnetic field is created between the pads at the fracture site.

B. Nationally Covered Indications

1. Noninvasive Stimulator

The noninvasive stimulator device is covered only for the following indications:

- Nonunion of long bone fractures;
- Failed fusion, where a minimum of 9 months has elapsed since the last surgery;
- Congenital pseudarthroses
- Effective July 1, 1996, as an adjunct to spinal fusion surgery for patients at high risk of pseudarthrosis due to previously failed spinal fusion at the same site or for those undergoing multiple level fusion. A multiple level fusion involves 3 or more vertebrae (e.g., L3-L5, L4-S1, etc.).
- Effective September 15, 1980, nonunion of long bone fractures is considered to exist only after 6 or more months have elapsed without healing of the fracture.
- Effective April 1, 2000, nonunion of long bone fractures is considered to exist only when serial radiographs have confirmed that fracture healing has ceased for 3 or more months prior to starting treatment with the electrical osteogenic stimulator. Serial radiographs must include a minimum of 2 sets of radiographs, each including multiple views of the fracture site, separated by a minimum of 90 days.

2. Invasive (Implantable) Stimulator

The invasive stimulator device is covered only for the following indications:

- Nonunion of long bone fractures;
- Effective July 1, 1996, as an adjunct to spinal fusion surgery for patients at high risk of pseudarthrosis due to previously failed spinal fusion at the same site or for those undergoing multiple level fusion. A multiple level fusion involves 3 or more vertebrae (e.g., L3-L5, L4-S1, etc.).
- Effective September 15, 1980, nonunion of long bone fractures is considered to exist only after 6 or more months have elapsed without healing of the fracture.
- Effective April 1, 2000, nonunion of long bone fractures is considered to exist only when serial radiographs have confirmed that fracture healing has ceased for 3 or more months prior to starting treatment with the electrical osteogenic stimulator. Serial radiographs must include a minimum of 2 sets of radiographs, each including multiple views of the fracture site, separated by a minimum of 90 days.

Ultrasonic Osteogenic Stimulators

A. General

An ultrasonic osteogenic stimulator is a noninvasive device that emits low intensity, pulsed ultrasound. The device is applied to the surface of the skin at the fracture site and ultrasound waves are emitted via a conductive coupling gel to stimulate fracture healing. The ultrasonic osteogenic stimulators are not be used concurrently with other non-invasive osteogenic devices.

B. Nationally Covered Indications

Effective January 1, 2001, ultrasonic osteogenic stimulators are covered as medically reasonable and necessary for the treatment of nonunion fractures. In demonstrating nonunion fractures, CMS expects:

- A minimum of 2 sets of radiographs, obtained prior to starting treatment with the osteogenic stimulator, separated by a minimum of 90 days. Each radiograph set must include multiple views of the fracture site accompanied with a written interpretation by a physician stating that

there has been no clinically significant evidence of fracture healing between the 2 sets of radiographs; and,
- Indications that the patient failed at least one surgical intervention for the treatment of the fracture.
- Effective April 27, 2005, upon reconsideration of ultrasound stimulation for nonunion fracture healing, CMS determines that the evidence is adequate to conclude that noninvasive ultrasound stimulation for the treatment of nonunion bone fractures prior to surgical intervention is reasonable and necessary. In demonstrating nonunion fractures, CMS expects:
- A minimum of 2 sets of radiographs, obtained prior to starting treatment with the osteogenic stimulator, separated by a minimum of 90 days. Each radiograph set must include multiple views of the fracture site accompanied with a written interpretation by a physician stating that there has been no clinically significant evidence of fracture healing between the 2 sets of radiographs.

C. Nationally Non-Covered Indications

Nonunion fractures of the skull, vertebrae and those that are tumor-related are excluded from coverage.

Ultrasonic osteogenic stimulators may not be used concurrently with other non-invasive osteogenic devices.

Ultrasonic osteogenic stimulators for fresh fractures and delayed unions remains non-covered.

(This NCD last reviewed June 2005.)

150.6—Vitamin B12 Injections to Strengthen Tendons, Ligaments, etc., of the Foot

(Rev. 1, 10-03-03)

CIM 45-4

Not Covered

Vitamin B12 injections to strengthen tendons, ligaments, etc., of the foot are not covered under Medicare because (1) there is no evidence that vitamin B12 injections are effective for the purpose of strengthening weakened tendons and ligaments, and (2) this is nonsurgical treatment under the subluxation exclusion. Accordingly, vitamin B12 injections are not considered reasonable and necessary within the meaning of §1862(a)(1) of the Act.

Cross reference:

The Medicare Benefit Policy Manual, Chapter 1, "Inpatient Hospital Services," §30.

The Medicare Benefit Policy Manual, Chapter 16, "General Exclusions from Coverage," §100.

150.7—Prolotherapy, Joint Sclerotherapy, and Ligamentous Injections with Sclerosing Agents

(Rev. 1, 10-03-03)

CIM 35-13

Not Covered

The medical effectiveness of the above therapies has not been verified by scientifically controlled studies. Accordingly, reimbursement for these modalities should be denied on the ground that they are not reasonable and necessary as required by §1862(a)(1) of the Act.

160.2—Treatment of Motor Function Disorders with Electric Nerve Stimulation

(Rev. 1, 10-03-03)

CIM 35-20

Not Covered

While electric nerve stimulation has been employed to control chronic intractable pain for some time, its use in the treatment of motor function disorders, such as multiple sclerosis, is a recent innovation, and the medical effectiveness of such therapy has not been verified by scientifically controlled studies. Therefore, where electric nerve stimulation is employed to treat motor function disorders, no reimbursement may be made for the stimulator or for the services related to its implantation since this treatment cannot be considered reasonable and necessary. See §§30.1 and 160.7.

NOTE: For Medicare coverage of deep brain stimulation for essential tremor and Parkinson's disease, see §160.25.

160.6—Carotid Sinus Nerve Stimulator

(Rev. 1, 10-03-03)

CIM 65-4

Implantation of the carotid sinus nerve stimulator is indicated for relief of angina pectoris in carefully selected patients who are refractory to medical therapy and who after undergoing coronary angiography study either are poor candidates for or refuse to have coronary bypass surgery. In such cases, Medicare reimbursement may be made for this device and for the related services required for its implantation.

However, the use of the carotid sinus nerve stimulator in the treatment of paroxysmal supraventricular tachycardia is considered investigational and is not in common use by the medical community. The device and related services in such cases cannot be considered as reasonable and necessary for the treatment of an illness or injury or to improve the functioning of a malformed body member as required by §1862(a)(1) of the Act.

Cross-reference:

The Medicare Benefit Policy Manual, Chapter 15, "Covered Medical and Other Services," §120

The Medicare Benefit Policy Manual, Chapter 1, "Inpatient Hospital Services," §40 and §120.

160.7—Electrical Nerve Stimulators

(Rev. 1, 10-03-03)

CIM 65-8

Two general classifications of electrical nerve stimulators are employed to treat chronic intractable pain: peripheral nerve stimulators and central nervous system stimulators.

A. Implanted Peripheral Nerve Stimulators

Payment may be made under the prosthetic device benefit for implanted peripheral nerve stimulators. Use of this stimulator involves implantation of electrodes around a selected peripheral nerve. The stimulating electrode is connected by an insulated lead to a receiver unit which is implanted under the skin at a depth not greater than 1/2 inch.

Stimulation is induced by a generator connected to an antenna unit which is attached to the skin surface over the receiver unit. Implantation of electrodes requires surgery and usually necessitates an operating room.

NOTE: Peripheral nerve stimulators may also be employed to assess a patient's suitability for continued treatment with an electric nerve stimulator. As explained in §160.7.1, such use of the stimulator is covered as part of the total diagnostic service furnished to the beneficiary rather than as a prosthesis.

B. Central Nervous System Stimulators (Dorsal Column and Depth Brain Stimulators)

The implantation of central nervous system stimulators may be covered as therapies for the relief of chronic intractable pain, subject to the following conditions:

1. Types of Implantations

There are two types of implantations covered by this instruction:

- Dorsal Column (Spinal Cord) Neurostimulation - The surgical implantation of neurostimulator electrodes within the dura mater (endodural) or the percutaneous insertion of electrodes in the epidural space is covered.
- Depth Brain Neurostimulation - The stereotactic implantation of electrodes in the deep brain (e.g., thalamus and periaqueductal gray matter) is covered.

2. Conditions for Coverage

No payment may be made for the implantation of dorsal column or depth brain stimulators or services and supplies related to such implantation, unless all of the conditions listed below have been met:

- The implantation of the stimulator is used only as a late resort (if not a last resort) for patients with chronic intractable pain;
- With respect to item a, other treatment modalities (pharmacological, surgical, physical, or psychological therapies) have been tried and did not prove satisfactory, or are judged to be unsuitable or contraindicated for the given patient;
- Patients have undergone careful screening, evaluation and diagnosis by a multidisciplinary team prior to implantation. (Such screening must include psychological, as well as physical evaluation);
- All the facilities, equipment, and professional and support personnel required for the proper diagnosis, treatment training, and follow up of the patient (including that required to satisfy item c) must be available; and
- Demonstration of pain relief with a temporarily implanted electrode precedes permanent implantation.

Contractors may find it helpful to work with Quality Improvement Organizations (QIOs) to obtain the information needed to apply these conditions to claims.

See the Medicare Benefit Policy Manual, Chapter 15, "Covered Medical and Other Health Services," §120, and the following sections in this manual, §§160.2 and 30.1.

160.7.1—Assessing Patients Suitability for Electrical Nerve Stimulation Therapy

(Rev. 48, Issued: 03-17-06; Effective/Implementation Dates: 06-19-06)

CIM 35-46

Electrical nerve stimulation is an accepted modality for assessing a patient's suitability for ongoing treatment with a transcutaneous or an implanted nerve stimulator.

Accordingly, program payment may be made for the following techniques when used to determine the potential therapeutic usefulness of an electrical nerve stimulator:

A. Transcutaneous Electrical Nerve Stimulation (TENS)

This technique involves attachment of a transcutaneous nerve stimulator to the surface of the skin over the peripheral nerve to be stimulated. It is used by the patient on a trial basis and its effectiveness in modulating pain is monitored by the physician, or physical therapist. Generally, the physician or physical therapist is able to determine whether the patient is likely to derive a significant therapeutic benefit from continuous use of a transcutaneous stimulator within a trial period of one month; in a few cases this determination may take longer to make. Document the medical necessity for such services which are furnished beyond the first month. (See §160.13 for an explanation of coverage of medically necessary supplies for the effective use of TENS.)

If TENS significantly alleviates pain, it may be considered as primary treatment; if it produces no relief or greater discomfort than the original pain electrical nerve stimulation therapy is ruled out. However, where TENS produces incomplete relief, further evaluation with percutaneous electrical nerve stimulation may be considered to determine whether an implanted peripheral nerve stimulator would provide significant relief from pain.

Usually, the physician or physical therapist providing the services will furnish the equipment necessary for assessment. Where the physician or physical therapist advises the patient to rent the TENS from a supplier during the trial period rather than supplying it himself/herself, program payment may be made for rental of the TENS as well as for the services of the physician or physical therapist who is evaluating its use. However, the combined program payment which is made for the physician's or physical therapist's services and the rental of the stimulator from a supplier should not exceed the amount which would be payable for the total service, including the stimulator, furnished by the physician or physical therapist alone.

B. Percutaneous Electrical Nerve Stimulation (PENS)

This diagnostic procedure which involves stimulation of peripheral nerves by a needle electrode inserted through the skin is performed only in a physician's office, clinic, or hospital outpatient department. Therefore, it is covered only when performed by a physician or incident to physician's service. If pain is effectively controlled by percutaneous stimulation, implantation of electrodes is warranted.

As in the case of TENS (described in subsection A), generally the physician should be able to determine whether the patient is likely to derive a significant therapeutic benefit from continuing use of an implanted nerve stimulator within a trial period of 1 month. In a few cases, this determination may take longer to make. The medical necessity for such diagnostic services which are furnished beyond the first month must be documented.

NOTE: Electrical nerve stimulators do not prevent pain but only alleviate pain as it occurs. A patient can be taught how to employ the stimulator, and once this is done, can use it safely and effectively without direct physician supervision. Consequently, it is inappropriate for a patient to visit his/her physician, physical therapist, or an outpatient clinic on a continuing basis for treatment of pain with electrical nerve stimulation. Once it is determined that electrical nerve stimulation should be continued as therapy and the patient has been trained to use the stimulator, it is expected that a stimulator will be implanted or the patient will employ the TENS on a continual basis in his/her home. Electrical nerve stimulation treatments furnished by a physician in his/her office, by a physical therapist or outpatient clinic are excluded from coverage by §1862(a)(1) of the Act. (See §160.7 for an explanation of coverage of the therapeutic use of implanted peripheral nerve stimulators under the prosthetic devices benefit. See §280.13 for an explanation of coverage of the therapeutic use of TENS under the durable medical equipment benefit.)

160.12—Neuromuscular Electrical Stimulator (NMES)

(Rev. 55, Issued: 05-05-06, Effective: 10-01-06, Implementation: 10-02-06)

Neuromuscular electrical stimulation (NMES) involves the use of a device which transmits an electrical impulse to the skin over selected muscle groups by way of electrodes. There are two broad categories of NMES. One type of device stimulates the muscle when the patient is in a resting state to treat muscle atrophy. The second type is used to enhance functional activity of neurologically impaired patients.

Treatment of Muscle Atrophy

Coverage of NMES to treat muscle atrophy is limited to the treatment of disuse atrophy where nerve supply to the muscle is intact, including brain, spinal cord and peripheral nerves, and other non-neurological reasons for disuse atrophy. Some examples would be casting or splinting of a limb, contracture due to scarring of soft tissue as in burn lesions, and hip replacement surgery (until orthotic training begins). (See §160.13 for an explanation of coverage of medically necessary supplies for the effective use of NMES.)

Use for Walking in Patients with Spinal Cord Injury (SCI)

The type of NMES that is use to enhance the ability to walk of SCI patients is commonly referred to as functional electrical stimulation (FES). These devices are surface units that use electrical impulses to activate paralyzed or weak muscles in precise sequence. Coverage for the use of NMES/FES is limited to SCI patients for walking, who have completed a training program which consists of at least 32 physical therapy sessions with the device over a period of three months.

The trial period of physical therapy will enable the physician treating the patient for his or her spinal cord injury to properly evaluate the person's ability to use these devices frequently and for the long term. Physical therapy necessary to perform this training must be directly performed by the physical therapist as part of a one-on-one training program.

The goal of physical therapy must be to train SCI patients on the use of NMES/FES devices to achieve walking, not to reverse or retard muscle atrophy.

Coverage for NMES/FES for walking will be covered in SCI patients with all of the following characteristics:

1. Persons with intact lower motor unite (L1 and below) (both muscle and peripheral nerve);
2. Persons with muscle and joint stability for weight bearing at upper and lower extremities that can demonstrate balance and control to maintain an upright support posture independently;
3. Persons that demonstrate brisk muscle contraction to NMES and have sensory perception electrical stimulation sufficient for muscle contraction;
4. Persons that possess high motivation, commitment and cognitive ability to use such devices for walking;
5. Persons that can transfer independently and can demonstrate independent standing tolerance for at least 3 minutes;
6. Persons that can demonstrate hand and finger function to manipulate controls;
7. Persons with at least 6-month post recovery spinal cord injury and restorative surgery;
8. Persons with hip and knee degenerative disease and no history of long bone fracture secondary to osteoporosis; and
9. Persons who have demonstrated a willingness to use the device long-term.

NMES/FES for walking will not be covered in SCI patient with any of the following:

1. Persons with cardiac pacemakers;
2. Severe scoliosis or severe osteoporosis;
3. Skin disease or cancer at area of stimulation;
4. Irreversible contracture; or
5. Autonomic dysflexia.

The only settings where therapists with the sufficient skills to provide these services are employed, are inpatient hospitals; outpatient hospitals; comprehensive outpatient rehabilitation facilities; and outpatient rehabilitation facilities. The physical therapy necessary to perform this training must be part of a one-on-one training program.

Additional therapy after the purchase of the DME would be limited by our general policies in converge of skilled physical therapy.

(Also reference the Medicare Benefit Policy Manual, Chapter 15, "Covered Medical and Other Health Services," §220 and 230, and the Medicare Claims Processing Manual, Chapter 5, "Part B Outpatient Rehabilitation and CORF Services," §10.1.)

160.13—Supplies Used in the Delivery of Transcutaneous Electrical Nerve Stimulation (TENS) and Neuromuscular Electrical Stimulation (NMES)

(Rev. 1, 10-03-03)

CIM 45-25

Transcutaneous Electrical Nerve Stimulation (TENS) and/or Neuromuscular Electrical Stimulation (NMES) can ordinarily be delivered to patients through the use of conventional electrodes, adhesive tapes and lead wires. There may be times, however, where it might be medically necessary for certain patients receiving TENS or NMES treatment to use, as an alternative to conventional electrodes, adhesive tapes and lead wires, a form-fitting conductive garment (i.e., a garment with conductive fibers which are separated from the patients' skin by layers of fabric).

A form-fitting conductive garment (and medically necessary related supplies) may be covered under the program only when:

1. It has received permission or approval for marketing by the Food and Drug Administration;
2. It has been prescribed by a physician for use in delivering covered TENS or NMES treatment; and
3. One of the medical indications outlined below is met:

- The patient cannot manage without the conductive garment because there is such a large area or so many sites to be stimulated and the stimulation would have to be delivered so frequently that it is not feasible to use conventional electrodes, adhesive tapes and lead wires;
- The patient cannot manage without the conductive garment for the treatment of chronic intractable pain because the areas or sites to be stimulated are inaccessible with the use of conventional electrodes, adhesive tapes and lead wires;
- The patient has a documented medical condition such as skin problems that preclude the application of conventional electrodes, adhesive tapes and lead wires;
- The patient requires electrical stimulation beneath a cast either to treat disuse atrophy, where the nerve supply to the muscle is intact, or to treat chronic intractable pain; or
- The patient has a medical need for rehabilitation strengthening (pursuant to a written plan of rehabilitation) following an injury where the nerve supply to the muscle is intact.

A conductive garment is not covered for use with a TENS device during the trial period specified in §160.3 unless:

4. The patient has a documented skin problem prior to the start of the trial period; and
5. The carrier's medical consultants are satisfied that use of such an item is medically necessary for the patient.

(See conditions for coverage of the use of TENS in the diagnosis and treatment of chronic intractable pain in §§160.3 and 160.13 and the use of NMES in the treatment of disuse atrophy in §150.4.)

160.23—Sensory Nerve Conduction Threshold Tests (sNCTs) (Effective April 1, 2004)

(Rev. 15, 06-18-04)

A. GENERAL

The sNCT is a psychophysical assessment of both central and peripheral nerve functions. It measures the detection threshold of accurately calibrated sensory stimuli. This procedure is intended to evaluate and quantify function in both large and small caliber fibers for the purpose of detecting neurologic disease. Sensory perception and threshold detection are dependent on the integrity of both the peripheral sensory apparatus and peripheral-central sensory pathways. In theory, an abnormality detected by this procedure may signal dysfunction anywhere in the sensory pathway from the receptors, the sensory tracts, the primary sensory cortex, to the association cortex.

This procedure is different and distinct from assessment of nerve conduction velocity, amplitude and latency. It is also different from short-latency somatosensory evoked potentials.

Effective October 1, 2002, CMS initially concluded that there was insufficient scientific or clinical evidence to consider the sNCT test and the device used in performing this test reasonable and necessary within the meaning of section 1862(a)(1)(A) of the law.

Therefore, sNCT was noncovered.

Effective April 1, 2004, based on a reconsideration of current Medicare policy for sNCT, CMS concludes that the use of any type of sNCT device (e.g., "current output" type device used to perform current perception threshold (CPT), pain perception threshold (PPT), or pain tolerance threshold (PTT) testing or "voltage input" type device used for voltage-nerve conduction threshold (v-NCT) testing) to diagnose sensory neuropathies or radiculopathies in Medicare beneficiaries is not reasonable and necessary.

B. Nationally Covered Indications

Not applicable.

C. Nationally Noncovered Indications

All uses of sNCT to diagnose sensory neuropathies or radiculopathies are noncovered.

(This NCD last reviewed June 2004.)

100-03 Part 3

170.3—Speech -*Language* Pathology Services for the Treatment of Dysphagia

(Rev. 55, Issued: 05-05-06, Effective: 10-01-06, Implementation: 10-02-06)

Dysphagia is a swallowing disorder that may be due to various neurological, structural, and cognitive deficits. Dysphagia may be the result of head trauma, cerebrovascular accident, neuromuscular degenerative diseases, head and neck cancer, or encephalopathies. While dysphagia can afflict any age group, it most often appears among the elderly. Speech-*language* pathology services are covered under Medicare for the treatment of dysphagia, regardless of the presence of a communication disability.

Patients who are motivated, moderately alert, and have some degree of deglutition and swallowing functions are appropriate candidates for dysphagia therapy. Elements of the therapy program can include thermal stimulation to heighten the sensitivity of the swallowing reflex, exercises to improve oral-motor control, training in laryngeal adduction and compensatory swallowing techniques, and positioning and dietary modifications. Design all programs to ensure swallowing safety of the patient during oral feedings and maintain adequate nutrition.

Cross-reference:

The Medicare Benefit Policy, Chapter 15, "Covered Medical and Other Health Services," §§220 and 230.*3*

180.2—Enteral and Parenteral Nutritional Therapy

(Rev. 1, 10-03-03)

CIM 65-10

Covered As Prosthetic Device

There are patients who, because of chronic illness or trauma, cannot be sustained through oral feeding. These people must rely on either enteral or parenteral nutritional therapy, depending upon the particular nature of their medical condition.

Coverage of nutritional therapy as a Part B benefit is provided under the prosthetic device benefit provision which requires that the patient must have a permanently inoperative internal body organ or function thereof. Therefore, enteral and parenteral nutritional therapy are not covered under Part B in situations involving temporary impairments.

Coverage of such therapy, however, does not require a medical judgment that the impairment giving rise to the therapy will persist throughout the patient's remaining years. If the medical record, including the judgment of the attending physician, indicates that the impairment will be of long and indefinite duration, the test of permanence is considered met.

If the coverage requirements for enteral or parenteral nutritional therapy are met under the prosthetic device benefit provision, related supplies, equipment and nutrients are also covered under the conditions in the following paragraphs and the Medicare Benefit Policy Manual, Chapter 15, "Covered Medical and Other Health Services," §120.

Parenteral Nutrition Therapy Daily parenteral nutrition is considered reasonable and necessary for a patient with severe pathology of the alimentary tract which does not allow absorption of sufficient nutrients to maintain weight and strength commensurate with the patient's general condition.

Since the alimentary tract of such a patient does not function adequately, an indwelling catheter is placed percutaneously in the subclavian vein and then advanced into the superior vena cava where intravenous infusion of nutrients is given for part of the day. The catheter is then plugged by the patient until the next infusion. Following a period of hospitalization, which is required to initiate parenteral nutrition and to train the patient in catheter care, solution preparation, and infusion technique, the parenteral nutrition can be provided safely and effectively in the patient's home by nonprofessional persons who have undergone special training. However, such persons cannot be paid for their services, nor is payment available for any services furnished by nonphysician professionals except as services furnished incident to a physician's service.

For parenteral nutrition therapy to be covered under Part B, the claim must contain a physician's written order or prescription and sufficient medical documentation to permit an independent conclusion that the requirements of the prosthetic device benefit are met and that parenteral nutrition therapy is medically necessary. An example of a condition that typically qualifies for coverage is a massive small bowel resection resulting in severe nutritional deficiency in spite of adequate oral intake. However, coverage of parenteral nutrition therapy for this and any other condition must be approved on an individual, case-by-case basis initially and at periodic intervals of no more than three months by the carrier's medical consultant or specially trained staff, relying on such medical and other documentation as the carrier may require. If the claim involves an infusion pump, sufficient evidence must be provided to support a determination of medical necessity for the pump. Program payment for the pump is based on the reasonable charge for the simplest model that meets the medical needs of the patient as established by medical documentation.

Nutrient solutions for parenteral therapy are routinely covered. However, Medicare pays for no more than one month's supply of nutrients at any one time. Payment for the nutrients is based on the reasonable charge for the solution components unless the medical record, including a signed statement from the attending physician, establishes that the beneficiary, due to his/her physical or mental state, is unable to safely or effectively mix the solution and there is no family member or other person who can do so. Payment will be on the basis of the reasonable charge for more expensive premixed solutions only under the latter circumstances.

Enteral Nutrition Therapy

Enteral nutrition is considered reasonable and necessary for a patient with a functioning gastrointestinal tract who, due to pathology to, or nonfunction of, the structures that normally permit food to reach the digestive tract, cannot maintain weight and strength commensurate with his or her general condition. Enteral therapy may be given by nasogastric, jejunostomy, or gastrostomy tubes and can be provided safely and effectively in the home by nonprofessional persons who have undergone special training. However, such persons cannot be paid for their services, nor is payment available for any services furnished by nonphysician professionals except as services furnished incident to a physician's service.

Typical examples of conditions that qualify for coverage are head and neck cancer with reconstructive surgery and central nervous system disease leading to interference with the neuromuscular mechanisms of ingestion of such severity that the beneficiary cannot be maintained with oral feeding. However, claims for Part B coverage of enteral nutrition therapy for these and any other conditions must be approved on an individual, case-by-case basis. Each claim must contain a physician's written order or prescription and sufficient medical documentation (e.g., hospital records, clinical findings from the attending physician) to permit an independent conclusion that the patient's condition meets the requirements of the prosthetic device benefit and that enteral nutrition therapy is medically necessary. Allowed claims are to be reviewed

at periodic intervals of no more than 3 months by the contractor's medical consultant or specially trained staff, and additional medical documentation considered necessary is to be obtained as part of this review.

Medicare pays for no more than one month's supply of enteral nutrients at any one time.

If the claim involves a pump, it must be supported by sufficient medical documentation to establish that the pump is medically necessary, i.e., gravity feeding is not satisfactory due to aspiration, diarrhea, dumping syndrome. Program payment for the pump is based on the reasonable charge for the simplest model that meets the medical needs of the patient as established by medical documentation.

Nutritional Supplementation

Some patients require supplementation of their daily protein and caloric intake. Nutritional supplements are often given as a medicine between meals to boost protein-caloric intake or the mainstay of a daily nutritional plan. Nutritional supplementation is not covered under Medicare Part B.

190.2—Diagnostic Pap Smears

(Rev. 48, Issued: 03-17-06; Effective/Implementation Dates: 06-19-06)

CIM 50-20, CIM 50-20.1

A diagnostic pap smear and related medically necessary services are covered under Medicare Part B when ordered by a physician under one of the following conditions:

- Previous cancer of the cervix, uterus, or vagina that has been or is presently being treated;
- Previous abnormal pap smear;
- Any abnormal findings of the vagina, cervix, uterus, ovaries, or adnexa;
- Any significant complaint by the patient referable to the female reproductive system; or
- Any signs or symptoms that might in the physician's judgment reasonably be related to a gynecologic disorder.

Screening Pap Smears and Pelvic Examinations for Early Detection of Cervical or Vaginal Cancer. (See section 210.2.)

100-03 Part 4

210.1—Prostate Cancer Screening Tests

(Rev. 48, Issued: 03-17-06; Effective/Implementation Dates: 06-19-06)

CIM 50-55

Covered

A—General

Section 4103 of the Balanced Budget Act of 1997 provides for coverage of certain prostate cancer screening tests subject to certain coverage, frequency, and payment limitations. Medicare will cover prostate cancer screening tests/procedures for the early detection of prostate cancer. Coverage of prostate cancer screening tests includes the following procedures furnished to an individual for the early detection of prostate cancer:

- Screening digital rectal examination; and
- Screening prostate specific antigen blood test.

B—Screening Digital Rectal Examinations

Screening digital rectal examinations are covered at a frequency of once every 12 months for men who have attained age 50 (at least 11 months have passed following the month in which the last Medicare-covered screening digital rectal examination was performed). Screening digital rectal examination means a clinical examination of an individual's prostate for nodules or other abnormalities of the prostate. This screening must be performed by a doctor of medicine or osteopathy (as defined in §1861(r)(1) of the Act), or by a physician assistant, nurse practitioner, clinical nurse specialist, or certified nurse mid-wife (as defined in §1861(aa) and §1861(gg) of the Act) who is authorized under State law to perform the examination, fully knowledgeable about the beneficiary's medical condition, and would be responsible for using the results of any examination performed in the overall management of the beneficiary's specific medical problem.

C—Screening Prostate Specific Antigen Tests

Screening prostate specific antigen tests are covered at a frequency of once every 12 months for men who have attained age 50 (at least 11 months have passed following the month in which the last Medicare-covered screening prostate specific antigen test was performed). Screening prostate specific antigen tests (PSA) means a test to detect the marker for adenocarcinoma of prostate. PSA is a reliable immunocytochemical marker for primary and metastatic adenocarcinoma of prostate. This screening must be ordered by the beneficiary's physician or by the beneficiary's physician assistant, nurse practitioner, clinical nurse specialist, or certified nurse midwife (the term "attending physician" is defined in §1861(r)(1) of the Act to mean a doctor of medicine or osteopathy and the terms "physician assistant, nurse practitioner, clinical nurse specialist, or certified nurse midwife" are defined in §1861(aa) and §1861(gg) of the Act) who is fully knowledgeable about the beneficiary's medical condition, and who would be responsible for using the results of any examination (test) performed in the overall management of the beneficiary's specific medical problem.

220.6—Positron Emission Tomography (PET) Scans

(Rev. 31, Issued: 04-04-05; Effective: 01-28-05; Implementation: 04-18-05)

CIM 50-36

I. General Description

Positron emission tomography (PET) is a noninvasive diagnostic imaging procedure that assesses the level of metabolic activity and perfusion in various organ systems of the [human] body. A positron camera (tomograph) is used to produce cross-sectional tomographic images, which are obtained from positron emitting radioactive tracer substances (radiopharmaceuticals) such as 2-[F-18] Fluoro-D-Glucose (FDG), that are administered intravenously to the patient.

The following indications may be covered for PET under certain circumstances. Details of Medicare PET coverage are discussed later in this section. Unless otherwise indicated, the clinical conditions below are covered when PET utilizes FDG as a tracer.

NOTE: This manual section 220.6 lists all Medicare-covered uses of PET scans. Except as set forth below in cancer indications listed as "Coverage with Evidence Development", a particular use of PET scans is not covered unless this manual specifically provides that such use is covered. Although this section lists some non-covered uses of PET scans, it does not constitute an exhaustive list of all non-covered uses.

Clinical Condition	Effective Date	Coverage
Solitary Pulmonary Nodules (SPNs)	January 1, 1998	Characterization
Lung Cancer (Non Small Cell)	January 1, 1998	Initial staging
Lung Cancer (Non Small Cell)	July 1, 2001	Diagnosis, staging, restaging
Esophageal Cancer	July 1, 2001	Diagnosis, staging, restaging
Colorectal Cancer	July 1, 1999	Determining location of tumors if rising CEA level suggests recurrence
Colorectal Cancer	July 1, 2001	Diagnosis, staging, restaging
Lymphoma	July 1, 1999	Staging and restaging only when used as alternative to Gallium scan
Lymphoma	July 1, 2001	Diagnosis, staging and restaging
Melanoma	July 1, 1999	Evaluating recurrence prior to surgery as alternative to Gallium scan
Melanoma	July 1, 2001	Diagnosis, staging, restaging; Non-covered for evaluating regional nodes
Breast Cancer	October 1, 2002	As an adjunct to standard imaging modalities for staging patients with distant metastasis or restaging patients with loco-regional recurrence or metastasis; as an adjunct to standard imaging modalities for monitoring tumor response to treatment for women with locally advanced and metastatic breast cancer when a change in therapy is anticipated
Head and Neck Cancers (excluding CNS and thyroid)	July 1, 2001	Diagnosis, staging, restaging
Thyroid Cancer	October 1, 2003	Restaging of recurrent or residual thyroid cancers of follicular cell origin previously treated by thyroidectomy and radioiodine ablation and have a serum thyroglobulin .10 ng/ml and negative I-131 whole body scan performed
Myocardial Viability	July 1, 2001, to September 30, 2002	Only following inconclusive SPECT
Myocardial Viability	October 1, 2002	Primary or initial diagnosis, or following an inconclusive SPECT prior to revascularization. SPECT may not be used following an inconclusive PET scan
Refractory Seizures	July 1, 2001	Pre-surgical evaluation only
Perfusion of the heart using Rubidium 82* tracer	March 14, 1995	Noninvasive imaging of the perfusion of the heart

Clinical Condition	Effective Date	Coverage
Perfusion of the heart using ammonia N-13* tracer	October 1, 2003	Noninvasive imaging of the perfusion of the heart

* Not FDG-PET.

EFFECTIVE JANUARY 28, 2005: This manual section lists Medicare-covered uses of PET scans effective for services performed on or after January 28, 2005. Except as set forth below in cancer indications listed as "coverage with evidence development", a particular use of PET scans is not covered unless this manual specifically provides that such use is covered. Although this section 220.6 lists some non-covered uses of PET scans, it does not constitute an exhaustive list of all non-covered uses.

For cancer indications listed as "coverage with evidence development" CMS determines that the evidence is sufficient to conclude that an FDG PET scan is reasonable and necessary only when the provider is participating in, and patients are enrolled in, one of the following types of prospective clinical studies that is designed to collect additional information at the time of the scan to assist in patient management:

- A clinical trial of FDG PET that meets the requirements of Food and Drug Administration (FDA) category B investigational device exemption (42 CFR 405.201);
- An FDG PET clinical study that is designed to collect additional information at the time of the scan to assist in patient management. Qualifying clinical studies must ensure that specific hypotheses are addressed; appropriate data elements are collected; hospitals and providers are qualified to provide the PET scan and interpret the results; participating hospitals and providers accurately report data on all enrolled patients not included in other qualifying trials through adequate auditing mechanisms; and, all patient confidentiality, privacy, and other Federal laws must be followed.

Effective January 28, 2005: For PET services identified as "Coverage with Evidence Development." Medicare shall notify providers and beneficiaries where these services can be accessed, as they become available, via the following:

- Federal Register Notice
- CMS coverage Web site at: www.cms.gov/coverage

Indication	Covered[1]	Nationally Non-covered[2]	Coverage with evidence development[3]
Brain			X
Breast			
—Diagnosis		X	
—Initial staging of axillary nodes		X	
—Staging of distant metastasis	X		
—Restaging, monitoring*	X		
Cervical			
—Staging as adjunct to conventional imaging	X		
—Other staging			X
—Diagnosis, restaging, monitoring*			X

Indication	Covered[1]	Nationally Non-covered[2]	Coverage with evidence development[3]
Colorectal			
—Diagnosis, staging, restaging	X		
—Monitoring*			X
Esophagus			
—Diagnosis, staging, restaging	X		
—Monitoring*			X
Head and Neck (non-CNS/thyroid)			
—Diagnosis, staging, restaging	X		
—Monitoring*			X
Lymphoma			
—Diagnosis, staging, restaging	X		
—Monitoring*			X
Melanoma			
—Diagnosis, staging, restaging	X		
—Monitoring*			X
Non-Small Cell Lung			
—Diagnosis, staging, restaging	X		
—Monitoring*			X
Ovarian			X
Pancreatic			X
Small Cell Lung			X
Soft Tissue Sarcoma			X
Solitary Pulmonary Nodule (characterization)	X		
Thyroid			
—Staging of follicular cell tumors	X		
—Restaging of medullary cell tumors			X
—Diagnosis, other staging & restaging			X
—Monitoring*			X
Testicular			X
All other cancers not listed herein (all indications)			X

[1] Covered nationally based on evidence of benefit. Refer to National Coverage Determination Manual Section 220.6 in its entirety for specific coverage language and limitations for each indication.
[2] Non-covered nationally based on evidence of harm or no benefit.
[3] Covered only in specific settings discussed above if certain patient safeguards are provided. Otherwise, non-covered nationally based on lack of evidence sufficient to establish either benefit or harm or no prior decision addressing this cancer. Medicare shall notify providers and beneficiaries where these services can be accessed, as they become available, via the following:
- Federal Register Notice
- CMS coverage Web site at: www.cms.gov/coverage
* Monitoring = monitoring response to treatment when a change in therapy is anticipated.

II. General Conditions of Coverage for FDG PET

Allowable FDG PET Systems

A. Definitions: For purposes of this section:
- "Any FDA-approved" means all systems approved or cleared for marketing by the Food and Drug Administration (FDA) to image radionuclides in the body.
- "FDA-approved" means that the system indicated has been approved or cleared for marketing by the FDA to image radionuclides in the body.
- "Certain coincidence systems" refers to the systems that have all the following features
  —Crystal at least 5/8-inch thick;
  —Techniques to minimize or correct for scatter and/or random; and
  —Digital detectors and iterative reconstruction.

Scans performed with gamma camera PET systems with crystals thinner than 5/8" will not be covered by Medicare. In addition, scans performed with systems with crystals greater than or equal to 5/8" in thickness, but that do not meet the other listed design characteristics are not covered by Medicare.

B. Allowable PET systems by covered clinical indication (see table):

C. Regardless of any other terms or conditions, all uses of FDG PET scans, in order to be covered by the Medicare program, must meet the following general conditions prior to June 30, 2001:
- Submission of claims for payment must include any information Medicare requires to ensure the PET scans performed were: (a) medically necessary, (b) did not unnecessarily duplicate other covered diagnostic tests, and (c) did not involve investigational drugs or procedures using investigational drugs, as determined by the FDA.
- The PET scan entity submitting claims for payment must keep such patient records as Medicare requires on file for each patient for whom a PET scan claim is made.

Regardless of any other terms or conditions, all uses of FDG PET scans, in order to be covered by the Medicare program, must meet the following general conditions as of July 1, 2001:

- The provider of the PET scan should maintain on file the doctor's referral and documentation that the procedure involved only FDA-approved drugs and devices, as is normal business practice.
- The ordering physician is responsible for documenting the medical necessity of the study and ensuring that it meets the conditions specified in the instructions. The physician should have documentation in the beneficiary's medical record to support the referral to the PET scan provider.

III. Covered Indications for PET Scans and Limitations/Requirements for Usage

For all uses of PET relating to malignancies the following conditions apply:

A. Diagnosis: PET is covered only in clinical situations in which: (1) the PET results may assist in avoiding an invasive diagnostic procedure, or in which (2) the PET results may assist in determining the optimal anatomical location to perform an invasive diagnostic procedure. In general, for most solid tumors, a tissue diagnosis is made prior to the performance of PET scanning. PET scans following a tissue diagnosis are generally performed for the purpose of staging rather than diagnosis. PET is not covered as a screening test (i.e., testing patients without specific signs and symptoms of disease).

B. Staging: PET is covered for staging in clinical situations in which: (1)(a) the stage of the cancer remains in doubt after completion of a standard diagnostic workup, including conventional imaging (computed tomography (CT), magnetic resonance imaging (MRI), or ultrasound), or (1)(b) it could potentially replace one or more conventional imaging studies when it is expected that conventional study information is insufficient for the clinical management of the patient, and (2) clinical management of the patient would differ depending on the stage of the cancer identified.

C. Restaging: PET is covered for restaging: (1) after completion of treatment for the purpose of detecting residual disease, (2) for detecting suspected recurrence, (3) to determine the extent of a known recurrence, or (4) if it could potentially replace one or more conventional imaging studies when it is expected that conventional study information is insufficient for the clinical management of the patient.

D. Monitoring: This refers to use of PET to monitor tumor response to treatment during the planned course of therapy (i.e., when a change in therapy is anticipated)

NOTE: In the absence of national frequency limitations, contractors, should, if necessary, develop frequency requirements on any or all of the indications covered on and after July 1, 2001.

(This NCD last reviewed December 2004.)

220.6.1—PET for Perfusion of the Heart (Various Effective Dates Below)

(Rev. 31, Issued: 04-04-05; Effective: 01-28-05; Implementation: 04-18-05)

1. Rubidium 82 (Effective March 14, 1995)

Effective for services performed on or after March 14, 1995, PET scans performed at rest or with pharmacological stress used for noninvasive imaging of the perfusion of the heart for the diagnosis and management of patients with known or suspected coronary artery disease using the FDA-approved radiopharmaceutical Rubidium 82 (Rb 82) are covered, provided the requirements below are met:

- The PET scan, whether at rest alone, or rest with stress, is performed in place of, but not in addition to, a single photon emission computed tomography (SPECT); or
- The PET scan, whether at rest alone or rest with stress, is used following a SPECT that was found to be inconclusive. In these cases, the PET scan must have been considered necessary in order to determine what medical or surgical intervention is required to treat the patient. (For purposes of this requirement, an inconclusive test is a test(s) whose results are equivocal, technically uninterpretable, or discordant with a patient's other clinical data and must be documented in the beneficiary's file.)

- For any PET scan for which Medicare payment is claimed for dates of services prior to July 1, 2001, the claimant must submit additional specified information on the claim form (including proper codes and/or modifiers), to indicate the results of the PET scan. The claimant must also include information on whether the PET scan was performed after an inconclusive non-invasive cardiac test. The information submitted with respect to the previous noninvasive cardiac test must specify the type of test performed prior to the PET scan and whether it was inconclusive or unsatisfactory. These explanations are in the form of special G codes used for billing PET scans using Rb 82. Beginning July 1, 2001, claims should be submitted with the appropriate codes.

2. Ammonia N-13 (Effective October 1, 2003)

Effective for services performed on or after October 1, 2003, PET scans performed at rest or with pharmacological stress used for noninvasive imaging of the perfusion of the heart for the diagnosis and management of patients with known or suspected coronary artery disease using the FDA-approved radiopharmaceutical ammonia N-13 are covered, provided the requirements below are met:

- The PET scan, whether at rest alone, or rest with stress, is performed in place of, but not in addition to, a SPECT; or
- The PET scan, whether at rest alone or rest with stress, is used following a SPECT that was found to be inconclusive. In these cases, the PET scan must have been considered necessary in order to determine what medical or surgical intervention is required to treat the patient. (For purposes of this requirement, an inconclusive test is a test whose results are equivocal, technically uninterpretable, or discordant with a patient's other clinical data and must be documented in the beneficiary's file.)

(This NCD last reviewed April 2003.)

Covered Clinical Condition	Allowable Type of FDG PET System		
	Prior to July 1, 2001	July 1, 2001, through December 31, 2001	On or after January 1, 2002
Characterization of single pulmonary nodules	Effective 1/1/1998, any FDA-approved	Any FDA-approved	FDA-approved: Full/Partial ring certain coincidence systems
Initial staging of lung cancer (non small cell)	Effective 1/1/1998, any FDA-approved	Any FDA-approved	FDA-approved: Full/Partial ring, certain coincidence systems
Determining location of colorectal tumors if rising CEA level suggests recurrence	Effective 7/1/1999, any FDA-approved	Any FDA-approved	FDA-approved: Full/Partial ring, certain coincidence systems
Staging or restaging of lymphoma only when used as alternative to gallium scan	Effective 7/1/1999, any FDA-approved	Any FDA-approved	FDA-approved: Full/Partial ring, certain coincidence systems
Evaluating recurrence of melanoma prior to surgery as alternative to a gallium scan	Effective 7/1/1999, any FDA-approved	Any FDA-approved	FDA-approved: Full/Partial ring, certain coincidence systems
Diagnosis, staging, restaging of colorectal cancer	Not covered by Medicare	Full ring	FDA-approved: Full/Partial ring
Diagnosis, staging, restaging of esophageal cancer	Not covered by Medicare	Full ring	FDA-approved: Full/Partial ring
Diagnosis, staging, restaging of head and neck cancers (excluding CNS and thyroid)	Not covered by Medicare	Full ring	FDA-approved: Full/Partial ring
Diagnosis, staging, restaging of lung cancer (non small cell)	Not covered by Medicare	Full ring	FDA-approved: Full/Partial ring
Diagnosis, staging, restaging of lymphoma	Not covered by Medicare	Full ring	FDA-approved: Full/Partial ring
Diagnosis, staging, restaging of melanoma (non-covered for evaluating regional nodes)	Not covered by Medicare	Full ring	FDA-approved: Full/Partial ring
Determination of myocardial viability only following inconclusive SPECT	Not covered by Medicare	Full ring	FDA-approved: Full/Partial ring
Pre-surgical evaluation of refractory seizures	Not covered by Medicare	Full ring	FDA-approved: Full ring
Breast Cancer	Not covered	Not covered	Effective October 1, 2002, Full/Partial ring
Thyroid Cancer	Not covered	Not covered	Effective October 1, 2003, Full/Partial ring
Myocardial Viability Primary or initial diagnosis prior to revascularization	Not covered	Not covered	Effective October 1, 2002, Full/Partial ring
All other oncology indications not previously specified	Not covered	Not covered	Effective January 28, 2005, Full/Partial ring

220.6.2—FDG PET for Lung Cancer (Various Effective Dates Below)

(Rev. 31, Issued: 04-04-05; Effective: 01-28-05; Implementation: 04-18-05)

1. Characterization of Single Pulmonary Nodules (SPNs) (Effective January 1, 1998)

Effective for services performed on or after January 1, 1998, Medicare covers regional FDG PET chest scans, on any FDA-approved scanner, for the characterization of SPNs. The primary purpose of such characterization should be to determine the likelihood of malignancy in order to plan future management and treatment for the patient.

Beginning July 1, 2001, documentation should be maintained in the beneficiary's medical record file at the referring physician's office to support the medical necessity of the procedure, as is normal business practice. The following documentation is required:

- There must be evidence of primary tumor. Claims for regional PET chest scans for characterizing SPNs should include evidence of the initial detection of a primary lung tumor, usually by computed tomography (CT). This should include, but is not restricted to, a report on the results of such CT or other detection method, indicating an indeterminate or possibly malignant lesion, not exceeding 4 centimeters (cm) in diameter.
- PET scan claims must include the results of concurrent thoracic CT (as noted above), which is necessary for anatomic information, in order to ensure that the PET scan is properly coordinated with other diagnostic modalities.
- In cases of serial evaluation of SPNs using both CT and regional PET chest scanning, such PET scans will not be covered if repeated within 90 days following a negative PET scan.

NOTE: A tissue sampling procedure (TSP) is not routinely covered in the case of a negative PET scan for characterization of SPNs, since the patient is presumed not to have a malignant lesion, based upon PET scan results. When there is a negative PET, the provider must submit additional information with the claim to support the necessity of a TSP, for review by the Medicare contractor.

2. Initial Staging of Non-Small-Cell Lung Carcinoma (LSCLC) (Effective January 1, 1998)

Effective for services performed from January 1, 1998, through June 30, 2001, Medicare approved coverage of FDG PET for initial staging of NSCLC.

Limitations: This service is covered only when the primary cancerous lung tumor has been pathologically confirmed; claims for PET must include a statement or other evidence of the detection of such primary lung tumor. The evidence should include, but is not restricted to, a surgical pathology report, which documents the presence of an NSCLC. Whole body PET scan results and results of concurrent CT and follow-up lymph node biopsy must be properly coordinated with other diagnostic modalities. Claims must include both:

- The results of concurrent thoracic CT, necessary for anatomic information, and

- The results of any lymph node biopsy performed to finalize whether the patient will be a surgical candidate. The ordering physician is responsible for providing this biopsy result to the PET facility.

NOTE: Where the patient is considered a surgical candidate, (given the presumed absence of metastatic NSCLC unless medical review supports a determination of medical necessity of a biopsy) a lymph node biopsy will not be covered in the case of a negative CT and negative PET. A lymph node biopsy will be covered in all other cases, i.e., positive CT 1 positive PET; negative CT 1 positive PET; positive CT 1 negative PET.

3. Diagnosis, Staging, and Restaging of NSCLC (Effective July 1, 2001)

Effective for serviced performed on or after July 1, 2001, Medicare covers FDG PET for diagnosis, staging, and restaging of NSCLC.

4. Monitoring response to treatment of NSCLC (Effective January 28, 2005)

Effective for services performed on or after January 28, 2005, Medicare only covers FDG PET for monitoring response to treatment for NSCLC as "coverage with evidence development".

Medicare shall notify providers and beneficiaries where these services can be accessed, as they become available, via the following:

- Federal Register Notice
- CMS coverage Web site at: www.cms.gov/coverage

Requirements: PET is covered in any/all of the following circumstances:

A. Diagnosis: PET is covered only in clinical situations in which: (1) the PET results may assist in avoiding an invasive diagnostic procedure, or in which (2) the PET results may assist in determining the optimal anatomical location to perform an invasive diagnostic procedure. In general, for most solid tumors, a tissue diagnosis is made prior to the performance of PET scanning. PET scans following a tissue diagnosis are generally performed for the purpose of staging, rather than diagnosis. Therefore, the use of PET in the diagnosis of lymphoma, esophageal, and colorectal cancers as well as in melanoma, should be rare.

B. Staging and/or Restaging: PET is covered for staging in clinical situations in which: (1)(a) the stage of the cancer remains in doubt after completion of a standard diagnostic workup, including conventional imaging (CT, magnetic resonance imaging, or ultrasound) or, (1)(b) the use of PET could potentially replace one or more conventional imaging studies when it is expected that conventional study information is insufficient for the clinical management of the patient, and (2) clinical management of the patient would differ depending on the stage of the cancer identified.

PET is covered for restaging after the completion of treatment for: (1) the purpose of detecting residual disease, (2) detecting suspected recurrence, (3) determining the extent of a known recurrence, or (4) potentially replacing one or more conventional imaging studies when it is expected that conventional study information is insufficient for the clinical management of the patient.

C. Monitoring Response to Treatment: PET is covered for monitoring response to treatment when a change in therapy is anticipated.

Documentation should be maintained in the beneficiary's medical record at the referring physician's office to support the medical necessity of the procedure, as is normal business practice.

(This NCD last reviewed March 2005.)

220.6.3—FDG PET for Esophageal Cancer (Various Effective Dates Below)

(Rev. 31, Issued: 04-04-05; Effective: 01-28-05; Implementation: 04-18-05)

Effective for services performed on or after July 1, 2001, Medicare covers FDG PET for the diagnosis, staging, and restaging of esophageal cancer.

Effective for services performed on or after January 28, 2005, Medicare only covers FDG PET for monitoring response to treatment for esophageal cancer as "coverage with evidence development".

Medicare shall notify providers and beneficiaries where these services can be accessed, as they become available, via the following:

• Federal Register Notice
• CMS coverage Web site at: www.cms.gov/coverage

Requirements: PET is covered in any/all of the following circumstances:

A. Diagnosis: PET is covered only in clinical situations in which: (1) the PET results may assist in avoiding an invasive diagnostic procedure, or (2) the PET results may assist in determining the optimal anatomical location to perform an invasive diagnostic procedure. In general, for most solid tumors, a tissue diagnosis is made prior to the performance of PET scanning. PET scans following a tissue diagnosis are generally performed for the purpose of staging rather than diagnosis.

B. Staging and/or Restaging: PET is covered for staging in clinical situations in which: (1)(a) the stage of the cancer remains in doubt after completion of a standard diagnostic workup, including conventional imaging (CT, magnetic resonance imaging, or ultrasound), or (1)(b) the use of PET could potentially replace one or more conventional imaging studies when it is expected that conventional study information is insufficient for the clinical management of the patient, and (2) clinical management of the patient would differ depending on the stage of the cancer identified.

PET is covered for restaging after the completion of treatment for: (1) the purpose of detecting residual disease, (2) detecting suspected recurrence, (3) determining the extent of a known recurrence, or (4) potentially replacing one or more conventional imaging studies when it is expected that conventional study information is insufficient for the clinical management of the patient.

C. Monitoring Response to Treatment: PET is covered for monitoring response to treatment when a change in therapy is anticipated.

Documentation should be maintained in the beneficiary's medical record at the referring physician's office to support the medical necessity of the procedure, as is normal business practice.

(This NCD last reviewed March 2005.)

220.6.4—FDG PET for Colorectal Cancer (Various Effective Dates Below)

(Rev. 31, Issued: 04-04-05; Effective: 01-28-05; Implementation: 04-18-05)

1. Recurrent Colorectal Carcinoma With Rising Levels of Biochemical Tumor Marker Carcinoembryonic Antigen (CEA) (Effective July 1, 1999)

Effective for services performed on or after July 1, 1999, Medicare covers FDG PET for patients with recurrent colorectal carcinomas, suggested by rising levels of the biochemical tumor marker CEA.

Frequency Limitations: Whole body PET scans for assessment of recurrence of colorectal cancer cannot be ordered more frequently than once every 12 months unless medical necessity documentation supports a separate reevelation of CEA within this period.

Limitations: Because this service is covered only in those cases in which there has been a recurrence of colorectal tumor, claims for PET should include a statement or other evidence of previous colorectal tumor, through June 30, 2001.

2. Diagnosis, Staging, and Re-Staging (Effective July 1, 2001)

Effective for services performed on or after July 1, 2001, Medicare covers FDG PET for colorectal carcinomas for diagnosis, staging, and re-staging. New medical evidence supports the use of FDG PET as a useful tool in determining the presence of hepatic/extra-hepatic metastases in the primary staging of colorectal carcinoma, prior to selecting a treatment regimen. Use of FDG PET is also supported in evaluating recurrent colorectal cancer beyond the limited presentation of a rising CEA level where the patient presents clinical signs/symptoms of recurrence.

3. Monitoring Response to Treatment (Effective January 28, 2005)

Effective for services performed on or after January 28, 2005, Medicare only covers FDG PET for monitoring response to treatment for colorectal cancer as "coverage with evidence development".

Medicare shall notify providers and beneficiaries where these services can be accessed, as they become available, via the following:

• Federal Register Notice
• CMS coverage Web site at: www.cms.gov/coverage

Requirements: PET is covered in any/all of the following circumstances:

A. **Diagnosis:** PET is covered only in clinical situations in which: (1) the PET results may assist in avoiding an invasive diagnostic procedure, or in which (2) the PET results may assist in determining the optimal anatomical location to perform an invasive diagnostic procedure. In general, for most solid tumors, a tissue diagnosis is made prior to the performance of PET scanning. PET scans following a tissue diagnosis are generally performed for the purpose of staging rather than diagnosis.

B. **Staging and/or Restaging:** PET is covered for staging in clinical situations in which: (1)(a) the stage of the cancer remains in doubt after completion of a standard diagnostic workup, including conventional imaging (computed tomography, magnetic resonance imaging, or ultrasound), or (1)(b) the use of PET could potentially replace one or more conventional imaging studies when it is expected that conventional study information is insufficient for the clinical management of the patient, and (2) clinical management of the patient would differ depending on the stage of the cancer identified.

The PET is covered for restaging after completion of treatment for the purpose of: (1) detecting residual disease, (2) detecting suspected recurrence, (3) determining the extent of a known recurrence, or (4) potentially replacing one or more conventional imaging studies when it is expected that conventional study information is insufficient for the clinical management of the patient.

C. **Monitoring Response to Treatment: PET is covered for monitoring response to treatment when a change in therapy is anticipated.**

Documentation that these conditions are met should be maintained by the referring physician in the beneficiary's medical record, as is normal business practice.

(This NCD last reviewed March 2005.)

220.6.5—FDG PET for Lymphoma (Various Effective Dates Below)

(Rev. 31, Issued: 04-04-05; Effective: 01-28-05; Implementation: 04-18-05)

1. Staging and Restaging as Alternative to Gallium Scan (Effective July 1, 1999)

Effective for services performed on or after July 1, 1999, FDG PET is covered for the staging and restaging of lymphoma.

Requirements:

- The PET is covered only for staging or follow-up restaging of lymphoma. Claims must include a statement or other evidence of previous diagnosis of lymphoma when used as an alternative to a Gallium scan
- To ensure that the PET scan is properly coordinated with other diagnostic modalities, claims must include the results of concurrent computed tomography (CT) and/or other diagnostic modalities necessary for additional anatomic information.
- In order to ensure that the PET scan is covered only as an alternative to a Gallium scan, no PET scan may be covered in cases where it is performed within 50 days of a Gallium scan performed by the same facility where the patient has remained during the 50-day period. Gallium scans performed by another facility less than 50 days prior to the PET scan will not be counted against this screen. The purpose of this screen is to ensure that PET scans are covered only as an alternative to a Gallium scan within the same facility. The CMS is aware that, in order to ensure proper patient care, the treating physician may conclude that previously performed Gallium scans are either inconclusive or not sufficiently reliable.

Frequency Limitation for Restaging: PET scans will be allowed for restaging no sooner than 50 days following the last staging PET scan or Gallium scan, unless sufficient evidence is presented to convince the Medicare contractor that restaging at an earlier date is medically necessary. Since PET scans for restaging are generally performed following cycles of chemotherapy, and since such cycles usually take at least 8 weeks, CMS believes this screen will adequately prevent medically unnecessary scans while allowing some adjustments for unusual cases. In all cases, the determination of the medical necessity for a PET scan for re-staging lymphoma is the responsibility of the local Medicare contractor.

Effective for services performed on or after July 1, 2001, documentation should be maintained in the beneficiary's medical record at the referring physician's office to support the medical necessity of the procedure, as is normal business practice.

2. Diagnosis, Staging, and Restaging (Effective July 1, 2001)

Effective for services performed on or after July 1, 2001, Medicare covers FDG PET for the diagnosis, staging and restaging of lymphoma.

3. Monitoring Response to Treatment (Effective January 28, 2005)

Effective for services performed on or after January 28, 2005, Medicare only covers FDG PET for monitoring response to treatment for lymphoma as "coverage with evidence development".

Medicare shall notify providers and beneficiaries where these services can be accessed, as they become available, via the following:

- Federal Register Notice
- CMS coverage Web site at: www.cms.gov/coverage

Requirements: PET is covered in any/all of the following circumstances:

A. **Diagnosis:** PET is covered only in clinical situations in which: (1) the PET results may assist in avoiding an invasive diagnostic procedure, or (2) the PET results may assist in determining the optimal anatomical location to perform an invasive diagnostic procedure. In general, for most solid tumors, a tissue diagnosis is made prior to the performance of PET scanning. PET scans following a tissue diagnosis are generally performed for the purpose of staging rather than diagnosis.

B. **Staging and/or Restaging:** PET is covered for staging in clinical situations in which: (1)(a) the stage of the cancer remains in doubt after completion of a standard diagnostic workup, including conventional imaging (CT, magnetic resonance imaging, or ultrasound), or (1)(b) the use of PET could potentially replace one or more conventional imaging studies when it is expected that conventional study information is insufficient for the clinical management of the patient, and (2) clinical management of the patient would differ depending on the stage of the cancer identified.

The PET is covered for restaging after completion of treatment for the purpose of: (1) detecting residual disease, (2) detecting suspected recurrence, (3) determining the extent of a known recurrence, or (4) potentially replacing one or more conventional imaging studies when it is expected that conventional study information is insufficient for the clinical management of the patient.

C. Monitoring Response to Treatment: PET is covered for monitoring response to treatment when a change in therapy is anticipated.

Documentation that these conditions are met should be maintained by the referring physician in the beneficiary's medical record, as is normal business practice.

(This NCD last reviewed March 2005.)

220.6.6—FDG PET for Melanoma (Various Effective Dates Below)

(Rev. 31, Issued: 04-04-05; Effective: 01-28-05; Implementation: 04-18-05)

1. Evaluation of Recurrent Melanoma Prior to Surgery As Alternative to Gallium Scan (Effective July 1, 1999)

Effective for services performed on or after July 1, 1999, FDG PET (when used as an alternative to a Gallium scan) is covered for patients with recurrent melanoma prior to surgery for tumor evaluation. FDG PET is not covered for the evaluation of regional nodes.

Frequency Limitations: Whole body PET scans cannot be ordered more frequently than once every 12 months, unless medical necessity documentation, maintained in the beneficiary's medical record, supports the specific need for anatomic localization of possible recurrent tumor within this period.

Limitations: The FDG PET scan is covered only as an alternative to a Gallium scan. PET scans can not be covered in cases where they are performed within 50 days of a Gallium scan performed by the same PET facility where the patient has remained under the care of the same facility during the 50-day period. Gallium scans performed by another facility less than 50 days prior to the PET scan will not be counted against this screen. The purpose of this screen is to ensure that PET scans are covered only as an alternative to a Gallium scan within the same facility. The CMS is aware that, in order to ensure proper patient care, the treating physician may conclude that previously performed Gallium scans are either inconclusive or not sufficiently reliable to make the determination covered by this provision. Therefore, CMS will apply this 50-day rule only to PET scans performed by the same facility that performed the Gallium scan.

Effective for services performed on or after July 1, 2001, documentation should be maintained in the beneficiary's

medical file at the referring physician's office to support the medical necessity of the procedure, as is normal business practice.

2. Diagnosis, Staging, and Restaging (Effective July 1, 2001)

Effective for services performed on or after July 1, 2001, FDG PET is covered for the diagnosis, staging, and restaging of melanoma. FDG PET is not covered for the evaluation of regional nodes.

3. Monitoring Response to Treatment (Effective January 28, 2005)

Effective for services performed on or after January 28, 2005, Medicare only covers FDG PET for monitoring response to treatment for melanoma as "coverage with evidence development".

Medicare shall notify providers and beneficiaries where these services can be accessed, as they become available, via the following:

- Federal Register Notice
- CMS coverage Web site at: www.cms.gov/coverage

Requirements: PET is covered in any/all of the following circumstances:

A. Diagnosis: PET is covered only in clinical situations in which: (1) the PET results may assist in avoiding an invasive diagnostic procedure, or (2) the PET results may assist in determining the optimal anatomical location to perform an invasive diagnostic procedure. In general, for most solid tumors, a tissue diagnosis is made prior to the performance of PET scanning. PET scans following a tissue diagnosis are generally performed for the purpose of staging rather than diagnosis.

B. Staging and/or Restaging: PET is covered for staging in clinical situations in which: (1) (a) the stage of the cancer remains in doubt after completion of a standard diagnostic workup, including conventional imaging (computed tomography, magnetic resonance imaging, or ultrasound), or (1)(b) the use of PET could potentially replace one or more conventional imaging studies when it is expected that conventional study information is insufficient for the clinical management of the patient, and (2) clinical management of the patient would differ depending on the stage of the cancer identified.

The PET is covered for restaging after the completion of treatment for the purpose of: (1) detecting residual disease, (2) detecting suspected recurrence, (3) determining the extent of a known recurrence, or (4) potentially replacing one or more conventional imaging studies when it is expected that conventional study information is insufficient for the clinical management of the patient.

C. Monitoring Response to Treatment: PET is covered for monitoring response to treatment when a change in therapy is anticipated.

Documentation that these conditions are met should be maintained by the referring physician in the beneficiary's medical file, as is normal business practice.

(This NCD last reviewed March 2005.)

220.6.7—FDG PET for Head and Neck Cancers (Various Effective Dates Below)

(Rev. 31, Issued: 04-04-05; Effective: 01-28-05; Implementation: 04-18-05)

Effective for services performed on or after July 1, 2001, Medicare covers FDG PET for diagnosis, staging and restaging of cancer of the head and neck, excluding the central nervous system (CNS) and thyroid. The head and neck cancers encompass a diverse set of malignancies of which the majority is squamous cell carcinomas. Patients may present with metastases to cervical lymph nodes but conventional forms of diagnostic imaging fail to identify the primary tumor. Patients that present with cancer of the head and neck are left with two options—either to have a neck dissection or to have radiation of both sides of the neck with random biopsies. PET scanning attempts to reveal the site of primary tumor to prevent the adverse effects of random biopsies or unnecessary radiation.

Limitations: **PET scans for head and neck cancers are not covered for CNS or thyroid cancers** prior to October 1, 2003. Refer to section 220.6.11 for coverage for thyroid cancer effective October 1, 2003.

Effective for services performed on or after January 28, 2005, Medicare only covers FDG PET for monitoring response to treatment for head and neck cancers as "coverage with evidence development".

Medicare shall notify providers and beneficiaries where these services can be accessed, as they become available, via the following:

• Federal Register Notice
• CMS coverage Web site at: www.cms.gov/coverage

Requirements: PET is covered in any/all both of the following circumstances:

A. **Diagnosis:** PET is covered only in clinical situations in which: (1) the PET results may assist in avoiding an invasive diagnostic procedure, or (2) the PET results may assist in determining the optimal anatomical location to perform an invasive diagnostic procedure. In general, for most solid tumors a tissue diagnosis is made prior to the performance of PET scanning. PET scans following a tissue diagnosis are generally performed for the purpose of staging rather than diagnosis.

B. **Staging and/or Restaging:** PET is covered for staging in clinical situations in which: (1)(a) the stage of the cancer remains in doubt after completion of a standard diagnostic workup, including conventional imaging (computed tomography, magnetic resonance imaging, or ultrasound), or (1)(b) the use of PET could potentially replace one or more conventional imaging studies when it is expected that conventional study information is insufficient for the clinical management of the patient, and (2) clinical management of the patient would differ depending on the stage of the cancer identified.

PET is covered for restaging after completion of treatment for the purpose of: (1) detecting residual disease, (2) detecting suspected recurrence, (3) determining the extent of a known recurrence, or (4) potentially replacing one or more conventional imaging studies when it is expected that conventional study information is insufficient for the clinical management of the patient.

C. **Monitoring Response to Treatment: PET is covered for monitoring response to treatment when a change in therapy is anticipated.**

Documentation that these conditions are met should be maintained by the referring physician in the beneficiary's medical record, as is normal business practice.

(This NCD last reviewed March 2005.)

220.6.8—FDG PET for Myocardial Viability (Various Effective Dates Below)

(Rev. 31, Issued: 04-04-05; Effective: 01-28-05; Implementation: 04-18-05)

The identification of patients with partial loss of heart muscle movement or hibernating myocardium is important in selecting candidates with compromised ventricular function to determine appropriateness for revascularization. Diagnostic tests such as FDG PET distinguish between dysfunctional but viable myocardial tissue and scar tissue in order to affect management decisions in patients with ischemic cardiomyopathy and left ventricular dysfunction.

1. FDG PET is covered for the determination of myocardial viability following an inconclusive single photon emission computed tomography (SPECT) test from July 1, 2001, through September 30, 2002. Only full ring PET scanners are covered from July 1, 2001, through December 31, 2001. However, as of January 1, 2002, full and partial ring scanners are covered.
2. Beginning October 1, 2002, Medicare covers FDG PET for the determination of myocardial viability as a primary or initial diagnostic study prior to revascularization, or following an inconclusive SPECT. Studies performed by full and partial ring scanners are covered.

Limitations: In the event a patient receives a SPECT test with inconclusive results, a PET scan may be covered. However, if a patient receives a FDG PET study with inconclusive results, a follow up SPECT test is not covered.

Documentation that these conditions are met should be maintained by the referring physician in the beneficiary's medical record, as is normal business practice.

(See §220.12 for SPECT coverage.)

(This NCD last reviewed September 2002.)

220.6.9—FDG PET for Refractory Seizures (Effective July 1, 2001)

(Rev. 31, Issued: 04-04-05; Effective: 01-28-05; Implementation: 04-18-05)

Beginning July 1, 2001, Medicare covers FDG-PET for presurgical evaluation for the purpose of localization of a focus of refractory seizure activity.

Limitations: Covered only for pre-surgical evaluation.

Documentation that these conditions are met should be maintained by the referring physician in the beneficiary's medical record, as is normal business practice.

(This NCD last reviewed June 2001.)

220.6.10—FDG PET for Breast Cancer (Effective October 1, 2002)

(Rev. 31, Issued: 04-04-05; Effective: 01-28-05; Implementation: 04-18-05)

Effective for services performed on or after October 1, 2002, Medicare covers FDG PET only as an adjunct to other imaging modalities for: (1) staging breast cancer patients with distant metastasis, (2) restaging patients with loco-regional recurrence or metastasis, or (3) monitoring tumor response to treatment for women with locally advanced and metastatic breast cancer when a change in therapy is contemplated.

Limitations: Medicare continues to nationally non-cover initial diagnosis of breast cancer and staging of axillary lymph nodes.

Documentation that these conditions are met should be maintained by the referring physician in the beneficiary's medical record, as is normal business practice.

(This NCD last reviewed September 2002.)

220.6.11—FDG PET for Thyroid Cancer (Various Effective Dates Below)

(Rev. 31, Issued: 04-04-05; Effective: 01-28-05; Implementation: 04-18-05)

1. Effective for services performed on or after October 1, 2003, Medicare covers the use of FDG PET for thyroid cancer only for restaging of recurrent or residual thyroid cancers of follicular cell origin that have been previously treated by thyroidectomy and radioiodine ablation and have a serum thyroglobulin >10 ng/ml and negative I-131 whole body scan performed.
2. Effective for services performed on or after January 28, 2005, Medicare only covers FDG PET for diagnosis, other staging and restaging, restaging of medullary cell tumors, and monitoring response to treatment as "coverage with evidence development."

Medicare shall notify providers and beneficiaries where these services can be accessed, as they become available, via the following:

- Federal Register Notice
- CMS coverage Web site at: www.cms.gov/coverage

Requirements: PET is covered in any/all of the following circumstances:

A. Diagnosis: PET is covered only in clinical situations in which: (1) the PET results may assist in avoiding an invasive diagnostic procedure, or (2) the PET results may assist in determining the optimal anatomical location to perform an invasive diagnostic procedure. In general, for most solid tumors a tissue diagnosis is made prior to the performance of PET scanning. PET scans following a tissue diagnosis are generally performed for staging rather than diagnosis.

B. Staging and/or Restaging: PET is covered for staging in clinical situations in which: (1)(a) the stage of the cancer remains in doubt after completion of a standard diagnostic workup, including conventional imaging (computed tomography, magnetic resonance imaging, or ultra-

sound), or (1)(b) the use of PET could potentially replace one or more conventional imaging studies when it is expected that conventional study information is insufficient for the clinical management of the patient, and (2) clinical management of the patient would differ depending on the stage of the cancer identified.

The PET is covered for restaging after completion of treatment for the purpose of: (1) detecting residual disease, (2) detecting suspected recurrence, (3) determining the extent of a known recurrence, or (4) potentially replacing one or more conventional imaging studies when it is expected that conventional study information is insufficient for the clinical management of the patient.

C. Monitoring Response to Treatment: PET is covered for monitoring response to treatment when a change in therapy is anticipated.

Documentation that these conditions are met should be maintained by the referring physician in the beneficiary's medical record, as is normal business practice.

(This NCD last reviewed March 2005.)

220.6.12—FDG PET for Soft Tissue Sarcoma (Various Effective Dates Below)

(Rev. 31, Issued: 04-04-05; Effective: 01-28-05; Implementation: 04-18-05)

Following a thorough review of the scientific literature, including a technology assessment on the topic, Medicare maintains its national non-coverage determination for all uses of FDG PET for soft tissue sarcoma.

1. Effective for services performed on or after October 1, 2003, FDG PET for soft tissue sarcoma is nationally non-covered.
2. Effective for services performed on or after January 28, 2005, Medicare only covers FDG PET for soft tissue sarcoma as "coverage with evidence development". Medicare shall notify providers and beneficiaries where these services can be accessed, as they become available, via the following:

- Federal Register Notice
- CMS coverage Web site at: www.cms.gov/coverage

(This NCD last reviewed March 2005.)

220.6.13—FDG PET for Dementia and Neurodegenerative Diseases (Effective September 15, 2004)

(Rev. 31, Issued: 04-04-05; Effective: 01-28-05; Implementation: 04-18-05)

A. General

Medicare covers FDG-PET scans for either the differential diagnosis of fronto-temporal dementia (FTD) and Alzheimer's disease (AD) under specific requirements; OR, its use in a Centers for Medicare & Medicaid Services (CMS)-approved practical clinical trial focused on the utility of FDG-PET in the diagnosis or treatment of dementing neurodegenerative diseases. Specific requirements for each indication are clarified below:

B. Nationally Covered Indications

1. FDG-PET Requirements for Coverage in the Differential Diagnosis of AD and FTD

An FDG-PET scan is considered reasonable and necessary in patients with a recent diagnosis of dementia and documented cognitive decline of at least 6 months, who meet diagnostic criteria for both AD and FTD. These patients have been evaluated for specific alternate neurodegenerative diseases or other causative factors, but the cause of the clinical symptoms remains uncertain.

The following additional conditions must be met before an FDG-PET scan will be covered:

a. The patient's onset, clinical presentation, or course of cognitive impairment is such that FTD is suspected as an alternative neurodegenerative cause of the cognitive decline. Specifically, symptoms such as social disinhibition, awkwardness, difficulties with language, or loss of executive function are more prominent early in the course of FTD than the memory loss typical of AD;

b. The patient has had a comprehensive clinical evaluation (as defined by the American Academy of Neurology (AAN)) encompassing a medical history from the patient and a well-acquainted informant (including assessment of activities of daily living), physical and mental status examination (including formal documentation of cognitive decline occurring over at least 6 months) aided by cognitive scales or neuropsychological testing, laboratory tests, and structural imaging such as magnetic resonance imaging (MRI) or computed tomography (CT);

c. The evaluation of the patient has been conducted by a physician experienced in the diagnosis and assessment of dementia;

d. The evaluation of the patient did not clearly determine a specific neurodegenerative disease or other cause for the clinical symptoms, and information available through FDG-PET is reasonably expected to help clarify the diagnosis between FTD and AD and help guide future treatment;

e. The FDG-PET scan is performed in a facility that has all the accreditation necessary to operate nuclear medicine equipment. The reading of the scan should be done by an expert in nuclear medicine, radiology, neurology, or psychiatry, with experience interpreting such scans in the presence of dementia;

f. A brain single photon emission computed tomography (SPECT) or FDG-PET scan has not been obtained for the same indication. (The indication can be considered to be different in patients who exhibit important changes in scope or severity of cognitive decline, and meet all other qualifying criteria listed above and below (including the judgment that the likely diagnosis remains uncertain). The results of a prior SPECT or FDG-PET scan must have been inconclusive or, in the case of SPECT, difficult to interpret due to immature or inadequate technology. In these instances, an FDG-PET scan may be covered after 1 year has passed from the time the first SPECT or FDG-PET scan was performed.)

g. The referring and billing provider(s) have documented the appropriate evaluation of the Medicare beneficiary. Providers should establish the medical necessity of an FDG-PET scan by ensuring that the following information has been collected and is maintained in the beneficiary medical record:

- Date of onset of symptoms;
- Diagnosis of clinical syndrome (normal aging; mild cognitive impairment or MCI; mild, moderate or severe dementia);
- Mini mental status exam (MMSE) or similar test score;
- Presumptive cause (possible, probable, uncertain AD);
- Any neuropsychological testing performed;
- Results of any structural imaging (MRI or CT) performed;
- Relevant laboratory tests (B12, thyroid hormone); and,
- Number and name of prescribed medications.

The billing provider must furnish a copy of the FDG-PET scan result for use by CMS and its contractors upon request. These verification requirements are consistent with federal requirements set forth in 42 Code of Federal Regulations section 410.32 generally for diagnostic x-ray tests, diagnostic laboratory tests, and other tests. In summary, section 410.32 requires the billing physician and the referring physician to maintain information in the medical record of each patient to demonstrate medical necessity [410.32(d) (2)] and submit the information demonstrating medical necessity to CMS and/or its agents upon request [410.32(d)(3)(I)] (OMB number 0938-0685).

2. FDG-PET Requirements for Coverage in the Context of a CMS-approved Practical Clinical Trial Utilizing a Specific Protocol to Demonstrate the Utility of FDG-PET in the Diagnosis, and Treatment of Neurodegenerative Dementing Diseases

An FDG-PET scan is considered reasonable and necessary in patients with mild cognitive impairment or early dementia (in clinical circumstances other than those specified in subparagraph 1) only in the context of an approved clinical trial that contains patient safeguards and protections to ensure proper administration, use and evaluation of the FDG-PET scan.

The clinical trial must compare patients who do and do not receive an FDG-PET scan and have as its goal to monitor, evaluate, and improve clinical outcomes. In addition, it must meet the following basic criteria:

a. Written protocol on file;
b. Institutional Review Board review and approval;
c. Scientific review and approval by two or more qualified individuals who are not part of the research team; and,
d. Certification that investigators have not been disqualified.

C. Nationally Non-covered Indications

All other uses of FDG-PET for patients with a presumptive diagnosis of dementia-causing neurodegenerative disease (e.g., possible or probable AD, clinically typical FTD, dementia of Lewy bodies, or Creutzfeld-Jacob disease) for which CMS has not specifically indicated coverage continue to be non-covered.

D. Other

Not applicable.

(This NCD last reviewed September 2004.)

220.6.14—FDG PET for Brain, Cervical, Ovarian, Pancreatic, Small Cell Lung, and Testicular Cancers (Effective January 28, 2005)

(Rev. 31, Issued: 04-04-05; Effective: 01-28-05; Implementation: 04-18-05)

A. Staging for Invasive Cervical Cancer as an Adjunct to Conventional Imaging

The CMS has determined that there is sufficient evidence to conclude that an FDG PET scan is reasonable and necessary for the detection of metastases during the pre-treatment management phase (i.e., staging) in patients with newly diagnosed and locally advanced cervical cancer with no extra-pelvic metastasis on conventional imaging tests, such as computed tomography (CT) or magnetic resonance imaging (MRI). Use of FDG PET as an adjunct may more accurately assist in the non-invasive detection of para-aortic, pelvic nodal involvement and other metastases in the pre-treatment phase of disease. The following conditions must be met:

- A pathologic diagnosis of cervical cancer must have already been made before the FDG PET scan is performed,
- The results of other imaging procedures used (e.g., MRI or CT) must be reported, and,
- The available conventional imaging tests are negative for extra-pelvic metastasis.

NOTE: Other staging utilizing FDG PET (e.g., as a substitute for conventional structural imaging; when a previous MRI or CT is positive or inconclusive for para-aortic metastasis and negative for supra-clavicular nodal metastasis) are only covered as "coverage with evidence development".

Medicare shall notify providers and beneficiaries where these services can be accessed, as they become available, via the following:

- Federal Register Notice
- The CMS coverage Web site at: www.cms.gov/coverage

A. Brain, Ovarian, Pancreatic, Small Cell Lung, and Testicular Cancers, and other indications of Cervical Cancer not mentioned in Section A above

"Coverage with evidence development" applies to all FDG PET indications for brain, ovarian, pancreatic, small cell lung, testicular cancers, and other indications of cervical cancer not mentioned in Section A above.

For cancer indications listed as "coverage with evidence development" CMS determines that the evidence is sufficient to conclude that an FDG PET scan is reasonable and necessary only when the provider is participating in, and patients are enrolled in, one of the following types of prospective clinical studies that is designed to collect additional information at the time of the scan to assist in patient management:

- A clinical trial of FDG PET that meets the requirements of Food and Drug Administration (FDA) category B investigational device exemption (42 CFR 405.201); or
- An FDG PET clinical study that is designed to collect additional information at the time of the scan to assist in patient management. Qualifying clinical studies must ensure that specific hypotheses are addressed; appropriate data elements are collected; hospitals and providers are qualified to provide the PET scan and interpret the results;

participating hospitals and providers accurately report data on all enrolled patients not included in other qualifying trials through adequate auditing mechanisms; and, all patient confidentiality, privacy, and other Federal laws must be followed.

Medicare shall notify providers and beneficiaries where these services can be accessed, as they become available, via the following:

- Federal Register Notice
- CMS coverage Web site at: www.cms.gov/coverage

(This NCD last reviewed March 2005.)

220.6.15—FDG PET for All Other Cancer Indications Not Previously Specified (Effective January 28, 2005)

(Rev. 31, Issued: 04-04-05; Effective: 01-28-05; Implementation: 04-18-05)

Effective for services performed on or after January 28, 2005: "coverage with evidence development" applies to all FDG PET indications for all other cancers not previously specified in Section 220.6 above in its entirety.

For cancer indications listed as "coverage with evidence development" CMS has determined that the evidence is sufficient to conclude that an FDG PET scan is reasonable and necessary only when the provider is participating in, and patients are enrolled in, one of the following types of prospective clinical studies that is designed to collect additional information at the time of the scan to assist in patient management:

- A clinical trial of FDG PET that meets the requirements of Food and Drug Administration (FDA) category B investigational device exemption (42 CFR 405.201); or
- An FDG PET clinical study that is designed to collect additional information at the time of the scan to assist in patient management. Qualifying clinical studies must ensure that specific hypotheses are addressed; appropriate data elements are collected; hospitals and providers are qualified to provide the PET scan and interpret the results; participating hospitals and providers accurately report data on all enrolled patients not included in other qualifying trials through adequate auditing mechanisms; and, all patient confidentiality, privacy, and other Federal laws must be followed.

Medicare shall notify providers and beneficiaries where these services can be accessed, as they become available, via the following:

- Federal Register Notice
- CMS coverage Web site at: www.cms.gov/coverage

(This NCD last reviewed March 2005.)

220.6.16—FDG PET for Infection and Inflammation (Effective March 19, 2008)

(Rev. 84; Issued: 06-27-08; Effective Date: 03-19-08; Implementation Date: 07-28-08)

A. General

The Centers for Medicare & Medicaid Services (CMS) received a formal, complete request to reconsider the current, de facto non-coverage for FDG PET imaging for the following off-label uses, each in lieu of bone, leukocyte, and/or gallium scintigraphy:

1. Suspected chronic osteomyelitis in patients with: (a) previously documented osteomyelitis with suspected recurrence, or, (b) symptoms of osteomyelitis for more than 6 weeks (including diabetic foot ulcers),
2. Investigation of patients with suspected infection of hip prosthesis, and,
3. Fever of unknown origin in patients with a febrile illness of >3 weeks duration, a temperature of >38.3 degrees Centigrade on at least two occasions, and uncertain diagnosis after a thorough history, physical examination, and one week of proper investigation.

B. Nationally Covered Indications

N/A

C. Nationally Non-Covered Indications

The CMS is continuing its national non-coverage of FDG PET for the requested indications. Based upon our review, CMS has determined that the evidence is inadequate to conclude that FDG PET for chronic osteomyelitis, infection of hip arthroplasty, and fever of unknown origin improves health outcomes in the Medicare populations, and therefore has determined that FDG PET for chronic osteomyelitis, infection of hip arthroplasty, and fever of unknown origin is not reasonable and necessary under section 1862(a)(1)(A) of the Social Security Act.

D. Other

The CMS has also determined that the request for coverage is not appropriate for the Coverage with Evidence Development (CED) paradigm.

(This NCD last reviewed March 2008.)

220.7—Xenon Scan

(Rev. 1, 10-03-03)

CIM 50-27

Program payment may be made for this diagnostic procedure which involves perfusion lung imaging with 133 xenon. However, review for evidence of abuse which might include absence of reasonable indications, inappropriate sequence, or excessive number of kinds of procedures used in the care of individual patients.

230.5—Gravlee Jet Washer

(Rev. 1, 10-03-03)

CIM 50-4

The Gravlee Jet Washer is a sterile, disposable, diagnostic device for detecting endometrial cancer. The use of this device is indicated where the patient exhibits clinical symptoms or signs suggestive of endometrial disease, such as irregular or heavy vaginal bleeding.

Program payment cannot be made for the washer or the related diagnostic services when furnished in connection with the examination of an asymptomatic patient. Payment for routine physical checkups is precluded under the statute. (See §1862(a)(7) of the Act.)

(See the Medicare Benefit Policy Manual, Chapter 16, "General Exclusions From Coverage," §90).

230.7—Water Purification and Softening Systems Used in Conjunction With Home Dialysis

(Rev. 1, 10-03-03)

CIM 55-1

A—Water Purification Systems

Water used for home dialysis should be chemically free of heavy trace metals and/or organic contaminants that could be hazardous to the patient. It should also be as free of bacteria as possible but need not be biologically sterile. Since the characteristics of natural water supplies in most areas of the country are such that some type of water purification system is needed, such a system used in conjunction with a home dialysis (either peritoneal or hemodialysis) unit is covered under Medicare.

There are two types of water purification systems that will satisfy these requirements:

- Deionization—The removal of organic substances, mineral salts of magnesium and calcium (causing hardness), compounds of fluoride and chloride from tap water using the process of filtration and ion exchange; or
- Reverse Osmosis—The process used to remove impurities from tap water utilizing pressure to force water through a porous membrane.

Use of both a deionization unit and reverse osmosis unit in series, theoretically to provide the advantages of both systems, has been determined medically unnecessary since either system can provide water which is both chemically and bacteriologically pure enough for acceptable use in home dialysis. In addition, spare deionization tanks are not covered since they are essentially a precautionary supply rather than a current requirement for treatment of the patient.

Activated carbon filters used as a component of water purification systems to remove unsafe concentrations of chlorine and chloramines are covered when prescribed by a physician.

B—Water Softening System

Except as indicated below, a water softening system used in conjunction with home dialysis is excluded from coverage under Medicare as not being reasonable and necessary within the meaning of §1862(a)(1) of the Act. Such a system, in conjunction with a home dialysis unit, does not adequately remove the hazardous heavy metal contaminants (such as arsenic) which may be present in trace amounts.

A water softening system may be covered when used to pretreat water to be purified by a reverse osmosis (RO) unit for home dialysis where:

The manufacturer of the RO unit has set standards for the quality of water entering the RO (e.g., the water to be purified by the RO must be of a certain quality if the unit is to perform as intended);

The patients water is demonstrated to be of a lesser quality than required; and

The softener is used only to soften water entering the RO unit, and thus, used only for dialysis. (The softener need not actually be built into the RO unit, but must be an integral part of the dialysis system.)

C—Developing Need When a Water Softening System is Re-placed with a Water Purification Unit in an Existing Home Dialysis System

The medical necessity of water purification units must be carefully developed when they replace water softening systems in existing home dialysis systems. A purification system may be ordered under these circumstances for a number of reasons. For example, changes in the medical community's opinions regarding the quality of water necessary for safe dialysis may lead the physician to decide the quality of water previously used should be improved, or the water quality itself may have deteriorated. Patients may have dialyzed using only an existing water softener previous to Medicare ESRD coverage because of inability to pay for a purification system. On the other hand, in some cases, the installation of a purification system is not medically necessary. Thus, when such a case comes to the contractor's attention, the contractor asks the physician to furnish the reason for the changes. Supporting documentation, such as the suppliers recommendations or water analysis, may be required. All such cases should be reviewed by the contractor's medical consultants.

Cross reference:

The Medicare Benefit Policy Manual, Chapter 15, "Covered Medical and Other Health Services,"§110.

230.8—Non-Implantable Pelvic Flood Electrical Stimulator

(Rev. 48, Issued: 03-17-06; Effective/Implementation Dates: 06-19-06)

CIM 60-24

Non-implantable pelvic floor electrical stimulators provide neuromuscular electrical stimulation through the pelvic floor with the intent of strengthening and exercising pelvic floor musculature. Stimulation is generally delivered by vaginal or anal probes connected to an external pulse generator.

The methods of pelvic floor electrical stimulation vary in location, stimulus frequency (Hz), stimulus intensity or amplitude (mA), pulse duration (duty cycle), treatments per day, number of treatment days per week, length of time for each treatment session, overall time period for device use and between clinic and home settings. In general, the stimulus frequency and other parameters are chosen based on the patient's clinical diagnosis.

Pelvic floor electrical stimulation with a non-implantable stimulator is covered for the treatment of stress and/or urge urinary incontinence in cognitively intact patients who have failed a documented trial of pelvic muscle exercise (PME) training.

A failed trial of PME training is defined as no clinically significant improvement in urinary continence after completing 4 weeks of an ordered plan of pelvic muscle exercises designed to increase periurethral muscle strength.

230.12—Dimethyl Sulfoxide (DMSO)

(Rev. 1, 10-03-03)

CIM 45-23

DMSO is an industrial solvent produced as a chemical by-product of paper production from wood pulp. The Food and Drug Administration has determined that the only purpose for which DMSO is safe and effective for humans is in the treatment of the bladder condition, interstitial cystitis. Therefore, the use of DMSO for all other indications is not considered to be reasonable and necessary. Payment may be made for its use only when reasonable and necessary for a patient in the treatment of interstitial cystitis.

230.16—Bladder Stimulators (Pacemakers)

(Rev. 1, 10-03-03)

CIM 65-11

Not Covered

There are a number of devices available to induce emptying of the urinary bladder by using electrical current which forces the muscles of the bladder to contract. These devices (commonly known as bladder stimulators or pacemakers) are characterized by the implantation of electrodes in the wall of the bladder, the rectal cones, or the spinal cord. While these treatments may effectively empty the bladder, the issue of safety involving the initiation of infection, erosion, placement, and material selection has not been resolved. Further, some facilities previously using electronic emptying have stopped using this method due to the pain experienced by the patient.

The use of spinal cord electrical stimulators, rectal electrical stim-ulators, and bladder wall stimulators is not considered reasonable and necessary. Therefore, no program payment may be made for these devices or for their implant.

230.17—Urinary Drainage Bags

(Rev. 1, 10-03-03)

CIM 65-17

Urinary collection and retention systems are covered as prosthetic devices that replace bladder function in the case of permanent urinary incontinence. Urinary drainage bags that can be used either as bedside or leg drainage bags may be either multi-use or single use systems. Both the multi-use and the single use bags have a system that prevents urine backflow. However, the single use system is non-drainable. There is insufficient evidence to support the medical necessity of a single use system bag rather than the multi-use bag. Therefore, a single use drainage system is subject to the same coverage parameters as the multi-use drainage bags.

240.2—Home Use of Oxygen

(Rev. 1, 10-03-03)

CIM 60-4

A—General

Medicare coverage of home oxygen and oxygen equipment under the durable medical equipment (DME) benefit (see §1861(s)(6)of the Act) is considered reasonable and necessary only for patients with significant hypoxemia who meet the medical documentation, laboratory evidence, and health conditions specified in subsections B, C, and D. This section also includes special coverage criteria for portable oxygen systems. Finally, a statement on the absence of coverage of the professional services of a respiratory therapist under the DME benefit is included in subsection F.

B—Medical Documentation

Initial claims for oxygen services must include a completed Form CMS-484 (Certificate of Medical Necessity: Oxygen) to establish whether coverage criteria are met and to ensure that the oxygen services provided are consistent with the physician's prescrip-tion or other medical documentation. The treating physician's prescription or other medical documentation must indicate that other forms of treatment (e.g., medical and physical therapy directed at secretions, bronchospasm and infection) have been tried, have not been sufficiently successful, and oxygen therapy is still required. While there is no substitute for oxygen therapy, each patient must receive optimum therapy before long-term home oxygen therapy is ordered. Use Form CMS-484 for recertifications. (See the Medicare Program Integrity Manual, Chapter 5, for completion of Form CMS-484.)

The medical and prescription information in section B of Form CMS-484 can be completed only by the treating physician, the physician's employee, or another clinician (e.g., nurse, respiratory therapist, etc.) as long as that person is not the DME supplier. Although hospital discharge coordinators and medical social workers may assist in arranging for physician-prescribed home oxygen, they do not have the authority to prescribe the services. Suppliers may not enter this information. While this section may be completed by non-physician clinician or a physician employee, it must be reviewed and the Form CMS-484 signed by the attending physician.

A physician's certification of medical necessity for oxygen equipment must include the results of specific testing before coverage can be determined.

Claims for oxygen must also be supported by medical documentation in the patient's record. Separate documentation is used with electronic billing. This documentation may be in the form of a prescription written by the patient's attending physician who has recently examined the patient (normally within a month of the start of therapy) and must specify:

- A diagnosis of the disease requiring home use of oxygen;
- The oxygen flow rate; and
- An estimate of the frequency, duration of use (e.g., 2 liters per minute, 10 minutes per hour, 12 hours per day), and duration of need (e.g., 6 months or lifetime).

NOTE: A prescription for "Oxygen PRN" or "Oxygen as needed" does not meet this last requirement. Neither provides any basis for determining if the amount of oxygen is reasonable and necessary for the patient.

A member of the carrier's medical staff should review all claims with oxygen flow rates of more than four liters per minute before payment can be made.

The attending physician specifies the type of oxygen delivery system to be used (i.e., gas, liquid, or concentrator) by signing the completed Form CMS-484. In addition, the supplier

or physician may use the space in section C for written confirmation of additional details of the physician's order. The additional order information contained in section C may include the means of oxygen delivery (mask, nasal, cannula, etc.), the specifics of varying flow rates, and/or the noncontinuous use of oxygen as appropriate. The physician confirms this order information with their signature in section D.

New medical documentation written by the patient's attending physician must be submitted to the carrier in support of revised oxygen requirements when there has been a change in the patient's condition and need for oxygen therapy.

Carriers are required to conduct periodic, continuing medical necessity reviews on patients whose conditions warrant these reviews and on patients with indefinite or extended periods of necessity as described in the Medicare Program Integrity Manual, Chapter 5, "Items and Services Having Special DMERC Review Considerations." When indicated, carriers may also request documentation of the results of a repeat arterial blood gas or oximetry study.

NOTE: Section 4152 of OBRA 1990 requires earlier recertification and retesting of oxygen patients who begin coverage with an arterial blood gas result at or above a partial pressure of 55 or an arterial oxygen saturation percentage at or above 89. (See the Medicare Claims Processing Manual, Chapter 20, "Durable Medical Equipment, Prosthetics and Orthotics, and Supplies (DMEPOS),"§100.2.3, for certification and retesting schedules.)

C—Laboratory Evidence

Initial claims for oxygen therapy must also include the results of a blood gas study that has been ordered and evaluated by the attending physician. This is usually in the form of a measurement of the partial pressure of oxygen (PO_2) in arterial blood. A measurement of arterial oxygen saturation obtained by ear or pulse oximetry, however, is also acceptable when ordered and evaluated by the attending and performed under his or her supervision or when performed by a qualified provider or supplier of laboratory services.

When the arterial blood gas and the oximetry studies are both used to document the need for home oxygen therapy and the results are conflicting, the arterial blood gas study is the preferred source of documenting medical need. A DME supplier is not considered a qualified provider or supplier of laboratory services for purposes of these guidelines.

This prohibition does not extend to the results of blood gas test conducted by a hospital certified to do such tests. The conditions under which the laboratory tests are performed must be specified in writing and submitted with the initial claim, i.e., at rest, during exercise, or during sleep.

The preferred sources of laboratory evidence are, existing physician and/or hospital records that reflect the patient's medical condition. Since it is expected that virtually all patients who qualify for home oxygen coverage for the first time under these guidelines have recently been discharged from a hospital where they submitted to arterial blood gas tests, the carrier needs to request that such test results be submitted in support of their initial claims for home oxygen. If more than one arterial blood gas test is performed during the patient's hospital stay, the test result obtained closest to, but no earlier than two days prior to the hospital discharge date is required as evidence of the need for home oxygen therapy.

For those patients whose initial oxygen prescription did not originate during a hospital stay, blood gas studies should be done while the patient is in the chronic stable state, i.e., not during a period of an acute illness or an exacerbation of their underlying disease.

Carriers may accept an attending physician's statement of recent hospital test results for a particular patient, when appropriate, in lieu of copies of actual hospital records.

A repeat arterial blood gas study is appropriate when evidence indicates that an oxygen recipient has undergone a major change in their condition relevant to home use of oxygen. If the carrier has reason to believe that there has been a major change in the patient's physical condition, it may ask for documentation of the results of another blood gas or oximetry study.

D—Health Conditions

Coverage is available for patients with significant hypoxemia in the chronic stable state, i.e, not during a period of acute illness or an exacerbation of their underlying disease, if:

1. The attending physician has determined that the patient has a health condition outlined in subsection D.1,
2. The patient meets the blood gas evidence requirements specified in subsection D.3, and
3. The patient has appropriately tried other treatment without complete success. (See subsection B.)

1—Conditions for Which Oxygen Therapy May Be Covered

- A severe lung disease, such as chronic obstructive pulmonary disease, diffuse interstitial lung disease, cystic fibrosis, bronchiectasis, widespread pulmonary neoplasm, or
- Hypoxia-related symptoms or findings that might be expected to improve with oxygen therapy. Examples of these symptoms and findings are pulmonary hypertension, recurring congestive heart failure due to chronic cor pulmonale, erythrocytosis, impairment of the cognitive process, nocturnal restlessness, and morning headache.

2—Conditions for Which Oxygen Therapy Is Not Covered

- Angina pectoris in the absence of hypoxemia. This condition is generally not the result of a low oxygen level in the blood, and there are other preferred treatments;
- Breathlessness without cor pulmonale or evidence of hypoxemia. Although intermittent oxygen use is sometimes prescribed to relieve this condition, it is potentially harmful and psychologically addicting;
- Severe peripheral vascular disease resulting in clinically evident desaturation in one or more extremities. There is no evidence that increased PO_2 improves the oxygenation of tissues with impaired circulation; or
- Terminal illnesses that do not affect the lungs.

3—Covered Blood Gas Values

If the patient has a condition specified in subsection D.1, the carrier must review the medical documentation and laboratory evidence that has been submitted for a particular patient (see subsections B and C) and determine if coverage is available under one of the three group categories outlined below.

(a)—Group I—Except as modified in subsection d, coverage is provided for patients with significant hypoxemia evidenced by any of the following:

- An arterial PO_2 at or below 55 mm Hg, or an arterial oxygen saturation at or below 88 percent, taken at rest, breathing room air.
- An arterial PO_2 at or below 55 mm Hg, or an arterial oxygen saturation at or below 88 percent, taken during sleep for a patient who demonstrates an arterial PO_2 at or above 56 mm Hg, or an arterial oxygen saturation at or above 89 percent, while awake; or a greater than normal fall in oxygen level during sleep (a decrease in arterial PO_2 more than 10 mm Hg, or decrease in arterial oxygen saturation more than 5 percent) associated with symptoms or signs reasonably attributable to hypoxemia (e.g., impairment of cognitive processes and nocturnal restlessness or insomnia). In either of these cases, coverage is provided only for use of oxygen during sleep, and then only one type of unit will be covered. Portable oxygen, therefore, would not be covered in this situation.
- An arterial PO_2 at or below 55 mm Hg or an arterial oxygen saturation at or below 88 percent, taken during exercise for a patient who demonstrates an arterial PO_2 at or above 56 mm Hg, or an arterial oxygen saturation at or above 89 percent, during the day while at rest. In this case, supplemental oxygen is provided for during exercise if there is evidence the use of oxygen improves the hypoxemia that was demonstrated during exercise when the patient was breathing room air.

(b)—Group II—Except as modified in subsection d, coverage is available for patients whose arterial PO_2 is 56-59 mm Hg or whose arterial blood oxygen saturation is 89 percent, if there is evidence of:

- Dependent edema suggesting congestive heart failure;
- Pulmonary hypertension or cor pulmonale, determined by measurement of pulmonary artery pressure, gated blood pool scan, echocardiogram, or "P" pulmonale on EKG (P wave greater than 3 mm in standard leads II, III, or AVF); or
- Erythrocythemia with a hematocrit greater than 56 percent.

(c)—Group III—Except as modified in subsection d, carriers must apply a rebuttable presumption that a home program of oxygen use is not medically necessary for patients with arterial PO2 levels at or above 60 mm Hg, or arterial blood oxygen saturation at or above 90 percent. In order for claims in this category to be reimbursed, the carrier's reviewing physician needs to review any documentation submitted in rebuttal of this presumption and grant specific approval of the claims.

The CMS expects few claims to be approved for coverage in this category.

(d)—Variable Factors That May Affect Blood Gas Values—In reviewing the arterial PO_2 levels and the arterial oxygen saturation percentages specified in subsections D. 3.a, b and c, the carrier's medical staff must take into account variations in oxygen measurements that may result from such factors as the patient's age, the altitude level, or the patient's decreased oxygen carrying capacity.

E—Portable Oxygen Systems

A patient meeting the requirements specified below may qualify for coverage of a portable oxygen system either (1) by itself or (2) to use in addition to a stationary oxygen system. Portable oxygen is not covered when it is provided only as a backup to a stationary oxygen system. A portable oxygen system is covered for a particular patient if:

- The claim meets the requirements specified in subsections A-D, as appropriate; and
- The medical documentation indicates that the patient is mobile in the home and would benefit from the use of a portable oxygen system in the home. Portable oxygen systems are not covered for patients who qualify for oxygen solely based on blood gas studies obtained during sleep

F—Respiratory Therapists

Respiratory therapists' services are not covered under the provisions for coverage of oxygen services under the Part B durable medical equipment benefit as outlined above. This benefit provides for coverage of home use of oxygen and oxygen equipment, but does not include a professional component in the delivery of such services.

(See §280.1, and the Medicare Benefit Policy Manual, Chapter 15, "Covered Medical and Other Health Services," §110)

240.2.1—Home Use of Oxygen in Approved Clinical Trials (Effective March 20, 2006)

(Rev. 57, Issued: 05-26-06; Effective: 03-20-06; Implementation: 10-03-06)

A—General

Oxygen is a colorless, odorless gas that comprises 21 percent of the atmospheric gases at sea level. Historically, long term supplemental oxygen has been administered in higher than atmospheric concentrations to patients with chronic hypoxemia, generally resulting from cardiac and/or pulmonary disease. The need for supplemental oxygen is assessed by direct or indirect measurement of the partial pressure of oxygen (conventionally expressed in millimeters of mercury, mmHg) and the oxygen saturation of hemoglobin in arterial blood (expressed as a percent). Chronic oxygen therapy is generally administered via nasal cannulae, face mask, or tracheostomy, from a stationary or portable oxygen tank or an oxygen concentrator.

The medical literature documents health benefits as well as serious adverse events associated with supplemental oxygen use. In this light, it is clear that the decision to initiate, continue, or discontinue the use of supplemental oxygen should be guided by high quality scientific evidence.

B—Nationally Covered Indications

Effective for services performed on or after March 20, 2006 the home use of oxygen is covered for those beneficiaries with arterial oxygen partial pressure measurements from 56 to 65 mmHg or oxygen saturation at or above 89% who are enrolled subjects in clinical trials approved by the Centers for Medicare & Medicaid Services and sponsored by the National Heart, Lung & Blood Institute (NHLBI).

C—Nationally Non-Covered Indications

N/A

D—Other

This policy does not alter Medicare coverage for items and service that may be covered or non-covered according to the existing national coverage determination for the home use of oxygen provided outside the context of approved clinical trials (National Coverage Determination Manual, section 240.2 and 310.1).

(This NCD was last reviewed April 2006)

250.1—Treatment of Psoriasis

(Rev. 1, 10-03-03)

CIM 35-66

Psoriasis is a chronic skin disease, for which several conventional methods of treatment have been recognized as covered. These include topical application of steroids or other drugs; ultraviolet light (actinotherapy); and coal tar alone or in combination with ultraviolet B light (Goeckerman treatment).

A newer treatment for psoriasis uses a psoralen derivative drug in combination with ultraviolet A light, known as PUVA. PUVA therapy is covered for treatment of intractable, disabling psoriasis, but only after the psoriasis has not responded to more conventional treatment. The contractor should document this before paying for PUVA therapy.

In addition, reimbursement for PUVA therapy should be limited to amounts paid for other types of photochemotherapy; ordinarily, payment should not be allowed for more than 30 days of treatment, unless improvement is documented.

260.3—Pancreas Transplants (Effective April 26, 2006)

(Rev. 56, Issued: 05-19-06, Effective: 04-26-06, Implementation: 07-03-06 Carriers/10-02-06 FIs)

A. General

Pancreas transplantation is performed to induce an insulin-independent, euglycemic state in diabetic patients. The procedure is generally limited to those patients with severe secondary complications of diabetes, including kidney failure. However, pancreas transplantation is sometimes performed on patients with labile diabetes and hypoglycemic unawareness.

B. Nationally Covered Indications

Effective for services performed on or after July 1, 1999, whole organ pancreas transplantation is nationally covered by Medicare when performed simultaneous with or after a kidney transplant. If the pancreas transplant occurs after the kidney transplant, immunosuppressive therapy begins with the date of discharge from the inpatient stay for the pancreas transplant.

Effective for services performed on or after April 26, 2006, pancreas transplants alone (PA) are reasonable and necessary for Medicare beneficiaries in the following limited circumstances:

1. PA will be limited to those facilities that are Medicare-approved for kidney transplantation. (Approved centers can be found at http://www.cms.hhs.gov/ESRDGeneralInformation/02_Data.asp#TopOfPage.)

2. Patients must have a diagnosis of type I diabetes:
   - Patient with diabetes must be beta cell autoantibody positive; or
   - Patient must demonstrate insulinopenia defined as a fasting C-peptide level that is less than or equal to 110% of the lower limit of normal of the laboratory's measurement method. Fasting C-peptide levels will only be considered valid with a concurrently obtained fasting glucose <225 mg/dL.
3. Patients must have a history of medically-uncontrollable labile (brittle) insulin-dependent diabetes mellitus with documented recurrent, severe, acutely lifethreatening metabolic complications that require hospitalization. Aforementioned complications include frequent hypoglycemia unawareness or recurring severe ketoacidosis, or recurring severe hypoglycemic attacks;
4. Patients must have been optimally and intensively managed by an endocrinologist for at least 12 months with the most medically-recognized advanced insulin formulations and delivery systems;
5. Patients must have the emotional and mental capacity to understand the significant risks associated with surgery and to effectively manage the lifelong need for immunosuppression; and,
6. Patients must otherwise be a suitable candidate for transplantation.

C. Nationally Non-Covered Indications

The following procedure is not considered reasonable and necessary within the meaning of section 1862(a)(1)(A) of the Social Security Act:

1. Transplantation of partial pancreatic tissue or islet cells (except in the context of a clinical trial (see section 260.3.1 of the National Coverage Determinations Manual).

D. Other

Not applicable.

(This NCD last reviewed April 2006.)

260.3.1—Islet Cell Transplantation in the Context of A Clinical Trial (Effective October 1, 2004)

(Rev. 18, Issued 07-30-04, Effective: 10-01-04, Implementation: 10-04-04)

A. General

As a result of section 733 of the Medicare Prescription Drug Improvement and Modernization Act of 2003 (P.L. 108-173), The Secretary of the Department of Health and Human Services, acting through the National Institute of Diabetes and Digestive and Kidney Disorders, shall conduct a clinical investigation of pancreatic islet cell transplantation that includes Medicare beneficiaries.

The transplant is performed on patients with Type I diabetes. A typical islet cell transplant requires over 500,000 islet cells, but varies depending on the recipient's weight. One of the desired patient outcomes is insulin independence. Elimination of clinically significant hypoglycemia episodes and improved glucose control are other important patient outcomes

One or more pancreata are obtained from donor(s). The islets must be removed within hours after the recovery of the donor pancreas to ensure viability. The islet cells are transplanted by injection into the portal vein of the recipient either using direct visualization, guided ultrasound or percutaneously. The islet cell transplant may be performed alone, in combination with a kidney transplant, or after a kidney transplant. Islet recipients require immunosuppressant therapy to prevent rejection of the transplanted islet cells. Routine follow-up care is necessary for each trial participant.

B. Nationally Covered Indications

Medicare will pay for the routine costs, as well as transplantation and appropriate related items and services, for Medicare beneficiaries participating in a National Institutes of Health (NIH)-sponsored clinical trial(s). The term 'routine costs' means reasonable and necessary routine patient care costs, including immunosuppressive drugs and other follow-up care, as defined in section 310.1 of the NCD Manual.

Specifically, Medicare will cover transplantation of pancreatic islet cells, the insulin producing cells of the pancreas. Coverage will include the costs of acquisition and delivery of the pancreatic islet cells, as well as clinically necessary inpatient and outpatient medical care and immunosuppressants.

C. Nationally Noncovered Indications

Partial pancreatic tissue transplantation or islet cell transplantation performed outside the context of a clinical trial continues to be noncovered.

D. Other

Not applicable.

(This NCD last reviewed July 2004.)

260.6—Dental Examination Prior to Kidney Transplantation

(Rev. 1, 10-03-03)

CIM 50-26

Despite the "dental services exclusion" in §1862(a)(12) of the Act (see the Medicare Benefit Policy Manual, Chapter 16, "General Exclusions From Coverage," §140;), an oral or dental examination performed on an inpatient basis as part of a comprehensive workup prior to renal transplant surgery is a covered service. This is because the purpose of the examination is not for the care of the teeth or structures directly supporting the teeth. Rather, the examination is for the identification, prior to a complex surgical procedure, of existing medical problems where the increased possibility of infection would not only reduce the chances for successful surgery but would also expose the patient to additional risks in undergoing such surgery.

Such a dental or oral examination would be covered under Part A of the program if performed by a dentist on the hospital's staff, or under Part B if performed by a physician. (When performing a dental or oral examination, a dentist is not recognized as a physician under §1861(r) of the Act.) (See the Medicare General Information, Eligibility, and Entitlement Manual, Chapter 5, "Definitions," §70.2, and the Medicare Benefit Policy Manual, Chapter 15, "Covered Medical and Other Health Services," §150.)

270.1—Electrical Stimulation (ES) and Electromagnetic Therapy for the Treatment of Wounds – (Effective July 1, 2004)

(Rev 7, 03-19-04)

Electrical stimulation (ES) and electromagnetic therapy have been used or studied for many different applications, one of which is accelerating wound healing. ES for the treatment of wounds is the application of electrical current through electrodes placed directly on the skin in close proximity to the wound. Electromagnetic therapy uses a pulsed magnetic field to induce current. CMS was asked to reconsider its national noncoverage determination for electromagnetic therapy. After thorough review, CMS determined that the results from the use of electromagnetic therapy for the treatment of wounds were similar to the results from the use of ES. Therefore, effective July 1, 2004, Medicare will cover electromagnetic therapy for the same settings and conditions for which ES is covered. This means Medicare will allow either one covered ES therapy or one covered electromagnetic therapy for the treatment of wounds.

A. Nationally Covered Indications

The use of ES and electromagnetic therapy for the treatment of wounds are considered adjunctive therapies, and will only be covered for chronic Stage III or Stage IV pressure ulcers, arterial ulcers, diabetic ulcers, and venous stasis ulcers. Chronic ulcers are defined as ulcers that have not healed within 30 days of occurrence. ES or electromagnetic therapy will be covered only after appropriate standard wound therapy has been tried for at least 30 days and there are no measurable signs of improved healing. This 30-day period may begin while the wound is acute.

Standard wound care includes: optimization of nutritional status, debridement by any means to remove devitalized tissue, maintenance of a clean, moist bed of granulation tissue with appropriate moist dressings, and necessary treatment to resolve any infection that may be present. Standard wound care based on the specific type of wound includes: frequent repositioning of a patient with pressure ulcers (usually every 2 hours), offloading of pressure and good glucose control for diabetic ulcers, establishment of adequate circulation for arterial ulcers, and the use of a compression system for patients with venous ulcers.

Measurable signs of improved healing include: a decrease in wound size (either surface area or volume), decrease in amount of exudates, and decrease in amount of necrotic tissue. ES or electromagnetic therapy must be discontinued when the wound demonstrates 100% epitheliliazed wound bed.

The ES and electromagnetic therapy services can only be covered when performed by a physician, physical therapist, or incident to a physician service. Evaluation of the wound is an integral part of wound therapy. When a physician, physical therapist, or a clinician incident to a physician, performs ES or electromagnetic therapy, the practitioner must evaluate the wound and contact the treating physician if the wound worsens. If ES or electromagnetic therapy is being used, wounds must be evaluated at least monthly by the treating physician.

B. Nationally Noncovered Indications

1. ES and electromagnetic therapy will not be covered as an initial treatment modality.

2. Continued treatment with ES or electromagnetic therapy is not covered if measurable signs of healing have not been demonstrated within any 30-day period of treatment.

3. Unsupervised use of ES or electromagnetic therapy for wound therapy will not be covered, as this use has not been found to be medically reasonable and necessary.

C. Other

All other uses of ES and electromagnetic therapy not otherwise specified for the treatment of wounds remain at local contractor discretion.

280.1—Durable Medical Equipment Reference List (Effective May 5, 2005)

(Rev. 37, Issued: 06-03-05; Effective: 05-05-05; Implementation: 07-05-05)

The durable medical equipment (DME) list that follows is designed to facilitate the contractor's processing of DME claims. This section is designed as a quick reference tool for determining the coverage status of certain pieces of DME and especially for those items commonly referred to by both brand and generic names. The information contained herein is applicable (where appropriate) to all DME national coverage determinations (NCDs) discussed in the DME portion of this manual. The list is organized into two columns. The first column lists alphabetically various generic categories of equipment on which NCDs have been made by the Centers for Medicare & Medicaid Services (CMS); the second column notes the coverage status.

In the case of equipment categories that have been determined by CMS to be covered under the DME benefit, the list outlines the conditions of coverage that must be met if payment is to be allowed for the rental or purchase of the DME by a particular patient, or cross-refers to another section of the manual where the applicable coverage criteria are described in more detail. With respect to equipment categories that cannot be covered as DME, the list includes a brief explanation of why the equipment is not covered. This DME list will be updated periodically to reflect any additional NDC that CMS may make with regard to other categories of equipment.

When the contractor receives a claim for an item of equipment which does not appear to fall logically into any of the generic categories listed, the contractor has the authority and responsibility for deciding whether those items are covered under the DME benefit.

These decisions must be made by each contractor based on the advice of its medical consultants, taking into account:

- The Medicare Claims Processing Manual, Chapter 20, "Durable Medical Equipment, Prosthetics and Orthotics, and Supplies (DMEPOS)."
- Whether the item has been approved for marketing by the Food and Drug Administration (FDA) and is otherwise generally considered to be safe and effective for the purpose intended; and
- Whether the item is reasonable and necessary for the individual patient.

The term durable medical equipment (DME) is defined as equipment which:

- Can withstand repeated use; i.e., could normally be rented, and used by successive patients;
- Is primarily and customarily used to serve a medical purpose;
- Generally is not useful to a person in the absence of illness or injury; and
- Is appropriate for use in a patient's home.

Durable Medical Equipment Reference List

Item	Coverage
Air Cleaners	Deny—environmental control equipment; not primarily medical in nature (§1861(n) of the Act).
Air Conditioners	Deny—environmental control equipment; not primarily medical in nature (§1861 (n) of the Act).
Air-Fluidized Beds	(See Air-Fluidized Beds §280.8 of this manual.)
Alternating Pressure Pads, Mattresses and Lambs Wool Pads	Covered if patient has, or is highly susceptible to, decubitus ulcers and the patient's physician specifies that he/she will be supervising the course of treatment.
Audible/Visible Signal/ Pacemaker Monitor	(See Self-Contained Pacemaker Monitors.)
Augmentative Communication Device	(See Speech Generating Devices, §50.1 of this manual.)
Bathtub Lifts	Deny—convenience item; not primarily medical in nature (§1861(n) of the Act).
Bathtub Seats	Deny—comfort or convenience item; hygienic equipment; not primarily medical in nature (§1861(n) of the Act).
Bead Beds	(See §280.8.)
Bed Baths (home type)	Deny—hygienic equipment; not primarily medical in nature ((§1861(n) of the Act).
Bed Lifters (bed elevators)	Deny—not primarily medical in nature (§1861(n) of the Act).
Bedboards	Deny—not primarily medical in nature (§1861(n) of the Act).
Bed Pans (autoclavable hospital type)	Covered if patient is bed confined.
Bed Side Rails	(See Hospital Beds, §280.7 of this manual.)
Beds-Lounges (power or manual)	Deny—not a hospital bed; comfort or convenience item; not primarily medical in nature (§1861(n) of the Act).
Beds—Oscillating	Deny—institutional equipment; inappropriate for home use.
Bidet Toilet Seat	(See Toilet Seats.)
Blood Glucose Analyzers—Reflectance Colorimeter	Deny—unsuitable for home use (see §40.2 of this manual).
Blood Glucose Monitors	Covered if patient meets certain conditions (see §40.2 of this manual).
Braille Teaching Texts	Deny—educational equipment; not primarily medical in nature (§1861(n) of the Act).
Canes	Covered if patient meets Mobility Assistive Equipment clinical criteria (see §280.3 of this manual).
Carafes	Deny—convenience item; not primarily medical in nature (§1861(n) of the Act)
Catheters	Deny—nonreusable disposable supply (§1861(n) of the Act). (See The Medicare Claims Processing Manual, Chapter 20, DMEPOS)
Commodes	Covered if patient is confined to bed or room. NOTE: The term "room confined" means that the patient's condition is such that leaving the room is medically contraindicated. The accessibility of bathroom facilities generally would not be a factor in this determination. However, confinement of a patient to his home in a case where there are no toilet facilities in the home may be equated to room confinement. Moreover, payment may also be made if a patient's medical condition confines him to a floor of his home and there is no bathroom located on that floor.

Item	Coverage
Communicator	(See §50.1 of this manual, "Speech Generating Devices.")
Continuous Passive Motion Devices	Continuous passive motion devices are devices Covered for patients who have received a total knee replacement. To qualify for coverage, use of the device must commence within 2 days following surgery. In addition, coverage is limited to that portion of the 3-week period following surgery during which the device is used in the patient's home. There is insufficient evidence to justify coverage of these devices for longer periods of time or for other applications.
Continuous Positive Airway Pressure (CPAP) Devices	(See §240.4 of this manual.)
Crutches	Covered if patient meets Mobility Assistive Equipment clinical criteria (see section 280.3 of this manual).
Cushion Lift Power Seats	(See Seat Lifts.)
Dehumidifiers (room or central heating system type)	Deny—environmental control equipment; not primarily medical in nature (§1861(n) of the Act).
Diathermy Machines (standard pulses wave types)	Deny—inappropriate for home use (see §150.5 of this manual).
Digital Electronic Pacemaker Monitors	(See Self-Contained Pacemaker Monitors.)
Disposable Sheets and Bags	Deny—nonreusable disposable supplies (§1861(n) of the Act)
Elastic Stockings	Deny—nonreusable supply; not rental-type items (§1861(n) of the Act) (See §270.5 of this manual)
Electric Air Cleaners	Deny—(See Air Cleaners.) (§1861(n) of the Act).
Electric Hospital Beds	(See Hospital Beds §280.7 of this manual.)
Electrical Stimulation for Wounds	Deny—inappropriate for home use. (See §270.1 of this manual)
Electrostatic Machines	Deny—(See Air Cleaners and Air Conditioners.) (§1861(n) of the Act).
Elevators	Deny—convenience item; not primarily medical in nature (§1861(n) of the Act).
Emesis Basins	Deny—convenience item; not primarily medical in nature (§1861(n) of the Act).
Esophageal Dilators	Deny—physician instrument; inappropriate for patient use.
Exercise Equipment	Deny—not primarily medical in nature (§1861(n) of the Act).
Fabric Supports	Deny—nonreusable supplies; not rental-type items (§1861(n) of the Act).
Face Masks (oxygen)	Covered if oxygen is Covered. (See §240.2 of this manual.)
Face Masks (surgical)	Deny—nonreusable disposable items (§1861(n) of the Act)
Flowmeters	(See Medical Oxygen Regulators.) (See §240.2 of this manual.)
Fluidic Breathing Assisters	(See Intermittent Positive Pressure Breathing Machines.)
Fomentation Device	(See Heating Pads.)
Gel Flotation Pads and Mattresses	(See Alternating Pressure Pads and Mattresses.)
Grab Bars	Deny—self-help device; not primarily medical in nature (§1861(n) of the Act).
Heat and Massage Foam Cushion Pads	Deny—not primarily medical in nature; personal comfort item (§1861(n) and 1862(a)(6) of the Act).
Heating and Cooling Plants	Deny—environmental control equipment not primarily; medical in nature (§1861(n) of the Act).

Item	Coverage
Heating Pads	Covered if the contractor's medical staff determines patient's medical condition is one for which the application of heat in the form of a heating pad is therapeutically effective.
Heat Lamps	Covered if the contractor's medical staff determines patient's medical condition is one for which the application of heat in the form of a heat lamp is therapeutically effective.
Hospital Beds	(See §280.7 of this manual.)
Hot Packs	(See Heating Pads.)
Humidifiers (oxygen)	(See Oxygen Humidifiers.)
Humidifiers (room or central heating system types)	Deny—environmental control equipment; not medical in nature (§1861(n) of the Act).
Hydraulic Lifts	(See Patient Lifts.)
Incontinent Pads	Deny—nonreusable supply; hygienic item (§1861(n) of the Act).
Infusion Pumps	For external and implantable pumps, see §40.2 of this manual. If the pump is used with an enteral or parenteral nutritional therapy system, see §180.2 of this manual for special coverage rules.
Injectors (hypodermic jet)	Deny—not covered self-administered drug supply pressure powered devices (§1861(s)(2)(A) of the Act) for injection of insulin.
Intermittent Positive Pressure Breathing Machines	Covered if patient's ability to breathe is severely impaired.
Iron Lungs	(See Ventilators.)
Irrigating Kits	Deny—nonreusable supply; hygienic equipment (§1861(n) of the Act).
Lambs Wool Pads	(See Alternating Pressure Pads, Mattresses, and Lambs Wool Pads)
Leotards	Deny—(See Pressure Leotards.) (§1861(n) of the Act).
Lymphedema Pumps	Covered (See Pneumatic Compression Devices, §280.6 of this manual.)
Massage Devices	Deny—personal comfort items; not primarily medical in nature (§1861(n) and 1862(a)(6) of the Act).
Mattresses	Covered only where hospital bed is medically necessary. (Separate Charge for replacement mattress should not be allowed where hospital bed with mattress is rented.) (See §280.7 of this manual.)
Medical Oxygen Regulators	Covered if patient's ability to breathe is severely impaired. (See §240.2 of this manual.)
Mobile Geriatric Chairs	Covered if patient meets Mobility Assistive Equipment clinical criteria (see §280.3 of this manual). (See Rolling Chairs)
Motorized Wheelchairs	Covered if patient meets Mobility Assistive Equipment clinical criteria (see §280.3 of this manual).
Muscle Stimulators	Covered for certain conditions. (See §250.4 of this manual.)
Nebulizers	Covered if patient's ability to breathe is severely impaired.
Oscillating Beds	Deny—institutional equipment—inappropriate for home use.
Overbed Tables	Deny—convenience item; not primarily medical in nature (§1861(n) of the Act).
Oxygen	Covered if the oxygen has been prescribed for use in connection with medically necessary DME. (See §240.2 of this manual.)
Oxygen Humidifiers	Covered if the oxygen has been prescribed for use in connection with medically necessary DME for purposes of moisturizing oxygen. (See §240.2 of this manual.)
Oxygen Regulators (Medical)	(See Medical Oxygen Regulators.)

Item	Coverage
Oxygen Tents	(See §240.2 of this manual.)
Paraffin Bath Units (Portable)	(See Portable Paraffin Bath Units.)
Paraffin Bath Units (Standard)	Deny—institutional equipment; inappropriate for home use.
Parallel Bars	Deny—support exercise equipment; primarily for institutional use; in the home setting other devices (e.g., walkers) satisfy the patient's need.
Patient Lifts	Covered if contractor's medical staff determines patient's condition is such that periodic movement is necessary to effect improvement or to arrest or retard deterioration in his condition.
Percussors	Covered for mobilizing respiratory tract secretions in patients with chronic obstructive lung disease, chronic bronchitis, or emphysema, when patient or operator of powered percussor has receives appropriate training by a physician or therapist, and no one competent to administer manual therapy is available.
Portable Oxygen Systems	1. Regulated covered (adjustable covered under conditions specified in a flow rate). Refer all claims to medical staff for this determination. 2. Preset Deny (flow rate deny emergency, first-aid, or not adjustable) precautionary equipment; essentially not therapeutic in nature.
Portable Paraffin Bath Units	Covered when the patient has undergone a successful trial period of paraffin therapy ordered by a physician and the patient's condition is expected to be relieved by long term use of this modality.
Portable Room Heaters	Deny—environmental control equipment; not primarily medical in nature (§1861(n) of the Act).
Portable Whirlpool Pumps	Deny—not primarily medical in nature; personal comfort items (§§1861(n) and 1862(a)(6) of the Act).
Postural Drainage Boards	Covered if patient has a chronic pulmonary condition.
Preset Portable Oxygen Units	Deny—emergency, first-aid, or precautionary equipment; essentially not therapeutic in nature.
Pressure Leotards	Deny—non-reusable supply, not rental-type item (§1861(n) of the Act).
Pulse Tachometers	Deny—not reasonable or necessary for monitoring pulse of homebound patient with or without a cardiac pacemaker.
Quad-Canes	Covered if patient meets Mobility Assistive Equipment clinical criteria (see §280.3 of this manual).
Raised Toilet Seats	Deny—convenience item; hygienic equipment; not primarily medical in nature (§1861(n) of the Act).
Reflectance Colorimeters	(See Blood Glucose Analyzers.)
Respirators	(See Ventilators.)
Rolling Chairs	Covered if patient meets Mobility Assistive Equipment clinical criteria (see §280.3 of this manual). Coverage is limited to those roll-about chairs having casters of at least 5 inches in diameter and specifically designed to meet the needs of ill, injured, or otherwise impaired individuals. Coverage is denied for the wide range of chairs with smaller casters as are found in general use in homes, offices, and institutions for many purposes not related to the care/treatment of ill/injured persons. This type is not primarily medical in nature. (§1861(n) of the Act.)

Item	Coverage
Safety Rollers	Covered if patient meets Mobility Assistive Equipment clinical criteria (see §280.3 of this manual).
Sauna Baths	Deny—not primarily medical in nature; personal comfort items (§§1861(n) and (1862(a)(6) of the Act).
Seat Lifts	Covered under the conditions specified in §280.4 of this manual. Refer all to medical staff for this determination.
Self Contained Pacemaker Monitors	Covered when prescribed by a physician for a patient with a cardiac pacemaker. (See §§20.8.1 and 280.2 of this manual.)
Sitz Baths	Covered if the contractor's medical staff determines patient has an infection or injury of the perineal area and the item has been prescribed by the patient's physician as a part of his planned regimen of treatment in the patient's home.
Spare Tanks of Oxygen	Deny—convenience or precautionary supply.
Speech Teaching Machines	Deny—education equipment; not primarily medical in nature (§1861(n) of the Act).
Stairway Elevators	Deny—(See Elevators.) (§1861(n) of the Act).
Standing Tables	Deny—convenience item; not primarily medical in nature (§1861(n) of the Act).
Steam Packs	These packs are Covered under the same conditions as a heating pads. (See Heating Pads.)
Suction Machines	Covered if the contractor's medical staff determines that the machine specified in the claim is medically required and appropriate for home use without technical or professional supervision.
Support Hose	Deny (See Fabric Supports.) (§1861(n) of the Act).
Surgical Leggings	Deny—non-reusable supply; not rental-type item (§1861(n) of the Act).
Telephone Alert Systems	Deny—these are emergency communications systems and do not serve a diagnostic or therapeutic purpose.
Toilet Seats	Deny—not medical equipment (§1861(n) of the Act).
Traction Equipment	Covered if patient has orthopedic impairment requiring traction equipment that prevents ambulation during the period of use (Consider covering devices usable during ambulation; e.g., cervical traction collar, under the brace provision).
Trapeze Bars	Covered if patient is bed confined and the patient needs a trapeze bar to sit up because of respiratory condition, to change body position for other medical reasons, or to get in and out of bed.
Treadmill Exercisers	Deny—exercise equipment; not primarily medical in nature (§1861(n) of the Act).
Ultraviolet Cabinets	Covered for selected patients with generalized intractable psoriasis. Using appropriate consultation, the contractor should determine whether medical and other factors justify treatment at home rather than at alternative sites, e.g., outpatient department of a hospital.
Urinals autoclavable	Covered if patient is bed confined hospital type.
Vaporizers	Covered if patient has a respiratory illness.
Ventilators	Covered for treatment of neuromuscular diseases, thoracic restrictive diseases, and chronic respiratory failure consequent to chronic obstructive pulmonary disease. Includes both positive and negative pressure types. (See also §240.5 of this manual.)

Item	Coverage
Walkers	Covered if patient meets Mobility Assistive Equipment clinical criteria (see §280.3 of this manual).
Water and Pressure Pads and Mattresses	(See Alternating Pressure Pads, Mattresses and Lamb Wool Pads.)
Wheelchairs (manual)	Covered if patient meets Mobility Assistive Equipment clinical criteria (see §280.3 of this manual).
Wheelchairs (power operated)	Covered if patient meets Mobility Assistive Equipment clinical criteria (see §280.3 of this manual).
Wheelchairs (scooter/POV)	Covered if patient meets Mobility Assistive Equipment clinical criteria (see §280.3 of this manual).
Wheelchairs (specially-sized)	Covered if patient meets Mobility Assis-tive Equipment clinical criteria (see §280.3 of this manual).
Whirlpool Bath Equipment	Covered if patient is homebound and has a (standard) condition for which the whirlpool bath can be expected to provide substantial therapeutic benefit justifying its cost. Where patient is not homebound but has such a condition, payment is restricted to the cost of providing the services elsewhere; e.g., an outpatient department of a participating hospital, if that alternative is less costly. In all cases, refer claim to medical staff for a determination.
Whirlpool Pumps	Deny—(See Portable Whirlpool Pumps.) (§1861(n) of the Act).
White Canes	Deny—(See §280.2 of this manual.) (Not considered Mobility Assistive Equipment)

Cross-reference:

Medicare Benefit Policy Manual, Chapters 13, "Rural Health Clinic (RHC) and Federally Qualified Health Center (FQHC) Services," 15, "Covered Medical and Other Health Services."

Medicare Claims Processing Manual, Chapters 12, "Physician/Practitioner Billing," 20, "Durable Medical Equipment, Prosthetics and Orthotics, and Supplies (DMEPOS)," 23, "Fee Schedule Administration and Coding Requirements."

280.2—White Cane for Use by a Blind Person

(Rev. 1, 10-03-03)

CIM 60-3

Not Covered

A white cane for use by a blind person is more an identifying and self-help device than an item which makes a meaningful contribution in the treatment of an illness or injury.

280.3—Mobility Assistive Equipment (MAE) (Effective May 5, 2005)

(Rev. 37, Issued: 06-03-05; Effective: 05-05-05; Implementation: 07-05-05)

A—General

The Centers for Medicare & Medicaid Services (CMS) addresses numerous items that it terms "mobility assistive equipment" (MAE) and includes within that category canes, crutches, walkers, manual wheelchairs, power wheelchairs, and scooters. This list, however, is not exhaustive.

Medicare beneficiaries may require mobility assistance for a variety of reasons and for varying durations because the etiology of the disability may be due to a congenital cause, injury, or disease. Thus, some beneficiaries experiencing temporary disability may need mobility assistance on a short-term basis, while in contrast, those living with chronic conditions or enduring disabilities will require mobility assistance on a permanent basis.

Medicare beneficiaries who depend upon mobility assistance are found in varied living situations. Some may live alone and independently while others may live with a caregiver or in a custodial care facility. The beneficiary's environment is relevant to the determination of the appropriate form of mobility assistance that should be employed. For many patients, a device of some sort is compensation for the mobility deficit. Many beneficiaries experience co-morbid conditions that can impact their ability to safely utilize MAE independently or to successfully regain independent function even with mobility assistance.

The functional limitation as experienced by a beneficiary depends on the beneficiary's physical and psychological function, the availability of other support, and the beneficiary's living environment. A few examples include muscular spasticity, cognitive deficits, the availability of a caregiver, and the physical layout, surfaces, and obstacles that exist in the beneficiary's living environment.

B—Nationally Covered Indications

Effective May 5, 2005, CMS finds that the evidence is adequate to determine that MAE is reasonable and necessary for beneficiaries who have a personal mobility deficit sufficient to impair their participation in mobility-related activities of daily living (MRADLs) such as toileting, feeding, dressing, grooming, and bathing in customary locations within the home. Determination of the presence of a mobility deficit will be made by an algorithmic process, Clinical Criteria for MAE Coverage, to provide the appropriate MAE to correct the mobility deficit.

Clinical Criteria for MAE Coverage

The beneficiary, the beneficiary's family or other caregiver, or a clinician, will usually initiate the discussion and consideration of MAE use. Sequential consideration of the questions below provides clinical guidance for the coverage of equipment of appropriate type and complexity to restore the beneficiary's ability to participate in MRADLs such as toileting, feeding, dressing, grooming, and bathing in customary locations in the home. These questions correspond to the numbered decision points on the accompanying flow chart. In individual cases where the beneficiary's condition clearly and unambiguously precludes the reasonable use of a device, it is not necessary to undertake a trial of that device for that beneficiary.

1. Does the beneficiary have a mobility limitation that significantly impairs his/her ability to participate in one or more MRADLs in the home? A mobility limitation is one that:
   a. Prevents the beneficiary from accomplishing the MRADLs entirely, or,
   b. Places the beneficiary at reasonably determined heightened risk of morbidity or mortality secondary to the attempts to participate in MRADLs, or,

   c. Prevents the beneficiary from completing the MRADLs within a reasonable time frame.
2. Are there other conditions that limit the beneficiary's ability to participate in MRADLs at home?
   a. Some examples are significant impairment of cognition or judgment and/or vision.
   b. For these beneficiaries, the provision of MAE might not enable them to participate in MRADLs if the comorbidity prevents effective use of the wheelchair or reasonable completion of the tasks even with MAE.
3. If these other limitations exist, can they be ameliorated or compensated sufficiently such that the additional provision of MAE will be reasonably expected to significantly improve the beneficiary's ability to perform or obtain assistance to participate in MRADLs in the home?
   a. A caregiver, for example a family member, may be compensatory, if consistently available in the beneficiary's home and willing and able to safely operate and transfer the beneficiary to and from the wheelchair and to transport the beneficiary using the wheelchair. The caregiver's need to use a wheelchair to assist the beneficiary in the MRADLs is to be considered in this determination.
   b. If the amelioration or compensation requires the beneficiary's compliance with treatment, for example medications or therapy, substantive non-compliance, whether willing or involuntary, can be grounds for denial of MAE coverage if it results in the beneficiary continuing to have a significant limitation. It may be determined that partial compliance results in adequate amelioration or compensation for the appropriate use of MAE.
4. Does the beneficiary or caregiver demonstrate the capability and the willingness to consistently operate the MAE safely?
   a. Safety considerations include personal risk to the beneficiary as well as risk to others. The determination of safety may need to occur several times during the process as the consideration focuses on a specific device.
   b. A history of unsafe behavior in other venues may be considered.
5. Can the functional mobility deficit be sufficiently resolved by the prescription of a cane or walker?
   a. The cane or walker should be appropriately fitted to the beneficiary for this evaluation.
   b. Assess the beneficiary's ability to safely use a cane or walker.
6. Does the beneficiary's typical environment support the use of wheelchairs including scooters/power-operated vehicles (POVs)?
   a. Determine whether the beneficiary's environment will support the use of these types of MAE.
   b. Keep in mind such factors as physical layout, surfaces, and obstacles, which may render MAE unusable in the beneficiary's home.
7. Does the beneficiary have sufficient upper extremity function to propel a manual wheelchair in the home to participate in MRADLs during a typical day? The manual wheelchair should be optimally configured (seating options, wheelbase, device weight, and other appropriate accessories) for this determination.
   a. Limitations of strength, endurance, range of motion, coordination, and absence or deformity in one or both upper extremities are relevant.

b. A beneficiary with sufficient upper extremity function may qualify for a manual wheelchair. The appropriate type of manual wheelchair, i.e. light weight, etc., should be determined based on the beneficiary's physical characteristics and anticipated intensity of use.

c. The beneficiary's home should provide adequate access, maneuvering space and surfaces for the operation of a manual wheelchair.

d. Assess the beneficiary's ability to safely use a manual wheelchair.

NOTE: If the beneficiary is unable to self-propel a manual wheelchair, and if there is a caregiver who is available, willing, and able to provide assistance, a manual wheelchair may be appropriate.

8. Does the beneficiary have sufficient strength and postural stability to operate a POV/scooter?

a. A POV is a 3- or 4-wheeled device with tiller steering and limited seat modification capabilities. The beneficiary must be able to maintain stability and position for adequate operation.

b. The beneficiary's home should provide adequate access, maneuvering space and surfaces for the operation of a POV.

c. Assess the beneficiary's ability to safely use a POV/scooter.

9. Are the additional features provided by a power wheelchair needed to allow the beneficiary to participate in one or more MRADLs?

a. The pertinent features of a power wheelchair compared to a POV are typically control by a joystick or alternative input device, lower seat height for slide transfers, and the ability to accommodate a variety of seating needs.

b. The type of wheelchair and options provided should be appropriate for the degree of the beneficiary's functional impairments.

c. The beneficiary's home should provide adequate access, maneuvering space and surfaces for the operation of a power wheelchair.

d. Assess the beneficiary's ability to safely use a power wheelchair.

NOTE: If the beneficiary is unable to use a power wheelchair, and if there is a caregiver who is available, willing, and able to provide assistance, a manual wheelchair is appropriate. A caregiver's inability to operate a manual wheelchair can be considered in covering a power wheelchair so that the caregiver can assist the beneficiary.

C—Nationally Non-Covered Indications

Medicare beneficiaries not meeting the clinical criteria for prescribing MAE as outlined above, and as documented by the beneficiary's physician, would not be eligible for Medicare coverage of the MAE.

D—Other

All other durable medical equipment (DME) not meeting the definition of MAE as described in this instruction will continue to be covered, or noncovered, as is currently described in the NCD Manual, in Section 280, Medical and Surgical Supplies. Also, all other sections not altered here and the corresponding policies regarding MAEs which have not been discussed here remain unchanged.

(This NCD last reviewed May 2005).

Cross-references: section 280.1 of the NCD Manual.

280.4—Seat Lift

(Rev. 1, 10-03-03)

CIM 60-8

Reimbursement may be made for the rental or purchase of a medically necessary seat lift when prescribed by a physician for a patient with severe arthritis of the hip or knee and patients with mus-cular dystrophy or other neuromuscular disease when it has been determined the patient can benefit therapeutically from use of the device. In establishing medical necessity for the seat lift, the evidence must show that the item is included in the physician's course of treatment, that it is likely to effect improvement, or arrest or retard deterioration in the patient's condition, and that the severity of the condition is such that the alternative would be chair or bed confinement.

Coverage of seat lifts is limited to those types which operate smoothly, can be controlled by the patient, and effectively assist a patient in standing up and sitting down without other assistance. Excluded from coverage is the type of lift which operates by a spring release mechanism with a sudden, catapult-like motion and jolts the patient from a seated to a standing position. Limit the payment for units which incorporate a recliner feature along with the seat lift to the amount payable for a seat lift without this feature.

Cross Reference:

The Medicare Claims Processing Manual, Chapter 20, "Durable Medical Equipment, Prosthetics and Orthotics, and Supplies (DMEPOS)," §90.

280.7—Hospital Beds

(Rev. 1, 10-03-03)

CIM 60-18

A—General Requirements for Coverage of Hospital Beds

A physician's prescription, and such additional documentation as the contractors' medical staffs may consider necessary, including medical records and physicians' reports, must establish the medical necessity for a hospital bed due to one of the following reasons:

- The patient's condition requires positioning of the body; e.g., to alleviate pain, promote good body alignment, prevent contractures, avoid respiratory infections, in ways not feasible in an ordinary bed; or
- The patient's condition requires special attachments that cannot be fixed and used on an ordinary bed.

B—Physician's Prescription

The physician's prescription which must accompany the initial claim, and supplementing documentation when required, must establish that a hospital bed is medically necessary. If the stated reason for the need for a hospital bed is the patient's condition requires positioning, the prescription or other documentation must describe the medical condition, e.g., cardiac disease, chronic obstructive pulmonary disease, quadriplegia or paraplegia, and also the severity and frequency of the symptoms of the condition, that necessitates a hospital bed for positioning.

If the stated reason for requiring a hospital bed is the patient's condition requires special attachments, the prescription must describe the patient's condition and specify the attachments that require a hospital bed.

C—Variable Height Feature

In well documented cases, the contractors' medical staffs may determine that a variable height feature of a hospital bed, approved for coverage under subsection A above, is medically necessary and, therefore, covered, for one of the following conditions:

Clinical Criteria for MAE Coverage

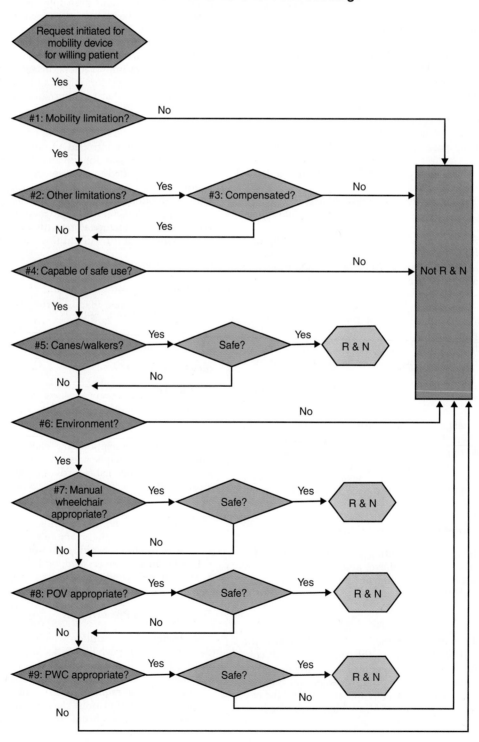

- Severe arthritis and other injuries to lower extremities; e.g., fractured hip—The condition requires the variable height feature to assist the patient to ambulate by enabling the patient to place his or her feet on the floor while sitting on the edge of the bed;
- Severe cardiac conditions—For those cardiac patients who are able to leave bed, but who must avoid the strain of "jumping" up or down;
- Spinal cord injuries, including quadriplegic and paraplegic patients, multiple limb amputee and stroke patients. For those patients who are able to transfer from bed to a wheelchair, with or without help; or
- Other severely debilitating diseases and conditions, if the variable height feature is required to assist the patient to ambulate.

D—Electric Powered Hospital Bed Adjustments

Electric powered adjustments to lower and raise head and foot may be covered when the contractor's medical staff determines that the patient's condition requires frequent change in body position and/or there may be an immediate need for a change in body position (i.e., no delay can be tolerated) and the patient can operate the controls and cause the adjustments. Exceptions may be made to this last requirement in cases of spinal cord injury and brain damaged patients.

E—Side Rails

If the patient's condition requires bed side rails, they can be covered when an integral part of, or an accessory to, a hospital bed.

280.11—Corset Used as Hernia Support

(Rev. 1, 10-03-03)

CIM 70-1

A hernia support (whether in the form of a corset or truss) which meets the definition of a brace is covered under Part B under §1861(s)(9) of the Act. See the Medicare Benefit Policy Manual, Chapter 15, "Covered Medical and Other Services,"§130.

280.12—Sykes Hernia Control

(Rev. 1, 10-03-03)

CIM 70-2

Based on professional advice, it has been determined that the sykes hernia control (a spring-type, U-shaped, strapless truss) is not functionally more beneficial than a conventional truss. Make program reimbursement for this device only when an ordinary truss would be covered. (Like all trusses, it is only of benefit when dealing with a reducible hernia.) Thus, when a charge for this item is substantially in excess of that which would be reasonable for a conventional truss used for the same condition, base reimbursement on the reasonable charges for the conventional truss. See the Medicare Benefit Policy Manual, Chapter 15, "Covered Medical and Other Services,"§130.

280.14—Infusion Pumps

(Rev. 27, Issued: 02-04-05, Effective: 12-17-04, Implementation: 02-18-05)

A—General

Infusion pumps are medical devices used to deliver solutions containing parenteral drugs under pressure at a regulated flow rate.

B—Nationally Covered Indications

The following indications for treatment using infusion pumps are covered under Medicare:

1. External Infusion Pumps

   a. Iron Poisoning—Effective for Services Performed On or After September 26, 1984.

When used in the administration of deferoxamine for the treatment of acute iron poisoning and iron overload, only external infusion pumps are covered.

   b. Thromboembolic Disease—Effective for Services Performed On or After September 26, 1984

When used in the administration of heparin for the treatment of thromboembolic disease and/or pulmonary embolism, only external infusion pumps used in an institutional setting are covered.

   c. Chemotherapy for Liver Cancer—Effective for Services Performed On or After January 29, 1985.

The external chemotherapy infusion pump is covered when used in the treatment of primary hepatocellular carcinoma or colorectal cancer where this disease is unresectable or where the patient refuses surgical excision of the tumor.

   d. Morphine for Intractable Cancer Pain—Effective for Services Performed On or After April 22, 1985.

Morphine infusion via an external infusion pump is covered when used in the treatment of intractable pain caused by cancer (in either an inpatient or outpatient setting, including a hospice).

   e. Continuous Subcutaneous Insulin Infusion (CSII) Pumps (Effective for Services Performed On or after December 17, 2004)

Continuous subcutaneous insulin infusion (CSII) and related drugs/supplies are covered as medically reasonable and necessary in the home setting for the treatment of diabetic patients who: (1) either meet the updated fasting C-Peptide testing requirement, or, are beta cell autoantibody positive; and, (2) satisfy the remaining criteria for insulin pump therapy as described below. Patients must meet either Criterion A or B as follows:

Criterion A: The patient has completed a comprehensive diabetes education program, and has been on a program of multiple daily injections of insulin (i.e. at least 3 injections per day), with frequent self-adjustments of insulin dose for at least 6 months prior to initiation of the insulin pump, and has documented frequency of glucose self-testing an average of at least 4 times per day during the 2 months prior to initiation of the insulin pump, and meets one or more of the following criteria while on the multiple daily injection regimen:

- Glycosylated hemoglobin level (HbAlc) > 7.0 percent
- History of recurring hypoglycemia

- Wide fluctuations in blood glucose before mealtime
- Dawn phenomenon with fasting blood sugars frequently exceeding 200 mg/dl
- History of severe glycemic excursions

Criterion B: The patient with diabetes has been on a pump prior to enrollment in Medicare and has documented frequency of glucose self-testing an average of at least 4 times per day during the month prior to Medicare enrollment.

General CSII Criteria

In addition to meeting Criterion A or B above, the following general requirements must be met:

The patient with diabetes must be insulinopenic per the updated fasting C-peptide testing requirement, or, as an alternative, must be beta cell autoantibody positive.

Updated fasting C-peptide testing requirement:

- Insulinopenia is defined as a fasting C-peptide level that is less than or equal to 110% of the lower limit of normal of the laboratory's measurement method.
- For patients with renal insufficiency and creatinine clearance (actual or calculated from age, gender, weight, and serum creatinine) ≤50 ml/minute, insulinopenia is defined as a fasting C-peptide level that is less than or equal to 200% of the lower limit of normal of the laboratory's measurement method.
- Fasting C-peptide levels will only be considered valid with a concurrently obtained fasting glucose ≤225 mg/dL.
- Levels only need to be documented once in the medical records.

Continued coverage of the insulin pump would require that the patient has been seen and evaluated by the treating physician at least every three months.

The pump must be ordered by and follow-up care of the patient must be managed by a physician who manages multiple patients with CSII and who works closely with a team including nurses, diabetes educators, and dietitians who are knowledgeable in the use of CSII.

Other Uses of CSII

The CMS will continue to allow coverage of all other uses of CSII in accordance with the Category B investigational device exemption (IDE) clinical trials regulation (42 CFR 405.201) or as a routine cost under the clinical trials policy (Medicare National Coverage Determinations (NCD) Manual 310.1).

f. Other Uses

Other uses of external infusion pumps are covered if the contractor's medical staff verifies the appropriateness of the therapy and of the prescribed pump for the individual patient.

NOTE: Payment may also be made for drugs necessary for the effective use of a covered external infusion pump as long as the drug being used with the pump is itself reasonable and necessary for the patient's treatment.

2. Implantable Infusion Pumps

a. Chemotherapy for Liver Cancer (Effective for Services Performed On or After September 26, 1984.)

The implantable infusion pump is covered for intra-arterial infusion of 5-FUdR for the treatment of liver cancer for patients with primary hepatocellular carcinoma or Duke's Class D colorectal cancer, in whom the metastases are limited to the liver, and where (1) the disease is unresectable or (2) where the patient refuses surgical excision of the tumor.

b. Anti-Spasmodic Drugs for Severe Spasticity

An implantable infusion pump is covered when used to administer anti-spasmodic drugs intrathecally (e.g., baclofen) to treat chronic intractable spasticity in patients who have proven unresponsive to less invasive medical therapy as determined by the following criteria:

As indicated by at least a 6-week trial, the patient cannot be maintained on noninvasive methods of spasm control, such as oral anti-spasmodic drugs, either because these methods fail to control adequately the spasticity or produce intolerable side effects, and prior to pump implantation, the patient must have responded favorably to a trial intrathecal dose of the anti-spasmodic drug.

c. Opioid Drugs for Treatment of Chronic Intractable Pain

An implantable infusion pump is covered when used to administer opioid drugs (e.g., morphine) intrathecally or epidurally for treatment of severe chronic intractable pain of malignant or non-malignant origin in patients who have a life expectancy of at least three months and who have proven unresponsive to less invasive medical therapy as determined by the following criteria:

The patient's history must indicate that he/she would not respond adequately to noninvasive methods of pain control, such as sys-temic opioids (including attempts to eliminate physical and behavioral abnormalities which may cause an exaggerated reaction to pain); and a preliminary trial of intraspinal opioid drug administration must be undertaken with a temporary intrathecal/epidural catheter to substantiate adequately acceptable pain relief and degree of side effects (including effects on the activities of daily living) and patient acceptance.

d. Coverage of Other Uses of Implanted Infusion Pumps

Determinations may be made on coverage of other uses of implanted infusion pumps if the contractor's medical staff verifies that:

- The drug is reasonable and necessary for the treatment of the individual patient;
- It is medically necessary that the drug be administered by an implanted infusion pump; and
- The Food and Drug Administration (FDA) approved labeling for the pump must specify that the drug being administered and the purpose for which it is administered is an indicated use for the pump.

e. Implantation of Infusion Pump Is Contraindicated

The implantation of an infusion pump is contraindicated in the following patients:

- With a known allergy or hypersensitivity to the drug being used (e.g., oral baclofen, morphine, etc.);

- Who have an infection;
- Whose body size is insufficient to support the weight and bulk of the device; and
- With other implanted programmable devices since crosstalk between devices may inadvertently change the prescription.

NOTE: Payment may also be made for drugs necessary for the effective use of an implantable infusion pump as long as the drug being used with the pump is itself reasonable and necessary for the patient's treatment.

C—Nationally Noncovered Indications

The following indications for treatment using infusion pumps are not covered under Medicare:

1. External Infusion Pumps

a. Vancomycin (Effective for Services Beginning On or After September 1, 1996)

Medicare coverage of vancomycin as a durable medical equipment infusion pump benefit is not covered. There is insufficient evidence to support the necessity of using an external infusion pump, instead of a disposable elastomeric pump or the gravity drip method, to administer vancomycin in a safe and appropriate manner.

2. Implantable Infusion Pump

a. Thromboembolic Disease (Effective for Services Performed On or After September 26, 1984.)

According to the Public Health Service, there is insufficient published clinical data to support the safety and effectiveness of the heparin implantable pump. Therefore, the use of an implantable infusion pump for infusion of heparin in the treatment of recurrent thromboembolic disease is not covered.

b. Diabetes

An implanted infusion pump for the infusion of insulin to treat diabetes is not covered. The data does not demonstrate that the pump provides effective administration of insulin.

D—Other

Not applicable.

(This NCD last reviewed January 2005.)

300.1—Obsolete or Unreliable Diagnostic Tests

(Rev. 48, Issued: 03-17-06; Effective/Implementation Dates: 06-19-06)

CIM 50-34

A. Diagnostic Tests

Do not routinely pay for the following diagnostic tests because they are obsolete and have been replaced by more advanced procedures. The listed tests may be paid for only if the medical need for the procedure is satisfactorily justified by the physician who performs it. When the services are subject to the Quality Improvement Organization (QIO) review, the QIO is responsible for determining that satisfactory medical justification exists.

When the services are not subject to QIO review, the intermediary or carrier is responsible for determining that satisfactory medical justification exists. This includes:

- Amylase, blood isoenzymes, electrophoretic,
- Chromium, blood,
- Guanase, blood,
- Zinc sulphate turbidity, blood,
- Skin test, cat scratch fever,
- Skin test, lymphopathia venereum,
- Circulation time, one test,
- Cephalin flocculation,
- Congo red, blood,
- Hormones, adrenocorticotropin quantitative animal tests,
- Hormones, adrenocorticotropin quantitative bioassay,
- Thymol turbidity, blood,
- Skin test, actinomycosis,
- Skin test, brucellosis,
- Skin test, psittacosis,
- Skin test, trichinosis,
- Calcium, feces, 24-hour quantitative,
- Starch, feces, screening,
- Chymotrypsin, duodenal contents,
- Gastric analysis, pepsin,
- Gastric analysis, tubeless,
- Calcium saturation clotting time,
- Capillary fragility test (Rumpel-Leede),
- Colloidal gold,
- Bendien's test for cancer and tuberculosis,
- Bolen's test for cancer,
- Rehfuss test for gastric acidity, and
- Serum seromucoid assay for cancer and other diseases.

B. Cardiovascular Tests

Do not pay for the following phonocardiography and vectorcardiography diagnostic tests because they have been determined to be outmoded and of little clinical value. They include:

- Phonocardiogram with or without ECG lead; with supervision during recording with interpretation and report (when equipment is supplied by the physician),
- Phonocardiogram; tracing only, without interpretation and report (e.g., when equipment is supplied by the hospital, clinic),
- Phonocardiogram; interpretation and report,
- Phonocardiogram with ECG lead, with indirect carotid artery and/or jugular vein tracing, and/or apex cardiogram; with interpretation and report,
- Phonocardiogram; without interpretation and report,
- Phonocardiogram; interpretation and report only,
- Intracardiac,
- Vectorcardiogram (VCG), with or without ECG; with interpretation and report,
- Vectorcardiogram; tracing only, without interpretation and report, and
- Vectorcardiogram; interpretation and report only.

100-04 Chapter 1

30.2.10—Payment Under Reciprocal Billing Arrangements—Claims Submitted to Carriers

(Rev. 1486, Issued: 04-04-08, Effective: 01-01-08, Implementation: 05-05-08)

The patient's regular physician may submit the claim, and (if assignment is accepted) receive the Part B payment, for covered visit services (including emergency visits and related services) which the regular physician arranges to be provided by a substitute physician on an occasional reciprocal basis, if:

- The regular physician is unavailable to provide the visit services;
- The Medicare patient has arranged or seeks to receive the visit services from the regular physician;
- The substitute physician does not provide the visit services to Medicare patients over a continuous period of longer than 60 days subject to the exception noted below; and
- The regular physician identifies the services as substitute physician services meeting the requirements of this section by entering in item 24d of Form CMS-1500 HCPCS code Q5 modifier (service furnished by a substitute physician under a reciprocal billing arrangement) after the procedure code. When Form CMS-1500 is next revised, provision will be made to identify the substitute physician by entering the unique physician identification number (UPIN) *or NPI when required* on the form and cross-referring the entry to the appropriate service line item(s) by number(s). Until further notice, the regular physician must keep on file a record of each service provided by the substitute physician, associated with the substitute physician's UPIN *or NPI when required,* and make this record available to the carrier upon request.

Exception: In accordance with section 116 of the "Medicare, Medicaid, and SCHIP Extension Act of 2007" (MMSE), enacted on December 29, 2007, the exception to the 60-day limit on substitute physician billing for physicians called to active duty in the Armed Forces has been extended for services furnished from January 1, 2008 through June 30, 2008. Thus, under this law, a physician called to active duty may bill for substitute physician services furnished from January 1, 2008 through June 30, 2008 for longer than the 60-day limit.

If the only substitution services a physician performs in connection with an operation are post-operative services furnished during the period covered by the global fee, these services need not be identified on the claim as substitution services.

A physician may have reciprocal arrangements with more than one physician. The arrangements need not be in writing.

The term **"covered visit service"** includes not only those services ordinarily characterized as a covered physician visit, but also any other covered items and services furnished by the substitute physician or by others as incident to the physician's services.

"Incident to" services furnished by staff of a substitute physician or regular physician are covered if furnished under the supervision of each.

A **"continuous period of covered visit services"** begins with the first day on which the substitute physician provides covered visit services to Medicare Part B patients of the regular physician, and ends with the last day the substitute physician provides services to these patients before the regular physician returns to work. This period continues without interruption on days on which no covered visit ser-

vices are provided to patients on behalf of the regular physician or are furnished by some other substitute physician on behalf of the regular physician. A new period of covered visit services can begin after the regular physician has returned to work.

EXAMPLE:

The regular physician goes on vacation on June 30, and returns to work on September 4. A substitute physician provides services to Medicare Part B patients of the regular physician on July 2, and at various times thereafter, including August 30 and September 2. The continuous period of covered visit services begins on July 2 and runs through September 2, a period of 63 days. Since the September 2 services are furnished after the expiration of 60 days of the period, the regular physician is not entitled to bill and receive direct payment for them. The substitute physician must bill for these services in his/her own name. The regular physician may, however, bill and receive payment for the services that the substitute physician provides on his/her behalf in the period July 2 through August 30.

The requirements for the submission of claims under reciprocal billing arrangements are the same for assigned and unassigned claims.

A—Physician Medical Group Claims Under Reciprocal Billing Arrangements

The requirements of this section generally do not apply to the substitution arrangements among physicians in the same medical group where claims are submitted in the name of the group. On claims submitted by the group, the group physician who actually performed the service must be identified in the manner described in §30.2.13 with one exception. When a group member provides services on behalf of another group member who is the designated attending physician for a hospice patient, the Q5 modifier may be used by the designated attending physician to bill for services related to a hospice patient's terminal illness that were performed by another group member.

For a medical group to submit assigned and unassigned claims for the covered visit services of a substitute physician who is **not** a member of the group and for an independent physician to submit assigned and unassigned claims for the substitution services of a physician who is a member of a medical group, the following requirements must be met:

- The regular physician is unavailable to provide the visit services;
- The Medicare patient has arranged or seeks to receive the visit services from the regular physician; and
- The substitute physician does not provide the visit services to Medicare patients over a continuous period of longer than 60 days.

Substitute billing services are billed for each entity as follows:

- The medical group must enter in item 24d of Form CMS-1500 the HCPCS code modifier Q5 after the procedure code.
- The independent physician must enter in item 24 of Form CMS-1500 HCPCS code modifier Q5 after the procedure code.

- The designated attending physician for a hospice patient (receiving services related to a terminal illness) bills the Q5 modifier in item 24 of Form CMS-1500 when another group member covers for the attending physician.
- A record of each service provided by the substitute physician must be kept on file and associated with the substitute physician's UPIN or NPI when required. This record must be made available to the carrier upon request.
- In addition, the medical group physician for whom the substitution services are furnished must be identified by his/her provider identification number (PIN) *or NPI when required* in block 24J of the appropriate line item.

Physicians who are members of a group but who bill in their own names are treated as independent physicians for purposes of applying the requirements of this section.

Carriers should inform physicians of the compliance requirements when billing for services of a substitute physician. The physician notification should state that, in entering the Q5 modifier, the regular physician (or the medical group, where applicable) is certifying that the services are covered visit services furnished by the substitute physician identified in a record of the regular physician which is available for inspection, and are services for which the regular physician (or group) is entitled to submit the claim. Carriers should include in the notice that penalty for false certifications may be civil or criminal penalties for fraud. The physician's right to receive payment or to submit claims or accept any assignments may be revoked. The revocation procedures are set forth in §40.

If a line item includes the code Q5 certification, carriers assume that the claim meets the requirements of this section in the absence of evidence to the contrary. Carriers need not track the 60-day period or validate the billing arrangement on a prepayment basis, absent postpayment findings that indicate that the certifications by a particular physician may not be valid.

When carriers make Part B payment under this section, they determine the payment amount as though the regular physician provided the services. The identification of the substitute physician is primarily for purposes of providing an audit trail to verify that the services were furnished, not for purposes of the payment or the limiting charge. Also, notices of noncoverage are to be given in the name of the regular physician.

30.2.11—Physician Payment Under Locum Tenens Arrangements—Claims Submitted to Carriers

(Rev. 1486, Issued: 04-04-08, Effective: 01-01-08, Implementation: 05-05-08)

A—Background

It is a longstanding and widespread practice for physicians to retain substitute physicians to take over their professional practices when the regular physicians are absent for reasons such as illness, pregnancy, vacation, or continuing medical education, and for the regular physician to bill and receive payment for the substitute physician's services as though he/she performed them. The substitute physician generally has no practice of his/her own and moves from area to area as needed. The regular physician generally pays the substitute physician a fixed amount per diem, with the substitute physician having the status of an independent contractor rather than of an employee. These substitute physicians are generally called "locum tenens" physicians.

Section 125(b) of the Social Security Act Amendments of 1994 makes this procedure available on a permanent basis. Thus, beginning January 1, 1995, a regular physician may bill for the services of a locum tenens physicians. A regular physician is the physician that is normally scheduled to see a patient. Thus, a regular physician may include physician specialists (such as a cardiologist, oncologist, urologist, etc.).

B—Payment Procedure

A patient's regular physician may submit the claim, and (if assignment is accepted) receive the Part B payment, for covered visit services (including emergency visits and related services) of a locum tenens physician who is not an employee of the regular physician and whose services for patients of the regular physician are not restricted to the regular physician's offices, if:

- The regular physician is unavailable to provide the visit services;
- The Medicare beneficiary has arranged or seeks to receive the visit services from the regular physician;
- The regular physician pays the locum tenens for his/her services on a per diem or similar fee-for-time basis;
- The substitute physician does not provide the visit services to Medicare patients over a continuous period of longer than 60 days subject to the exception noted below; and
- The regular physician identifies the services as substitute physician services meeting the requirements of this section by entering HCPCS code modifier Q6 (service furnished by a locum tenens physician) after the procedure code. When Form CMS-1500 is next revised, provision will be made to identify the substitute physician by entering his/her unique physician identification number (UPIN) or NPI when required to the carrier upon request.

Exception: In accordance with section 116 of the "Medicare, Medicaid, and SCHIP Extension Act of 2007" (MMSE), enacted on December 29, 2007, the exception to the 60-day limit on substitute physician billing for physicians called to active duty in the Armed Forces has been extended for services furnished from January 1, 2008 through June 30, 2008. Thus, under this law, a physician called to active duty may bill for substitute physician services furnished from January 1, 2008 through June 30, 2008 for longer than the 60-day limit.

If the only substitution services a physician performs in connection with an operation are post-operative services furnished during the period covered by the global fee, these services need not be identified on the claim as substitution services.

The requirements for the submission of claims under reciprocal billing arrangements are the same for assigned and unassigned claims.

C—Medical Group Claims Under Locum Tenens Arrangements

For a medical group to submit assigned and unassigned claims for the services a locum tenens physician provides for patients of the regular physician who is a member of the group, the requirements of subsection B must be met. For purposes of these requirements, per diem or similar fee-for-time compensation which the group pays the locum tenens physician is considered paid by the regular physician. Also, a physician who has left the group and for whom the group has engaged a locum tenens physician as a temporary replacement may bill for the temporary physician for up to 60 days. The group must enter in item 24d of Form CMS-1500 the HCPCS modifier Q6 after the procedure code. Until further notice, the group must keep on file a record of each service provided by the substitute physician, associated with the substitute physician's UPIN *or NPI when required,* and make this record available to the carrier upon request. In addition, the medical group physician for whom the substitution services are furnished must be identified by his/her provider identification number (PIN) *or NPI when required* on block 24J of the appropriate line item.

Physicians who are members of a group but who bill in their own names are generally treated as independent physicians for purposes of applying the requirements of subsection A for payment of locum tenens physician services. Compensation paid by the group to the locum tenens physician is considered paid by the regular physician for purposes of those requirements. The term "regular physician" includes a physician who has left the group and for whom the group has hired the locum tenens physician as a replacement.

30.3.5—Effect of Assignment Upon Purchase of Cataract Glasses From Participating Physician or Supplier on Claims Submitted to Carriers

(Rev. 1, 10-01-03)

B3-3045.4

A pair of cataract glasses is comprised of two distinct products: a professional product (the prescribed lenses) and a retail commercial product (the frames). The frames serve not only as a holder of lenses but also as an article of personal apparel. As such, they are usually selected on the basis of personal taste and style. Although Medicare will pay only for standard frames, most patients want deluxe frames. Participating physicians and suppliers cannot profitably furnish such deluxe frames unless they can make an extra (noncovered) charge for the frames even though they accept assignment.

Therefore, a participating physician or supplier (whether an ophthalmologist, optometrist, or optician) who accepts assignment on cataract glasses with deluxe frames may charge the Medicare patient the difference between his/her usual charge to private pay patients for glasses with standard frames and his/her usual charge to such patients for glasses with deluxe frames, in addition to the applicable deductible and coinsurance on glasses with standard frames, if all of the following requirements are met:

A. The participating physician or supplier has standard frames available, offers them for sale to the patient, and issues and ABN to the patient that explains the price and other differences between standard and deluxe frames. Refer to Chapter 30.

B. The participating physician or supplier obtains from the patient (or his/her representative) and keeps on file the following signed and dated statement:

| Name of Patient | Medicare Claim Number |

Having been informed that an extra charge is being made by the physician or supplier for deluxe frames, that this extra charge is not covered by Medicare, and that standard frames are available for purchase from the physician or supplier at no extra charge, I have chosen to purchase deluxe frames.

| Signature | Date |

C. The participating physician or supplier itemizes on his/her claim his/her actual charge for the lenses, his/her actual charge for the standard frames, and his/her actual extra charge for the deluxe frames (charge differential).

Once the assigned claim for deluxe frames has been processed, the carrier will follow the ABN instructions as described in §60.

100-04 Chapter 3

10.4—Payment of Nonphysician Services for Inpatients

(Rev. 1, 10-01-03)

HO-407

All items and nonphysician services furnished to inpatients must be furnished directly by the hospital or billed through the hospital under arrangements. This provision applies to all hospitals, regardless of whether they are subject to PPS.

A. Other Medical Items, Supplies, and Services

The following medical items, supplies, and services furnished to inpatients are covered under Part A. Consequently, they are covered by the prospective payment rate or reimbursed as reasonable costs under Part A to hospitals excluded from PPS.

- Laboratory services (excluding anatomic pathology services and certain clinical pathology services);
- Pacemakers and other prosthetic devices including lenses, and artificial limbs, knees, and hips;
- Radiology services including computed tomography (CT) scans furnished to inpatients by a physician's office, other hospital, or radiology clinic;
- Total parenteral nutrition (TPN) services; and
- Transportation, including transportation by ambulance, to and from another hospital or freestanding facility to receive specialized diagnostic or therapeutic services not available at the facility where the patient is an inpatient.

The hospital must include the cost of these services in the appropriate ancillary service cost center, i.e., in the cost of the diagnostic or therapeutic service. It must not show them separately under revenue code 0540.

EXCEPTIONS:

- **Pneumococcal Vaccine** - is payable under Part B only and is billed by the hospital on the Form CMS-1450.

- **Ambulance Service** - For purposes of this section "hospital inpatient" means a beneficiary who has been formally admitted it does not include a beneficiary who is in the process of being transferred from one hospital to another. Where the patient is transferred from one hospital to another, and is admitted as an inpatient to the second, the ambulance service is payable under only Part B. If transportation is by a hospital owned and operated ambulance, the hospital bills separately on Form CMS-1450 as appropriate. Similarly, if the hospital arranges for the ambulance transportation with an ambulance operator, including paying the ambulance operator, it bills separately. However, if the hospital does not assume any financial responsibility, the billing is to the carrier by the ambulance operator or beneficiary, as appropriate, if an ambulance is used for the transportation of a hospital inpatient to another facility for diagnostic tests or special treatment the ambulance trip is considered part of the DRG, and not separately billable, if the resident hospital is under PPS.
- **Part B Inpatient Services** - Where Part A benefits are not payable, payment may be made to the hospital under Part B for certain medical and other health services. See Chapter 4 for a description of Part B inpatient services.
- **Anesthetist Services "Incident to" Physician Services** - If a physician's practice was to employ anesthetists and to bill on a reasonable charge basis for these services and that practice was in effect as of the last day of the hospital's most recent 12-month cost reporting period ending before September 30, 1983, the physician may continue that practice through cost reporting periods beginning October 1, 1984. However, if the physician chooses to continue this practice, the hospital may not add costs of the anesthetist's service to its base period costs for purposes of its transition payment rates. If it is the existing or new practice of the physician to employ certified registered nurse anesthetists (CRNAs) and other qualified anesthetists and include charges for their services in the physician bills for anesthesiology services for the hospital's cost report periods beginning on or after October 1, 1984, and before October 1, 1987, the physician may continue to do so.

B. Exceptions/Waivers

These provisions were waived before cost reporting periods beginning on or after October 1, 1986, under certain circumstances. The basic criteria for waiver was that services furnished by outside suppliers are so extensive that a sudden change in billing practices would threaten the stability of patient care. Specific criteria for waiver and processing procedures are in §2804 of the Provider Reimbursement Manual (CMS Pub. 15-1).

40.3—Outpatient Services Treated as Inpatient Services

(Rev. 1429; Issued: 02-01-08; Effective: 07-01-08; Implementation: 07-07-08)

A3-3610.3, HO-415.6, HO-400D, A-03-008, A-03-013, A-03-054

A. Outpatient Services Followed by Admission Before Midnight of the Following Day

(Effective For Services Furnished Before October 1, 1991)

When a beneficiary receives outpatient hospital services during the day immediately preceding the hospital admission, the outpatient hospital services are treated as inpatient services if the beneficiary has Part A coverage. Hospitals and FIs apply this provision only when the beneficiary is admitted to the hospital before midnight of the day following receipt of outpatient services. The day on which the patient is formally admitted as an inpatient is counted as the first inpatient day.

When this provision applies, services are included in the applicable PPS payment and not billed separately. When this provision applies to hospitals and units excluded from the hospital PPS, services are shown on the bill and included in the Part A payment. See Chapter 1 for FI requirements for detecting duplicate claims in such cases.

B. Preadmission Diagnostic Services (Effective for Services Furnished On or After January 1, 1991)

Diagnostic services (including clinical diagnostic laboratory tests) provided to a beneficiary by the admitting hospital, or by an entity wholly owned or wholly operated by the admitting hospital (or by another entity under arrangements with the admitting hospital), within 3 days prior to and including the date of the beneficiary's admission are deemed to be inpatient services and included in the inpatient payment, unless there is no Part A coverage. For example, if a patient is admitted on a Wednesday, outpatient services provided by the hospital on Sunday, Monday, Tuesday, or Wednesday are included in the inpatient Part A payment.

This provision does not apply to ambulance services and maintenance renal dialysis services (see the Medicare Benefit Policy Manual, Chapters 10 and 11, respectively). Additionally, Part A services furnished by skilled nursing facilities, home health agencies, and hospices are excluded from the payment window provisions.

For services provided before October 31, 1994, this provision applies to both hospitals subject to the hospital inpatient prospective payment system (IPPS) as well as those hospitals and units excluded from IPPS.

For services provided on or after October 31, 1994, for hospitals and units excluded from IPPS, this provision applies only to services furnished within one day prior to and including the date of the beneficiary's admission. The hospitals and units that are excluded from IPPS are: psychiatric hospitals and units; inpatient rehabilitation facilities (IRF) and units; long-term care hospitals (LTCH); children's hospitals; and cancer hospitals.

Critical access hospitals (CAHs) are not subject to the 3-day (nor 1-day) DRG payment window.

An entity is considered to be "wholly owned or operated" by the hospital if the hospital is the **sole** owner or operator. A hospital need not exercise administrative control over a facility in order to operate it. A hospital is considered the sole operator of the facility if the hospital has exclusive responsibility for implementing facility policies (i.e., conducting or overseeing the facility's routine operations), regardless of whether it also has the authority to make the policies.

For this provision, diagnostic services are defined by the presence on the bill of the following revenue and/or HCPCS codes:

0254	Drugs incident to other diagnostic services
0255	Drugs incident to radiology
030X	Laboratory
031X	Laboratory pathological
032X	Radiology diagnostic
0341	Nuclear medicine, diagnostic
035X	CT scan
0371	Anesthesia incident to Radiology
0372	Anesthesia incident to other diagnostic services
040X	Other imaging services
046X	Pulmonary function
0471	Audiology diagnostic
048X	Cardiology, with HCPCS codes 93015, 93307, 93308, 93320, 93501, 93503, 93505, 93510, 93526, 93541, 93542, 93543, 93544 – 93552, 93561, or 93562
053X	Osteopathic services
061X	MRT
062X	Medical/surgical supplies, incident to radiology or other diagnostic services
073X	EKG/ECG
074X	EEG
092X	Other diagnostic services

The CWF rejects services furnished January 1, 1991, or later when outpatient bills for diagnostic services with through dates or last date of service (occurrence span code 72) fall on the day of admission or any of the 3 days immediately prior to admission to an IPPS or IPPS-excluded hospital. This reject applies to the bill in process, regardless of whether the outpatient or inpatient bill is processed first. Hospitals must analyze the two bills and report appropriate corrections. For services on or after October 31, 1994, for hospitals and units excluded from IPPS, CWF will reject outpatient diagnostic bills that occur on the day of or one day before admission. For IPPS hospitals, CWF will continue to reject outpatient diagnostic bills for services that occur on the day of or any of the 3 days prior to admission.

Hospitals in Maryland that are under the jurisdiction of the Health Services Cost Review Commission are subject to the 3-day payment window.

C. Other Preadmission Services (Effective for Services Furnished On or After October 1, 1991)

Nondiagnostic outpatient services that are related to a patient's hospital admission and that are provided by the hospital, or by an entity wholly owned or wholly operated by the admitting hospital (or by another entity under arrangements with the admitting hospital), to the patient during the 3 days immediately preceding and including the date of the patient's admission are deemed to be inpatient services and are included in the inpatient payment. Effective March 13, 1998, we defined nondiagnostic preadmission services as being related to the admission only when there is an exact match (for all digits) between the ICD-9-CM principal diagnosis code assigned for both the preadmission services and the inpatient stay. Thus, whenever Part A covers an admission, the hospital may bill nondiagnostic preadmission services to Part B as outpatient services **only** if they are **not** related to the admission. The FI shall assume, in the absence of evidence to the contrary, that such bills are not admission related and, therefore, are not deemed to be inpatient (Part A) services. If there are both diagnostic and nondiagnostic preadmission services and the nondiagnostic services are unrelated to the admission, the hospital may separately bill the nondiagnostic preadmission services to Part B. This provision applies only when the patient has Part A coverage. This provision does not apply to ambulance services and maintenance renal dialysis. Additionally, Part A services furnished by skilled nursing facilities, home health agencies, and hospices are excluded from the payment window provisions.

For services provided before October 31, 1994, this provision applies to both hospitals subject to IPPS as well as those hospitals and units excluded from IPPS (see section B above).

For services provided on or after October 31, 1994, for hospitals and units excluded from IPPS, this provision applies only to services furnished within one day prior to and including the date of the beneficiary's admission.

Critical access hospitals (CAHs) are not subject to the 3-day (nor 1-day) DRG payment window.

Hospitals in Maryland that are under the jurisdiction of the Health Services Cost Review Commission are subject to the 3-day payment window.

Effective for dates of service on or after July 1, 2008, CWF will reject therapeutic services when the line item date of service (LIDOS) falls on the day of admission or any of the 3 days immediately prior to an admission to an IPPS hospital or on the day of admission or one day prior to admission for hospitals excluded from IPPS.

40.3.1—Billing Procedures to Avoid Duplicate Payments

(Rev. 1, 10-01-03)

HO-400H

The hospital must install adequate billing procedures to avoid submission of duplicate claims. This includes duplicate claims for the same service and outpatient bills for nonphysician services considered included in the DRG for a related inpatient admission in the facility or in another hospital.

Where the hospital bills separately for nonphysician services provided to a patient either on the day before admission to a PPS hospital or during a patient's inpatient stay, the claim will be rejected by the FI as a duplicate and the hospital may be subject to sanction penalties per §1128A of the Act.

100-04 Chapter 4

20—Reporting Hospital Outpatient Services Using Healthcare Common Procedure Coding System (HCPCS)

(Rev. 1, 10-03-03)

A3-3626.4, HO-442.6

20.1—General

(Rev. 1, 10-03-03)

HO-442.6

Reporting of HCPCS codes is required of acute care hospitals including those paid under alternate payment systems, e.g., Maryland, long-term care hospitals. HCPCS codes are also required of rehabilitation hospitals, psychiatric hospitals, hospital-based RHCs, hospital-based FQHCs, and CAHs reimbursed under Method II (HCPCS required to be billed for fee reimbursed services). This also includes all-inclusive rate hospitals.

HCPCS includes the American Medical Association's "Current Procedural Terminology," 4th Edition, (CPT-4) for physician services and CMS developed codes for certain nonphysician services. All of the CPT-4 is contained within HCPCS, and is identified as Level I CPT codes consist of five numeric characters. The CMS developed codes are known as Level II. Level II codes are five-character codes that begin with an alpha character that is followed by either numeric or alpha characters.

Hospital-based and independent ESRD facilities must use HCPCS to bill for blood and blood products, and to bill for drugs and clinical laboratory services paid outside the composite rate. In addition, the hospital is required to report modifiers as applicable and as described in §20.6.

The CAHs are required to report HCPCS only for Part B services not paid to them on a reasonable cost basis, e.g., screening mammographies and bone mass measurements.

The HCPCS codes are required for all outpatient hospital services unless specifically excepted in manual instructions. This means that codes are required on surgery, radiology, other diagnostic procedures, clinical diagnostic laboratory, durable medical equipment, orthotic-prosthetic devices, take-home surgical dressings, therapies, preventative services, immunosuppressive drugs, other covered drugs, and most other services.

Claims with required HCPCS coding missing will be returned to the hospital for correction.

20.1.1 – Elimination of 90-day Grace Period for HCPCS (Level I and Level II)

(Rev. 89, 02-06-04)

The CMS had permitted a 90-day grace period for the use of discontinued codes for dates of service January through March 31 that were submitted to Medicare contractors by April 1 of the current year.

The Health Insurance Portability and Accountability Act (HIPAA) requires that medical code sets must be date of service compliant. Since HCPCS is a medical code set, effective January 1, 2005, CMS will no longer provide a 90-day grace period for discontinued HCPCS. The elimination of the grace period applies to the annual HCPCS update and to any mid-year coding changes. Any codes discontinued mid-year will no longer have a 90-day grace period.

The FIs must eliminate the 90-day grace period from their system effective with the January 1, 2005 HCPCS update. FIs will no longer accept discontinued HCPCS codes for dates of service January 1 through March 31 submitted prior to April 1. Hospitals can purchase the American Medical Association's CPT-4 coding book that is published each October that contains new, revised, and discontinued CPT-4 codes for the upcoming year. CMS posts on its Web site the annual alpha-numeric HCPCS file for the upcoming year at the end of each October. Hospitals are encouraged to access CMS Web site to see the new, revised, and discontinued alpha-numeric codes for the upcoming year. The CMS web site to view the annual HCPCS update is http://www.cms.hhs.gov/providers/pufdownload/anhcpcdl.asp

The FIs must continue to return to the provider (RTP) claims containing deleted codes.

20.2—Applicability of OPPS to Specific HCPCS Codes

(Rev. 1536, Issued: 06-19-08; Effective: 07-01-08; Implementation: 07-07-08)

The CPT codes generally are created to describe and report physician services, but are also used by other providers/suppliers to describe and report services that they provide. Therefore, the CPT code descriptors do not necessarily reflect the facility component of a service furnished by the hospital. Some CPT code descriptors include reference to a physician performing a service. For OPPS purposes, unless indicated otherwise, the usage of the term "physician" does not restrict the reporting of the code or application of related policies to physicians only, but applies to all practitioners, hospitals, providers, or suppliers eligible to bill the relevant CPT codes pursuant to applicable portions of the Social Security Act (SSA) of 1965, the Code of Federal Regulations (CFR), and Medicare rules. In cases where there are separate codes for the technical component, professional component, and/or complete procedure, hospitals should report the code that represents the technical component for their facility services. If there is no separate technical component code for the service, hospitals should report the code that represents the complete procedure. Tables describing the treatment of HCPCS codes for OPPS are published in the Federal Register annually.

20.3—Line Item Dates of Service

(Rev. 1, 10-03-03)

Where HCPCS is required a line item date of service is also required. (FL 45 on Form CMS-1450).

The FI will return claims to hospitals where a line item date of service is not entered for each HCPCS code reported or if the line item dates of service reported are outside of the statement-covers period.

20.4—Reporting of Service Units

(Rev. 1, 10-03-03)

The definition of service units (FL 46 on the Form CMS-1450) where HCPCS code reporting is required is the number of times the service or procedure being reported was performed.

EXAMPLES:

If the following codes are performed once on a specific date of service, the entry in the service units field is as follows:

HCPCS Code	Service Units
90849 - Multiple-family group psychotherapy	Units > 1
92265 - Needle oculoelectromyography, one or more extraocular muscles, one or both eyes, with interpretation and report	Units > 1
95004 - Percutaneous tests (scratch, puncture, prick) with allergenic extracts, immediate type reaction, specify number of tests.	Units = no. of tests performed
95861 - Needle electromyography two extremities with or without related paraspinal areas	Units > 1
	6 Units > 83 min. to < 98 min.
	7 Units > 98 min. to < 113 min.
	8 Units > 113 min. to < 128 min.

The pattern remains the same for treatment times in excess of two hours. Hospitals should not bill for services performed for less than eight minutes. The expectation (based on the work values for these codes) is that a provider's time for each unit will average 15 minutes in length. If hospitals have a practice of billing less than 15 minutes for a unit, their FI will highlight these situations for review.

The above schedule of times is intended to provide assistance in rounding time into 15-minute increments. It does not imply that any minute until the eighth should be excluded from the total count as the timing of active treatment counted includes time.

The beginning and ending time of the treatment should be recorded in the patient's medical record along with the note describing the treatment. (The total length of the treatment to the minute could be recorded instead.) If more than one CPT code is billed during a calendar day, then the total number of units that can be billed is constrained by the total treatment time. For example, if 24 minutes of code 97112 and 23 minutes of code 97110 were furnished, then the total treatment time was 47 minutes; so only 3 units can be billed for the treatment. The correct coding is two units of code 97112 and one unit of code 97110, assigning more units to the service that took more time.

20.5—Clarification of HCPCS Code to Revenue Code Reporting

(Rev. 1487, Issued: 04-08-08, Effective: 04-01-08, Implementation: 04-07-08))

Generally, CMS does not instruct hospitals on the assignment of HCPCS codes to revenue codes for services provided under OPPS since hospitals' assignment of cost vary. Where explicit instructions are not provided, providers should report their charges under the revenue code that will result in the charges being assigned to the same cost center to which the cost of those services are assigned in the cost report.

20.5.14—Revenue Codes for "Sometimes Therapy" Services

(Rev. 1445, Issued: 02-08-08; Effective: 01-01-08; Implementation: 03-10-08)

Certain wound care services described by CPT codes are classified as "sometimes therapy" services that may be appropriately provided under either a certified therapy plan of care or without a certified therapy plan of care.

Hospitals receive separate payment under the OPPS when they bill for certain wound care services that are furnished to hospital outpatients independent of a certified therapy plan of care.

When billing for wound care services under the OPPS that are furnished independent of a certified plan of care, providers should neither attach a therapy modifier (that is, GP for physical therapy, GO for occupational therapy, and GN for speech language pathology) to the wound care CPT codes nor report their charges under a therapy revenue code (that is, 042x, 043x, or 044x, to receive paymet under the OPPS.

20.6—Use of Modifiers

(Rev. 1487, Issued: 04-08-08, Effective: 04-01-08, Implementation: 04-07-08)

The Integrated Outpatient Code Editor (I/OCE) accepts all valid CPT and HCPCS modifiers on OPPS claims. Definitions for the following modifiers may be found in the CPT and HCPCS guides:

Level I (CPT) Modifiers

-25, -27, -50, -52, -58, -59, -73, -74, -76, -77, -78, -79, -91

Level II (HCPCS) Modifiers

-CA, -E1, -E2, -E3, -E4, -FA, -FB, -FC, -F1, -F2, -F3, -F4, -F5, -F6, -F7, -F8, -F9, -GA, -GG, -GH, -GY, -GZ, -LC, -LD, -LT, -QL, -QM, -RC, -RT, -TA, -T1, -T2, -T3, -T4, -T5, -T6, -T7, -T8, -T9

As indicated in §20.6.2, modifier -50, while it may be used with diagnostic and radiology procedures as well as with surgical procedures, should be used to report bilateral procedures that are performed at the same operative session as a single line item. Modifiers RT and LT are not used when modifier -50 applies. A bilateral procedure is reported on one line using modifier -50. Modifier -50 applies to any bilateral procedure performed on both sides at the same session.

NOTE: Use of modifiers applies to services/procedures performed on the same calendar day.

Other valid modifiers that are used under other payment methods are still valid and should continue to be reported, e.g., those that are used to report outpatient rehabilitation and ambulance services. Modifiers may be applied to surgical, radiology, and other diagnostic procedures. Providers must use any applicable modifier where appropriate. Providers do not use a modifier if the narrative definition of a code indicates multiple occurrences.

EXAMPLES:

The code definition indicates two to four lesions. The code indicates multiple extremities.

Modifiers Used for Outpatient Prospective Payment System											
Level I (CPT) Modifiers				Level II (HCPCS) Modifiers							
-25	-50	-73	-91	-CA	-E1	-FA	-GA	-LC	-QL	-RC	-TA
-27	-52	-74			-E2	-F1	-GG	-LD	-QM	-RT	-T1
	-58	-76			-E3	-F2	-GH	-LT			-T2
	-59	-77			-E4	-F3	-GY				-T3
		-78				-F4	-GZ				-T4
		-79				-F5					-T5
						-F6					-T6
						-F7					-T7
						-F8					-T8
						-F9					-T9

Providers do not use a modifier if the narrative definition of a code indicates that the procedure applies to different body parts.

EXAMPLES:

Code 11600 (Excision malignant lesion, trunks, arms, or legs; lesion diameter 0.5 cm. or less)

Code 11640 (Excision malignant lesion, face, ears, eyelids, nose, lips; lesion diameter 0.5 cm. or less)

Modifiers -GN, -GO, and -GP must be used to identify the therapist performing speech language therapy, occupational therapy, and physical therapy respectively.

Modifier -50 (bilateral) applies to diagnostic, radiological, and surgical procedures.

Modifier -52 applies to radiological procedures.

Modifiers -73, and -74 apply only to certain diagnostic and surgical procedures that require anesthesia.

Following are some general guidelines for using modifiers. They are in the form of questions to be considered. If the answer to any of the following questions is yes, it is appropriate to use the applicable modifier.

1. **Will the modifier add more information regarding the anatomic site of the procedure?**

EXAMPLE: Cataract surgery on the right or left eye.

2. **Will the modifier help to eliminate the appearance of duplicate billing?**

EXAMPLES: Use modifier 77 to report the same procedure performed more than once on the same date of service but at different encounters.

Use modifier 25 to report significant, separately identifiable evaluation and management service by the same physician on the same day of the procedure or other service.

Use modifier 58 to report staged or related procedure or service by the same physician during the postoperative period.

Use modifier 78 to report a return to the operating room for a related procedure during the postoperative period.

Use modifier 79 to report an unrelated procedure or service by the same physician during the postoperative period.

3. **Would a modifier help to eliminate the appearance of unbundling?**

EXAMPLE: CPT codes 90765 (Intravenous infusion, for therapy, prophylaxis, or diagnosis (specify substance or drug); intital, up to 1 hour) and 36000 (Introduction of needle or intra catheter, vein): If procedure 36000 was performed for a reason other than as part of the IV infusion, modifier -59 would be appropriate.

20.6.1—Where to Report Modifiers on the UB-92 (Form CMS-1450) and ANSI X12N Formats

(Rev. 1472, Issued: 03-06-08, Effecive: 05-23-07, Implementation: 04-07-08))

Modifiers are reported on the hardcopy CMS-1450 and the HIPAA X12N 837 corresponding to the HCPCS code. There is space for four modifiers on the harcopy form.

The dash that is often seen preceding a modifier should never be reported.

When it is appropriate to use a modifier, the most specific modifier should be used first. That is, when modifiers E1 through E4, FA through F9, LC, LD, RC, and TA through T9 apply, they should be used before modifiers LT, RT, or -59.

Note: Information regarding the claim form locators that correspond with these fields and a table to crosswalk the CMS-1450 form locators to the 837 transaction is found in Chapter 25.

20.6.2—Use of Modifiers -50, -LT, and -RT

(Rev. 1, 10-03-03)

Modifier -50 is used to report bilateral procedures that are performed at the same operative session as a single line item. Do not use modifiers RT and LT when modifier -50 applies. Do not submit two line items to report a bilateral procedure using modifier -50.

Modifier -50 applies to any bilateral procedure performed on both sides at the same operative session.

The bilateral modifier -50 is restricted to operative sessions only.

Modifier -50 may not be used:

- To report surgical procedures identified by their terminology as "bilateral," or
- To report surgical procedures identified by their terminology as "unilateral or bilateral".

The unit entry to use when modifier -50 is reported is one.

20.6.3—Modifiers -LT and -RT

(Rev. 1, 10-03-03)

Modifiers -LT or -RT apply to codes, which identify procedures, which can be performed on paired organs, e.g., ears, eyes, nostrils, kidneys, lungs, and ovaries.

Modifiers -LT and -RT should be used whenever a procedure is performed on only one side. Hospitals use the appropriate -RT or -LT modifier to identify which of the paired organs was operated upon.

These modifiers are required whenever they are appropriate.

20.6.4—Use of Modifiers for Discontinued Services

(Rev. 1445, Issued: 02-08-08; Effective: 01-01-08; Implementation: 03-10-08)

A. General

Modifiers provide a way for hospitals to report and be paid for expenses incurred in preparing a patient for surgery and scheduling a room for performing the procedure where the service is subsequently discontinued. This instruction is applicable to both outpatient hospital departments and to ambulatory surgical centers.

Modifier -73 is used by the facility to indicate that a surgical or diagnostic procedure requiring anesthesia was terminated due to extenuating circumstances or to circumstances that threatened the well being of the patient after the patient had been prepared for the procedure (including procedural premedication when provided), and been taken to the room where the procedure was to be performed, but prior to administration of anesthesia. For purposes of billing for services furnished in the hospital outpatient department, anesthesia is defined to include local, regional block(s), moderate sedation/analgesia ("conscious sedation"), deep sedation/analgesia, or general anesthesia. This modifier code was created so that the costs incurred by the hospital to prepare the patient for the procedure and the resources expended in the procedure room and recovery room (if needed) could be recognized for payment even though the procedure was discontinued. Prior to January 1, 1999, modifier -52 was used for reporting these discontinued services.

Modifier -74 is used by the facility to indicate that a surgical or diagnostic procedure requiring anesthesia was terminated after the induction of anesthesia or after the procedure was started (e.g., incision made, intubation started, scope inserted) due to extenuating circumstances or circumstances that threatened the well being of the patient. For purposes of billing for services furnished in the hospital outpatient department, anesthesia is defined to include local, regional block(s), moderate sedation/analgesia ("conscious sedation"), deep sedation/analgesia, and general anesthesia. This modifier code was created so that the costs incurred by the hospital to initiate the procedure (preparation of the patient, procedure room, recovery room) could be recognized for payment even though the procedure was discontinued prior to completion. Prior to January 1, 1999, modifier -53 was used for reporting these discontinued services.

Modifiers -52 and -53 are no longer accepted as modifiers for certain diagnostic and surgical procedures under the hospital outpatient prospective payment system. Coinciding with the addition of the modifiers -73 and -74, modifiers -52 and -53 were revised. Modifier -52 is used to indicate partial reduction or discontinuation of radiology procedures and other services that do not require anesthesia. The modifier provides a means for reporting reduced services without disturbing the identification of the basic service. Modifier -53 is used to indicate discontinuation of physician services and is not approved for use for outpatient hospital services.

The elective cancellation of a procedure should not be reported.

Modifiers -73 and -74 are used to indicate discontinued surgical and certain diagnostic procedures only. They are not used to indicate discontinued radiology procedures.

B. Effect on Payment

Procedures that are discontinued after the patient has been prepared for the procedure and taken to the procedure room but before anesthesia is provided will be paid at 50 percent of the full OPPS payment amount. Modifier -73 is used for these procedures.

Procedures that are discontinued after the procedure has been initiated and/or the patient has received anesthesia will be paid at the full OPPS payment amount. Modifier -74 is used for these procedures.

Procedures for which anesthesia is not planned that are discontinued after the patient is prepared and taken to the room where the procedure is to be performed will be paid at 50 percent of the full OPPS payment amount. Modifier -52 is used for these procedures.

C. Termination Where Multiple Procedures Planned

When one or more of the procedures planned is completed, the completed procedures are reported as usual. The other(s) that were planned, and not started, are not reported. When none of the procedures that were planned are completed, and the patient has been prepared and taken to the procedure room, the first procedure that was planned, but not ompleted is reported with modifier -73. If the first procedure has been started (scope inserted, intubation started, incision made, etc.) and/or the patient has received anesthesia, modifier -74 is used. The other procedures are not reported.

If the first procedure is terminated prior to the induction of anesthesia and before the patient is wheeled into the procedure room, the procedure should not be reported. The patient has to be taken to the room where the procedure is to be performed in order to report modifier -73 or -74.

20.6.5—Modifiers for Repeat Procedures

(Rev. 1, 10-03-03)

Two repeat procedure modifiers are applicable for hospital use:

- Modifier -76 is used to indicate that the same physician repeated a procedure or service in a separate operative session on the same day.
- Modifier -77 is used to indicate that another physician repeated a procedure or service in a separate operative session on the same day.

If there is a question regarding who the ordering physician was and whether or not the same physician ordered the second procedure, the code selected is based on whether or not the physician performing the procedure is the same.

The procedure must be the same procedure. It is listed once and then listed again with the appropriate modifier.

20.6.6—Modifiers for Radiology Services

(Rev. 1599, Issued: 09-19-08, Effective: 10-01-08, Implementation: 10-06-08)

Modifiers -52 (Reduced Services), -59, -76, and -77, and the Level II modifiers apply to radiology services.

When a radiology procedure is reduced, the correct reporting is to code to the extent of the procedure performed. If no HCPCS code exists for the service that has been completed, report the intended HCPCS code with modifier -52 appended.

EXAMPLE: CPT code 71020 (Radiologic examination, chest, two views, frontal and lateral) is ordered. Only one frontal view is performed. CPT code 71010 (Radiologic examination, chest: single view, frontal) is reported. The service is not reported as CPT code 71020-52.

20.6.7—CA Modifier

(Rev. 1, 10-03-03)

Definition:

Procedure payable only in the inpatient setting when performed emergently on an outpatient who expires prior to admission.

20.6.8—HCPCS Level II Modifiers

(Rev. 1, 10-03-03)

Generally, these codes are required to add specificity to the reporting of procedures performed on eyelids, fingers, toes, and arteries.

They may be appended to CPT codes.

If more than one level II modifier applies, the HCPCS code is repeated on another line with the appropriate level II modifier:

EXAMPLE: Code 26010 (drainage of finger abscess; simple) done on the left thumb and second finger would be coded:

26010FA

26010F1

The Level II modifiers apply whether Medicare is the primary or secondary payer.

20.6.9—Use of HCPCS Modifier -FB

(Rev. 1103, Issued: 11-03-06, Effective: 01-01-07, Implementation: 01-02-07)

Effective January 1, 2007, the definition of modifier -FB is **"Item Provided Without Cost to Provider, Supplier or Practitioner, or Credit Received for Replacement Device (Examples, but not Limited to: Covered Under Warranty, Replaced Due to Defect, Free Samples)"**. See the Medicare Claims Processing Manual, Pub 100-04, Chapter 4, §61.3 for instructions regarding charges for items billed with the -FB modifier.

The OPPS hospitals must report modifier - FB on the same line as the procedure code (not the device code) for a service that requires a device for which neither the hospital, nor the beneficiary, is liable to the manufacturer. Hospitals must report modifier -FB on the same line as the procedure code for a service that requires a device when the manufacturer gives credit for a device being replaced with a more costly device.

20.6.10—Use of HCPCS Modifier -FC

(Rev. 1487, Issued: 04-08-08, Effective: 04-01-08, Implementation: 04-07-08)

Effective January 1, 2008, the definition of modifier -FC is **"Partial credit received for replaced device."** See the Medicare Claims Processing Manual, Pub 100-04, Chapter 4, §61.3 for instructions regarding charges for items billed with the -FC modifier.

OPPS hospitals must report the -FC modifier for cases in which the hospital receives a partial credit of 50 percent or more of the cost of a new replacement device under warranty, recall, or field action. The hospital must append the -FC modifier to the procedure code (not the device code) that reports the services provided to replace the device.

20.7 – Billing of 'C' HCPCS Codes by Non-OPPS Providers

(Rev. 976, Issued: 06-09-06, Effective: 10-01-06, Implementation: 10-02-06)

Prior to October 1, 2006, the "C" series of HCPCS codes were used exclusively by hospitals subject to OPPS to identify items that may have qualified for transitional pass through payment under OPPS or items or services for which an appropriate HCPCS code did not exist for the purposes of implementing the OPPS. The C-codes could not be used to bill services payable under other payment systems. CMS realized that these C-codes evolved and also target services that are uniquely hospital services that may be provided by an OPPS provider, other providers, or be paid under other payment systems.

Effective October 1, 2006, the following non-OPPS providers may elect to bill using the C-codes or an appropriate CPT code on Types of Bill (TOBs) 12X, 13X, or 85X:

- Critical Access Hospitals (CAHs);
- Indian Health Service Hospitals (IHS);
- Hospitals located in American Samoa, Guam, Saipan or the Virgin Islands; and
- Maryland waiver hospitals.

The OPPS providers shall continue to receive pass-through payment on items or services that qualify for pass through payment. Non-OPPS providers are not eligible for pass through payments.

The C-codes shall be replaced with permanent codes. Whenever a permanent code is established to replace a temporary code, the temporary code is deleted and crossreferenced to the new permanent code. Upon deletion of a temporary code, providers shall bill using the new permanent code.

Providers are encouraged to access the CMS Web site to view the quarterly HCPCS Code updates. The URL to view the quarterly updates is http://www.cms.hhs.gov/HCPCSReleaseCodeSets/.

The billing of C-codes by Method I and Method II Critical Access Hospitals (CAHs) is limited to the billing for facility (technical) services. The C-codes shall not be billed by Method II CAHs for professional services with revenue codes 96X, 97X, or 98X.

230.1—Coding and Payment for Drugs and Biologicals, and Radiopharmaceuticals

(Rev. 1445, Issued: 02-08-08; Effective: 01-01-08; Implementation: 03-10-08)

This section provides hospitals with coding instructions and payment information for drugs paid under OPPS. For additional information on coding and payment for drugs and biologicals under the OPPS, see the Medicare Claims Processing Manual, Chapter 17 "Drugs and Biologicals."

230.2—Coding and Payment for Drug Administration

(Rev. 1445, Issued: 02-08-08; Effective: 01-01-08; Implementation: 03-10-08)

A. Overview

Drug administration services furnished under the Hospital Outpatient Prospective Payment System (OPPS) during CY 2005 were reported using CPT codes 90780, 90781, and 96400-96459.

Effective January 1, 2006, some of these CPT codes were replaced with more detailed CPT codes incorporating specific procedural concepts, as defined and described by the CPT manual, such as initial, concurrent, and sequential.

Hospitals are instructed to use the full set of CPT codes, including those codes referencing concepts of initial, concurrent, and sequential, to bill for drug administration services furnished in the hospital outpatient department beginning January 1, 2007. In addition, hospitals are instructed to continue billing the HCPCS codes that most accurately describe the service(s) provided.

Hospitals are reminded to bill a separate Evaluation and Management code (with modifier 25) only if a significant, separately identifiable E/M service is performed in the same encounter with OPPS drug administration services.

B. Billing for Infusions and Injections

Beginning in CY 2007, hospitals were instructed to use the full set of drug administration CPT codes (90760-90779; 96401-96549), (96413-96523 beginning in CY 2008) when billing for drug administration services provided in the hospital outpatient department. In addition, hospitals are to continue to bill HCPCS code C8957 (Intravenous infusion for therapy/diagnosis; initiation of prolonged infusion (more than 8 hours), requiring use of portable or implantable pump) when appropriate. Hospitals are expected to report all drug administration CPT codes in a manner consistent with their descriptors, CPT instructions, and correct coding principles. Hospitals should note the conceptual changes between CY 2006 drug administration codes effective under the OPPS and the CPT codes in effect beginning January 1, 2007, in order to ensure accurate billing under the OPPS. Hospitals should report all HCPCS codes that describe the drug administration services provided, regardless of whether or not those services are separately paid or their payment is packaged.

Medicare's general policy regarding physician supervision within hospital outpatient department meets the physician supervision requirements for use of CPT codes 90760-90779, 96401-96549, (96413-96523 beginning in CY 2008) (Reference: Medicare Benefit Policy Manual, Pub. 100-02, chapter 6, §20.4.1)

C. Payments For Drug Administration Services

For CY 2007, OPPS drug administration APCs were restructured, resulting in a six-level hierarchy where active HCPCS codes have been assigned according to their clinical coherence and resource use. Contrary to the CY 2006 payment structure that bundled payment for several instances of a type of service (non-chemotherapy, chemotherapy by infusion, non-infusion chemotherapy) into a per-encounter APC payment, structure introduced in CY 2007 provides a separate APC payment for each reported unit of a separately payable HCPCS code.

Hospitals should note that the transition to the full set of CPT drug administration codes provides for conceptual differences when reporting, such as those noted below.

- In CY 2006, hospitals were instructed to bill for the first hour (and any additional hours) by each type of infusion service (non-chemotherapy, chemotherapy by infusion, non-infusion chemotherapy). Beginning in CY 2007, the first hour concept no longer exists. CPT codes in CY 2007 and beyond allow for only one initial service per encounter, for each vascular access site, no matter how many types of infusion services are provided; however, hospitals will receive an APC payment for the initial service and separate APC payment(s) for additional hours of infusion or other drug administration services provided they are separately payable.
- In CY 2006, hospitals providing infusion services of different types (non-chemotherapy, chemotherapy by infusion, non-infusion chemotherapy) received payment for the associated per-encounter infusion APC even if these infusions occurred during the same time period. Beginning in CY 2007, CPT instructions allow reporting of only one initial drug administration service, including infusion services, per encounter for each distinct vascular access site, with other services through the same vascular access site being reported via the sequential, concurrent or additional hour codes.

(**NOTE:** This list above provides a brief overview of a limited number of the conceptual changes between CY 2006 OPPS drug administration codes and CY 2007 OPPS drug administration codes - this list is not comprehensive and does not include all items hospitals will need to consider during this transition).

For APC payment rates, refer to the most current quarterly version of Addendum B on the CMS Web site at http://www.cms.hhs.gov/HospitalOutpatientPPS/.

D. Infusions Started Outside the Hospital

Hospitals may receive Medicare beneficiaries for outpatient services who are in the process of receiving an infusion at their time of arrival at the hospital (e.g., a patient who arrives via ambulance with an ongoing intravenous infusion initiated by paramedics during transport). Hospitals are reminded to bill for all services provided using the HCPCS code(s) that most accurately describe the service(s) they provided. This includes hospitals reporting an initial hour of infusion, even if the hospital did not initiate the infusion, and additional HCPCS codes for additional or sequential infusion services if needed.

240—Inpatient Part B Hospital Services

(Rev. 980, Issued: 06-14-06, Effective: 10-01-06, Implementation: 10-02-06)

Inpatient Part B services which are paid under OPPS include:

- Diagnostic x-ray tests, and other diagnostic tests (excluding clinical diagnostic laboratory tests);
- X-ray, radium, and radioactive isotope therapy, including materials and services of technicians;
- Surgical dressings applied during an encounter at the hospital and splints, casts, and other devices used for reduction of fractures and dislocations (splints and casts, etc., include dental splints);
- Implantable prosthetic devices;
- Hepatitis B vaccine and its administration, and certain preventive screening services (pelvic exams, screening sigmoidoscopies, screening colonoscopies, bone mass measurements, and prostate screening.)
- Bone Mass measurements;
- Prostate screening;
- Immunosuppressive drugs;
- Oral anti-cancer drugs;
- Oral drug prescribed for use as an acute anti-emetic used as part of an anti-cancer chemotherapeutic regimen; and
- Epoetin Alfa (EPO)

NOTE: Payment for some of these services is packaged into the payment rate of other separately payable services.

Inpatient Part B services paid under other payment methods include:

- Clinical diagnostic laboratory tests, prosthetic devices other than implantable ones and other than dental which replace all or part of an internal body organ (including contiguous tissue), or all or part of the function of a permanently inoperative or malfunctioning internal body organ, including replacement or repairs of such devices;
- Leg, arm, back and neck braces; trusses and artificial legs; arms and eyes including adjustments, repairs, and replacements required because of breakage, wear, loss, or a change in the patient's physical condition; take home surgi-

cal dressings; outpatient physical therapy; outpatient occupational therapy; and outpatient speech-language pathology services;
- Ambulance services;
- Screening pap smears, screening colorectal tests, and screening mammography;
- Influenza virus vaccine and its administration, pneumococcal vaccine and its administration;
- Diabetes self-management;
- Hemophilia clotting factors for hemophilia patients competent to use these factors without supervision).

See Chapter 6 of the Medicare Benefit Policy Manual for a discussion of the circumstances under which the above services may be covered as Part B Inpatient services.

240.1 – Editing Of Hospital Part B Inpatient Services

(Rev. 351, Issued: 10-29-04, Effective: 01-01-05, Implementation: 01-03-05)

Medicare pays under Part B for physician services and for non-physician medical and other health services listed in Section 240 above when furnished by a participating hospital to an inpatient of the hospital when patients are not eligible or entitled to Part A benefits or the patient has exhausted their Part A benefits.

The SSM shall edit to prevent payment on Type of Bill 12x for claims containing the revenue codes listed in the table below.

When denying lines containing the above revenue codes on TOB 12x, the FI shall use MSN message 21.21– This service was denied because Medicare only covers this service under certain circumstances.

The FIs shall place reason code M28 on the remittance advice when denying services on the specified revenue codes.

240.2 – Indian Health Service/Tribal Hospital Inpatient Social Admits

(Rev. 1446, Issued: 02-08-08; Effective: 07-01-08; Implementation: 07-07-08)

There may be situations when an American Indian/Alaskan Native (AI/AN) beneficiary is admitted to an IHS/Tribal facility for social reasons. These social admissions are for patient and family convenience and are not billable to Medicare. There are also occasions where IHS/Tribal hospitals elect to admit patients prior to a scheduled day of surgery, or place a patient in a room after an inpatient discharge. These services are also considered to be social admissions as well.

For patients in a social admission status requiring out patient services at another facility, Medicare disallows payment for inpatient Part B ancillary services. Type of Bill (TOB) 12X during a social admission stay when there is another bill from a different facility for an outpatient service, TOB 13X or 72X. The Common Working File (CWF) returns an A/B crossover edit and creates an unsolicited response (IUR) in this situation.

The CWF also creates an IUR when a line item date of service on TOB 12X is equal to or one day following the discharge date on TOB 11X for the same provider.

010x	011x	012x	013x	014x	015x	016x	017x
018x	019x	020x	021x	022x	023x	0250	0251
0252	0253	0256	0257	0258	0259	0261	0269
0270	0273	0277	0279	029x	0339	036x	0370
0374	041x	045x	0472	0479	049x	050x	051x
052x	053x	0541	0542	0543	0544	0546	0547
0548	0549	055x	057x	058x	059x	060x	0630
0631	0632	0633	0637	064x	065x	066x	067x
068x	072x	0762	078x	079x	093x	0940	0941
0943	0944	0945	0946	0947	0949	095x	0960
0961	0962	0969	097x	098x	099x	100x	210x
310x							

The CWF bypasses both of these edits when the beneficiary is not entitled to Medicare Part A at the time the services on TOB 12X are rendered.

250 – Special Rules for Critical Access Hospital Outpatient Billing

(Rev. 1111, Issued: 11-09-06, Effective: 04-01-07, Implementation: 04-02-07)

For cost reporting periods beginning before October 1, 2000, a CAH will be paid for outpatient services under the method in §250.1. The BIPA legislation on payment for professional services at 115 percent of what would otherwise be paid under the fee schedule is effective for services furnished on or after July 1, 2001. This provision was implemented with respect to cost reporting periods starting on or after October 1, 2001.

For cost reporting period beginning on or after October 1, 2001, the CAH will be paid under the method in item 1 below unless it elects to be paid under the method in §250.1.

If a CAH elects payment under the elective method (cost-based facility payment plus fee schedule for professional services) for a cost reporting period, that election is effective for the entire cost reporting period to which it applies. If the CAH wishes to make a new election or change a previous election, that election should be made in writing, made on an annual basis and delivered to the appropriate FI, at least 30 days in advance of the beginning of the affected cost reporting period.

All outpatient CAH services, other than pneumococcal pneumonia vaccines, influenza vaccines, administration of the vaccines, screening mammograms, and clinical diagnostic laboratory tests are subject to Part B deductible and coinsurance. Regardless of the payment method applicable for a period, payment for outpatient CAH services is not subject to the following payment principles:

- Lesser of cost or charges,
- Reasonable compensation equivalent (RCE) limits,
- Any type of reduction to operating or capital costs under 42 CFR 413.124 or 413.30(j)(7), or

- Blended payment rates for ASC-type, radiology, and other diagnostic services.

See §250.4 below regarding payment for screening mammography services.

250.1—Standard Method - Cost-Based Facility Services, With Billing of Carrier for Professional Services

(Rev. 976, Issued: 06-09-06, Effective: 10-01-06, Implementation: 10-02-06)

Effective for cost reporting periods beginning on or after January 1, 2004, payment for outpatient CAH services under this method will be made for the lesser of: 1) 80 percent of 101 percent of the reasonable cost of the CAH in furnishing those services, or 2) 101 percent of the reasonable cost of the CAH in furnishing those services, less applicable Part B deductible and coinsurance amounts.

Payment for professional medical services furnished in a CAH to CAH outpatients is made by the carrier on a fee schedule, charge, or other fee basis, as would apply if the services had been furnished in a hospital outpatient department. For purposes of CAH payment, professional medical services are defined as services provided by a physician or other practitioner, e.g., a physician assistant that could be billed directly to a carrier under Part B of Medicare or a nurse practitioner that could be billed directly to a carrier under Part B of Medicare.

In general, payment for professional medical services, under the cost-based CAH payment plus professional services billed to the carrier method should be made on the same basis as would apply if the services had been furnished in the outpatient department of a hospital.

Bill type 85X is used for all outpatient services including services approved as ASC services. Non-patient laboratory specimens (those not meeting the criteria for reasonable cost payment in §250.6) will be billed on a 14X type of bill.

(See Section 260.6 – Clinical Diagnostic Laboratory Tests Furnished by CAHs.)

100-04 Chapter 8

60.4.2—Epoetin Alfa (EPO) Supplier Billing Requirements (Method II) on the Form CMS-1500 and Electronic Equivalent

(Rev 118, 03-05-04)

A. Claims with dates of service prior to January 1, 2004:

For claims with dates of service prior to January 1, 2004, the correct EPO code to use is the one that indicates the patient's most recent hematocrit (HCT) (rounded to the nearest whole percent) or hemoglobin (Hgb) (rounded to the nearest g/dl) prior to the date of service of the EPO. For example, if the patient's most recent hematocrit was 20.5 percent, bill Q9921; if it was 28.4 percent, bill Q9928.

To convert actual hemoglobin to corresponding hematocrit for Q code reporting, multiply the Hgb value by 3 and round to the nearest whole number. For example, if Hgb = 8.4, report as Q9925 (8.4 × 3 = 25.2, rounded down to 25).

One unit of service of EPO is reported for each 1000 units dispensed. For example if 20,000 units are dispensed, bill 20 units. If the dose dispensed is not an even multiple of 1,000, rounded down for 1–499 units (e.g. 20,400 units dispensed = 20 units billed), round up for 500–999 units (e.g. 20,500 units dispensed = 21 units billed).

Q9920	Injection of EPO, per 1,000 units, at patient HCT of 20 or less
Q9921	Injection of EPO, per 1,000 units, at patient HCT of 21
Q9922	Injection of EPO, per 1,000 units, at patient HCT of 22
Q9923	Injection of EPO, per 1,000 units, at patient HCT of 23
Q9924	Injection of EPO, per 1,000 units, at patient HCT of 24
Q9925	Injection of EPO, per 1,000 units, at patient HCT of 25
Q9926	Injection of EPO, per 1,000 units, at patient HCT of 26
Q9927	Injection of EPO, per 1,000 units, at patient HCT of 27
Q9928	Injection of EPO, per 1,000 units, at patient HCT of 28
Q9929	Injection of EPO, per 1,000 units, at patient HCT of 29
Q9930	Injection of EPO, per 1,000 units, at patient HCT of 30
Q9931	Injection of EPO, per 1,000 units, at patient HCT of 31
Q9932	Injection of EPO, per 1,000 units, at patient HCT of 32
Q9933	Injection of EPO, per 1,000 units, at patient HCT of 33
Q9934	Injection of EPO, per 1,000 units, at patient HCT of 34
Q9935	Injection of EPO, per 1,000 units, at patient HCT of 35
Q9936	Injection of EPO, per 1,000 units, at patient HCT of 36
Q9937	Injection of EPO, per 1,000 units, at patient HCT of 37
Q9938	Injection of EPO, per 1,000 units, at patient HCT of 38
Q9939	Injection of EPO, per 1,000 units, at patient HCT of 39
Q9940	Injection of EPO, per 1,000 units, at patient HCT of 40 or above.

B. Claims with Dates of Service January 1, 2004 and after

The above codes were replaced effective January 1, 2004 by Q4055. This Q code is for the injection of EPO furnished to ESRD Beneficiaries on Dialysis. The new code does not include the hematocrit. See §60.7.

Q4055—Injection, Epoetin alfa, 1,000 units (for ESRD on Dialysis).

The DMERC shall return to provider (RTP) assigned claims for EPO, Q4055, that do not contain a HCT value. For unassigned claims, the DMERC shall deny claims for EPO, Q4055 that do not contain a HCT value.

DMERCs must use the following messages when payment for the injection (Q4055) does not meet the coverage criteria and is denied:

MSN Message 6.5—English: Medicare cannot pay for this injection because one or more requirements for coverage were not met

MSN Message 6.5—Spanish: Medicare no puede pagar por esta inyeccion porque uno o mas requisitos para la cubierta no fueron cumplidos. (MSN Message 6.5 in Spanish).

Adjustment Reason Code B:5 Payment adjusted because coverage/program guidelines were not met or were exceeded.

The DMERCs shall use the following messages when returning as unprocessable assigned claims without a HCT value:

ANSI Reason Code 16—Claim/service lacks information, which is needed for adjudication.

Additional information is supplied using remittance advice remarks codes whenever appropriate.

Remark Code M58—Missing/incomplete/invalid claim information. Resubmit claim after corrections.

Deductibles and coinsurance apply.

60.4.2.1—Other Information Required on the Form CMS-1500

(Rev 118, 03-05-04)

The following information is required for EPO. Incomplete assigned claims are returned to providers for completion. Incomplete unassigned claims are rejected. The rejection will be due to a lack of a HCT value. Note that when a claim is submitted on paper Form CMS-1500, these items are submitted on a separate document. It is not necessary to enter them into the claims processing system. This information is used in utilization review.

A. **Diagnoses**—The diagnoses must be submitted according to ICD-9-CM and correlated to the procedure. This information is in Item 21, of the Form CMS-1500.

B. **Hematocrit (HCT)/Hemoglobin (Hgb)**—There are special HCPCS codes for reporting the injection of EPO for claims with dates of service prior to January 1, 2004. These allow the simultaneous reporting of the patient's latest HCT or Hgb reading before administration of EPO.

The physician and/or staff are instructed to enter a separate line item for injections of EPO at different HCT/Hgb levels. The Q code for each line items is entered in Item 24D.

1. Code Q9920—Injection of EPO, per 1,000 units, at patient HCT of 20 or less/Hgb of 6.8 or less.
2. Codes Q9921 through Q9939—Injection of EPO, per 1,000 units, at patient HCT of 21 to 39/Hgb of 6.9 to 13.1. For HCT levels of 21 or more, up to a HCT of 39/Hgb of 6.9 to 13.1, a Q code that includes the actual HCT levels is used. To convert actual Hgb to corresponding HCT values for Q code reporting, multiply the Hgb value by 3 and round to the nearest whole number.

Use the whole number to determine the appropriate Q code.

EXAMPLES: If the patient's HCT is 25/Hgb is 8.2-8.4, Q9925 must be entered on the claim. If the patient's HCT is 39/Hgb is 12.9-13.1, Q9939 is entered.

3. Code Q9940—Injection of EPO, per 1,000 units at patient HCT of 40 or above.

A single line item may include multiple doses of EPO administered while the patient's HCT level remained the same.

Codes Q9920-Q9940 will no longer be recognized by the system if submitted after March 31, 2004. If claims for dates of service prior to January 1, 2004 are submitted after March 31, 2004, then code Q4055 must be used.

C. Units Administered—The standard unit of EPO is 1,000. The number of 1,000 units administered per line item is included on the claim. The physician's office enters 1 in the units field for each multiple of 1,000 units. For example, if 12,000 units are administered, 12 is entered. This information is shown in Item 24G (Days/Units) on Form CMS-1500.

In some cases, the dosage for a single line item does not total an even multiple of 1,000. If this occurs, the physician's office rounds down supplemental dosages of 0 to 499 units to the prior 1,000 units. Supplemental dosages of 500 to 999 are rounded up to the next 1,000 units.

EXAMPLES

A patient's HCT reading on August 6 was 22/Hgb was 7.3. The patient received 5,000 units of EPO on August 7, August 9, and August 11, for a total of 15,000 units. The first line of Item 24 of Form CMS-1500 shows:

Dates of Service	Procedure Code	Days or Units
8/7–8/11	Q9922	15

On September 13, the patient's HCT reading increased to 27/Hgb increased to 9. The patient received 5,100 units of EPO on September 13, September 15, and September 17, for a total of 15,300 units. Since less than 15,500 units were given, the figure is rounded down to 15,000. This line on the claim form shows:

Dates of Service	Procedure Code	Days or Units
9/13–9/17	Q9927	15

On October 16, the HCT level increased to 33/Hgb increased to 11. The patient received doses of 4,850 units on October 16, October 18, and October 20 for a total of 14,550 units. Since more than 14,500 units were administered, the figure is rounded up to 15,000. Form CMS-1500 shows:

Dates of Service	Procedure Code	Days or Units
10/16–10/20	Q9933	15

NOTE: Creatinine and weight identified below are required on EPO claims as applicable.

D. Date of the Patient's most recent HCT or Hgb.
E. Most recent HCT or Hgb level—(prior to initiation of EPO therapy).
F. Date of most recent HCT or Hgb level—(prior to initiation of EPO therapy).
G. Patient's most recent serum creatinine—(within the last month, prior to initiation of EPO therapy).
H. Date of most recent serum creatinine—(prior to initiation of EPO therapy).
I. Patient's weight in kilograms
J. Patient's starting dose per kilogram—(The usual starting dose is 50-100 units per kilogram.)

60.4.2.2—Completion of Subsequent Form CMS-1500 Claims for EPO

(Rev 118, 03-05-04)

Subsequent claims are completed as initial claims in §60.4.2, except the following fields:

A. Diagnoses.
B. Hematocrit or Hemoglobin—For dates of service prior to January 1, 2004, this is indicated by the appropriate Q code. For dates of service January 1, 2004, and after, suppliers must indicate the beneficiary's hematocrit on the claim. (See 60.4.2.) Claims include an EJ modifier to the Q code. This allows the contractor to identify subsequent claims, which do not require as much information as initial claims and prevent unnecessary development.

Number of Units Administered—Subsequent claims may be submitted electronically.

90.1—DMERC Denials for Beneficiary Submitted Claims Under Method II

(Rev. 1, 10-01-03)

A3-3170.6, A3-3644.3, A3-3644.3.A - E, HO-238.2.C, HO-238.3, HO-238.3.A, B3-2231.3.A AND B, B3-2231, B3-4270.1, PRM-1-2709.2.A

Under Method II, beneficiaries may not submit any claims and cannot receive payment for any benefits for home dialysis equipment and supplies. DMERCs must deny unassigned and beneficiary submitted claims with the following MSN messages.

MSN # 16.6: "This item or service cannot be paid unless the provider accepts assignment."

Spanish: "Este articulo o servicio no se pagará a menos de que el proveedor acepte asignación."

MSN # 16.7: "Your provider must complete and submit your claim."

Spanish: "Su proveedor debe completar y someter su reclamación."

MSN # 16.36: "If you have already paid it, you are entitled to a refund from this provider."

Spanish: "Si usted ya lo ha pagado, tiene derecho a un reembolso de su proveedor."

100-04 Chapter 12

30.4—Cardiovascular System (Codes 92950-93799)

(Rev. 979, Issued: 06-09-06, Effective: 07-10-06, Implementation: 07-10-06)

A. Echocardiography Contrast Agents

Effective October 1, 2000, physicians may separately bill for contrast agents used in echocardiography. Physicians should use HCPCS Code A9700 (Supply of Injectable Contrast Material for Use in Echocardiography, per study). The type of service code is 9. This code will be carrier-priced.

B. Electronic Analyses of Implantable Cardioverter-defibrillators and Pacemakers

The CPT codes 93731, 93734, 93741 and 93743 are used to report electronic analyses of single or dual chamber pacemakers and single or dual chamber implantable cardioverter-defibrillators. In the office, a physician uses a device called a programmer to obtain information about the status and performance of the device and to evaluate the patient's cardiac rhythm and response to the implanted device.

Advances in information technology now enable physicians to evaluate patients with implanted cardiac devices without requiring the patient to be present in the physician's office. Using a manufacturer's specific monitor/transmitter, a patient can send complete device data and specific cardiac data to a distant receiving station or secure Internet server. The electronic analysis of cardiac device data that is remotely obtained provides immediate and long-term data on the device and clinical data on the patient's cardiac functioning equivalent to that obtained during an in-office evaluation. Physicians should report the electronic analysis of an implanted cardiac device using remotely obtained data as described above with CPT code 93731, 93734, 93741 or 93743, depending on the type of cardiac device implanted in the patient.

30.6—Evaluation and Management Service Codes - General (Codes 99201 - 99499)

(Rev. 178, 05-14-04)

B3-15501-15501.1

30.6.1—Selection of Level of Evaluation and Management Service

(Rev. 178, 05-14-04)

A. Use of CPT Codes

Advise physicians to use CPT codes (level 1 of HCPCS) to code physician services, including evaluation and management services. Medicare will pay for E/M services for specific non-physician practitioners (i.e., nurse practitioner (NP), clinical nurse specialist (CNS) and certified nurse midwife (CNM)) whose Medicare benefit permits them to bill these services. A physician assistant (PA) may also provide a physician service, however, the physician collaboration and general supervision rules as well as all billing rules apply to all the above non-physician practitioners. The service provided must be medically necessary and the service must be within the scope of practice for a nonphysician practitioner in the State in which he/she practices. Do not pay for CPT evaluation and management codes billed by physical therapists in independent practice or by occupational therapists in independent practice.

Medical necessity of a service is the overarching criterion for payment in addition to the individual requirements of a CPT code. It would not be medically necessary or appropriate to bill a higher level of evaluation and management service when a lower level of service is warranted. The volume of documentation should not be the primary influence upon which a specific level of service is billed. Documentation should support the level of service reported. The service should be documented during, or as soon as practicable after it is provided in order to maintain an accurate medical record.

B. Selection of Level Of Evaluation and Management Service

Instruct physicians to select the code for the service based upon the content of the service. The duration of the visit is an ancillary factor and does not control the level of the service to be billed unless more than 50 percent of the face-to-face time (for non-inpatient services) or more than 50 percent of the floor time (for inpatient services) is spent providing counseling or coordination of care as described in subsection C.

Any physician or non-physician practitioner (NPP) authorized to bill Medicare services will be paid by the carrier at the appropriate physician fee schedule amount based on the rendering UPIN/PIN. "Incident to" Medicare Part B payment policy is applicable for office visits when the requirements for "incident to" are met (refer to sections 60.1, 60.2, and 60.3, chapter 15 in IOM 100-02).

SPLIT/SHARED E/M SERVICE

Office/Clinic Setting

In the office/clinic setting when the physician performs the E/M service the service must be reported using the physician's UPIN/PIN. When an E/M service is a shared/split encounter between a physician and a non-physician practitioner (NP, PA, CNS or CNM), the service is considered to have been performed "incident to" if the requirements for "incident to" are met and the patient is an established patient. If "incident to" requirements are not met for the shared/split E/M service, the service must be billed under the NPP's UPIN/PIN, and payment will be made at the appropriate physician fee schedule payment.

Hospital Inpatient/Outpatient/Emergency Department Setting

When a hospital inpatient/hospital outpatient or emergency department E/M is shared between a physician and an NPP from the same group practice and the physician provides any face-to-face portion of the E/M encounter with the patient, the service may be billed under either the physician's or the NPP's UPIN/PIN number. However, if there was no face-to-face encounter between the patient and the physician (e.g., even if the physician participated in the service by only reviewing the patient's medical record) then the service may only be billed under the NPP's UPIN/PIN. Payment will be made at the appropriate physician fee schedule rate based on the UPIN/PIN entered on the claim.

EXAMPLES OF SHARED VISITS

1. If the NPP sees a hospital inpatient in the morning and the physician follows with a later face-to-face visit with the patient on the same day, the physician or the NPP may report the service.
2. In an office setting the NPP performs a portion of an E/M encounter and the physician completes the E/M service. If the "incident to" requirements are met, the physician reports the service. If the "incident to" requirements are not met, the service must be reported using the NPP's UPIN/PIN.

In the rare circumstance when a physician (or NPP) provides a service that does not reflect a CPT code description, the service must be reported as an unlisted service with CPT code 99499. A description of the service provided must accompany the claim. The carrier has the discretion to value the service when the service does not meet the full terms of a CPT code description (e.g., only a history is performed). The carrier also determines the payment based on the applicable percentage of the physician fee schedule depending on whether the claim is paid at the physician rate or the non-physician practitioner rate. CPT modifier -52 (reduced services) must not be used with an evaluation and management service. Medicare does not recognize modifier -52 for this purpose.

C. Selection Of Level Of Evaluation and Management Service Based On Duration Of Coordination Of Care and/or Counseling

Advise physicians that when counseling and/or coordination of care dominates (more than 50 percent) the face-to-face physician/patient encounter or the floor time (in the case of inpatient services), time is the key or controlling factor in selecting the level of service. In general, to bill an E/M code, the physician must complete at least 2 out of 3 criteria applicable to the type/level of service provided. However, the physician may document time spent with the patient in conjunction with the medical decision-making involved and a description of the coordination of care or counseling provided. Documentation must be in sufficient detail to support the claim.

EXAMPLE: A cancer patient has had all preliminary studies completed and a medical decision to implement chemotherapy. At an office visit the physician discusses the treatment options and subsequent lifestyle effects of treatment the patient may encounter or is experiencing. The physician need not complete a history and physical examination in order to select the level of service. The time spent in counseling/coordination of care and medical decision-making will determine the level of service billed.

The code selection is based on the total time of the face-to-face encounter or floor time, not just the counseling time. The medical record must be documented in sufficient detail to justify the selection of the specific code if time is the basis for selection of the code.

In the office and other outpatient setting, counseling and/or coordination of care must be provided in the presence of the patient if the time spent providing those services is used to determine the level of service reported. Face-to-face time refers to the time with the physician only. Counseling by other staff is not considered to be part of the face-to-face physi-

cian/patient encounter time. Therefore, the time spent by the other staff is not considered in selecting the appropriate level of service. The code used depends upon the physician service provided.

In an inpatient setting, the counseling and/or coordination of care must be provided at the bedside or on the patient's hospital floor or unit that is associated with an individual patient. Time spent counseling the patient or coordinating the patient's care after the patient has left the office or the physician has left the patient's floor or begun to care for another patient on the floor is not considered when selecting the level of service to be reported.

The duration of counseling or coordination of care that is provided face-to-face or on the floor may be estimated but that estimate, along with the total duration of the visit, must be recorded when time is used for the selection of the level of a service that involves predominantly coordination of care or counseling.

D. Use of Highest Levels of Evaluation and Management Codes

Carriers must advise physicians that to bill the highest levels of visit and consultation codes, the services furnished must meet the definition of the code (e.g., to bill a Level 5 new patient visit, the history must meet CPT's definition of a comprehensive history).

The comprehensive history must include a review of all the systems and a complete past (medical and surgical) family and social history obtained at that visit. In the case of an established patient, it is acceptable for a physician to review the existing record and update it to reflect only changes in the patient's medical, family, and social history from the last encounter, but the physician must review the entire history for it to be considered a comprehensive history.

The comprehensive examination may be a complete single system exam such as cardiac, respiratory, psychiatric, or a complete multi-system examination.

30.6.1.1 – Initial Preventive Physical Examination (HCPCS Codes G0344, G0366, G0367 and G0368)

(Rev. 417, Issued: 12-22-04, Effective: 01-01-05, Implementation: 01-03-05)

A. Definition

The initial preventive physical examination (IPPE), or "Welcome to Medicare Visit", is a preventive evaluation and management service (E/M) that includes: (1) review of the individual's medical and social history with attention to modifiable risk factors for disease detection, (2) review of the individual's potential (risk factors) for depression or other mood disorders, (3) review of the individual's functional ability and level of safety; (4) a physical examination to include measurement of the individual's height, weight, blood pressure, a visual acuity screen, and other factors as deemed appropriate by the examining physician or qualified nonphysician practitioner (NPP), (5) performance and interpretation of an electrocardiogram (EKG); (6) education, counseling, and referral, as deemed appropriate, based on the results of the review and evaluation services described in the previous 5 elements, and (7) education, counseling, and referral including a brief written plan (e.g., a checklist or alternative) provided to the individual for obtaining the appropriate screening and other preventive services, which are separately covered under Medicare Part B benefits. (For billing requirements, refer to Pub. 100-04, Chapter 18, Section 80.)

B. Who May Perform

The IPPE may be performed by a doctor of medicine or osteopathy as defined in section 1861 (r)(1) of the Social Security Act or by a qualified NPP (nurse practitioner, physician assistant and clinical nurse specialist). The carrier will pay the appropriate physician fee schedule amount based on the rendering UPIN/PIN.

C. Eligibility

Medicare will pay for one IPPE per beneficiary per lifetime. A beneficiary is eligible when he first enrolls in Medicare Part B on or after January 1, 2005, and receives the IPPE benefit within the first 6 months of the effective date of the initial Part B coverage period.

D. The EKG Component

If the physician or qualified NPP is not able to perform both the examination and the screening EKG, an arrangement may be made to ensure that another physician or entity performs the screening EKG and reports the EKG separately using the appropriate HCPCS G code. The primary physician or qualified NPP shall document the results of the screening EKG into the beneficiary's medical record to complete and bill for the IPPE benefit. **NOTE:** Both components of the IPPE (the examination and the screening EKG) must be performed before the claims can be submitted by the physician, qualified NPP and/or entity.

E. Codes Used to Bill the IPPE

The physician or qualified NPP shall bill HCPCS code G0344 for the physical examination performed face-to-face and HCPCS code G0366 for performing a screening EKG that includes both the interpretation and report. If the primary physician or qualified NPP performs only the examination, he/she shall bill HCPCS code G0344 only. The physician or entity that performs the screening EKG that includes both the interpretation and report shall bill HCPCS code G0366. The physician or entity that performs the screening EKG tracing only (without interpretation and report) shall bill HCPCS code G0367. The physician or entity that performs the interpretation and report only (without the EKG tracing) shall bill HCPCS code G0368. Medicare will pay for a screening EKG only as part of the IPPE. **NOTE:** For an IPPE performed during the global period of surgery refer to section 30.6.6, chapter 12, Pub 100-04 for reporting instructions.

F. Documentation

The physician and qualified NPP shall use the appropriate screening tools typically used in routine physician practice. As for all E/M services, the 1995 and 1997 E/M documentation guidelines (http://www.cms.hhs.gov/medlearn/emdoc. asp) should be followed for recording the appropriate clinical information in the beneficiary's medical record. All referrals and a written medical plan must be included in this documentation.

G. Reporting A Medically Necessary E/M at Same IPPE Visit

When the physician or qualified NPP provide a medically necessary E/M service in addition to the IPPE, CPT codes 99201 – 99215 may be used depending on the clinical appropriateness of the circumstances. CPT Modifier –25 shall be appended to the medically necessary E/M service identifying this service as a separately identifiable service from the IPPE code G0344 reported. **NOTE:** Some of the components of a medically necessary E/M service (e.g., a portion of history or physical exam portion) may have been part of the IPPE and should not be included when determining the most appropriate level of E/M service to be billed for the medically necessary E/M service.

30.6.2—Billing for Medically Necessary Visit on Same Occasion as Preventive Medicine Service

(Rev. 1, 10-01-03)

See Chapter 18 for payment for covered preventive services.

When a physician furnishes a Medicare beneficiary a covered visit at the same place and on the same occasion as a noncovered preventive medicine service (CPT codes 99381- 99397), consider the covered visit to be provided in lieu of a part of the preventive medicine service of equal value to the visit. A preventive medicine service (CPT codes 99381-99397) is a noncovered service. The physician may charge the beneficiary, as a charge for the noncovered remainder of the service, the amount by which the physician's current established charge for the preventive medicine service exceeds his/her current established charge for the covered visit. Pay for the covered visit based on the lesser of the fee schedule amount or the physician's actual charge for the visit. The physician is not required to give the beneficiary written advance notice of noncoverage of the part of the visit that constitutes a routine preventive visit. However, the physician is responsible for notifying the patient in advance of his/her liability for the charges for services that are not medically necessary to treat the illness or injury.

There could be covered and noncovered procedures performed during this encounter (e.g., screening x-ray, EKG, lab tests.). These are considered individually. Those procedures which are for screening for asymptomatic conditions are considered noncovered and, therefore, no payment is made. Those procedures ordered to diagnose or monitor a symptom, medical condition, or treatment are evaluated for medical necessity and, if covered, are paid.

30.6.3—Payment for Immunosuppressive Therapy Management

(Rev. 1, 10-01-03)

B3-4820-4824

Physicians bill for management of immunosuppressive therapy using the office or subsequent hospital visit codes that describe the services furnished. If the physician who is managing the immunotherapy is also the transplant surgeon, he or she bills these visits with modifier "-24" indicating that the visit during the global period is not related to the original procedure if the physician also performed the transplant surgery and submits documentation that shows that the visit is for immunosuppressive therapy.

30.6.4—Evaluation and Management (E/M) Services Furnished Incident to Physician's Service by Nonphysician Practitioners

(Rev. 1, 10-01-03)

When evaluation and management services are furnished incident to a physician's service by a nonphysician practitioner, the physician may bill the CPT code that describes the evaluation and management service furnished.

When evaluation and management services are furnished incident to a physician's service by a nonphysician employee of the physician, not as part of a physician service, the physician bills code 99211 for the service.

A physician is not precluded from billing under the "incident to" provision for services provided by employees whose services cannot be paid for directly under the Medicare program. Employees of the physician may provide services incident to the physician's service, but the physician alone is permitted to bill Medicare.

Services provided by employees as "incident to" are covered when they meet all the requirements for incident to and are medically necessary for the individual needs of the patient.

30.6.5—Physicians in Group Practice

(Rev. 1, 10-01-03)

Physicians in the same group practice who are in the same specialty must bill and be paid as though they were a single physician. If more than one evaluation and management (face-to-face) service is provided on the same day to the same patient by the same physician or more than one physician in the same specialty in the same group, only one evaluation and management service may be reported unless the evaluation and management services are for unrelated problems. Instead of billing separately, the physicians should select a level of service representative of the combined visits and submit the appropriate code for that level.

Physicians in the same group practice but who are in different specialties may bill and be paid without regard to their membership in the same group.

30.6.6—Payment for Evaluation and Management Services Provided During Global Period of Surgery

(Rev. 954, Issued: 05-19-06, Effective: 06-01-06, Implementation: 08-20-06)

A. CPT Modifier "-24" - Unrelated Evaluation and Management Service by Same Physician During Postoperative Period

Carriers pay for an evaluation and management service other than inpatient hospital care before discharge from the hospital following surgery (CPT codes 99221-99238) if it was provided during the postoperative period of a surgical procedure, furnished by the same physician who performed the procedure, billed with CPT modifier "-24," and accompanied by documentation that supports that the service is not related to the postoperative care of the procedure. They do not pay for inpatient hospital care that is furnished during the hospital stay in which the surgery occurred unless the doctor is also treating another medical condition that is unrelated to the surgery. All care provided during the inpatient stay in which the surgery occurred is compensated through the global surgical payment.

B. CPT Modifier "-25" - Significant Evaluation and Management Service by Same Physician on Date of Global Procedure

Medicare requires that Current Procedural Terminology (CPT) modifier -25 should only be used on claims for evaluation and management (E/M) services, and only when these services are provided by the same physician (or same qualified nonphysician practitioner) to the same patient on the same day as another procedure or other service. Carriers pay for an E/M service provided on the day of a procedure with a global fee period if the physician indicates that the service is for a significant, separately identifiable E/M service that is above and beyond the usual pre- and post-operative work of the procedure. Different diagnoses are not required for reporting the E/M service on the same date as the procedure or other service. Modifier -25 is added to the E/M code on the claim.

Both the medically necessary E/M service and the procedure must be appropriately and sufficiently documented by the physician or qualified nonphysician practitioner in the patient's medical record to support the claim for these services, even though the documentation is not required to be submitted with the claim.

If the physician bills the service with the CPT modifier "-25," carriers pay for the service in addition to the global fee without any other requirement for documentation unless one of the following conditions is met:

- When inpatient dialysis services are billed (CPT codes 90935, 90945, 90947, and 93937), the physician must document that the service was unrelated to the dialysis and could not be performed during the dialysis procedure;
- When preoperative critical care codes are being billed on the date of the procedure, the diagnosis must support that the service is unrelated to the performance of the procedure; or
- When a carrier has conducted a specific medical review process and determined, after reviewing the data, that an individual or a group has high use of modifier "-25" compared to other physicians, has done a case-by-case review of the records to verify that the use of modifier was inappropriate, and has educated the individual or group, the carrier may impose prepayment screens or documentation requirements for that provider or group. When a carrier has completed a review and determined that a high usage rate of modifier "-57," the carrier must complete a case-by-case review of the records. Based upon this review, the carrier will educate providers regarding the appropriate use of modifier "-57." If high usage rates continue, the carrier may impose prepayment screens or documentation requirements for that provider or group.

Carriers may not permit the use of CPT modifier "-25" to generate payment for multiple evaluation and management services on the same day by the same physician, notwithstanding the CPT definition of the modifier.

C. CPT Modifier "-57" - Decision for Surgery Made Within Global Surgical Period

Carriers pay for an evaluation and management service on the day of or on the day before a procedure with a 90-day global surgical period if the physician uses CPT modifier "-57" to indicate that the service resulted in the decision to perform the procedure. Carriers may no pay for an evaluation and management service billed with the CPT modifier "-57" if it was provided on the day of or the day before a procedure with a 0 or 10-day global surgical period.

30.6.7—Payment for Office or Other Outpatient Evaluation and Management (E/M) Visits (Codes 99201 - 99215)

(Rev. 731, Issued: 10-28-05, Effective: 01-01-04 Chemotherapy and Non-Chemotherapy drug infusion codes/01-01-05 Therapeutic and Diagnostic injection codes, Implementation: 01-03-06)

A. Definition of New Patient for Selection of E/M Visit Code

Interpret the phrase "new patient" to mean a patient who has not received any professional services, i.e., E/M service or other face-to-face service (e.g., surgical procedure) from the physician or physician group practice (same physician specialty) within the previous 3 years. For example, if a professional component of a previous procedure is billed in a 3 year time period, e.g., a lab interpretation is billed and no E/M service or other face-to-face service with the patient is performed, then this patient remains a new patient for the initial visit. An interpretation of a diagnostic test, reading an x-ray or EKG etc., in the absence of an E/M service or other face-to-face service with the patient does not affect the designation of a new patient.

B. Office/Outpatient E/M Visits Provided on Same Day for Unrelated Problems

As for all other E/M services except where specifically noted, carriers may not pay two E/M office visits billed by a physician (or physician of the same specialty from the same group practice) for the same beneficiary on the same day unless the physician documents that the visits were for unrelated problems in the office or outpatient setting which could not be provided during the same encounter (e.g., office visit for blood pressure medication evaluation, followed five hours later by a visit for evaluation of leg pain following an accident).

C. Office/Outpatient or Emergency Department E/M Visit on Day of Admission to Nursing Facility

Carriers may not pay a physician for an emergency department visit or an office visit and a comprehensive nursing facility assessment on the same day. Bundle E/M visits on the same date provided in sites other than the nursing facility into the initial nursing facility care code when performed on the same date as the nursing facility admission by the same physician.

D. Drug Administration Services and E/M Visits Billed on Same Day of Service

Carriers must advise physicians that CPT code 99211 cannot be paid if it is billed with a drug administration service such as a chemotherapy or nonchemotherapy drug infusion code (effective January 1, 2004). This drug administration policy was expanded in the Physician Fee Schedule Final Rule, November 15, 2004, to also include a therapeutic or diagnostic injection code (effective January 1, 2005). Therefore, when a medically necessary, significant and separately identifiable E/M service (which meets a higher complexity

level than CPT code 99211) is performed, in addition to one of these drug administration services, the appropriate E/M CPT code should be reported with modifier -25. Documentation should support the level of E/M service billed. For an E/M service provided on the same day, a different diagnosis is not required.

30.6.8—Payment for Hospital Observation Services (Codes 99217 - 99220) and Observation or Inpatient Care Services (Including Admission and Discharge Services – (Codes 99234 – 99236))

(Rev. 1466, Issued: 02-22-08, Effective: 04-01-08, Implementation: 04-07-08)

A. Who May Bill Initial Observation Care

Contractors pay for initial observation care billed by only the physician who admitted the patient to hospital observation and was responsible for the patient during his/her stay in observation. A physician who does not have inpatient admitting privileges but who is authorized to admit a patient to observation status may bill these codes.

For a physician to bill the initial observation care codes, there must be a medical observation record for the patient which contains dated and timed physician's admitting orders regarding the care the patient is to receive while in observation, nursing notes, and progress notes prepared by the physician while the patient was in observation status. This record must be in addition to any record prepared as a result of an emergency department or outpatient clinic encounter.

Payment for an initial observation care code is for all the care rendered by the admitting physician on the date the patient was admitted to observation. All other physicians who see the patient while he or she is in observation must bill the office and other outpatient service codes or outpatient consultation codes as appropriate when they provide services to the patient.

For example, if an internist admits a patient to observation and asks an allergist for a consultation on the patient's condition, only the internist may bill the initial observation care code. The allergist must bill using the outpatient consultation code that best represents the services he or she provided. The allergist cannot bill an inpatient consultation since the patient was not a hospital inpatient.

B. Physician Billing for Observation Care Following Admission to Observation

When a patient is admitted for observation care for less than 8 hours on the same calendar date, the Initial Observation Care, from CPT code range 99218 – 99220, shall be reported by the physician. The Observation Care Discharge Service, CPT code 99217, shall not be reported for this scenario.

When a patient is admitted for observation care and then discharged on a different calendar date, the physician shall report Initial Observation Care, from CPT code range 99218 – 99220 and CPT observation care discharge CPT code 99217.

When a patient has been admitted for observation care for a minimum of 8 hours, but less than 24 hours and discharged on the same calendar date, Observation or Inpatient Care

Services (Including Admission and Discharge Services) from CPT code range 99234 – 99236, shall be reported. The observation discharge, CPT code 99217, cannot also be reported for this scenario.

C. Documentation Requirements for Billing Observation or Inpatient Care Services (Including Admission and Discharge Services (Codes 99234 – 99236))

The physician shall satisfy the E/M documentation guidelines for admission to and discharge from observation care or inpatient hospital care. In addition to meeting the documentation requirements for history, examination, and medical decision making documentation in the medical record shall include:

- Documentation stating the stay for observation care or inpatient hospital care involves 8 hours, but less than 24 hours;
- Documentation identifying the billing physician was present and personally performed the services; and
- Documentation identifying the admission and discharge notes were written by the billing physician.

In the rare circumstance when a patient is held in observation status for more than 2 calendar dates, the physician shall bill a visit furnished before the discharge date using the outpatient/office visit codes. The physician may not use the subsequent hospital care codes since the patient is not an inpatient of the hospital.

D. Admission to Inpatient Status from Observation

If the same physician who admitted a patient to observation status also admits the patient to inpatient status from observation before the end of the date on which the patient was admitted to observation, pay only an initial hospital visit for the evaluation and management services provided on that date. Medicare payment for the initial hospital visit includes all services provided to the patient on the date of admission by that physician, regardless of the site of service. The physician may not bill an initial observation care code for services on the date that he or she admits the patient to inpatient status. If the patient is admitted to inpatient status from observation subsequent to the date of admission to observation, the physician must bill an initial hospital visit for the services provided on that date. The physician may not bill the hospital observation discharge management code (code 99217) or an outpatient/office visit for the care provided in observation on the date of admission to inpatient status.

E. Hospital Observation During Global Surgical Period

The global surgical fee includes payment for hospital observation (codes 99217, 99218, 99219, and 99220, 99234, 99235, 99236) services unless the criteria for use of CPT modifiers "-24," "-25," or "-57" are met. Contractors must pay for these services in addition to the global surgical fee only if both of the following requirements are met:

- The hospital observation service meets the criteria needed to justify billing it with CPT modifiers "-24," "-25," or "-57" (decision for major surgery); and
- The hospital observation service furnished by the surgeon meets all of the criteria for the hospital observation code billed.

Examples of the decision for surgery during a hospital observation period are:

- A patient is admitted by an emergency department physician to an observation unit for observation of a head injury. A neurosurgeon is called in to do a consultation on the need for surgery while the patient is in the observation unit and decides that the patient requires surgery. The surgeon would bill an outpatient consultation with the "-57" modifier to indicate that the decision for surgery was made during the consultation. The surgeon must bill an outpatient consultation because the patient in an observation unit is not an inpatient of the hospital. Only the physician who admitted the patient to hospital observation may bill for initial observation care.
- A patient is admitted by a neurosurgeon to a hospital observation unit for observation of a head injury. During the observation period, the surgeon makes the decision for surgery. The surgeon would bill the appropriate level of hospital observation code with the "-57" modifier to indicate that the decision for surgery was made while the surgeon was providing hospital observation care.

Examples of hospital observation services during the postoperative period of a surgery are:

- A patient at the 80th day following a TURP is admitted to observation by the surgeon who performed the procedure with abdominal pain from a kidney stone. The surgeon decides that the patient does not require surgery. The surgeon would bill the observation code with CPT modifier "-24" and documentation to support that the observation services are unrelated to the surgery.
- A patient at the 80th day following a TURP is admitted to observation with abdominal pain by the surgeon who performed the procedure. While the patient is in hospital observation, the surgeon decides that the patient requires kidney surgery. The surgeon would bill the observation code with HCPCS modifier "-57" to indicate that the decision for surgery was made while the patient was in hospital observation. The subsequent surgical procedure would be reported with modifier "-79."
- A patient at the 20th day following a resection of the colon is admitted to observation for abdominal pain by the surgeon who performed the surgery. The surgeon determines that the patient requires no further colon surgery and discharges the patient. The surgeon may not bill for the observation services furnished during the global period because they were related to the previous surgery.

An example of a billable hospital observation service on the same day as a procedure is a patient is admitted to the hospital observation unit for observation of a head injury by a physician who repaired a laceration of the scalp in the emergency department. The physician would bill the observation code with a CPT modifier 25 and the procedure code.

30.6.9—Payment for Inpatient Hospital Visits - General (Codes 99221 - 99239)

(Rev. 1473; Issued: 03-07-08; Effective: 04-01-08; Implementation: 04-07-08)

A. Hospital Visit and Critical Care on Same Day

When a hospital inpatient (or emergency department, or office/outpatient) evaluation and management service (E/M) is furnished on a calendar date at which time the patient does not require critical care and the patient subsequently requires critical care, both the critical Care Services (CPT codes 99291 and 99292) and the previous E/M service may be paid on the same date of service. During critical care management of a patient those services that do not meet the level of critical care shall be reported using an inpatient hospital care service with CPT Subsequent Hospital Care using a code from CPT code range 99231 – 99233.

Both Initial Hospital Care (CPT codes 99221 – 99223) and Subsequent Hospital Care codes are "per diem" services and may be reported only once per day by the same physician or physicians of the same specialty from the same group practice.

Physicians and qualified nonphysician practitioners (NPPs) are advised to retain documentation for discretionary contractor review should claims be questioned for both hospital care and critical care claims. The retained documentation shall support claims for critical care when the same physician or physicians of the same specialty in a group practice report critical care services for the same patient on the same calendar date as other E/M services.

B. Two Hospital Visits Same Day

Contractors pay a physician for only one hospital visit per day for the same patient, whether the problems seen during the encounters are related or not. The inpatient hospital visit descriptors contain the phrase "per day" which means that the code and the payment established for the code represent all services provided on that date. The physician should select a code that reflects all services provided during the date of the service.

C. Hospital Visits Same Day But by Different Physicians

In a hospital inpatient situation involving one physician covering for another, if physician A sees the patient in the morning and physician B, who is covering for A, sees the same patient in the evening, carriers do not pay physician B for the second visit. The hospital visit descriptors include the phrase "per day" meaning care for the day.

If the physicians are each responsible for a different aspect of the patient's care, pay both visits if the physicians are in different specialties and the visits are billed with different diagnoses. There are circumstances where concurrent care may be billed by physicians of the same specialty.

D. Visits to Patients in Swing Beds

If the inpatient care is being billed by the hospital as inpatient hospital care, the hospital care codes apply. If the inpatient care is being billed by the hospital as nursing facility care, then the nursing facility codes apply.

30.6.9.1—Payment for Initial Hospital Care Services (Codes 99221 - 99223) and Observation or Inpatient Care Services (Including Admission and Discharge Services) (Codes 99234 – 99236)

(Rev. 1465, Issued: 02-22-08, Effective: 04-01-08, Implementation: 04-07-08)

(Rev. 1, 10-01-03)

A. Initial Hospital Care From Emergency Room

Contractors pay for an initial hospital care service or an initial inpatient consultation if a physician sees his/her patient in the emergency room and decides to admit the person to the hospital. They do not pay for both E/M services. Also, they do not pay for an emergency department visit by the same physician on the same date of service. When the patient is admitted to the hospital via another site of service (e.g., hospital emergency department, physician's office, nursing facility), all services provided by the physician in conjunction with that admission are considered part of the initial hospital care when performed on the **same date** as the admission.

B. Initial Hospital Care on Day Following Visit

Contractors pay both visits if a patient is seen in the office on one date and admitted to the hospital on the next date, even if fewer than 24 hours has elapsed between the visit and the admission.

C. Initial Hospital Care and Discharge on Same Day

When the patient is admitted to inpatient hospital care for less than 8 hours on the same date, then Initial Hospital Care, from CPT code range 99221 – 99223, shall be reported by the physician. The Hospital Discharge Day Management service, CPT codes 99238 or 99239, shall not be reported for this scenario.

When a patient is admitted to inpatient initial hospital care and then discharged on a different calendar date, the physician shall report an Initial Hospital Care from CPT code range 99221 – 99223 and a Hospital Discharge Day Management service, CPT code 99238 or 99239.

When a patient has been admitted to inpatient hospital care for a minimum of 8 hours but less than 24 hours and discharged on the same calendar date, Observation or Inpatient Hospital Care Services (Including Admission and Discharge Services), from CPT code range 99234 – 99236, shall be reported.

D. Documentation Requirements for Billing Observation or Inpatient Care Services (Including Admission and Discharge Services), CPT codes 99234 - 99236

The physician shall satisfy the E/M documentation guidelines for admission to and discharge from inpatient observation or hospital care. In addition to meeting the documentation requirements for history, examination and medical decision making documentation in the medical record shall include:

- Documentation stating the stay for hospital treatment or observation care status involves 8 hours but less than 24 hours;
- Documentation identifying the billing physician was present and personally performed the services; and
- Documentation identifying the admission and discharge notes were written by the billing physician.

E. Physician Services Involving Transfer From One Hospital to Another; Transfer Within Facility to Prospective Payment System (PPS) Exempt Unit of Hospital; Transfer From One Facility to Another Separate Entity Under Same Ownership and/or Part of Same Complex; or Transfer From One Department to Another Within Single Facility

Physicians may bill both the hospital discharge management code and an initial hospital care code when the discharge and admission do not occur on the same day if the transfer is between:

1. Different hospitals;
2. Different facilities under common ownership which do not have merged records; or
3. Between the acute care hospital and a PPS exempt unit within the same hospital when there are no merged records.

In all other transfer circumstances, the physician should bill only the appropriate level of subsequent hospital care for the date of transfer.

F. Initial Hospital Care Service History and Physical That Is Less Than Comprehensive

When a physician performs a visit or consultation that meets the definition of a Level 5 office visit or consultation several days prior to an admission and on the day of admission performs less than a comprehensive history and physical, he or she should report the office visit or consultation that reflects the services furnished and also report the lowest level initial hospital care code (i.e., code 99221) for the initial hospital admission. Contractors pay the office visit as billed and the Level 1 initial hospital care code.

G. Initial Hospital Care Visits by Two Different M.D.s or D.O.s When They Are Involved in Same Admission

Physicians use the initial hospital care codes (codes 99221-99223) to report the first hospital inpatient encounter with the patient when he or she is the admitting physician.

Contractors consider only one M.D. or D.O. to be the admitting physician and permit only the admitting physician to use the initial hospital care codes. Physicians that participate in the care of a patient but are not the admitting physician of record should bill the inpatient evaluation and management services codes that describe their participation in the patient's care (i.e., subsequent hospital visit or inpatient consultation).

H. Initial Hospital Care and Nursing Facility Visit on Same Day

Pay only the initial hospital care code if the patient is admitted to a hospital following a nursing facility visit on the same date by the same physician. Instruct physicians that they may not report a nursing facility service and an initial hospital care service on the same day. Payment for the initial hospital care service includes all work performed by the physician in all sites of service on that date.

30.6.9.2—Subsequent Hospital Visit and Hospital Discharge Day Management (Codes 99231 - 99239)

(Rev. 1460, Issued: 02-22-08, Effective: 04-01-08, Implementation: 04-07-08)

A. Subsequent Hospital Visits During the Global Surgery Period

(Refer to §§40-40.4 on global surgery)

The Medicare physician fee schedule payment amount for surgical procedures includes all services (e.g., evaluation and management visits) that are part of the global surgery payment; therefore, contractors shall not pay more than that amount when a bill is fragmented for staged procedures.

B. Hospital Discharge Day Management Service

Hospital Discharge Day Management Services, CPT code 99238 or 99239 is a face-to-face evaluation and management (E/M) service between the attending physician and the patient. The E/M discharge day management visit shall be reported for the date of the actual visit by the physician or qualified nonphysician practitioner even if the patient is discharged from the facility on a different calendar date. Only one hospital discharge day management service is payable per patient per hospital stay.

Only the attending physician of record reports the discharge day management service. Physicians or qualified nonphysician practitioners, other than the attending physician, who have been managing concurrent health care problems not primarily managed by the attending physician, and who are not acting on behalf of the attending physician, shall use Subsequent Hospital Care (CPT code range 99231 – 99233) for a final visit.

Medicare pays for the paperwork of patient discharge day management through the pre- and post- service work of an E/M service.

C. Subsequent Hospital Visit and Discharge Management on Same Day

Pay only the hospital discharge management code on the day of discharge (unless it is also the day of admission, in which case, refer to §30.6.9.1 C for the policy on Observation or Inpatient Care Services (Including Admission and Discharge Services CPT Codes 99234 - 99236). Contractors do not pay both a subsequent hospital visit in addition to hospital discharge day management service on the same day by the same physician. Instruct physicians that they may not bill for both a hospital visit and hospital discharge management for the same date of service.

D. Hospital Discharge Management (CPT Codes 99238 and 99239) and Nursing acility Admission Code When Patient Is Discharged From Hospital and Admitted to Nursing Facility on Same Day

Contractors pay the hospital discharge code (codes 99238 or 99239) in addition to a nursing facility admission code when they are billed by the same physician with the same date of service.

If a surgeon is admitting the patient to the nursing facility due to a condition that is not as a result of the surgery during the postoperative period of a service with the global surgical period, he/she bills for the nursing facility admission and care with a modifier "-24" and provides documentation that the service is unrelated to the surgery (e.g., return of an elderly patient to the nursing facility in which he/she has resided for five years following discharge from the hospital for cholecystectomy).

Contractors do not pay for a nursing facility admission by a surgeon in the postoperative period of a procedure with a global surgical period if the patient's admission to the nursing facility is to receive post operative care related to the surgery (e.g., admission to a nursing facility to receive physical therapy following a hip replacement). Payment for the nursing facility admission and subsequent nursing facility services are included in the global fee and cannot be paid separately.

E. Hospital Discharge Management and Death Pronouncement

Only the physician who personally performs the pronouncement of death shall bill for the face-to-face Hospital Discharge Day Management Service, CPT code 99238 or 99239. The date of the pronouncement shall reflect the calendar date of service on the day it was performed even if the paperwork is delayed to a subsequent date.

30.6.10—Consultation Services (Codes 99241 - 99255)

(Rev. 788, Issued: 12-20-05, Effective: 01-01-06, Implementation: 01-17-06)

A. Consultation Services versus Other Evaluation and Management (E/M) Visits

Carriers pay for a reasonable and medically necessary consultation service when all of the following criteria for the use of a consultation code are met:

- Specifically, a consultation service is distinguished from other evaluation and management (E/M) visits because it is provided by a physician or qualified nonphysician practitioner (NPP) whose opinion or advice regarding evaluation and/or management of a specific problem is requested by another physician or other appropriate source. The qualified NPP may perform consultation services within the scope of practice and licensure requirements for NPPs in the State in which he/she practices. Applicable collaboration and general supervision rules apply as well as billing rules;
- A request for a consultation from an appropriate source and the need for consultation (i.e., the reason for a consultation service) shall be documented by the consultant in the patient's medical record and included in the requesting physician or qualified NPP's plan of care in the patient's medical record; and
- After the consultation is provided, the consultant shall prepare a written report of his/her findings and recommendations, which shall be provided to the referring physician.

The intent of a consultation service is that a physician or qualified NPP or other appropriate source is asking another physician or qualified NPP for advice, opinion, a recommendation, suggestion, direction, or counsel, etc. in evaluating or treating a patient because that individual has expertise in a specific medical area beyond the requesting professional's knowledge. Consultations may be billed based on time if the counseling/coordination of care constitutes more than 50 percent of the face-to-face encounter between the physician or qualified NPP and the patient. The preceding requirements (request, evaluation (or counseling/coordination) and written report) shall also be met when the consultation is based on time for counseling/coordination.

A consultation shall not be performed as a split/shared E/M visit.

B. Consultation Followed by Treatment

A physician or qualified NPP consultant may initiate diagnostic services and treatment at the initial consultation service or subsequent visit. Ongoing management, following the initial consultation service by the consultant physician, shall not be reported with consultation service codes. These services shall be reported as subsequent visits for the appropriate place of service and level of service. Payment for a consultation service shall be made regardless of treatment initiation unless a transfer of care occurs.

Transfer of Care

A transfer of care occurs when a physician or qualified NPP requests that another physician or qualified NPP take over the responsibility for managing the patients' complete care for the condition and does not expect to continue treating or caring for the patient for that condition.

When this transfer is arranged, the requesting physician or qualified NPP is not asking for an opinion or advice to personally treat this patient and is not expecting to continue treating the patient for the condition. The receiving physician or qualified NPP shall document this transfer of the patient's care, to his/her service, in the patient's medical record or plan of care.

In a transfer of care the receiving physician or qualified NPP would report the appropriate new or established patient visit code according to the place of service and level of service performed and shall not report a consultation service.

C. Initial and Follow-Up Consultation Services

Initial Consultation Service

In the hospital setting, the consulting physician or qualified NPP shall use the appropriate Initial Inpatient Consultation codes (99251 – 99255) for the initial consultation service.

In the nursing facility setting, the consulting physician or qualified NPP shall use the appropriate Initial Inpatient Consultation codes (99251 – 99255) for the initial consultation service.

The Initial Inpatient Consultation may be reported only once per consultant per patient per facility admission.

In the office or other outpatient setting, the consulting physician or qualified NPP shall use the appropriate Office or Other Outpatient Consultation (new or established patient) codes (99241 – 99245) for the initial consultation service.

If an additional request for an opinion or advice, regarding the same or a new problem with the same patient, is received from the same or another physician or qualified NPP and documented in the medical record, the Office or Other Outpatient Consultation (new or established patient) codes (99241 – 99245) may be used again. However, if the consultant continues to care for the patient for the original condition following his/her initial consultation, repeat consultation services shall not be reported by this physician or qualified NPP during his/her ongoing management of this condition.

Follow-Up Consultation Service

Effective January 1, 2006, the follow-up inpatient consultation codes (99261 – 99263) are deleted.

In the hospital setting, following the initial consultation service, the Subsequent Hospital Care codes (99231 – 99233) shall be reported for additional follow-up visits.

In the nursing facility setting, following the initial consultation service, the Subsequent Nursing Facility (NF) Care codes (new CPT codes 99307 – 99310) shall be reported for additional follow-up visits. Effective January 1, 2006, CPT codes 99311 – 99313 are deleted and not valid for Subsequent NF visits.

In the office or other outpatient setting, following the initial consultation service, the Office or Other Outpatient Established Patient codes (99212 – 99215) shall be reported for additional follow-up visits. The CPT code 99211 shall not be reported as a consultation service. The CPT code 99211 is not included by Medicare for a consultation service since this service typically does not require the presence of a physician or qualified NPP and would not meet the consultation service criteria.

D. Second Opinion E/M Service Requests

Effective January 1, 2006, the Confirmatory Consultation codes (99271 – 99275) are deleted.

A second opinion E/M service is a request by the patient and/or family or mandated (e.g., by a third-party payer) and is not requested by a physician or qualified NPP. A consultation service requested by a physician, qualified NPP or other appropriate source that meets the requirements stated in Section A shall be reported using the initial consultation service codes as discussed in Section C. A written report is not required by Medicare to be sent to a physician when an evaluation for a second opinion has been requested by the patient and/or family.

A second opinion, for Medicare purposes, is generally performed as a request for a second or third opinion of a previously recommended medical treatment or surgical procedure. A second opinion E/M service initiated by a patient and/or family is not reported using the consultation codes.

In both the inpatient hospital setting and the NF setting, a request for a second opinion would be made through the attending physician or physician of record. If an initial consultation is requested of another physician or qualified NPP by the attending physician and meets the requirements for a consultation service (as identified in Section A) then the appropriate Initial Inpatient Consultation code shall be reported by the consultant. If the service does not meet the consultation requirements, then the E/M service shall be reported using the Subsequent Hospital Care codes (99231 – 99233) in the inpatient hospital setting and the Subsequent NF Care codes (99307 – 99310) in the NF setting.

A second opinion E/M service performed in the office or other outpatient setting shall be reported using the Office or Other Outpatient new patient codes (99201 – 99205) for a new patient and established patient codes (99212 – 99215) for an established patient, as appropriate. The 3 year rule regarding "new patient" status applies. Any medically necessary follow-up visits shall be reported using the appropriate subsequent visit/established patient E/M visit codes.

The CPT modifier -32 (Mandated Services) is not recognized as a payment modifier in Medicare. A second opinion evaluation service to satisfy a requirement for a third party payer is not a covered service in Medicare.

E. Consultations Requested by Members of Same Group

Carriers pay for a consultation if one physician or qualified NPP in a group practice requests a consultation from another physician in the same group practice when the consulting physician or qualified NPP has expertise in a specific medical area beyond the requesting professional's knowledge. A consultation service shall not be reported on every patient as a routine practice between physicians and qualified NPPs within a group practice setting.

F. Documentation for Consultation Services

Consultation Request

A written request for a consultation from an appropriate source and the need for a consultation must be documented in the patient's medical record. The initial request may be a verbal interaction between the requesting physician and the consulting physician; however, the verbal conversation shall be documented in the patient's medical record, indicating a request for a consultation service was made by the requesting physician or qualified NPP.

The reason for the consultation service shall be documented by the consultant (physician or qualified NPP) in the patient's medical record and included in the requesting physician or qualified NPP's plan of care. The consultation service request may be written on a physician order form by the requestor in a shared medical record.

Consultation Report

A written report shall be furnished to the requesting physician or qualified NPP.

In an emergency department or an inpatient or outpatient setting in which the medical record is shared between the referring physician or qualified NPP and the consultant, the request may be documented as part of a plan written in the requesting physician or qualified NPP's progress note, an order in the medical record, or a specific written request for the consultation. In these settings, the report may consist of an appropriate entry in the common medical record.

In an office setting, the documentation requirement may be met by a specific written request for the consultation from the requesting physician or qualified NPP or if the consultant's records show a specific reference to the request. In this setting, the consultation report is a separate document communicated to the requesting physician or qualified NPP.

In a large group practice, e.g., an academic department or a large multi-specialty group, in which there is often a shared medical record, it is acceptable to include the consultant's report in the medical record documentation and not require a separate letter from the consulting physician or qualified NPP to the requesting physician or qualified NPP. The written request and the consultation evaluation, findings and recommendations shall be available in the consultation report.

G. Consultation for Preoperative Clearance

Preoperative consultations are payable for new or established patients performed by any physician or qualified NPP at the request of a surgeon, as long as all of the requirements for performing and reporting the consultation codes are met and the service is medically necessary and not routine screening.

H. Postoperative Care by Physician Who Did Preoperative Clearance Consultation

If subsequent to the completion of a preoperative consultation in the office or hospital, the consultant assumes responsibility for the management of a portion or all of the patient's condition(s) during the postoperative period, the consultation codes should not be used postoperatively. In the hospital setting, the physician or qualified NPP who has performed a preoperative consultation and assumes responsibility for the management of a portion or all of the patient's condition(s) during the postoperative period should use the appropriate subsequent hospital care codes to bill for the concurrent care he or she is providing. In the office setting, the appropriate established patient visit codes should be used during the postoperative period.

A physician (primary care or specialist) or qualified NPP who performs a postoperative evaluation of a new or established patient at the request of the surgeon may bill the appropriate consultation code for evaluation and management services furnished during the postoperative period following surgery when all of the criteria for the use of the consultation codes are met and that same physician has not already performed a preoperative consultation.

I. Surgeon's Request That Another Physician Participate In Postoperative Care

If the surgeon asks a physician or qualified NPP who had been treating the patient preoperatively or who had not seen the patient for a preoperative consultation to take responsibility for the management of an aspect of the patient's condition during the postoperative period, the physician or qualified NPP may not bill a consultation because the surgeon is not asking the physician or qualified NPP's opinion or advice for the surgeon's use in treating the patient. The physician or qualified NPP's services would constitute concurrent care and should be billed using the appropriate subsequent hospital care codes in the hospital inpatient setting, subsequent NF care codes in the SNF/NF setting or the appropriate office or other outpatient visit codes in the office or outpatient settings.

J. Examples That Meet the Criteria for Consultation Services

For brevity, the consultation request and the consultation written report is not repeated in each of these examples. Criteria for consultation services shall always include a request and a written report in the medical record as described above.

EXAMPLE 1:

An internist sees a patient that he has followed for 20 years for mild hypertension and diabetes mellitus. He identifies a questionable skin lesion and asks a dermatologist to evaluate the lesion. The dermatologist examines the patient and decides the lesion is probably malignant and needs to be removed. He removes the lesion which is determined to be an early melanoma. The dermatologist dictates and forwards a report to the internist regarding his evaluation and treatment of the patient. Modifier -25 shall be used with the consultation service code in addition to the procedure code. Modifier -25 is required to identify the consultation service as a significant, separately identifiable E/M service in addition to the procedure code reported for the incision/removal of lesion. The internist resumes care of the patient and continues surveillance of the skin on the advice of the dermatologist.

EXAMPLE 2:

A rural family practice physician examines a patient who has been under his care for 20 years and diagnoses a new onset of atrial fibrillation. The family practitioner sends the patient to a cardiologist at an urban cardiology center for advice on his care and management. The cardiologist examines the patient, suggests a cardiac catheterization and other diagnostic tests which he schedules and then sends a written report to the requesting physician. The cardiologist subsequently periodically sees the patient once a year as follow-up. Subsequent visits provided by the cardiologist should be billed as an established patient visit in the office or other outpatient setting, as appropriate. Following the advice and intervention by the cardiologist the family practice physician resumes the general medical care of the patient.

EXAMPLE 3:

A family practice physician examines a female patient who has been under his care for some time and diagnoses a breast mass. The family practitioner sends the patient to a general surgeon for advice and management of the mass and related patient care. The general surgeon examines the patient and recommends a breast biopsy, which he schedules, and then sends a written report to the requesting physician. The general surgeon subsequently performs a biopsy and then periodically sees the patient once a year as follow-up. Subsequent visits provided by the surgeon should be billed as an established patient visit in the office or other outpatient setting, as appropriate. Following the advice and intervention by the surgeon the family practice physician resumes the general medical care of the patient.

I. Examples That Do Not Meet the Criteria for Consultation Services

EXAMPLE 1: Standing orders in the medical record for consultations.

EXAMPLE 2: No order for a consultation.

EXAMPLE 3: No written report of a consultation.

EXAMPLE 4: The emergency room physician treats the patient for a sprained ankle. The patient is discharged and instructed to visit the orthopedic clinic for follow-up. The physician in the orthopedic clinic shall not report a consultation service because advice or opinion is not required by the emergency room physician. The orthopedic physician shall report the appropriate office or other outpatient visit code.

30.6.11—Emergency Department Visits (Codes 99281 - 99288)

(Rev. 1, 10-01-03)

B3-15507

A. Use of Emergency Department Codes by Physicians Not Assigned to Emergency Department

Any physician seeing a patient registered in the emergency department may use emergency department visit codes (for services matching the code description). It is not required that the physician be assigned to the emergency department.

B. Use of Emergency Department Codes In Office

Emergency department coding is not appropriate if the site of service is an office or outpatient setting or any sight of service other than an emergency department. The emergency department codes should only be used if the patient is seen in the emergency department and the services described by the HCPCS code definition are provided. The emergency department is defined as an organized hospital-based facility for the provision of unscheduled or episodic services to patients who present for immediate medical attention.

C. Use of Emergency Department Codes to Bill Nonemergency Services

Services in the emergency department may not be emergencies. However the codes (99281 - 99288) are payable if the described services are provided.

However, if the physician asks the patient to meet him or her in the emergency department as an alternative to the physician's office and the patient is not registered as a patient in the emergency department, the physician should bill the appropriate office/outpatient visit codes. Normally a lower level emergency department code would be reported for a non-emergency condition.

D. Emergency Department or Office/Outpatient Visits on Same Day As Nursing Facility Admission

Emergency department visit provided on the same day as a comprehensive nursing facility assessment are not paid. Payment for evaluation and management services on the same date provided in sites other than the nursing facility are included in the payment for initial nursing facility care when performed on the same date as the nursing facility admission.

E. Physician Billing for Emergency Department Services Provided to Patient by Both Patient's Personal Physician and Emergency Department Physician

If a physician advises his/her own patient to go to an emergency department (ED) of a hospital for care and the physician subsequently is asked by the ED physician to come to the hospital to evaluate the patient and to advise the ED physician as to whether the patient should be admitted to the hospital or be sent home, the physicians should bill as follows:

- If the patient is admitted to the hospital by the patient's personal physician, then the patient's regular physician should bill only the appropriate level of the initial hospital care (codes 99221 - 99223) because all evaluation and management services provided by that physician in conjunction with that admission are considered part of the initial hospital care when performed on the same date as the admission. The ED physician who saw the patient in the emergency department should bill the appropriate level of the ED codes.
- If the ED physician, based on the advice of the patient's personal physician who came to the emergency department to see the patient, sends the patient home, then the ED physician should bill the appropriate level of emergency department service. The patient's personal physician should also bill the level of emergency department code that describes the service he or she provided in the emergency department. The patient's personal physician would not bill a consultation because he or she is not providing information to the emergency department physician for his or her use in treating the patient. If the patient's personal physician does not come to the hospital to see the patient, but only advises the emergency department physician by telephone, then the patient's personal physician may not bill.

F. Emergency Department Physician Requests Another Physician to See the Patient in Emergency Department or Office/Outpatient Setting

If the emergency department physician requests that another physician evaluate a given patient, the other physician should bill a consultation if the criteria for consultation are met. If the criteria for a consultation are not met and the patient is discharged from the Emergency Department or admitted to the hospital by another physician, the physician contacted by the Emergency Department physician should bill an emergency department visit. If the consulted physician admits the patient to the hospital and the criteria for a consultation are not met, he/she should bill an initial hospital care code.

30.6.12—Critical Care Visits and Neonatal Intensive Care (Codes 99291 - 99292)

(Rev. 1548, Issued: 07-089-08; Effective Date: 07-01-08; Implementation Date: 07-07-08)

CRITICAL CARE SERVICES (CODES 99291-99292)

A. Use of Critical Care Codes

Pay for services reported with CPT codes 99291 and 99292 when all the criteria for critical care and critical care services are met. Critical care is defined as the direct delivery by a physician(s) medical care for a critically ill or critically injured patient. A critical illness or injury acutely impairs one or more vital organ systems such that there is a high probability of imminent or life threatening deterioration in the patient's condition.

Critical care involves high complexity decision making to assess, manipulate, and support vital system functions(s) to treat single or multiple vital organ system failure and/or to prevent further life threatening deterioration of the patient's condition.

Examples of vital organ system failure include, but are not limited to: central nervous system failure, circulatory failure, shock, renal, hepatic, metabolic, and/or respiratory failure. Although critical care typically requires interpretation of multiple physiologic parameters and/or application of advanced technology(s), critical care may be provided in life threatening situations when these elements are not present.

Providing medical care to a critically ill, injured, or post-operative patient qualifies as a critical care service only if both the illness or injury and the treatment being provided meet the above requirements.

Critical care is usually, but not always, given in a critical care area such as a coronary care unit, intensive care unit, respiratory care unit, or the emergency department. However, payment may be made for critical care services provided in any location as long as the care provided meets the definition of critical care.

Consult the American Medical Association (AMA) CPT Manual for the applicable codes and guidance for critical care services provided to neonates, infants and children.

B. Critical Care Services and Medical Necessity

Critical care services must be medically necessary and reasonable. Services provided that do not meet critical care services or services provided for a patient who is not critically ill or injured in accordance with the above definitions and criteria but who happens to be in a critical care, intensive care, or other specialized care unit should be reported using another appropriate E/M code (e.g., subsequent hospital care, CPT codes 99231 - 99233).

As described in Section A, critical care services encompass both treatment of "vital organ failure" and "prevention of further life threatening deterioration of the patient's condition." Therefore, although critical care may be delivered in a moment of crisis or upon being called to the patient's bedside emergently, this is not a requirement for providing critical care service. The treatment and management of the patient's condition, while not necessarily emergent, shall be required, based on the threat of imminent deterioration (i.e., the patient shall be critically ill or injured at the time of the physician's visit).

Chronic Illness and Critical Care:

Examples of patients whose medical condition may not warrant critical care services:

1. Daily management of a patient on chronic ventilator therapy does not meet the criteria for critical care unless the critical care is separately identifiable from the chronic long term management of the ventilator dependence.
2. Management of dialysis or care related to dialysis for a patient receiving ESRD hemodialysis does not meet the criteria for critical care unless the critical care is separately identifiable from the chronic long term management of the dialysis dependence (refer to Chapter 8, §160.4). When a separately identifiable condition (e.g., management of seizures or pericardial tamponade related to renal failure) is being managed, it may be billed as critical care if critical care requirements are met. Modifier –25 should be appended to the critical care code when applicable in this situation.

Examples of patients whose medical condition may warrant critical care services:

1. An 81 year old male patient is admitted to the intensive care unit following abdominal aortic aneurysm resection. Two days after surgery he requires fluids and pressors to maintain adequate perfusion and arterial pressures. He remains ventilator dependent.
2. A 67 year old female patient is 3 days status post mitral valve repair. She develops petechiae, hypotension and hypoxia requiring respiratory and circulatory support.
3. A 70 year old admitted for right lower lobe pneumococcal pneumonia with a history of COPD becomes hypoxic and hypotensive 2 days after admission.
4. A 68 year old admitted for an acute anterior wall myocardial infarction continues to have symptomatic ventricular tachycardia that is marginally responsive to antiarrhythmic therapy.

Examples of patients who may not satisfy Medicare medical necessity criteria, or do not meet critical care criteria or who do not have a critical care illness or injury and therefore not eligible for critical care payment:

1. Patients admitted to a critical care unit because no other hospital beds were available;
2. Patients admitted to a critical care unit for close nursing observation and/or frequent monitoring of vital signs (e.g., drug toxicity or overdose); and

3. Patients admitted to a critical care unit because hospital rules require certain treatments (e.g., insulin infusions) to be administered in the critical care unit.

Providing medical care to a critically ill patient should not be automatically deemed to be a critical care service for the sole reason that the patient is critically ill or injured. While more than one physician may provide critical care services to a patient during the critical care episode of an illness or injury each physician must be managing one or more critical illness(es) or injury(ies) in whole or in part.

> **EXAMPLE:** A dermatologist evaluates and treats a rash on an ICU patient who is maintained on a ventilator and nitroglycerine infusion that are being managed by an intensivist. The dermatologist should not report a service for critical care.

C. Critical Care Services and Full Attention of the Physician

The duration of critical care services to be reported is the time the physician spent evaluating, providing care and managing the critically ill or injured patient's care. That time must be spent at the immediate bedside or elsewhere on the floor or unit so long as the physician is immediately available to the patient.

For example, time spent reviewing laboratory test results or discussing the critically ill patient's care with other medical staff in the unit or at the nursing station on the floor may be reported as critical care, even when it does not occur at the bedside, if this time represents the physician's full attention to the management of the critically ill/injured patient.

For any given period of time spent providing critical care services, the physician must devote his or her full attention to the patient and, therefore, cannot provide services to any other patient during the same period of time.

D. Critical Care Services and Qualified Non-Physician Practitioners (NPP)

Critical care services may be provided by qualified NPPs and reported for payment under the NPP's National Provider Identifier (NPI) when the services meet the definition and requirements of critical care services in Sections A and B. The provision of critical care services must be within the scope of practice and licensure requirements for the State in which the qualified NPP practices and provides the service(s). Collaboration, physician supervision and billing requirements must also be met. A physician assistant shall meet the general physician supervision requirements.

E. Critical Care Services and Physician Time

Critical care is a time- based service, and for each date and encounter entry, the physician's progress note(s) shall document the total time that critical care services were provided. More than one physician can provide critical care at another time and be paid if the service meets critical care, is medically necessary and is not duplicative care. Concurrent care by more than one physician (generally representing different physician specialties) is payable if these requirements are met (refer to the Medicare Benefit Policy Manual, Pub. 100-02, Chapter 15, §30 for concurrent care policy discussion).

The CPT critical care codes 99291 and 99292 are used to report the total duration of time spent by a physician providing critical care services to a critically ill or critically injured patient, even if the time spent by the physician on that date is not continuous. Non-continuous time for medically necessary critical care services may be aggregated. Reporting CPT code 99291 is a prerequisite to reporting CPT code 99292. Physicians of the same specialty within the same group practice bill and are paid as though they were a single physician (§30.6.5).

1. Off the Unit/Floor

   Time spent in activities (excluding those identified previously in Section C) that occur outside of the unit or off the floor (i.e., telephone calls, whether taken at home, in the office, or elsewhere in the hospital) may not be reported as critical care because the physician is not immediately available to the patient. This time is regarded as pre- and post service work bundled in evaluation and management services.

2. Split/Shared Service

   A split/shared E/M service performed by a physician and a qualified NPP of the same group practice (or employed by the same employer) cannot be reported as a critical care service. Critical care services are reflective of the care and management of a critically ill or critically injured patient by an individual physician or qualified non-physician practitioner for the specified reportable period of time.

   Unlike other E/M services where a split/shared service is allowed the critical care service reported shall reflect the evaluation, treatment and management of a patient by an individual physician or qualified non-physician practitioner and shall not be representative of a combined service between a physician and a qualified NPP.

   When CPT code time requirements for both 99291 and 99292 and critical care criteria are met for a medically necessary visit by a qualified NPP the service shall be billed using the appropriate individual NPI number. Medically necessary visit(s) that do not meet these requirements shall be reported as subsequent hospital care services.

3. Unbundled Procedures

   Time involved performing procedures that are not bundled into critical care (i.e., billed and paid separately) may not be included and counted toward critical care time. The physician's progress note(s) in the medical record should document that time involved in the performance of separately billable procedures was not counted toward critical care time.

4. Family Counseling/Discussions

   Critical care CPT codes 99291 and 99292 include pre and post service work. Routine daily updates or reports to family members and or surrogates are considered part of this service. However, time involved with family members or other surrogate decision makers, whether to obtain a history or to discuss treatment options (as described in CPT), may be counted toward critical care time when these specific criteria are met:

   a) The patient is unable or incompetent to participate in giving a history and/or making treatment decisions, and
   b) The discussion is necessary for determining treatment decisions.

For family discussions, the physician should document:

a. The patient is unable or incompetent to participate in giving history and/or making treatment decisions
b. The necessity to have the discussion (e.g., "no other source was available to obtain a history" or "because the patient was deteriorating so rapidly I needed to immediately discuss treatment options with the family",
c. Medically necessary treatment decisions for which the discussion was needed, and
d. A summary in the medical record that supports the medical necessity of the discussion

   All other family discussions, no matter how lengthy, may not be additionally counted towards critical care. Telephone calls to family members and or surrogate decision-makers may be counted towards critical care time, but only if they meet the same criteria as described in the aforementioned paragraph.

5. Inappropriate Use of Time for Payment of Critical Care Services.

Time involved in activities that do not directly contribute to the treatment of the critically ill or injured patient may not be counted towards the critical care time, even when they are performed in the critical care unit at a patient's bedside (e.g., review of literature, and teaching sessions with physician residents whether conducted on hospital rounds or in other venues).

F. Hours and Days of Critical Care that May Be Billed

Critical care service is a time-based service provided on an hourly or fraction of an hour basis. Payment should not be restricted to a fixed number of hours, a fixed number of physicians, or a fixed number of days, on a per patient basis, for medically necessary critical care services. Time counted towards critical care services may be continuous or intermittent and aggregated in time increments (e.g., 50 minutes of continuous clock time or (5) 10 minute blocks of time spread over a given calendar date). Only one physician may bill for critical care services during any one single period of time even if more than one physician is providing care to a critically ill patient.

For Medicare Part B physician services paid under the physician fee schedule, critical care is not a service that is paid on a "shift" basis or a "per day" basis. Documentation may be requested for any claim to determine medical necessity. Examples of critical care billing that may require further review could include: claims from several physicians submitting multiple units of critical care for a single patient, and submitting claims for more than 12 hours of critical care time by a physician for one or more patients on the same given calendar date. Physicians assigned to a critical care unit (e.g., hospitalist, intensivist, etc.) may not report critical care for patients based on a 'per shift" basis.

The CPT code 99291 is used to report the first 30 - 74 minutes of critical care on a given calendar date of service. It should only be used once per calendar date per patient by the same physician or physician group of the same specialty. CPT code 99292 is used to report additional block(s) of time, of up to 30 minutes each beyond the first 74 minutes of critical care (See table below). Critical care of less than 30 minutes total duration on a given calendar date is not reported separately using the critical care codes. This service should be reported using another appropriate E/M code such as subsequent hospital care.

Clinical Example of Correct Billing of Time:

A patient arrives in the emergency department in cardiac arrest. The emergency department physician provides 40 minutes of critical care services. A cardiologist is called to the ED and assumes responsibility for the patient, providing 35 minutes of critical care services. The patient stabilizes and is transferred to the CCU. In this instance, the ED physician provided 40 minutes of critical care services and reports only the critical care code (CPT code 99291) and not also emergency department services. The cardiologist may report the 35 minutes of critical care services (also CPT code 99291) provided in the ED. Additional critical care services by the cardiologist in the CCU may be reported on the same calendar date using 99292 or another appropriate E/M code depending on the clock time involved.

G. Counting of Units of Critical Care Services

The CPT code 99291 (critical care, first hour) is used to report the services of a physician providing full attention to a critically ill or critically injured patient from 30-74 minutes on a given date. Only one unit of CPT code 99291 may be billed by a physician for a patient on a given date. Physicians of the same specialty within the same group practice bill and are paid as though they were a single physician and would not each report CPT 99291on the same date of service.

The following illustrates the correct reporting of critical care services:

TOTAL DURATION OF CRITICAL CARE CODES	
Less than 30 minutes	99232 or 99233 or other appropriate E/M code
30 - 74 minutes	99291 x 1
75 - 104 minutes	99291 x 1 and 99292 x 1
105 - 134 minutes	99291 x1 and 99292 x 2
135 - 164 minutes	99291 x 1 and 99292 x 3
165 - 194 minutes	99291 x 1 and 99292 x 4
194 minutes or longer	99291 – 99292 as appropriate (per the above illustrations)

H. Critical Care Services and Other Evaluation and Management Services Provided on Same Day

When critical care services are required upon the patient's presentation to the hospital emergency department, only critical care codes 99291 - 99292 may be reported. An emergency department visit code may not also be reported.

When critical care services are provided on a date where an inpatient hospital or office/outpatient evaluation and management service was furnished earlier on the same date at which time the patient did not require critical care, both the critical care and the previous evaluation and management service may be paid. Hospital emergency department services are not payable for the same calendar date as critical care services when provided by the same physician to the same patient.

Physicians are advised to submit documentation to support a claim when critical care is additionally reported on the same calendar date as when other evaluation and management services are provided to a patient by the same physician or physicians of the same specialty in a group practice.

I. Critical Care Services Provided by Physicians in Group Practice(s)

Medically necessary critical care services provided on the same calendar date to the same patient by physicians representing different medical specialties that are not duplicative services are payable. The medical specialists may be from the same group practice or from different group practices.

Critically ill or critically injured patients may require the care of more than one physician medical specialty. Concurrent critical care services provided by each physician must be medically necessary and not provided during the same instance of time. Medical record documentation must support the medical necessity of critical care services provided by each physician (or qualified NPP). Each physician must accurately report the service(s) he/she provided to the patient in accordance with any applicable global surgery rules or concurrent care rules. (Refer to Medicare Claims Processing Manual, Pub. 100-04, Chapter 12, §40, and the Medicare Benefit Policy Manual, Pub. 100-02, Chapter 15, §30.)

CPT Code 99291

The initial critical care time, billed as CPT code 99291, must be met by a single physician or qualified NPP. This may be performed in a single period of time or be cumulative by the same physician on the same calendar date. A history or physical exam performed by one group partner for another group partner in order for the second group partner to make a medical decision would not represent critical care services.

CPT Code 99292

Subsequent critical care visits performed on the same calendar date are reported using CPT code 99292. The service may represent aggregate time met by a single physician or physicians in the same group practice with the same medical specialty in order to meet the duration of minutes required for CPT code 99292. The aggregated critical care visits must be medically necessary and each aggregated visit must meet the definition of critical care in order to combine the times.

Physicians in the same group practice who have the same specialty may not each report CPT initial critical care code 99291 for critical care services to the same patient on the same calendar date. Medicare payment policy states that physicians in the same group practice who are in the same specialty must bill and be paid as though each were the single physician. (Refer to the Medicare Claims Processing Manual, Pub. 100-04, Chapter 12, §30.6.)

Physician specialty means the self-designated primary specialty by which the physician bills Medicare and is known to the contractor that adjudicates the claims. Physicians in the same group practice who have different medical specialties may bill and be paid without regard to their membership in the same group. For example, if a cardiologist and an endocrinologist are group partners and the critical care services of each are medically necessary and not duplicative, the critical care services may be reported by each regardless of their group practice relationship.

Two or more physicians in the same group practice who have different specialties and who provide critical care to a critically ill or critically injured patient may not in all cases each report the initial critical care code (CPT 99291) on the same date. When the group physicians are providing care that is unique to his/her individual medical specialty and managing at least one of the patient's critical illness(es) or critical injury(ies) then the initial critical care service may be payable to each.

However, if a physician or qualified NPP within a group provides "staff coverage" or "follow-up" for each other after the first hour of critical care services was provided on the same calendar date by the previous group clinician (physician or qualified NPP), the subsequent visits by the "covering" physician or qualified NPP in the group shall be billed using CPT critical care add-on code 99292. The appropriate individual NPI number shall be reported on the claim. The services will be paid at the specific physician fee schedule rate for the individual clinician (physician or qualified NPP) billing the service.

Clinical Examples of Critical Care Services

1. Drs. Smith and Jones, pulmonary specialists, share a group practice. On Tuesday Dr. Smith provides critical care services to Mrs. Benson who is comatose and has been in the intensive care unit for 4 days following a motor vehicle accident. She has multiple organ dysfunction including cerebral hematoma, flail chest and pulmonary contusion. Later on the same calendar date Dr. Jones covers for Dr. Smith and provides critical care services. Medically necessary critical care services provided at the different time periods may be reported by both Drs. Smith and Jones. Dr. Smith would report CPT code 99291 for the initial visit and Dr. Jones, as part of the same group practice would report CPT code 99292 on the same calendar date if the appropriate time requirements are met.

2. Mr. Marks, a 79 year old comes to the emergency room with vague joint pains and lethargy. The ED physician evaluates Mr. Marks and phones his primary care physician to discuss his medical evaluation. His primary care physician visits the ER and admits Mr. Marks to the observation unit for monitoring, and diagnostic and laboratory tests. In observation Mr. Marks has a cardiac arrest. His primary care physician provides 50 minutes of critical care services. Mr. Marks' is admitted to the intensive care unit. On the same calendar day Mr. Marks' condition deteriorates and he requires intermittent critical care services. In this scenario the ED physician should report an emergency department visit and the primary care physician should report both an initial hospital visit and critical care services.

J. Critical Care Services and Other Procedures Provided on the Same Day by the Same Physician as Critical Care Codes 99291 – 99292

The following services when performed on the day a physician bills for critical care are included in the critical care service and should not be reported separately:

- The interpretation of cardiac output measurements (CPT 93561, 93562);

- Chest x-rays, professional component (CPT 71010, 71015, 71020);
- Blood draw for specimen (CPT 36415);
- Blood gases, and information data stored in computers (e.g., ECGs, blood pressures, hematologic data-CPT 99090);
- Gastric intubation (CPT 43752, 91105);
- Pulse oximetry (CPT 94760, 94761, 94762);
- Temporary transcutaneous pacing (CPT 92953);
- Ventilator management (CPT 94002 – 94004, 94660, 94662); and
- Vascular access procedures (CPT 36000, 36410, 36415, 36591, 36600).

No other procedure codes are bundled into the critical care services. Therefore, other medically necessary procedure codes may be billed separately.

K. Global Surgery

Critical care services shall not be paid on the same calendar date the physician also reports a procedure code with a global surgical period unless the critical care is billed with CPT modifier -25 to indicate that the critical care is a significant, separately identifiable evaluation and management service that is above and beyond the usual pre and post operative care associated with the procedure that is performed.

Services such as endotracheal intubation (CPT code 31500) and the insertion and placement of a flow directed catheter e.g., Swan-Ganz (CPT code 93503) are not bundled into the critical care codes. Therefore, separate payment may be made for critical care in addition to these services if the critical care was a significant, separately identifiable service and it was reported with modifier -25. The time spent performing the pre, intra, and post procedure work of these unbundled services, e.g., endotracheal intubation, shall be excluded from the determination of the time spent providing critical care.

This policy applies to any procedure with a 0, 10 or 90 day global period including cardiopulmonary resuscitation (CPT code 92950). CPR has a global period of 0 days and is not bundled into critical care codes. Therefore, critical care may be billed in addition to CPR if critical care was a significant, separately identifiable service and it was reported with modifier -25. The time spent performing CPR shall be excluded from the determination of the time spent providing critical care. In this instance it must be the physician who performs the resuscitation who bills for this service. Members of a code team must not each bill Medicare Part B for this service.

When postoperative critical care services (for procedures with a global surgical period) are provided by a physician other than the surgeon, no modifier is required unless all surgical postoperative care has been officially transferred from the surgeon to the physician performing the critical care services. In this situation, CPT modifiers "-54" (surgical care only) and "-55"(postoperative management only) must be used by the surgeon and intensivist who are submitting claims. Medical record documentation by the surgeon and the physician who assumes a transfer (e.g., intensivist) is required to support claims for services when CPT modifiers -54 and -55 are used indicating the transfer of care from the surgeon to the intensivist. Critical care services must meet all the conditions previously described in this manual section.

L. Critical Care Services Provided During Preoperative Portion and Postoperative Portion of Global Period of Procedure with 90 Day Global Period in Trauma and Burn Cases

Preoperative

Preoperative critical care may be paid in addition to a global fee if the patient is critically ill and requires the full attention of the physician, and the critical care is unrelated to the specific anatomic injury or general surgical procedure performed. Such patients may meet the definition of being critically ill and criteria for conditions where there is a high probability of imminent or life threatening deterioration in the patient's condition.

Preoperatively, in order for these services to be paid, two reporting requirements must be met. Codes 99291 - 99292 and modifier -25 (significant, separately identifiable evaluation and management services by the same physician on the day of the procedure) must be used, and documentation identifying that the critical care was unrelated to the specific anatomic injury or general surgical procedure performed shall be submitted. An ICD-9-CM code in the range 800.0 through 959.9 (except 930.0 – 939.9), which clearly indicates that the critical care was unrelated to the surgery, is acceptable documentation.

Postoperative

Postoperatively, in order for critical care services to be paid, two reporting requirements must be met. Codes 99291 - 99292 and modifier -24 (unrelated evaluation and management service by the same physician during a postoperative period) must be used, and documentation that the critical care was unrelated to the specific anatomic injury or general surgical procedure performed must be submitted. An ICD-9-CM code in the range 800.0 through 959.9 (except 930.0 – 939.9), which clearly indicates that the critical care was unrelated to the surgery, is acceptable documentation.

Medicare policy allows separate payment to the surgeon for postoperative critical care services during the surgical global period when the patient has suffered trauma or burns. When the surgeon provides critical care services during the global period, for reasons unrelated to the surgery, these are separately payable as well.

M. Teaching Physician Criteria

In order for the teaching physician to bill for critical care services the teaching physician must meet the requirements for critical care described in the preceding sections. For CPT codes determined on the basis of time, such as critical care, the teaching physician must be present for the entire period of time for which the claim is submitted. For example, payment will be made for 35 minutes of critical care services only if the teaching physician is present for the full 35 minutes. (See IOM, Pub 100-04, Chapter12, § 100.1.4)

1. Teaching

Time spent teaching may not be counted towards critical care time. Time spent by the resident, in the absence of the teaching physician, cannot be billed by the teaching physician as critical care or other time-based services. Only time spent by the resident and teaching physician together with the patient or the teaching physician alone with the patient can be counted toward critical care time.

2. Documentation

A combination of the teaching physician's documentation and the resident's documentation may support critical care services. Provided that all requirements for critical care services are met, the teaching physician documentation may tie into the resident's documentation. The teaching physician may refer to the resident's documentation for specific patient history, physical findings and medical assessment. However, the teaching physician medical record documentation must provide substantive information including: (1) the time the teaching physician spent providing critical care, (2) that the patient was critically ill during the time the teaching physician saw the patient, (3) what made the patient critically ill, and (4) the nature of the treatment and management provided by the teaching physician. The medical review criteria are the same for the teaching physician as for all physicians. (See the Medicare Claims Processing, Pub. 100-04, Chapter 12, §100.1.1 for teaching physician documentation guidance.)

Unacceptable Example of Documentation:

"I came and saw (the patient) and agree with (the resident)".

Acceptable Example of Documentation:

"Patient developed hypotension and hypoxia; I spent 45 minutes while the patient was in this condition, providing fluids, pressor drugs, and oxygen. I reviewed the resident's documentation and I agree with the resident's assessment and plan of care."

N. Ventilator Management

Medicare recognizes the ventilator codes (CPT codes 94002 - 94004, 94660 and 94662) as physician services payable under the physician fee schedule. Medicare Part B under the physician fee schedule does not pay for ventilator management services in addition to an evaluation and management service (e.g., critical care services, CPT codes 99291 - 99292) on the same day for the patient even when the evaluation and management service is billed with CPT modifier -25.

30.6.13—Nursing Facility Services (Codes 99304 - 99318)

(Rev. 1489, Issued: 04-11-08, Effective: 07-01-08, Implementation: 07-07-08)

A. Visits to Perform the Initial Comprehensive Assessment and Annual Assessments

The distinction made between the delegation of physician visits and tasks in a skilled nursing facility (SNF) and in a nursing facility (NF) is based on the Medicare Statute. Section 1819 (b) (6) (A) of the Social Security Act (the Act) governs SNFs while section 1919 (b) (6) (A) of the Act governs NFs. For further information refer to Medlearn Matters article number SE0418 at www.cms.hhs.gov/medlearn/matters

The initial visit in a SNF and NF must be performed by the physician except as otherwise permitted (42 CFR 483.40 (c) (4)). The initial visit is defined in S&C-04-08 (see www.cms.hhs.gov/medlearn/matters) as the initial comprehensive assessment visit during which the physician completes a thorough assessment, develops a plan of care and writes or verifies admitting orders for the nursing facility resident. For

Survey and Certification requirements, a visit must occur no later than 30 days after admission.

Further, per the Long Term Care regulations at 42 CFR 483.40 (c)(4) and (e) (2), the physician may not delegate a task that the physician must personally perform. Therefore, as stated in S&C-04-08 the physician may not delegate the initial visit in a SNF. This also applies to the NF with one exception.

The only exception, as to who performs the initial visit, relates to the NF setting. In the NF setting, a qualified NPP (i.e., a nurse practitioner (NP), physician assistant (PA), or a clinical nurse specialist (CNS), who is not employed by the facility, may perform the initial visit when the State law permits this. The evaluation and management (E/M) visit shall be within the State scope of practice and licensure requirements where the E/M visit is performed and the requirements for physician collaboration and physician supervision shall be met.

Under Medicare Part B payment policy, other medically necessary E/M visits may be performed and reported prior to and after the initial visit, if the medical needs of the patient require an E/M visit. A qualified NPP may perform medically necessary E/M visits prior to and after the initial visit if all the requirements for collaboration, general physician supervision, licensure and billing are met.

The CPT Nursing Facility Services codes shall be used with place of service (POS) 31 (SNF) if the patient is in a Part A SNF stay. They shall be used with POS 32 (nursing facility) if the patient does not have Part A SNF benefits or if the patient is in a NF or in a non-covered SNF stay (e.g., there was no preceding 3-day hospital stay). The CPT Nursing Facility code definition also includes POS 54 (Intermediate Care Facility/Mentally Retarded) and POS 56 (Psychiatric Residential Treatment Center). For further guidance on POS codes and associated CPT codes refer to §30.6.14.

Effective January 1, 2006, the Initial Nursing Facility Care codes 99301– 99303 are deleted.

Beginning January 1, 2006, the new CPT codes, Initial Nursing Facility Care, per day, (99304 – 99306) shall be used to report the initial visit. Only a physician may report these codes for an initial visit performed in a SNF or NF (with the exception of the qualified NPP in the NF setting who is not employed by the facility and when State law permits, as explained above).

A readmission to a SNF or NF shall have the same payment policy requirements as an initial admission in both the SNF and NF settings.

A physician who is employed by the SNF/NF may perform the E/M visits and bill independently to Medicare Part B for payment. An NPP who is employed by the SNF or NF may perform and bill Medicare Part B directly for those services where it is permitted as discussed above. The employer of the PA shall always report the visits performed by the PA. A physician, NP or CNS has the option to bill Medicare directly or to reassign payment for his/her professional service to the facility.

As with all E/M visits for Medicare Part B payment policy, the E/M documentation guidelines apply.

B. Visits to Comply With Federal Regulations (42 CFR 483.40 (c) (1)) in the SNF and NF

Payment is made under the physician fee schedule by Medicare Part B for federally mandated visits. Following the initial visit by the physician, payment shall be made for federally mandated visits that monitor and evaluate residents at least once every 30 days for the first 90 days after admission and at least once every 60 days thereafter. Effective January 1, 2006, the Subsequent Nursing Facility Care, per day, codes 99311– 99313 are deleted.

Beginning January 1, 2006, the new CPT codes, Subsequent Nursing Facility Care, per day, (99307 – 99310) shall be used to report federally mandated physician E/M visits and medically necessary E/M visits.

Carriers shall not pay for more than one E/M visit performed by the physician or qualified NPP for the same patient on the same date of service. The Nursing Facility Services codes represent a "per day" service.

The federally mandated E/M visit may serve also as a medically necessary E/M visit if the situation arises (i.e., the patient has health problems that need attention on the day the scheduled mandated physician E/M visit occurs). The physician/qualified NPP shall bill only one E/M visit.

Beginning January 1, 2006, the new CPT code, Other Nursing Facility Service (99318), may be used to report an annual nursing facility assessment visit on the required schedule of visits on an annual basis. For Medicare Part B payment policy, an annual nursing facility assessment visit code may substitute as meeting one of the federally mandated physician visits if the code requirements for CPT code 99318 are fully met and in lieu of reporting a Subsequent Nursing Facility Care, per day, service (codes 99307 – 99310). It shall not be performed in addition to the required number of federally mandated physician visits. The new CPT annual assessment code does not represent a new benefit service for Medicare Part B physician services.

Qualified NPPs, whether employed or not by the SNF, may perform alternating federally mandated physician visits, at the option of the physician, after the initial visit by the physician in a SNF.

Qualified NPPs in the NF setting, who are not employed by the NF, may perform federally mandated physician visits, at the option of the State, after the initial visit by the physician.

Medicare Part B payment policy does not pay for additional E/M visits that may be required by State law for a facility admission or for other additional visits to satisfy facility or other administrative purposes. E/M visits, prior to and after the initial physician visit, that are reasonable and medically necessary to meet the medical needs of the individual patient (unrelated to any State requirement or administrative purpose) are payable under Medicare Part B.

C. Visits by Qualified Nonphysician Practitioners

All E/M visits shall be within the State scope of practice and licensure requirements where the visit is performed and all the requirements for physician collaboration and physician supervision shall be met when performed and reported by qualified NPPs. General physician supervision and employer billing requirements shall be met for PA services in addition to the PA meeting the State scope of practice and licensure requirements where the E/M visit is performed.

Medically Necessary Visits

Qualified NPPs may perform medically necessary E/M visits prior to and after the physician's initial visit in both the SNF and NF. Medically necessary E/M visits for the diagnosis or treatment of an illness or injury or to improve the functioning of a malformed body member are payable under the physician fee schedule under Medicare Part B. CPT codes, Subsequent Nursing Facility Care, per day (99307 - 99310), shall be reported for these E/M visits even if the visits are provided prior to the initial visit by the physician.

SNF Setting--Place of Service Code 31

Following the initial visit by the physician, the physician may delegate alternate federally mandated physician visits to a qualified NPP who meets collaboration and physician supervision requirements and is licensed as such by the State and performing within the scope of practice in that State.

NF Setting--Place of Service Code 32

Per the regulations at 42 CFR 483.40 (f), a qualified NPP, who meets the collaboration and physician supervision requirements, the State scope of practice and licensure requirements, and who is not employed by the NF, may at the option of the State, perform the initial visit in a NF, and may perform any other federally mandated physician visit in a NF in addition to performing other medically necessary E/M visits.

Questions pertaining to writing orders or certification and recertification issues in the SNF and NF settings shall be addressed to the appropriate State Survey and Certification Agency departments for clarification.

D. Medically Complex Care

Payment is made for E/M visits to patients in a SNF who are receiving services for medically complex care upon discharge from an acute care facility when the visits are reasonable and medically necessary and documented in the medical record. Physicians and qualified NPPs shall report E/M visits using the Subsequent Nursing Facility Care, per day (codes 99307 - 99310) for these E/M visits even if the visits are provided prior to the initial visit by the physician.

E. Incident to Services

Where a physician establishes an office in a SNF/NF, the "incident to" services and requirements are confined to this discrete part of the facility designated as his/her office. "Incident to" E/M visits, provided in a facility setting, are not payable under the Physician Fee Schedule for Medicare Part B. Thus, visits performed outside the designated "office" area in the SNF/NF would be subject to the coverage and payment rules applicable to SNF/NF setting and shall not be reported using the CPT codes for office or other outpatient visits or use place of service code 11.

F. Use of the Prolonged Services Codes and Other Time-Related Services

Beginning January 1, 2008, typical/average time units for E/M visits in the SNF/NF settings are reestablished. Medically necessary prolonged services for E/M visits (codes 99356 and 99357) in a SNF or NF may be billed with the Nursing Facility Services in the code ranges (99304 – 99306, 99307 – 99310 and 99318).

Counseling and Coordination of Care Visits

With the reestablishment of typical/average time units, medically necessary E/M visits for counseling and coordination of care, for Nursing Facility Services in the code ranges (99304 – 99306, 99307 – 99310 and 99318) that are time-based services, may be billed with the appropriate prolonged services codes (99356 and 99357).

G. Gang Visits

The complexity level of an E/M visit and the CPT code billed must be a covered and medically necessary visit for each patient (refer to §§1862 (a)(1)(A) of the Act). Claims for an unreasonable number of daily E/M visits by the same physician to multiple patients at a facility within a 24-hour period may result in medical review to determine medical necessity for the visits. The E/M visit (Nursing Facility Services) represents a "per day" service per patient as defined by the CPT code. The medical record must be personally documented by the physician or qualified NPP who performed the E/M visit and the documentation shall support the specific level of E/M visit to each individual patient.

H. Split/Shared E/M Visit

A split/shared E/M visit cannot be reported in the SNF/NF setting. A split/shared E/M visit is defined by Medicare Part B payment policy as a medically necessary encounter with a patient where the physician and a qualified NPP each personally perform a substantive portion of an E/M visit face-to-face with the same patient on the same date of service. A substantive portion of an E/M visit involves all or some portion of the history, exam or medical decision making key components of an E/M service. The physician and the qualified NPP must be in the same group practice or be employed by the same employer. The split/shared E/M visit applies only to selected E/M visits and settings (i.e., hospital inpatient, hospital outpatient, hospital observation, emergency department, hospital discharge, office and non facility clinic visits, and prolonged visits associated with these E/M visit codes). The split/shared E/M policy does not apply to consultation services, critical care services or procedures.

I. SNF/NF Discharge Day Management Service

Medicare Part B payment policy requires a face-to-face visit with the patient provided by the physician or the qualified NPP to meet the SNF/NF discharge day management service as defined by the CPT code. The E/M discharge day management visit shall be reported for the date of the actual visit by the physician or qualified NPP even if the patient is discharged from the facility on a different calendar date. The CPT codes 99315 – 99316 shall be reported for this visit. The Discharge Day Management Service may be reported using CPT code 99315 or 99316, depending on the code requirement, for a patient who has expired, but only if the physician or qualified NPP personally performed the death pronouncement.

30.6.14—Home Care and Domiciliary Care Visits (Codes 99324-99350)

(Rev. 775, Issued: 12-02-05, Effective: 01-01-06, Implementation: 01-03-06)

Physician Visits to Patients Residing in Various Places of Service

The American Medical Association's Current Procedural Terminology (CPT) 2006 new patient codes 99324 – 99328 and established patient codes 99334 - 99337 (new codes beginning January 2006), for Domiciliary, Rest Home (e.g., Boarding Home), or Custodial Care Services, are used to report evaluation and management (E/M) services to residents residing in a facility which provides room, board, and other personal assistance services, generally on a long-term basis. These CPT codes are used to report E/M services in facilities assigned places of service (POS) codes 13 (Assisted Living Facility), 14 (Group Home), 33 (Custodial Care Facility) and 55 (Residential Substance Abuse Facility). Assisted living facilities may also be known as adult living facilities.

Physicians and qualified nonphysician practitioners (NPPs) furnishing E/M services to residents in a living arrangement described by one of the POS listed above must use the level of service code in the CPT code range 99324 – 99337 to report the service they provide. The CPT codes 99321 – 99333 for Domiciliary, Rest Home (e.g., Boarding Home), or Custodial Care Services are deleted beginning January, 2006.

Beginning in 2006, reasonable and medically necessary, face-to-face, prolonged services, represented by CPT codes 99354 – 99355, may be reported with the appropriate companion E/M codes when a physician or qualified NPP, provides a prolonged service involving direct (face-to-face) patient contact that is beyond the usual E/M visit service for a Domiciliary, Rest Home (e.g., Boarding Home) or Custodial Care Service. All the requirements for prolonged services at §30.6.15.1 must be met.

The CPT codes 99341 through 99350, Home Services codes, are used to report E/M services furnished to a patient residing in his or her own private residence (e.g., private home, apartment, town home) and not residing in any type of congregate/shared facility living arrangement including assisted living facilities and group homes. The Home Services codes apply only to the specific 2-digit POS 12 (Home). Home Services codes may not be used for billing E/M services provided in settings other than in the private residence of an individual as described above.

Beginning in 2006, E/M services provided to patients residing in a Skilled Nursing Facility (SNF) or a Nursing Facility (NF) must be reported using the appropriate CPT level of service code within the range identified for Initial Nursing Facility Care (new CPT codes 99304 – 99306) and Subsequent Nursing Facility Care (new CPT codes 99307 – 99310). Use the CPT code, Other Nursing Facility Services (new CPT code 99318), for an annual nursing facility assessment. Use CPT codes 99315 – 99316 for SNF/NF discharge services. The CPT codes 99301 – 99303 and 99311 – 99313 are deleted beginning January, 2006. The Home Services codes should not be used for these places of service.

The CPT SNF/NF code definition includes intermediate care facilities (ICFs) and long term care facilities (LTCFs). These codes are limited to the specific 2-digit POS 31 (SNF), 32 (Nursing Facility), 54 (Intermediate Care Facility/Mentally Retarded) and 56 (Psychiatric Residential Treatment Center).

The CPT nursing facility codes should be used with POS 31 (SNF) if the patient is in a Part A SNF stay and POS 32 (nursing facility) if the patient does not have Part A SNF benefits. There is no longer a different payment amount for a Part A or Part B benefit period in these POS settings.

30.6.14.1—Home Services (Codes 99341 - 99350)

(Rev. 1, 10-01-03)

B3-15515, B3-15066

A. Requirement for Physician Presence

Home services codes 99341-99350 are paid when they are billed to report evaluation and management services provided in a private residence. A home visit cannot be billed by a physician unless the physician was actually present in the beneficiary's home.

B. Homebound Status

Under the home health benefit the beneficiary must be confined to the home for services to be covered. For home services provided by a physician using these codes, the beneficiary does not need to be confined to the home. The medical record must document the medical necessity of the home visit made in lieu of an office or outpatient visit.

C. Fee Schedule Payment for Services to Homebound Patients under General Supervision

Payment may be made in some medically underserved areas where there is a lack of medical personnel and home health services for injections, EKGs, and venipunctures that are performed for homebound patients under general physician supervision by nurses and paramedical employees of physicians or physician-directed clinics. Section 10 provides additional information on the provision of services to homebound Medicare patients.

30.6.15—Prolonged Services and Standby Services (Codes 99354 - 99360)

(Rev. 1, 10-01-03)

B3-15511-15511.3

30.6.15.1—Prolonged Services (Codes 99354 - 99357) (ZZZ codes)

(Rev. 1490, Issued: 04-11-08, Effective: 07-01-08, Implementation: 07-07-08)

A. Definition

Prolonged physician services (CPT code 99354) in the office or other outpatient setting with direct face-to-face patient contact which require one hour beyond the usual service are payable when billed on the same day by the same physician or qualified nonphysician practitioner (NPP) as the companion evaluation and management codes. The time for usual service refers to the typical/average time units associated with the companion evaluation and management service as noted in the CPT code. Each additional 30 minutes of direct face-to-face patient contact following the first hour of prolonged services may be reported by CPT code 99355.

Prolonged physician services (code 99356) in the inpatient setting, with direct face-to-face patient contact which require one hour beyond the usual service are payable when they are billed on the same day by the same physician or qualified NPP as the companion evaluation and management codes. Each additional 30 minutes of direct face-to-face patient contact following the first hour of prolonged services may be reported by CPT code 99357.

Prolonged service of less than 30 minutes total duration on a given date is not separately reported because the work involved is included in the total work of the evaluation and management codes.

Code 99355 or 99357 may be used to report each additional 30 minutes beyond the first hour of prolonged services, based on the place of service. These codes may be used to report the final 15 – 30 minutes of prolonged service on a given date, if not otherwise billed. Prolonged service of less than 15 minutes beyond the first hour or less than 15 minutes beyond the final 30 minutes is not reported separately.

B. Required Companion Codes

- The companion evaluation and management codes for 99354 are the Office or Other Outpatient visit codes (99201 - 99205, 99212 – 99215), the Office or Other Outpatient Consultation codes (99241 – 99245), the Domiciliary, Rest Home, or Custodial Care Services codes (99324 – 99328, 99334 – 99337), the Home Services codes (99341 - 99345, 99347 – 99350);
- The companion codes for 99355 are 99354 and one of the evaluation and management codes required for 99354 to be used;
- The companion evaluation and management codes for 99356 are the Initial Hospital Care codes and Subsequent Hospital Care codes (99221 - 99223, 99231 – 99233), the Inpatient Consultation codes (99251 – 99255); Nursing Facility Services codes (99304 -99318) or
- The companion codes for 99357 are 99356 and one of the evaluation and management codes required for 99356 to be used.

Prolonged services codes 99354 – 99357 are not paid unless they are accompanied by the companion codes as indicated.

C. Requirement for Physician Presence

Physicians may count only the duration of direct face-to-face contact between the physician and the patient (whether the service was continuous or not) **beyond** the typical/average time of the visit code billed to determine whether prolonged services can be billed and to determine the prolonged services codes that are allowable. In the case of prolonged office services, time spent by office staff with the patient, or time the patient remains unaccompanied in the office cannot be billed. In the case of prolonged hospital services, time spent reviewing charts or discussion of a patient with house medical staff and not with direct face-to-face contact with the patient, or waiting for test results, for changes in the patient's condition, for end of a therapy, or for use of facilities cannot be billed as prolonged services.

D. Documentation

Documentation is not required to accompany the bill for prolonged services unless the physician has been selected for medical review. Documentation is required in the medical record about the duration and content of the medically necessary evaluation and management service and prolonged services billed. The medical record must be appropriately and sufficiently documented by the physician or qualified NPP to show that the physician or qualified NPP personally furnished the direct face-to-face time with the patient specified in the CPT code definitions. The start and end times of the visit shall be documented in the medical record along with the date of service.

E. Use of the Codes

Prolonged services codes can be billed only if the total duration of all physician or qualified NPP direct face-to-face service (including the visit) equals or exceeds the threshold time for the evaluation and management service the physician or qualified NPP provided (typical/average time associated with the CPT E/M code plus 30 minutes). If the total duration of direct face-to-face time does not equal or exceed the threshold time for the level of evaluation and management service the physician or qualified NPP provided, the physician or qualified NPP may not bill for prolonged services.

F. Threshold Times for Codes 99354 and 99355 (Office or Other Outpatient Setting)

If the total direct face-to-face time equals or exceeds the threshold time for code 99354, but is less than the threshold time for code 99355, the physician should bill the evaluation and management visit code and code 99354. No more than one unit of 99354 is acceptable. If the total direct face-to-face time equals or exceeds the threshold time for code 99355 by no more than 29 minutes, the physician should bill the visit code 99354 and one unit of code 99355. One additional unit of code 99355 is billed for each additional increment of 30 minutes extended duration. Contractors use the following threshold times to determine if the prolonged services codes 99354 and/or 99355 can be billed with the office or other outpatient settings including outpatient consultation services and domiciliary, rest home, or custodial care services and home services codes.

Threshold Time for Prolonged Visit Codes 99354 and/or 99355

Billed with Office/Outpatient and Consultation Codes

Code	Typical Time for Code	Threshold Time to Bill Code 99354	Threshold Time to Bill Codes 99354 and 99355
99201	10	40	85
99202	20	50	95
99203	30	60	105
99204	45	75	120
99205	60	90	135
99212	10	40	85
99213	15	45	90
99214	25	55	100
99215	40	70	115

Code	Typical Time for Code	Threshold Time to Bill Code 99354	Threshold Time to Bill Codes 99354 and 99355
99241	15	45	90
99242	30	60	105
99243	40	70	115
99244	60	90	135
99245	80	110	155
99341	20	50	95
99342	30	60	105
99343	45	75	120
99344	60	90	135
99345	75	105	150
99347	15	45	90
99348	25	55	100
99349	40	70	115
99350	60	90	135

Add 30 minutes to the threshold time for billing codes 99354 and 99355 to get the threshold time for billing code 99354 and 2 units of code 99355. For example, to bill code 99354 and 2 units of code 99355 when billing a code 99205, the threshold time is 150 minutes.

G. Threshold Times for Codes 99356 and 99357 (Inpatient Setting)

If the total direct face-to-face time equals or exceeds the threshold time for code 99356, but is less than the threshold time for code 99357, the physician should bill the visit and code 99356. Carriers do not accept more than 1 unit of code 99356. If the total direct face-to-face time equals or exceeds the threshold time for code 99356 by no more than 29 minutes, the physician bills the visit code 99356 and one unit of code 99357. One additional unit of code 99357 is billed for each additional increment of 30 minutes extended duration. Carriers use the following threshold times to determine if the prolonged services codes 99356 and/or 99357 can be billed with the office/outpatient visit and consultation codes.

Threshold Time for Prolonged Visit Codes 99356 and/or 99357

Billed with Office/Outpatient and Consultation Codes

Code	Typical Time for Code	Threshold Time to Bill Code 99356	Threshold Time to Bill Codes 99356 and 99357
99221	30	60	105
9222	50	80	125
99223	70	100	145
99231	15	45	90
99232	25	55	100
99233	35	65	110
99251	20	50	95

Code	Typical Time for Code	Threshold Time to Bill Code 99356	Threshold Time to Bill Codes 99356 and 99357
99252	40	70	115
99253	55	85	130
99254	80	110	155
99255	110	140	185
99304	25	55	100
99305	35	65	110
99306	45	75	120
99307	10	40	85
99308	15	45	90
99309	25	55	100
99310	35	65	110
99318	30	60	105

Add 30 minutes to the threshold time for billing codes 99356 and 99357 to get the threshold time for billing code 99356 and two units of 99357.

H. Prolonged Services Associated With Evaluation and Management Services Based on Counseling and/or Coordination of Care (Time-Based)

When an evaluation and management service is dominated by counseling and/or coordination of care (the counseling and/or coordination of care represents more than 50% of the total time with the patient) in a face-to-face encounter between the physician or qualified NPP and the patient in the office/clinic or the floor time (in the scenario of an inpatient service), then the evaluation and management code is selected based on the typical/average time associated with the code levels. The time approximation must meet or exceed the specific CPT code billed (determined by the typical/average time associated with the evaluation and management code) and should not be "rounded" to the next higher level.

In those evaluation and management services in which the code level is selected based on time, prolonged services may only be reported with the highest code level in that family of codes as the companion code.

I. Examples of Billable Prolonged Services

EXAMPLE 1

A physician performed a visit that met the definition of visit code 99213 and the total duration of the direct face-to-face services (including the visit) was 65 minutes. The physician bills code 99213 and 1 unit of code 99354.

EXAMPLE 2

A physician performed a visit that met the definition of visit code 99303 and the total duration of the direct face-to-face contact (including the visit) was 115 minutes. The physician bills codes 99303, 99356, and 1 unit of code 99357.

EXAMPLE 3

A physician performed an office visit to an established patient that was predominantly counseling, spending 75 minutes (direct face-to-face) with the patient. The physician should report CPT code 99215 and one unit of code 99354.

J. Examples of Nonbillable Prolonged Services

EXAMPLE 1

A physician performed a visit that met the definition of visit code 99212 and the total duration of the direct face-to-face contact (including the visit) was 35 minutes. The physician cannot bill prolonged services because the total duration of direct face-to-face service did not meet the threshold time for billing prolonged services.

EXAMPLE 2

A physician performed a visit that met the definition of code 99213 and, while the patient was in the office receiving treatment for 4 hours, the total duration of the direct face-to-face service of the physician was 40 minutes. The physician cannot bill prolonged services because the total duration of direct face-to-face service did not meet the threshold time for billing prolonged services.

EXAMPLE 3

A physician provided a subsequent office visit that was predominantly counseling, spending 60 minutes (face-to-face) with the patient. The physician cannot code 99214, which has a typical time of 25 minutes, and one unit of code 99354. The physician must bill the highest level code in the code family (99215 which has 40 minutes typical/average time units associated with it). The additional time spent beyond this code is 20 minutes and does not meet the threshold time for billing prolonged services.

30.6.15.2—Prolonged Services Without Face to Face Service (Codes 99358 - 99359)

(Rev. 1490, Issued: 04-11-08, Effective: 07-01-08, Implementation: 07-07-08)

Contractors may not pay prolonged services codes 99358 and 99359, which do not require any direct patient contact. Payment for these services is included in the payment for direct face-to-face services that physicians bill. The physician cannot bill the patient for these services since they are Medicare covered services and payment is included in the payment for other billable services.

30.6.15.3—Physician Standby Service (Code 99360) (Rev. 1, 10-01-03)

Standby services are not payable to physicians. Physicians may not bill Medicare or beneficiaries for standby services. Payment for standby services is included in the Part A payment to the facility. Such services are a part of hospital costs to provide quality care. If hospitals pay physicians for standby services, such services are part of hospital costs to provide quality care.

30.6.15.4 – Power Mobility Devices (PMDs) (Code G0372)

(Rev. 748, Issued: 11-04-05; Effective/Implementation Dates: 10-25-05)

Section 302(a)(2)(E)(iv) of the Medicare Prescription Drug, Improvement, and Modernization Act of 2003 (MMA) sets forth revised conditions for Medicare payment of Power Mobility Devices (PMDs). This section of the MMA states that payment for motorized or power wheelchairs may not be made unless a physician (as defined in §1861(r)(1) of the Act), a physician assistant, nurse practitioner, or a clinical nurse specialist (as those terms are defined in §1861(aa)(5)) has conducted a face-to-face examination of the beneficiary and written a prescription for the PMD.

Payment for the history and physical examination will be made through the appropriate evaluation and management (E&M) code corresponding to the history and physical examination of the patient. Due to the MMA requirement that the physician or treating practitioner create a written prescription and a regulatory requirement that the physician or treating practitioner prepare pertinent parts of the medical record for submission to the durable medical equipment supplier, code G0372 (physician service required to establish and document the need for a power mobility device) has been established to recognize additional physician services and resources required to establish and document the need for the PMD.

The G code indicates that all of the information necessary to document the PMD prescription is included in the medical record, and the prescription and supporting documentation is delivered to the PMD supplier within 30 days after the face-to-face examination.

Effective October 25, 2005, G0372 will be used to recognize additional physician services and resources required to establish and document the need for the PMD and will be added to the Medicare physician fee schedule.

30.6.16—Case Management Services (Codes 99362 and 99371 - 99373)

(Rev. 1, 10-01-03)

B3-15512

A. Team Conferences

Team conferences (codes 99361-99362) may not be paid separately. Payment for these services is included in the payment for the services to which they relate.

B. Telephone Calls

Telephone calls (codes 99371-99373) may not be paid separately. Payment for telephone calls is included in payment for billable services (e.g., visit, surgery, diagnostic procedure results).

70—Payment Conditions for Radiology Services

(Rev. 1, 10-01-03)

B3-15022

See chapter 13, for claims processing instructions for radiology.

90—Physicians Practicing in Special Settings

(Rev. 1, 10-01-03)

90.1—Physicians in Federal Hospitals

(Rev. 1, 10-01-03)

B3-2020.5

There are many physicians performing services in hospitals operated by the Federal Government, e.g., military, Veterans Administration, and Public Health Service hospitals. Normally Medicare does not pay for the services provided by a physician in a Federal hospital except when the hospital provides services to the public generally as a community institution. Such a physician working in the scope of his Federal employment may be considered as coming within the statutory definition of physician even though he may not have a license to practice in the State in which he is employed.

90.2—Physician Billing for End-Stage Renal Disease Services

(Rev. 1, 10-01-03)

See the Medicare Benefit Policy Manual, Chapter 11, for a description of ESRD policy.

See chapter 8, for billing requirements for physicians and facilities.

90.2.1—Inpatient Hospital Visits With Dialysis Patients

(Rev. 1, 10-01-03)

B3-15062-15062.1

Global billing practices that involve the submission of charges for each day that a patient is hospitalized are allowed. Therefore, carriers may make payment for inpatient hospital visits that are specified relative to time, place, day, and services directly provided to inpatients. This guideline may, however, differ with respect to daily visit charges for inpatient hospital visits with dialysis inpatients. When an ESRD patient is hospitalized, the hospitalization may or may not be due to a renal-related condition. In either case, the patient must continue to be dialyzed.

Chapter 8 provides policy and payment instructions for physicians' services furnished to dialysis inpatients. It also provides instructions for billing physicians' renal-related medical services furnished on dialysis days and for dialysis and evaluation and management services performed on the same day.

90.3—Physicians' Services Performed in Ambulatory Surgical Centers (ASC)

(Rev. 1, 10-01-03)

B3-2265, B3-2265.4

See Chapter 14, for a description of services that may be billed by an ASC and services separately billed by physicians.

The ASC payment does not include the professional services of the physician. These are billed separately by the physician. Physicians' services include the services of anesthesiologists administering or supervising the administration of anesthesia to ASC patients and the patients' recovery from the anesthesia. The term physicians' services also includes any routine pre- or postoperative services, such as office visits, consultations, diagnostic tests, removal of stitches, changing

of dressings, and other services which the individual physician usually performs.

The physician must enter the place of service code (POS) 24 on the claim to show that the procedure was performed in an ASC.

The carrier pays the "facility" fee from the MPFSDB to the physician. The facility fee is for services done in a facility other than the physician's office and is less then the nonfacility fee for services performed in the physician's office.

90.4—Billing and Payment in a Health Professional Shortage Area (HPSA)

(Rev. 1273; Issued: 06-29-07; Effective/Implementation Dates: 10-01-07)

In accordance with §1833(m) of the Act, physicians who provide covered professional services in any rural or urban HPSA are entitled to an incentive payment. Beginning January 1, 1989, physicians providing services in certain classes of rural HPSAs were entitled to a 5-percent incentive payment. Effective January 1, 1991, physicians providing services in either rural or urban HPSAs are eligible for a 10-percent incentive payment.

Eligibility for receiving the 10 percent bonus payment is based on whether the specific location at which the service is furnished is within an area that is designated (under section 332(a)(1)(A) of the Public Health Services Act) as a HPSA. The Health Resources and Services Administration (HRSA), within the Department of Health & Human Services, is responsible for designating shortage areas.

HRSA designates three types of HPSAs: geographic, population, and facility-based. Geographic-based HPSAs are areas with shortages of primary care physicians, dentists or psychiatrists. Population-based HPSAs are designations based on underserved populations within an area. Facility-based HPSAs are designations based on a public or non-profit private facility that is providing services to an underserved area or population and has an insufficient capacity to meet their needs.

Section 1833(m) of the Social Security Act (the Act) provides incentive payments for physicians who furnish services in areas designated as HPSAs under section 332 (a)(1)(A) of the Public Health Service (PHS) Act. This section of the PHS Act pertains to geographic-based HPSAs. Consequently, Medicare incentive payments are available only in geographic HPSAs.

Although section 1833(m) of the Act provides the authority to recognize the three types of geographic-based HPSAs (primary medical care, dental and mental health), only physicians, including psychiatrists, furnishing services in a primary medical care HPSA are eligible to receive bonus payments. In addition, effective for claims with dates of service on or after July 1, 2004, psychiatrists furnishing services in mental health HPSAs are eligible to receive bonus payments. CMS does not recognize dental HPSAs for the bonus payment program.

It is not enough for the physician merely to have his/her office or primary service location in a HPSA, nor must the beneficiary reside in a HPSA, although frequently this will be the case. The key to eligibility is where the service is actually provided (place of service). For example, a physician providing a service in his/her office, the patient's home, or in a hospital qualifies for the incentive payment as long as the specific location of the service is within an area designated as a HPSA. On the other hand, a physician may have an office in a HPSA but go outside the office (and the designated HPSA area) to provide the service. In this case, the physician would not be eligible for the incentive payment. Carrier responsibilities include:

Informing the physician community of these provisions;
Providing a link to the CMS Web site to access the HPSA automated ZIP code files;
Providing a direct link to HRSA's HPSA database
Modifying the claims processing system to recognize and appropriately handle eligible claims;
Paying physicians the incentive payments; and
Performing post-payment reviews of samples of paid claims submitted using the AQ modifier.

90.4.1 – Provider Education

(Rev. 1273; Issued: 06-29-07; Effective/Implementation Dates: 10-01-07)

Prior to 2005, at the time carriers are notified that an area has been classified (or declassified) as a HPSA, they inform the applicable physician community of the status of the area, the requirements for eligibility for the incentive payment, and the mechanism for claiming payment. To assure that all physicians understand these requirements, carriers publish a general summary bulletin on an annual basis.

Effective January 1, 2005, payment files for the automated payment of the HPSA bonus payment will be developed and updated annually. Once the annual designations are made, no interim changes will be made to the automated payment files to account for HRSA updates to designations throughout the year. New designations and withdrawals of HPSA designations during a calendar year will be included in the next annual update.

For newly designated HPSA areas, physicians will be able to receive the bonus by selfdesignating through the use of the QB or QU modifier for claims with dates of service prior to January 1, 2006. For claims with dates of service on or after January 1, 2006, the AQ modifier (Physician providing a service in a Health Professional Shortage Area (HPSA)) must be submitted. They will also need to submit the modifier for any designated areas not included in the automated file due to the cut off date of the data used. This will only be necessary if the zip code of where they provide their service is not already on the list of zip codes that will automatically receive the bonus payment. Physicians must not continue to self-designate through the use of the modifiers for HPSA designations that are withdrawn during the year, but are not part of the automated files.

Prior to the beginning of each calendar year beginning with 2005, CMS will post on its Web site zip codes that are eligible to automatically receive the bonus payment as well as information on how to determine when the modifier is needed to receive the bonus payment. Through regularly scheduled bulletins and list servs, carriers must notify all physicians to verify their zip code eligibility via the CMS Web site or the HRSA Web site for the area where they provide physician services.

90.4.1.1 – Carrier Web Pages

(Rev. 1273; Issued: 06-29-07; Effective/Implementation Dates: 10-01-07)

Carrier Web pages shall direct the physician community to a direct link to the CMS Web site to access the automated HPSA bonus payment files, and a direct link to the HRSA/HPSA designations database.

90.4.2—HPSA Designations

(Rev. 1273; Issued: 06-29-07; Effective/Implementation Dates: 10-01-07)

HPSA designations are made by the Division of Shortage Designation (DSD) of the Public Health Service (PHS). Prior to January 1, 2005, upon receipt from DSD, CMS sends carriers individual notices of HPSA status changes (initial classification of HPSA areas or deletion of existing ones). Carriers must effectuate these changes as of the first day of the second month after carriers receive them. For example, any notice carriers receive during August is effective for physician services provided on or after October 1. Before effectuating these changes, carriers must ready the system for acceptance of the change and notify all physicians providing services in the impacted area who may be eligible for the incentive payment. Each quarter, CMS also provides carriers with an updated DSD comprehensive listing of all HPSAs in their jurisdiction. Carriers use this listing as a control to assure that all changes are accounted for and effectuated.

Although some HPSAs span entire counties (or other territorial subdivisions within a State), typically, they represent only sections of counties. For partial-county HPSAs, carriers prepare and distribute to physicians local maps which clearly delineate the HPSA areas. Carriers must notify physicians about HPSA areas by:

Publishing a list of HPSAs and allowing physicians to call carriers if they need assistance in determining whether their practice locale falls within the boundaries of a HPSA; and

Issuing maps of partial-county HPSAs that make it easier for physicians to determine if they provide services within designated HPSA areas.

Beginning with 2005, an automated file of designations will be updated on an annual basis and will be effective for services rendered with dates of service on or after January 1 of each calendar year beginning January 1, 2005, through December 31, 2005. Physicians will be allowed to self-designate throughout the year for newly designated HPSAs and HPSAs not included in the automated file based on the date of the data run used to create the file. The bonus will be effective for services rendered on or after the date of designation by HRSA. Designation letters from HRSA will continue to be forwarded from the CMS Central Office to the Regional Offices to send to carriers. Carriers must use the letters when verification is necessary to determine the designation date or removal date of the HPSA bonus payment status. The carriers and standard systems will be provided with a file at the appropriate time prior to the beginning of the calendar year for which it is effective. This file will contain zip codes that fully fall within a HPSA bonus area for both mental health and primary care services. After the implementation of this new process effective January 1, 2005, a recurring update notification will be issued for each annual update. Carriers will be informed of the availability of the file and the file name via an email notice.

Carriers will automatically pay bonuses for services rendered in zip code areas that fully fall within a designated primary care or mental health full county HPSA; are considered to fully fall in the county based on a determination of dominance made by the United States Postal Service (USPS); or are fully within a partial county HPSA area. Should a zip code fall within both a primary care and mental health HPSA, only one bonus will be paid on the service. Bonuses for mental health HPSAs will only be paid when performed by the provider specialty of 26 – psychiatry.

For services rendered in zip code areas that do not fall within a designated full county HPSA; are not considered to fall within the county based on a determination of dominance made by the USPS; are partially within a partial county HPSA; or are designated after the annual update is made to the automated file, physicians must still submit a AQ modifier to receive payment.

To determine whether a modifier is needed, physicians must review the information provided on the CMS Web or the HRSA Web site for HPSA designations to determine if the location where they render services is, indeed, within a HPSA bonus area. Physicians may also base the determinations on letters of designations received from HRSA. They must be prepared to provide these letters as documentation upon the request of the carrier and should verify the eligibility of their area for a bonus with their carrier before submitting services with a HPSA modifier.

For services rendered in zip code areas that cannot automatically receive the bonus, it will be necessary to know the census tract of the area to determine if a bonus should be paid and a modifier submitted. Census tract data can be retrieved by visiting the U.S. Census Bureau website at www.Census.gov or the Federal Financial Institutions Examination Council (FFIEC) website at www.ffiec.gov/geocode/default.htm. Instructions on how to use these web sites can be found on the CMS web site at http://new.cms.hhs.gov/HPSAPSAPhysicianBonuses. Neither CMS nor the Medicare carriers can provide information on the functionality of these Web sites.

90.4.3—Claims Coding Requirements

(Rev. 608, Issued: 07-22-05; Effective: 01-01-06; Implementation: 01-03-06)

For services with dates of service prior to January 1, 2005, physicians must indicate that their services were provided in an incentive-eligible rural or urban HPSA by using one of the following modifiers:

QB—physician providing a service in a rural HPSA; or
QU—physician providing a service in an urban HPSA.

Effective for claims with dates of service on or after January 1, 2006, the QB and QU modifiers will no longer be accepted. Claims with prior dates of service must still be submitted with those modifiers. The AQ modifier, Physician providing a service in a Health Professional Shortage Area (HPSA), will replace the QB and QU modifiers and will be effective for claims with dates of service on or after January 1, 2006.

For services with dates of service on or after January 1, 2005, the bonus will automatically be paid without the submission of a modifier for the following:

- When services are provided in a zip code area that fully falls within a full county HPSA.
- When services are provided in a zip code area that partially falls within a full county HPSA and has been determined to be dominant for the county by the USPS; and
- When services are provided within a zip code that fully falls within a partial county HPSA.

The submission of the QB or QU modifier, or the AQ modifier for claims with dates of service on or after January 1, 2006, will be required for the following:

- When services are provided in zip code areas that do not fully fall within a designated full county HPSA bonus area.
- When services are provided in a zip code area that partially falls within a full county HPSA but is not considered to be in that county based on the dominance decision made by the USPS.
- When services are provided in a zip code area that partially falls within a partial county HPSA.
- When services are provided in a zip code area that was not included in the automated file based on the date of the data run used to create the file.

In order to be considered for the bonus payment, the name, address, and zip code of where the service was rendered must be included on all electronic and paper claims submissions.

90.4.4—Payment

(Rev. 1, 10-01-03)

B3-3350.4

The incentive payment is 10 percent of the amount actually paid, not the approved amount. Carriers pay the incentive payment for services identified on either assigned or unassigned claims.

They do not include the incentive payment with each claim payment. Carriers should:

- Establish a quarterly schedule for issuing incentive payments. These payments are taxable and must be reported to the IRS.
- Prepare a list to accompany each payment. Include a line item for each assigned claim represented in the incentive check and a "summary" item showing the number of unassigned claims represented. The sum of the line items and the "summary" item should equal the amount of the check.

90.4.5—Services Eligible for HPSA and Physician Scarcity Bonus Payments

(Rev. 906, Issued: 04-14-06, Effective: 07-01-06, Implementation: 07-03-06)

A—Information in the Professional Component/Technical Component (PC/TC) Indicator Field of the Medicare Physician Fee Schedule Database

Carriers use the information in the Professional Component/Technical Component (PC/TC) indicator field of the Medicare Physician Fee Schedule Database to identify professional services eligible for HPSA and physician scarcity bonus payments.

The following are the rules to apply in determining whether to pay the bonus on services furnished within a geographic HPSA or physician scarcity bonus area.

Should carriers receive notification from physicians that they have chosen to forego the bonus payments, the carriers shall make no bonus payments to that physician for any service.

PC/TC Indicator	Bonus Payment Policy
0	Pay bonus
1	Globally billed. Only the professional component of this service qualifies for the bonus payment. The bonus cannot be paid on the technical component of globally billed services. ACTION: Effective for claims received prior to October 1, 2005, carriers return the service as unprocessable and notify the physician that the professional component must be re-billed if it is performed within a qualifying bonus area. If the technical component is the only component of the service that was performed in the bonus area, there wouldn't be a qualifying service. Effective for claims received on or after October 1, 2005, carriers shall accept claims with services with a PC/TC indicator of 1 that are eligible for the HPSA or PSA bonus. They shall pay the bonus only on the professional component of the service.
1	Professional Component (modifier 26). Carriers pay the bonus.
1	Technical Component (modifier TC). Carriers do not pay the bonus.
2	Professional Component only. Carriers pay the bonus.
3	Technical Component only. Carriers do not pay the bonus.
4	Global test only. Only the professional component of this service qualifies for the bonus payment. ACTION: Effective for claims received prior to July 1, 2006, carriers return the service as unprocessable. They instruct the provider to re-bill the service as separate professional and technical component procedure codes. Effective for claims received on or after July 1, 2006, except for 93015, carriers shall accept claims with services with a PC/TC indicator of 4 that are eligible for the HPSA or PSA bonus. They shall pay the bonus only on the associated professional component of the service. Since 93015 has two associated professional components, carriers will not be able to make a determination as to which would be the correct component to use to calculate the bonuses. Therefore, carriers shall continue to treat 93015 as unprocessable.
5	Incident to codes. Carriers do not pay the bonus.
6	Laboratory physician interpretation codes. Carriers pay the bonus.
7	Physical therapy service. Carriers do not pay the bonus.
8	Physician interpretation codes. Carriers pay the bonus.
9	Concept of PC/TC does not apply. Carriers do not pay the bonus.

NOTE: Codes that have a status of "X" on the Medicare Physician Fee Schedule Database (MFSDB) have been assigned PC/TC indicator 9 and are not considered physician services for MFSDB payment purposes. Therefore, neither the HPSA bonus payment nor the physician scarcity area will be paid for these codes.

B—Anesthesia Codes (CPT Codes 00100 Through 01999) That Do Not Appear on the MFSDB

Anesthesia codes (CPT codes 00100 through 01999) do not appear on the MFSDB. However, when a medically necessary anesthesia service is furnished within a HPSA or physician scarcity area by a physician, a HPSA bonus and/or physician scarcity bonus is payable.

To claim a bonus payment for anesthesia, physicians bill codes 00100 through 01999 with modifiers QY, QK, AD, AA, or GC to signify that the anesthesia service was performed by a physician along with the QB or QU modifier or the AQ modifier for claims with dates of service on or after January 1, 2006, when required per §90.4.3 or the AR modifier as required per §90.5.3.

C—Mental Health Services

Physicians' professional mental health services rendered by the provider specialty of 26—psychiatry, are eligible for a HPSA bonus when rendered in a mental health HPSA. The service must have a PC/TC designation per the chart above. Should a zip code fall within both a primary care and mental health HPSA, only one bonus must be paid on the service.

90.4.6—Remittance Messages

(Rev. 280, Issued 08-13-04, Effective/Implementation: October 1, 2004 for the analysis and design phases for the MCS Maintainer and Contractors January 1, 2005 for the coding, testing, and implementation phases for the MCS Maintainer and Contractors January 1, 2005 for all phases for the VIPS Maintainers and Contractors)

B3-3350.6

Carriers use the following messages for services on which the HPSA/physician scarcity bonus is claimed.

A - Services Where the HPSA/Physician Scarcity Bonus Can Only Be Paid on a Portion of the Billed Service at the Service/Line Level

Claim adjustment reason code 16, "Claim/service lacks information which is needed for adjudication. Additional information is supplied using remittance advice remarks codes whenever appropriate."

Line level remark code M73, "The HPSA/Physician Scarcity bonus can only be paid on the professional component of this service. Rebill as separate professional and technical components."

B. Services That Are Not Eligible for HPSA/Physician Scarcity Payments at the Service/Line Level

Line level remark code M74, "This service does not qualify for a HPSA/Physician Scarcity bonus payment."

NOTE: This is an informational message only.

90.4.7 – Post-payment Review

(Rev. 608, Issued: 07-22-05; Effective: 01-01-06; Implementation: 01-03-06)

On a post-payment basis, services submitted with the QB or QU modifier, or the AQ modifier for claims with dates of service on or after January 1, 2006, will be subject to validation.

90.4.8—Reporting

(Rev. 1, 10-01-03)

B3-3350.8, B3-13320, B3-13320.1, B3-13322.3

Reporting instructions are included in Chapter 6 of the Medicare Financial Management Manual.

90.4.9—HPSA Incentive Payments for Physician Services Rendered in a Critical Access Hospital (CAH)

(Rev. 608, Issued: 07-22-05; Effective: 01-01-06; Implementation: 01-03-06)

If a CAH electing the Optional Method (Method II) is located within a mental health HPSA, the psychiatrists providing (outpatient) professional services in the CAH are eligible for the Mental Health and Primary Care HPSA bonus payments. When billing for this service, the CAH must bill using Revenue code 961 plus the applicable HCPCS. This Mental Health HPSA bonus will be paid to the CAH on a quarterly basis by the FI. If an area is designated as both a mental health HPSA and a primary medical HPSA, only one 10% bonus will be paid for the service.

Refer to §250.2 in the Claims Processing Manual, Chapter 4 for additional information.

90.4.10 – Administrative and Judicial Review

(Rev. 280, Issued 08-13-04, Effective/Implementation: October 1, 2004 for the analysis and design phases for the MCS Maintainer and Contractors January 1, 2005 for the coding, testing, and implementation phases for the MCS Maintainer and Contractors January 1, 2005 for all phases for the VIPS Maintainers and Contractors)

Per Section 413(b)(1) of the Medicare Prescription Drug, Improvement, and Modernization Act of 2003, there shall be no administrative or judicial review respecting:

- The identification of a county or area;
- The assignment of a specialty of any physician;
- The assignment of a physician to a county; or
- The assignment of a postal zip code to a county or other area.

170—Clinical Psychologist Services

(Rev. 1, 10-01-03)

B3-2150

See Medicare Benefit Policy Manual, Chapter 15, for general coverage requirements.

Direct payment may be made under Part B for professional services. However, services furnished incident to the professional services of CPs to hospital patients remain bundled. Therefore, payment must continue to be made to the hospital (by the FI) for such "incident to" services.

170.1—Payment

(Rev. 1, 10-01-03)

B3-2150, B3-17001.1

All covered therapeutic services furnished by qualified CPs are subject to the outpatient mental health services limitation (i.e., only 62 1/2 percent of expenses for these services are considered incurred expenses for Medicare purposes). The limitation does not apply to diagnostic services. Refer to §210 below for a discussion of the outpatient mental health limitation.

Payment for the services of CPs is made on the basis of a fee schedule or the actual charge, whichever is less, and only on the basis of assignment.

CPs are identified by specialty code 68 and provider type 27. Modifier "AH" is required on CP services.

190—Medicare Payment for Telehealth Services

(Rev. 1, 10-01-03)

A3-3497, A3-3660.2, B3-4159, B3-15516

190.1—Background

(Rev. 1026, Issued: 08-11-06: Effective: 01-01-07; Implementation: 01-02-07)

Section 223 of the Medicare, Medicaid and SCHIP Benefits Improvement and Protection Act of 2000 (BIPA) - Revision of Medicare Reimbursement for Telehealth Services amended §1834 of the Act to provide for an expansion of Medicare payment for telehealth services.

Effective October 1, 2001, coverage and payment for Medicare telehealth includes consultation, office visits, individual psychotherapy, and pharmacologic management delivered via a telecommunications system. Eligible geographic areas include rural health professional shortage areas (HPSA) and counties not classified as a metropolitan statistical area (MSA). Additionally, Federal telemedicine demonstration projects as of December 31, 2000, may serve as the originating site regardless of geographic location.

An interactive telecommunications system is required as a condition of payment; however, BIPA does allow the use of asynchronous "store and forward" technology in delivering these services when the originating site is a Federal telemedicine demonstration program in Alaska or Hawaii. BIPA does not require that a practitioner present the patient for interactive telehealth services.

With regard to payment amount, BIPA specified that payment for the professional service performed by the distant site practitioner (i.e., where the expert physician or practitioner is physically located at time of telemedicine encounter) is equal to what would have been paid without the use of tele-medicine. Distant site practitioners include only a physician as described in §1861(r) of the Act and a medical practitioner as described in §1842(b)(18)(C) of the Act. BIPA also expanded payment under Medicare to include a $20 originating site facility fee (location of beneficiary).

Previously, the Balanced Budget Act of 1997 (BBA) limited the scope of Medicare telehealth coverage to consultation services and the implementing regulation prohibited the use of an asynchronous, 'store and forward' telecommunications system. BBA 1997 also required the professional fee to be shared between the referring and consulting practitioners, and prohibited Medicare payment for facility fees and line charges associated with the telemedicine encounter.

BIPA required that Medicare Part B (Supplementary Medical Insurance) pay for this expansion of telehealth services beginning with services furnished on October 1, 2001.

Time limit for teleconsultation provision.

The teleconsultation provision as authorized by §4206 (a) and (b) of the BBA of 1997 and implemented in 42 CFR 410.78 and 414.65 applies only to teleconsultations provided on or after January 1, 1999, and before October 1, 2001.

190.2—Eligibility Criteria

(Rev. 1, 10-01-03)

1. Beneficiaries eligible for telehealth services

Medicare beneficiaries are eligible for telehealth services only if they are presented from an originating site located in either a rural health professional shortage area (HPSA) as defined by §332(a)(1) (A) of the Public Health Services Act or in a county outside of a MSA as defined by §1886(d)(2)(D) of the Act.

2. Exception to rural HPSA and non MSA geographic requirements

Entities participating in a Federal telemedicine demonstration project that were approved by or were receiving funding from the Secretary of Health and Human Services as of December 31, 2000, qualify as originating sites regardless of geographic location. Such entities are not required to be in a rural HPSA or non- MSA.

3. Originating site defined

The term originating site means the location of an eligible Medicare beneficiary at the time the service being furnished via a telecommunications system occurs. Originating sites authorized by law are listed below:

    The office of a physician or practitioner;
    A hospital (inpatient or outpatient);
    A critical access hospital (CAH);
    A rural health clinic (RHC); and
    A federally qualified health center (FQHC);

For asynchronous, store and forward telecommunications technologies, an originating site is only a Federal telemedicine demonstration program conducted in Alaska or Hawaii.

190.3—List of Medicare Telehealth Services

(Rev. 1277, Issued: 06-29-07, Effective: 01-01-08, Implementation: 01-07-08)

The use of a telecommunications system may substitute for a face-to-face, "hands on" encounter for consultation, office visits, individual psychotherapy, pharmacologic management, psychiatric diagnostic interview examination, end stage renal disease related services, and individual medical nutrition therapy. These services and corresponding current procedure terminology (CPT) or Healthcare Common Procedure Coding System (HCPCS) codes are listed below.

- Consultations (CPT codes 99241 - 99275) - Effective October 1, 2001 – December 31, 2005;
- Consultations (CPT codes 99241 - 99255) - Effective January 1, 2006;
- Office or other outpatient visits (CPT codes 99201 - 99215);
- Individual psychotherapy (CPT codes 90804 - 90809);
- Pharmacologic management (CPT code 90862); and
- Psychiatric diagnostic interview examination (CPT code 90801) – Effective March 1, 2003.
- End Stage Renal Disease (ESRD) related services (HCPCS codes G0308, G0309, G0311, G0312, G0314, G0315, G0317, and G0318) – Effective January 1, 2005.
- Individual Medical Nutrition Therapy (HCPCS codes G0270, 97802, and 97803) (Effective January 1, 2006).
- Neurobehavioral status exam (CPT code 96116) (Effective January 1, 2008).

190.4—Conditions of Payment

(Rev. 1, 10-01-03)

1. Technology

For Medicare payment to occur, interactive audio and video telecommunications must be used, permitting real-time communication between the distant site physician or practitioner and the Medicare beneficiary. As a condition of payment, the patient must be present and participating in the telehealth visit.

2. Exception to the interactive telecommunications requirement

In the case of Federal telemedicine demonstration programs conducted in Alaska or Hawaii, Medicare payment is permitted for telemedicine when asynchronous "store and forward technology" in single or multimedia formats is used as a substitute for an interactive telecommunications system. The originating site and distant site practitioner must be included within the definition of the demonstration program.

3. "Store and forward" defined

For purposes of this instruction, "store and forward" means the asynchronous transmission of medical information to be reviewed at a later time by physician or practitioner at the distant site. A patient's medical information may include, but not limited to, video clips, still images, x-rays, MRIs, EKGs and EEGs, laboratory results, audio clips, and text. The physician or practitioner at the distant site reviews the case without the patient being present. Store and forward substitutes for an interactive encounter with the patient present; the patient is not present in real-time.

NOTE: Asynchronous telecommunications system in single media format does not include telephone calls, images transmitted via facsimile machines and text messages without visualization of the patient (electronic mail). Photographs must be specific to the patients' condition and adequate for rendering or confirming a diagnosis and or treatment plan. Dermatological photographs, e.g., a photograph of a skin lesion, may be considered to meet the requirement of a single media format under this instruction.

4. Telepresenters

A medical professional is not required to present the beneficiary to physician or practitioner at the distant site unless medically necessary. The decision of medical necessity will be made by the physician or practitioner located at the distant site.

190.5—Payment Methodology for Physician/Practitioner at the Distant Site

(Rev. 790, Issued: 12-23-05; Effective: 01-01-06; Implementation: 04-03-06)

1. Distant Site Defined

The term "distant site" means the site where the physician or practitioner, providing the professional service, is located at the time the service is provided via a telecommunications system.

2. Payment Amount (professional fee)

The payment amount for the professional service provided via a telecommunications system by the physician or practitioner at the distant site is equal to the current fee schedule amount for the service provided. Payment for an office visit, consultation, individual psychotherapy or pharmacologic management via a telecommunications system should be made at the same amount as when these services are furnished without the use of a telecommunications system. For Medicare payment to occur, the service must be within a practitioner's scope of practice under State law. The beneficiary is responsible for any unmet deductible amount and applicable coinsurance.

3. Medicare Practitioners Who May Receive Payment at the Distant Site (i.e., at a site other than where beneficiary is)

As a condition of Medicare Part B payment for telehealth services, the physician or practitioner at the distant site must be licensed to provide the service under State law. When the physician or practitioner at the distant site is licensed under State law to provide a covered telehealth service (i.e., professional consultation, office and other outpatient visits, individual psychotherapy, and pharmacologic management) then he or she may bill for and receive payment for this service when delivered via a telecommunications system. If the physician or practitioner at the distant site is located in a critical access hospital (CAH) that has elected Method II, and the physician or practitioner has reassigned his/her benefits to the CAH, the CAH bills its regular FI for the professional services provided at the distant site via a telecommunications system, in any of the revenue codes 096x, 097x or 098x. All requirements for billing distant site telehealth services apply.

4. Medicare Practitioners Who May Bill for Covered Telehealth Services are Listed Below (subject to State law)

Physician.
Nurse practitioner.
Physician assistant.
Nurse-midwife.
Clinical nurse specialist.
Clinical psychologist.*
Clinical social worker.*
Registered dietitian or nutrition professional.

*Clinical psychologists and clinical social workers cannot bill for psychotherapy services that include medical evaluation and management services under Medicare. These practitioners may not bill or receive payment for the following CPT codes: 90805, 90807, and 90809.

190.6—Originating Site Facility Fee Payment Methodology

(Rev. 1026, Issued: 08-11-06: Effective: 01-01-07; Implementation: 01-02-07)

1. Originating site defined

The term originating site means the location of an eligible Medicare beneficiary at the time the service being furnished via a telecommunications system occurs. For asynchronous, store and forward telecommunications technologies, an originating site is only a Federal telemedicine demonstration program conducted in Alaska or Hawaii.

2. Facility fee for originating site (See B, above, for definition of originating site.)

The originating site facility fee is a Part B payment. The contractor pays it outside of the current fee schedule or other payment methodologies (e.g., FIs make payment in addition to the DRG, or OPPS). For telehealth services furnished from October 1, 2001, through December 31, 2002, the originating site fee is the lesser of $20 or the actual charge. For services furnished on or after January 1 of each subsequent year, the Medicare Economic Index (MEI) will update the facility site fee for the originating site annually. This fee is subject to post payment verification.

3. Payment amount:

For telehealth services furnished from October 1, 2001, through December 31, 2002, the payment amount to the originating site is the lesser of the actual charge or the originating site facility fee of $20. The beneficiary is responsible for any unmet deductible amount and Medicare coinsurance. The originating site facility fee payment methodology for each type of facility is clarified below.

Hospital outpatient department. When the originating site is a hospital outpatient department, payment for the originating site facility fee must be made as described above and not under the outpatient prospective payment system. Payment is not based on current fee schedules or other payment methodologies.

Hospital inpatient. For hospital inpatients, payment for the originating site facility fee must be made outside the diagnostic related group (DRG) payment, since this is a Part B benefit, similar to other services paid separately from the DRG payment, (e.g., hemophilia blood clotting factor).

Critical access hospitals. When the originating site is a critical access hospital, make payment as described above, separately from the cost-based reimbursement methodology.

Federally qualified health centers (FQHCs) and rural health clinics (RHCs). The originating site facility fee for telehealth services is not an FQHC or RHC service. When an FQHC or RHC serves as the originating site, the originating site facility fee must be paid separately from the center or clinic all-inclusive rate.

Physicians' and practitioners' offices. When the originating site is a physician's or practitioner's office, the payment amount, in accordance with the law, is the lesser of the actual charge or $20 regardless of geographic location. The carrier shall not apply the geographic practice cost index (GPCI) to the originating site facility fee. This fee is statutorily set and is not subject to the geographic payment adjustments authorized under the physician fee schedule.

To receive the originating facility site fee, the provider submits claims with HCPCS code "Q3014, telehealth originating site facility fee"; short description "telehealth facility fee." The type of service for the telehealth originating site facility fee is "9, other items and services." For carrier-processed claims, the "office" place of service (code 11) is the only payable setting for code Q3014. There is no participation payment differential for code Q3014 and it is not priced off of the MPFS Database file. Deductible and coinsurance rules apply to Q3014. By submitting Q3014 HCPCS code, the originating site authenticates they are located in either a rural HPSA or non-MSA county.

This benefit may be billed on bill types 12X, 13X, 71X, 73X, and 85X. The originating site can be located in a number of revenue centers within a facility, such as an emergency room (0450), operating room (0360), or clinic (0510). Report this service under the revenue center where the service was performed and include HCPCS code "Q3014, telehealth originating site facility fee."

Hospitals and critical access hospitals bill their intermediary for the originating site facility fee. Telehealth bills originating in inpatient hospitals must be submitted on a 12X TOB using the date of discharge as the line item date of service. Independent and provider-based RHCs and FQHCs bill the appropriate intermediary using the RHC or FQHC bill type and billing number. HCPCS code Q3014 is the only non-RHC/FQHC service that is billed using the clinic/center bill type and provider number. All RHCs and FQHCs must use revenue code 078x when billing for the originating site facility fee. For all other non-RHC/FQHC services, provider based RHCs and FQHCs must bill using the base provider's bill type and billing number. Independent RHCs and FQHCs must bill the carrier for all other non-RHC/FQHC services. If an RHC/FQHC visit occurs on the same day as a telehealth service, the RHC/FQHC serving as an originating site must bill for HCPCS code Q3014 telehealth originating site facility fee on a separate revenue line from the RHC/FQHC visit using revenue code 078x.

The beneficiary is responsible for any unmet deductible amount and Medicare coinsurance.

190.6.1—Submission of Telehealth Claims for Distant Site Practitioners

(Rev. 1026, Issued: 08-11-06: Effective: 01-01-07; Implementation: 01-02-07)

Claims for telehealth services are submitted to the contractors that process claims for the performing physician/practitioner's service area. Physicians/practitioners submit the ap-

propriate HCPCS procedure code for covered professional telehealth services along with the "GT" modifier ("via interactive audio and video telecommunications system"). By coding and billing the "GT" modifier with a covered telehealth procedure code, the distant site physician/practitioner certifies that the beneficiary was present at an eligible originating site when the telehealth service was furnished. By coding and billing the "GT" modifier with a covered ESRD-related service telehealth code (HCPCS codes G0308, G0309, G0311, G0312, G0314, G0315, G0317, and G0318), the distant site physician/practitioner certifies that 1 visit per month was furnished face-to-face "hands on" to examine the vascular access site. Refer to Pub. 100-02, Chapter 15, Section 270.4.1 for the conditions of telehealth payment for ESRD-related services.

In situations where a CAH has elected payment Method II for CAH outpatients, and the practitioner has reassigned his/her benefits to the CAH, FIs should make payment for telehealth services provided by the physician or practitioner at 80 percent of the MPFS amount for the distant site service. In all other cases, except for MNT services as discussed in 190.7-Contractor Editing of Telehealth Claims, telehealth services provided by the physician or practitioner at the distant site are billed to the carrier.

Physicians and practitioners at the distant site bill their local Medicare carrier for covered telehealth services, for example, "99245 GT." Physicians' and practitioners' offices serving as a telehealth originating site bill their local Medicare carrier for the originating site facility fee.

190.6.2—Exception for Store and Forward (Noninteractive) Telehealth

(Rev. 1, 10-01-03)

In the case of Federal telemedicine demonstration programs conducted in Alaska or Hawaii, store and forward technologies may be used as a substitute for an interactive telecommunications system. Covered store and forward telehealth services are billed with the "GQ" modifier, "via asynchronous telecommunications system." By using the "GQ" modifier, the distant site physician/practitioner certifies that the asynchronous medical file was collected and transmitted to them at their distant site from a Federal telemedicine demonstration project conducted in Alaska or Hawaii.

190.7—Contractor Editing of Telehealth Claims

(Rev. 997, Issued: 07-07-06; Effective: 01-01-06; Implementation: 08-07-06)

Medicare telehealth services (as listed in section 190.3) are billed with either the "GT" or "GQ" modifier. The contractor shall approve covered telehealth services if the physician or practitioner is licensed under State law to provide the service. Contractors must familiarize themselves with licensure provisions of States for which they process claims and disallow telehealth services furnished by physicians or practitioners who are not authorized to furnish the applicable telehealth service under State law. For example, if a nurse practitioner is not licensed to provide individual psychotherapy under State law, he or she would not be permitted to receive payment for individual psychotherapy under Medicare. The contractor shall install edits to ensure that only properly licensed physicians and practitioners are paid for covered telehealth services.

If a contractor receives claims for professional telehealth services coded with the "GQ" modifier (representing "via asynchronous telecommunications system"), it shall approve/pay for these services only if the physician or practitioner is affiliated with a Federal telemedicine demonstration conducted in Alaska or Hawaii. The contractor may require the physician or practitioner at the distant site to document his or her participation in a Federal telemedicine demonstration program conducted in Alaska or Hawaii prior to paying for telehealth services provided via asynchronous, store and forward technologies.

If a contractor denies telehealth services because the physician or practitioner may not bill for them, the contractor uses MSN message 21.18: "This item or service is not covered when performed or ordered by this practitioner." The contractor uses remittance advice message 52 when denying the claim based upon MSN message 21.18.

If a service is billed with one of the telehealth modifiers and the procedure code is not designated as a covered telehealth service, the contractor denies the service using MSN message 9.4: "This item or service was denied because information required to make payment was incorrect." The remittance advice message depends on what is incorrect, e.g., B18 if procedure code or modifier is incorrect, 125 for submission billing errors, 4-12 for difference inconsistencies. The contractor uses B18 as the explanation for the denial of the claim.

The only claims from institutional facilities that FIs shall pay for telehealth services at the distant site, except for MNT services, are for physician or practitioner services when the distant site is located in a CAH that has elected Method II, and the physician or practitioner has reassigned his/her benefits to the CAH. The CAH bills its regular FI for the professional services provided at the distant site via a telecommunications system, in any of the revenue codes 096x, 097x or 098x. All requirements for billing distant site telehealth services apply.

Claims from hospitals or CAHs for MNT services are submitted to the hospital's or CAH's regular FI. Payment is based on the non-facility amount on the Medicare Physician Fee Schedule for the particular HCPCS codes.

210.1—Application of Limitation

(Rev. 1, 10-01-03)

B3-2472 - 2472.5

A. Status of Patient

The limitation is applicable to expenses incurred in connection with the treatment of an individual who is not an inpatient of a hospital. Thus, the limitation applies to mental health services furnished to a person in a physician's office, in the patient's home, in a skilled nursing facility, as an outpatient, and so forth. The term "hospital" in this context means an institution, which is primarily engaged in providing to inpatients, by or under the supervision of physician(s):

- Diagnostic and therapeutic services for medical diagnosis, treatment and care of injured, disabled, or sick persons;

- Rehabilitation services for injured, disabled, or sick persons; or
- Psychiatric services for the diagnosis and treatment of mentally ill patients.

B. Disorders Subject to Limitation

The term "mental, psychoneurotic, and personality disorders" is defined as the specific psychiatric conditions described in the American Psychiatric Association's (APA) "Diagnostic and Statistical Manual of Mental Disorders, Third Edition - Revised (DSMIII- R)."

When the treatment services rendered are both for a psychiatric condition as defined in the DSM-III-R and one or more nonpsychiatric conditions, separate the expenses for the psychiatric aspects of treatment from the expenses for the nonpsychiatric aspects of treatment. However, in any case in which the psychiatric treatment component is not readily distinguishable from the nonpsychiatric treatment component, all of the expenses are allocated to whichever component constitutes the primary diagnosis.

1. Diagnosis Clearly Meets Definition - If the primary diagnosis reported for a particular service is the same as or equivalent to a condition described in the APA's DSM-III-R, the expense for the service is subject to the limitation except as described in subsection D.
2. Diagnosis Does Not Clearly Meet Definition - When it is not clear whether the primary diagnosis reported meets the definition of mental, psychoneurotic, and personality disorders, it may be necessary to contact the practitioner to clarify the diagnosis. In deciding whether contact is necessary in a given case, give consideration to such factors as the type of services rendered, the diagnosis, and the individual's previous utilization history.

C. Services Subject to Limitation

Carriers apply the limitation to claims for professional services that represent mental health treatment furnished to individuals who are not hospital inpatients by physicians, clinical psychologists, clinical social workers, and other allied health professionals. Items and supplies furnished by physicians or other mental health practitioners in connection with treatment are also subject to the limitation. (The limitation also applies to CORF claims processed by intermediaries.)

Carriers apply the limitation only to treatment services. It does not apply to diagnostic services as described in subsection D. Testing services performed to evaluate a patient's progress during treatment are considered part of treatment and are subject to the limitation.

D. Services Not Subject to Limitation

1. Diagnosis of Alzheimer's Disease or Related Disorder - When the primary diagnosis reported for a particular service is Alzheimer's Disease (coded 331.0 in the "International Classification of Diseases, 9th Revision") or Alzheimer's or other disorders coded 290.XX in the APA's DSM-III-R, carriers look to the nature of the service that has been rendered in determining whether it is subject to the limitation. Typically, treatment provided to a patient with a diagnosis of Alzheimer's Dis-

ease or a related disorder represents medical management of the patient's condition (rather than psychiatric treatment) and is not subject to the limitation. However, when the primary treatment rendered to a patient with such a diagnosis is psychotherapy, it is subject to the limitation.

2. Brief Office Visits for Monitoring or Changing Drug Prescriptions - Brief office visits for the sole purpose of monitoring or changing drug prescriptions used in the treatment of mental, psychoneurotic and personality disorders are not subject to the limitation. These visits are reported using HCPCS code M0064 (brief office visit for the sole purpose of monitoring or changing drug prescriptions used in the treatment of mental, psychoneurotic, and personality disorders). Claims where the diagnosis reported is a mental, psychoneurotic, or personality disorder (other than a diagnosis specified in subsection A) are subject to the limitation except for the procedure identified by HCPCS code M0064.

3. Diagnostic Services - Carriers do not apply the limitation to tests and evaluations performed to establish or confirm the patient's diagnosis. Diagnostic services include psychiatric or psychological tests and interpretations, diagnostic consultations, and initial evaluations.

An initial visit to a practitioner for professional services often combines diagnostic evaluation and the start of therapy. Such a visit is neither solely diagnostic nor solely therapeutic. Therefore, carriers deem the initial visit to be diagnostic so that the limitation does not apply. Separating diagnostic and therapeutic components of a visit is not administratively feasible, unless the practitioner already has separately identified them on the bill. Determining the entire visit to be therapeutic is not justifiable since some diagnostic work must be done before even a tentative diagnosis can be made and certainly before therapy can be instituted. Moreover, the patient should not be disadvantaged because therapeutic as well as diagnostic services were provided in the initial visit. In the rare cases where a practitioner's diagnostic services take more than one visit, carriers do not apply the limitation to the additional visits. However, it is expected such cases are few. Therefore, when a practitioner bills for more than one visit for professional diagnostic services, carriers request documentation to justify the reason for more than one diagnostic visit.

4. Partial Hospitalization Services Not Directly Provided by Physician - The limitation does not apply to partial hospitalization services that are not directly provided by a physician. These services are billed by hospitals and community mental health centers (CMHCs) to intermediaries.

E. Computation of Limitation

Carriers determine the Medicare allowed payment amount for services subject to the limitation. They:

- Multiply this amount by 0.625;
- Subtract any unsatisfied deductible; and,
- Multiply the remainder by 0.8 to obtain the amount of Medicare payment.

The beneficiary is responsible for the difference between the amount paid by Medicare and the full allowed amount.

EXAMPLE A:

A beneficiary is referred to a Medicare participating psychiatrist who performs a diagnostic evaluation that costs $350. Those services are not subject to the limitation, and they satisfy the deductible. The psychiatrist then conducts 10 weekly therapy sessions for which he/she charges $125 each. The Medicare allowed amount is $90 each, for a total of $900.

Apply the limitation by multiplying 0.625 times $900, which equals $562.50.

Apply regular 20 percent coinsurance by multiplying 0.8 times $562.50, which equals $450 (the amount of Medicare payment).

The beneficiary is responsible for $450 (the difference between Medicare payment and the allowed amount).

EXAMPLE B:

A beneficiary was an inpatient of a psychiatric hospital and was discharged on January 1, 1992. During his/her inpatient stay he/she was diagnosed and therapy was begun under a treatment team that included a clinical psychologist. He/she received post-discharge therapy from the psychologist for 12 sessions, at which point the psychologist administered testing that showed the patient had recovered sufficiently to warrant termination of therapy. The allowed amount for the therapy sessions was $80 each, and the amount for the testing was $125, for a total of $1085. All services in 1992 were subject to the limitation, since the diagnosis had been completed in the hospital and the subsequent testing was a part of therapy.

Apply the limitation by multiplying 0.625 times $1085, which gives $678.13.

Since the deductible must be met for 1992, subtract $100 from $678.13, for a remainder of $578.13.

Determine Medicare payment by multiplying the remainder by 0.8, which equals $462.50.

The beneficiary is responsible for $622.50.

100-04 Chapter 13

20—Payment Conditions for Radiology Services

(Rev. 1, 10-01-03)

B3-15022

20.1—Professional Component (PC)

(Rev. 1, 10-01-03)

Carriers must pay for the PC of radiology services furnished by a physician to an individual patient in all settings under the fee schedule for physician services regardless of the specialty of the physician who performs the service. For services furnished to hospital patients, carriers pay only if the services meet the conditions for fee schedule payment and are identifiable, direct, and discrete diagnostic or therapeutic services to an individual patient, such as an interpretation of diagnostic procedures and the PC of therapeutic procedures. The interpretation of a diagnostic procedure includes a written report.

20.2—Technical Component (TC)

(Rev. 1, 10-01-03)

20.2.1—Hospital and Skilled Nursing Facility (SNF) Patients

(Rev. 1221, Issued: 04-18-07, Effective: 04-01-07, Implementation: 04-02-07)

Carriers may not pay for the technical component (TC) of radiology services furnished to hospital patients. Payment for physicians' radiological services to the hospital, e.g., administrative or supervisory services, and for provider services needed to produce the radiology service, is made by the fiscal intermediary (FI) as a provider service.

FIs include the TC of radiology services for hospital inpatients except Critical Access Hospitals (CAH) in the prospective payment system (PPS) payment to hospitals.

Hospital bundling rules exclude payment to suppliers of the Technical Component (TC) of a radiology service for beneficiaries in a hospital inpatient stay. CWF performs reject edits to incoming claims from suppliers of radiology services.

Upon receipt of a hospital inpatient claim at the CWF, CWF searches paid claim history and compares the period between the hospital inpatient admission and discharge dates to the line item service date on a line item TC of a radiology service billed by a supplier. The CWF will generate an unsolicited response when the line item service date falls within the admission and discharge dates of the hospital inpatient claim.

Upon receipt of an unsolicited response, the carrier will adjust the TC of the radiology service and recoup the payment.

For CAHs, payment is made by the FI based on reasonable cost.

Radiology and other diagnostic services furnished to hospital outpatients are paid under the Outpatient Prospective Payment System (OPPS) to the hospital. This applies to bill types 12X and 13X that are submitted to the FI. Effective 4/1/06, type of bill 14X is for non-patient laboratory specimens and is no longer applicable for radiology services.

As a result of SNF Consolidated Billing (Section 4432(b) of the Balanced Budget Act (BBA) of 1997), carriers may not pay for the TC of radiology services furnished to Skilled Nursing Facility (SNF) inpatients during a Part A covered stay. The SNF must bill radiology services furnished its inpatients in a Part A covered stay and payment is included in the SNF Prospective Payment System (PPS).

Radiology services furnished to outpatients of SNFs may be billed by the supplier performing the service or by the SNF under arrangements with the supplier. If billed by the SNF, FIs pay according to the Medicare Physician Fee Schedule. SNFs submit claims to the FI with type of bill 22X or 23X.

20.2.2—Services Not Furnished in Hospitals

(Rev. 1, 10-01-03)

Carriers must pay under the fee schedule for the TC of radiology services furnished to beneficiaries who are not patients of any hospital, and who receive services in a physician's office, a freestanding imaging or radiation oncology center, or other setting that is not part of a hospital.

20.2.3—Services Furnished in Leased Departments

(Rev. 1, 10-01-03)

In the case of procedures furnished in a leased hospital radiology department to a beneficiary who is neither an inpatient nor an outpatient of any hospital, e.g., the patient is referred by an outside physician and is not registered as a hospital outpatient, both the PC and the TC of the services are payable under the fee schedule by the carrier.

20.2.4—Purchased Diagnostic Tests - Carriers

(Rev. 1, 10-01-03)

B3-15048

Section 1842(n) of the Social Security Act (the Act) establishes payment rules for diagnostic tests billed by a physician but performed by an outside supplier. For this purpose, diagnostic tests are tests covered under §1861(s)(3) of the Act other than clinical diagnostic laboratory tests. These include, but are not limited to, such tests as x-rays, EKGs, EEGs, cardiac monitoring, ultrasound, and the technical component of physician pathology services furnished on or after January 1, 1994. (Note that screening mammography services are covered under another provision of the Act and are not subject to the purchased services limitation.) These rules apply to the purchased test itself (the TC) and not to physicians' services associated with the test.

20.2.4.1—Carrier Payment Rules

(Rev. 135, 04-02-04)

If a test is personally performed by a physician or is supervised by a physician, such physician may bill under the normal physician fee schedule rules. This includes situations in which the test is performed or supervised by another physician with whom the billing physician shares a practice. Section 80, chapter 15, of Pub. 100-02, Medicare Benefit Polity, sets forth the various levels of physician supervision required for diagnostic tests. The supervision requirement for physician billing is not met when the test is administered by supplier personnel regardless of whether the test is performed at the physician's office or at another location.

If a physician bills for a diagnostic test performed by an outside supplier, the fee schedule amount for the purchased service equals the lower of the billing physician's fee schedule or the price he or she paid for the service. The lower figure is the fee schedule amount for purposes of the limiting charge. (See §30.3.12.1, chapter 1 of this publication.) The billing physician must identify the supplier (including the supplier's provider number) and the amount the supplier charged the billing physician (net of any discounts). A physician who accepts assignment is permitted to bill and collect from the beneficiary only the applicable deductible and coinsurance for the purchased test. A physician who does not accept assignment is permitted to bill and collect from the beneficiary only the fee schedule amount (as defined above) for the purchased test. The limiting charge provision is not applicable.

If the physician does not identify the supplier and provide the other required information, no payment is allowed, and the physician may not bill the beneficiary any amount for the test.

20.2.4.2—Payment to Physician for Purchased Diagnostic Tests

(Rev. 135, 04-02-04)

A physician or a medical group may submit the claim and (if assignment is accepted) receive the Part B payment, for the technical component of diagnostic tests which the physician or group purchases from an independent physician, medical group, or other supplier. (This claim and payment procedure does not extend to clinical diagnostic laboratory tests.) The purchasing physician or group may be the same physician or group as ordered the tests or may be a different physician or group. An example of the latter situation is when the attending physician orders radiology tests from a radiologist and the radiologist purchases the tests from an imaging center. The purchasing physician or group may not mark up the charge for a test from the purchase price and must accept the lowest of the fee schedule amount if the supplier had billed directly; the physician's actual charge; or the supplier's net charge to the purchasing physician or group, as full payment for the test even if assignment is not accepted.

In order to purchase a diagnostic test, the purchaser must perform the interpretation. The physician or other supplier that furnished the technical component must be enrolled in the Medicare program. No formal reassignment is necessary.

A. Purchased TC Services

Carriers must apply the purchased services limitation to the TC of radiologic services other than screening mammography procedures.

B. Payment to Supplier of Diagnostic Tests for Purchased Interpretations

A person or entity that provides diagnostic tests may submit the claim, and (if assignment is accepted) receive the Part B payment, for diagnostic test interpretations which that person or entity purchases from an independent physician or medical group if:

- The tests are initiated by a physician or medical group which is independent of the person or entity providing the tests and of the physician or medical group providing the interpretations;
- The physician or medical group providing the interpretations does not see the patient; and
- The purchaser (or employee, partner, or owner of the purchaser) performs the technical component of the test. The interpreting physician must be enrolled in the Medicare program. No formal reassignment is necessary.

The purchaser must keep on file the name, the provider identification number and address of the interpreting physician. The rules permitting claims by a facility or clinic for services of an independent contractor physician on the physical premises of the facility or clinic are set forth in Chapter 1.

C. Sanctions

Physicians who knowingly and willfully, in repeated cases, bill Medicare beneficiaries amounts beyond those outlined in this chapter are subject to the penalties contained under §1842(j)(2) of the Act. Penalties are assigned after post-pay review depending on the severity.

D. Questionable Business Arrangements

No special charge or payment constraints are imposed on tests performed by a physician or a technician under the physician's supervision. There are two requirements for all diagnostic tests under §1861(s)(3) of the Act, as implemented by 42 CFR §410.32 and section 10 of chapter13 of this publication and section 80, chapter 15 of Pub. 100-02BP. Namely, the test must be ordered by the treating practitioner, and the test must be supervised by a physician. However, attempts may be made by the medical diagnostic community to adjust or establish arrangements which continue to allow physicians to profit from other's work or by creating the appearance that the physician has performed or supervised his/her technicians who are employed, contracted, or leased. Some of these arrangements may involve cardiac scanning services and mobile ultrasound companies leasing their equipment to physicians for the day the equipment is used, and hiring out their staff to the physicians to meet the supervision requirement.

The bonafides of such arrangements may be suspect and could be an attempt to circumvent the prohibition against the mark-up on purchased diagnostic tests. If you have any doubt that a particular arrangement is a valid relationship where the physician is performing or supervising the services, this should be investigated. The Office of the Inspector General (OIG) has responsibility for investigating violations of §1842(n) of the Act.

Another arrangement to circumvent the purchased diagnostic service provision is for the ordering physician to reassign his/her payment for the interpretation of the test to the supplier. The supplier, in turn, bills for both the test and the interpretation and pays the ordering physician a fee for the interpretation. This arrangement violates §1842(b)(6) of the Act, which prohibits Medicare from paying benefits due the person that furnished the service to any other person, subject to limited exceptions discussed in §3060.D. Also, this arrangement could constitute a violation of §1128 B (b) of the Act, which prohibits remuneration for referrals (i.e., kickbacks).

Violations of §1128B (b) of the Act may subject the physician or supplier to criminal penalties or exclusion from the Medicare and Medicaid programs. Illegal remuneration for referrals can be found even when the ordering physician performs some service for the remuneration.

90—Services of Portable X-Ray Suppliers

(Rev. 1, 10-01-03)

B3-2070.4, B3-15022.G, B3-4131, B3-4831

Services furnished by portable x-ray suppliers may have as many as four components. Carriers must follow the following rules.

90.1—Professional Component

(Rev. 1, 10-01-03)

Pay the PC of radiologic services furnished by portable x-ray suppliers on the same basis as other physician fee schedule services.

90.2—Technical Component

(Rev. 1, 10-01-03)

Pay the TC of radiology services furnished by portable x-ray suppliers under the fee schedule on the same basis as TC services generally.

90.3—Transportation Component (HCPCS Codes R0070 - R0076)

(Rev. 343, Issued: 10-29-04, Effective: 04-01-05, Implementation: 04-04-05)

This component represents the transportation of the equipment to the patient. Establish local RVUs for the transportation R codes based on carrier knowledge of the nature of the service furnished. Carriers shall allow only a single transportation payment for each trip the portable x-ray supplier makes to a particular location. When more than one Medicare patient is x-rayed at the same location, e.g., a nursing home, prorate the single fee schedule transportation payment among all patients receiving the services. For example, if two patients at the same location receive x-rays, make one-half of the transportation payment for each.

R0075 must be billed in conjunction with the CPT radiology codes (7000 series) and only when the x-ray equipment used was actually transported to the location where the x-ray was taken. R0075 would not apply to the x-ray equipment stored in the location where the x-ray was done (e.g., a nursing home) for use as needed.

Below are the definitions for each modifier that must be reported with R0075. Only one of these five modifiers shall be reported with R0075. **NOTE:** If only one patient is served, R0070 should be reported with no modifier since the descriptor for this code reflects only one patient seen.

UN - Two patients served
UP - Three patients served
UQ - Four patients served
UR - Five Patients served
US - Six or more patients served

Payment for the above modifiers must be consistent with the definition of the modifiers. Therefore, for R0075 reported with modifiers, -UN, -UP, -UQ, and –UR, the total payment for the service shall be divided by 2, 3, 4, and 5 respectively. For modifier –US, the total payment for the service shall be divided by 6 regardless of the number of patients served. For example, if 8 patients were served, R0075 would be reported with modifier –US and the total payment for this service would be divided by 6.

The units field for R0075 shall always be reported as "1" except in extremely unusual cases. The number in the units field should be completed in accordance with the provisions of 100-04, chapter 23, section 10.2 item 24 G which defines the units field as the number of times the patient has received the itemized service during the dates listed in the from/to field. The units field must never be used to report the number of patients served during a single trip. Specifically, the units field must reflect the number of services that the specific beneficiary received, not the number of services received by other beneficiaries.

As a carrier priced service, carriers must initially determine a payment rate for portable x-ray transportation services that is associated with the cost of providing the service. In order to determine an appropriate cost, the carrier should, at a minimum, cost out the vehicle, vehicle modifications, gasoline and the staff time involved in only the transportation for a portable x-ray service. A review of the pricing of this service should be done every five years.

Direct costs related to the vehicle carrying the x-ray machine are fully allocable to determining the payment rate. This includes the cost of the vehicle using a recognized depreciation method, the salary and fringe benefits associated with the staff who drive the vehicle, the communication equipment used between the vehicle and the home office, the salary and fringe benefits of the staff who determine the vehicles route (this could be proportional of office staff), repairs and maintenance of the vehicle(s), insurance for the vehicle(s), operating expenses for the vehicles and any other reasonable costs associated with this service as determined by the carrier. The carrier will have discretion for allocating indirect costs (those costs that cannot be directly attributed to portable x-ray transportation) between the transportation service and the technical component of the x-ray tests.

Suppliers may send carriers unsolicited cost information. The carrier may use this cost data as a comparison to its carrier priced determination. The data supplied should reflect a year's worth (either calendar or corporate fiscal) of information. Each provider who submits such data is to be informed that the data is subject to verification and will be used to supplement other information that is used to determine Medicare's payment rate.

Carriers are required to update the rate on an annual basis using independently determined measures of the cost of providing the service. A number of readily available measures (e.g., ambulance inflation factor, the Medicare economic index) that are used by the Medicare program to adjust payment rates for other types of services may be appropriate to use to update the rate for years that the carrier does not recalibrate the payment. Each carrier has the flexibility to identify the index it will use to update the rate. In addition, the carrier can consider locally identified factors that are measured independently of CMS as an adjunct to the annual adjustment.

NOTE: No transportation charge is payable unless the portable x-ray equipment used was actually transported to the location where the x-ray was taken. For example, carriers do not allow a transportation charge when the x-ray equipment is stored in a nursing home for use as needed. However, a set-up payment (see §90.4, below) is payable in such situations. Further, for services furnished on or after January 1, 1997, carriers may not make separate payment under HCPCS code R0076 for the transportation of EKG equipment by portable x-ray suppliers or any other entity.

90.4—Set-Up Component (HCPCS Code Q0092)

(Rev. 1, 10-01-03)

Carriers must pay a set-up component for each radiologic procedure (other than retakes of the same procedure) during both single patient and multiple patient trips under Level II HCPCS code Q0092. Carriers do not make the set-up payment for EKG services furnished by the portable x-ray supplier.

90.5—Transportation of Equipment Billed by a SNF to an FI

(Rev. 716, Issued: 10-21-05; Effective Date: 04-01-06; Implementation Date: 04-03-06)

SNF 533.1.J

When a SNF bills for portable x-ray equipment transported to a site by van or other vehicle, the SNF should bill for the transportation costs using one of the following HCPCS codes along with the appropriate revenue code:

R0070   Transportation of Portable x-ray Equipment and Personnel to Home or Nursing Home, Per Trip to Facility or Location, One Patient Seen.

R0075   Transportation of Portable x-ray Equipment and Personnel to Home of Nursing Home, Per Trip to Facility or Location, More than One Patient Seen, Per Patient.

These HCPCS codes are subject to the fee schedule.

Effective April 1, 2006, SNFs are required to report the appropriate modifiers to identify the number of patients served when billing for R0075. See section 90.3, of this chapter for the list of modifiers used to identify on the claim the number of patients served.

Fiscal intermediaries shall ensure that payment for R0075 is consistent with the definition of the modifiers.

100-04 Chapter 15

50—Carrier Disclosure to Suppliers

(Rev. 1, 10-01-03)

B-02-048

Beginning February 28, 2003, and continuing through 2005 (the transition period) carriers must disclose to each ambulance supplier the supplier's reasonable charge allowance for the forthcoming year (e.g., the full amount that would have been payable under reasonable charge for all ambulance services). Carriers must:

- For each supplier, prepare a reasonable charge disclosure package that includes, at a minimum, the reasonable charge amounts for each procedure code that the supplier is eligible to bill. Carriers do not need to disclose the reasonable charge amount for procedure codes that the supplier does not routinely bill. The disclosure package may include other reasonable charge amounts (e.g., prevailing rate, prevailing IIC, customary charge, customary IIC). However, carriers must indicate the reasonable charge allowed amount, e.g., the principle payment amount of the prevailing, prevailing IIC, customary, or customary IIC, and the corresponding HCPCS code.

- Provide the data for only those procedure codes that apply to each supplier's particular billing method. For Method 2 and Method 3 ambulance suppliers, carriers provide the reasonable charge amounts for codes A0425 through A0436. If providing the reasonable charge amounts for the old HCPCS codes, carriers use A0300 - A0370 and provide a crosswalk to the new codes. For Method 3 and 4 suppliers, carriers also include the applicable item/supply codes (e.g., the reasonable charge amounts for A0384, A0392, A0394, A0396, and A0398).

- Wherever possible, use the new HCPCS codes. They must clearly indicate that the corresponding amounts are the full reasonable charge amounts, e.g., the 100 percent reasonable charge amounts, and specify what portion of the charge is reimbursable within the current transition year. (For 2002, 80 percent of the total reasonable charge amount is reimbursable.) If old or deleted HCPCS codes are used, carriers must include a crosswalk in the disclosure package that maps each HCPCS code to the new replacement procedure code. The crosswalk may be provided as part of the disclosure statement or as a separate insert included as an enclosure with the disclosure.

- Send each supplier its disclosure package in accordance with the timetable specified below. Publication of the reasonable charge disclosure is contingent upon the release of the ambulance inflation factor (AIF). If multiple AIFs are issued in the same calendar year, carriers must prepare a separate disclosure package to notify suppliers of the appropriate amounts and dates of service for each AIF.

- Assure that ambulance suppliers are aware of the ambulance fee schedule yearly payment blend percentages and the location of the ambulance fee schedule on the CMS Web site http://www.cms.hhs.gov/medlearn/refamb.asp.

Carriers must adhere to the following schedule of disclosure activities:

- **For CY 2003, on or before February 28, 2003** - Mail to each ambulance supplier, the supplier's 2002 reasonable charge allowance, updated by the 2003 AIF. If applicable, include a crosswalk that maps each HCPCS code to the new replacement procedure code.

- (**NOTE:** Publication of the reasonable charge disclosure is contingent upon the release of the AIF.)

- **For CY 2004, on or before December 31, 2003** - Mail to each ambulance supplier, the supplier's reasonable charge allowance for 2003, updated by the 2004 AIF. If applicable, include a crosswalk that maps each HCPCS code to the new replacement procedure code.

- (**NOTE:** Publication of the reasonable charge disclosure is contingent upon the release of the AIF.)

- **For CY 2005, on or before December 31, 2004** - Mail to each ambulance supplier, the supplier's reasonable charge allowance for 2004, updated by the 2005 AIF. If applicable, include a crosswalk that maps each HCPCS code to the new replacement procedure code.

- (**NOTE:** Publication of the reasonable charge disclosure is contingent upon the release of the AIF.)

100-04 Chapter 16

10—Background

(Rev. 1, 10-01-03)

B3-2070, B3-2070.1, B3-4110.3, B3-5114

Diagnostic X-ray, laboratory, and other diagnostic tests, including materials and the services of technicians, are covered under the Medicare program. Some clinical laboratory procedures or tests require Food and Drug Administration (FDA) approval before coverage is provided.

A diagnostic laboratory test is considered a laboratory service for billing purposes, regardless of whether it is performed in:

- A physician's office, by an independent laboratory;
- By a hospital laboratory for its outpatients or nonpatients;
- In a rural health clinic; or
- In an HMO or Health Care Prepayment Plan (HCPP) for a patient who is not a member.

When a hospital laboratory performs laboratory tests for nonhospital patients, the laboratory is functioning as an independent laboratory, and still bills the fiscal intermediary (FI). Also, when physicians and laboratories perform the same test, whether manually or with automated equipment, the services are deemed similar.

Laboratory services furnished by an independent laboratory are covered under SMI if the laboratory is an approved Independent Clinical Laboratory. However, as is the case of all diagnostic services, in order to be covered these services must be related to a patient's illness or injury (or symptom or complaint) and ordered by a physician. A small number of laboratory tests can be covered as a preventive screening service.

See the Medicare Benefit Policy Manual, Chapter 15, for detailed coverage requirements.

See the Medicare Program Integrity Manual, Chapter 10, for laboratory/supplier enrollment guidelines.

See the Medicare State Operations Manual for laboratory/supplier certification requirements.

10.1 – Definitions

(Rev. 85, 02-06-04)

B3-2070.1, B3-2070.1.B, RHC-406.4

"Independent Laboratory" - An independent laboratory is one that is independent both of an attending or consulting physician's office and of a hospital that meets at least the requirements to qualify as an emergency hospital as defined in §1861(e) of the Social Security Act (the Act.) (See the Medicare Benefits Policy Manual, Chapter 15, for detailed discussion.)

"Physician Office Laboratory" – A physician office laboratory is a laboratory maintained by a physician or group of physicians for performing diagnostic tests in connection with the physician practice.

"Clinical Laboratory" - See the Medicare Benefits Policy Manual, Chapter 15.

"Qualified Hospital Laboratory" - A qualified hospital laboratory is one that provides some clinical laboratory tests 24 hours a day, 7 days a week, to serve a hospital's emergency room that is also available to provide services 24 hours a day, 7 days a week. For the qualified hospital laboratory to meet this requirement, the hospital must have physicians physically present or available within 30 minutes through a medical staff call roster to handle emergencies 24 hours a day, 7 days a week; and hospital laboratory technologists must be on duty or on call at all times to provide testing for the emergency room.

"Hospital Outpatient" - See the Medicare Benefit Policy Manual, Chapter 2.

"Referring laboratory" - A Medicare-approved laboratory that receives a specimen to be tested and that refers the specimen to another laboratory for performance of the laboratory test.

"Reference laboratory" - A Medicare-enrolled laboratory that receives a specimen from another, referring laboratory for testing and that actually performs the test.

"Billing laboratory" - The laboratory that submits a bill or claim to Medicare.

"Service" - A clinical diagnostic laboratory test. Service and test are synonymous.

"Test" - A clinical diagnostic laboratory service. Service and test are synonymous.

"CLIA" - The Clinical Laboratory Improvement Act and CMS implementing regulations and processes.

"Certification" - A laboratory that has met the standards specified in the CLIA.

"Draw Station' - A place where a specimen is collected but no Medicare-covered clinical laboratory testing is performed on the drawn specimen.

"Medicare-approved laboratory - A laboratory that meets all of the enrollment standards as a Medicare provider including the certification by a CLIA certifying authority.

10.2—General Explanation of Payment

(Rev. 795, Issued: 12-30-05; Effective: 10-01-04; Implementation: 04-03-06)

Outpatient laboratory services can be paid in different ways:

- Physician Fee Schedule;
- Reasonable costs (Critical Access Hospitals (CAH) only);

NOTE : When the CAH bills a 14X bill type as a non-patient laboratory specimen, the CAH is paid under the laboratory fee schedule.

- Laboratory Fee Schedule;
- Outpatient Prospective Payment System, (OPPS) except for most hospitals in the state of Maryland that are subject to waiver; or
- Reasonable Charge

Annually, CMS distributes a list of codes and indicates the payment method. Carriers and FIs pay as directed by this list. Neither deductible nor coinsurance applies to HCPCS codes paid under the laboratory fee schedule; further, deductible and coinsurance do not apply to HCPCS laboratory codes paid via reasonable cost to CAHs. The majority of outpatient laboratory services are paid under the laboratory fee schedule or the OPPS.

Carriers and FIs are responsible for applying the correct fee schedule for payment of clinical laboratory tests. FIs must determine which hospitals meet the criteria for payment at the 62 percent fee schedule. Only sole community hospitals with qualified hospital laboratories are eligible for payment under the 62 percent fee schedule. Generally, payment for diagnostic laboratory tests that are not subject to the clinical laboratory fee schedule is made in accordance with the reasonable charge or physician fee schedule methodologies (or reasonable costs for CAHs).

For Clinical Diagnostic Laboratory services denied due to frequency edits contractors must use standard health care adjustment reason code 151—"Payment adjusted because the payer deems the information submitted does not support this many services."

60—Specimen Collection Fee and Travel Allowance

(Rev. 1, 10-01-03)

B3-5114.1

60.1—Specimen Collection Fee

(Rev. 1, 10-01-03)

B3-5114.1, A3-3628

In addition to the amounts provided under the fee schedules, the Secretary shall provide for and establish a nominal fee to cover the appropriate costs of collecting the sample on which a clinical laboratory test was performed and for which payment is made with respect to samples collected in the same encounter.

A specimen collection fee is allowed in circumstances such as drawing a blood sample through venipuncture (i.e., inserting into a vein a needle with syringe or vacutainer to draw the specimen) or collecting a urine sample by catheterization. A specimen collection fee is not allowed for blood samples where the cost of collecting the specimen is minimal (such as a throat culture or a routine capillary puncture for clotting or bleeding time). This fee will not be paid to anyone who has not extracted the specimen. Only one collection fee is allowed for each type of specimen for each patient encounter, regardless of the number of specimens drawn. When a series of specimens is required to complete a single test (e.g., glucose tolerance test), the series is treated as a single encounter.

60.1.1—Physician Specimen Drawing

(Rev. 1, 10-01-03)

HO-437, A3-3628, B3-5114.1

Medicare allows a specimen collection fee for physicians only when (1) it is the accepted and prevailing practice among physicians in the locality to make separate charges for drawing or collecting a specimen, and (2) it is the customary practice of the physician performing such services to bill separate charges for drawing or collecting the specimen.

60.1.2—Independent Laboratory Specimen Drawing

(Rev. 1, 10-01-03)

B3-4110.4, HO-437, A3-3628

Medicare allows separate charges made by laboratories for drawing or collecting specimens whether or not the specimens are referred to hospitals or independent laboratories. The laboratory does not bill for routine handling charges where a specimen is referred by one laboratory to another.

Medicare allows a specimen collection fee when it is medically necessary for a laboratory technician to draw a specimen from either a nursing home patient or homebound patient. The technician must personally draw the specimen, e.g., venipuncture or urine sample by catheterization. Medicare does not allow a specimen collection fee to the visiting technician if a patient in a facility is (a) not confined to the facility, or (b) the facility has personnel on duty qualified to perform the specimen collection. Medical necessity for such services exists, for example, where a laboratory technician draws a blood specimen from a homebound or an institutionalized patient. A patient need not be bedridden to be homebound. However, where the specimen is a type that would require only the services of a messenger and would not require the skills of a laboratory technician, e.g., urine or sputum, a specimen pickup service would not be considered medically necessary. (See Chapters 7 and 15 of the Medicare Benefit Policy Manual for a discussion of "homebound" and a more complete definition of a medically necessary laboratory service to a homebound or an institutional patient.)

In addition to the usual information required on claim forms (including the name of the prescribing physician), all independent laboratory claims for such specimen drawing or EKG services prescribed by a physician should be appropriately annotated, e.g., "patient confined to home," "patient homebound," or "patient in nursing home, no qualified person on duty to draw specimen." Carriers must assure the validity of the annotation through scientific claims samples as well as through regular bill review techniques. (This could be done by use of the information in carrier files, and where necessary, contact with the prescribing physician.)

If a physician requests an independent laboratory to obtain specimens in situations which do not meet, or without regard to whether they meet, the medical necessity criteria in Chapter 15 of the Medicare Benefit Policy Manual, an educational contact with the prescribing physician is warranted and, where necessary, corroborating documentation should be obtained on claims until the carrier is assured that the physician prescribes such services only when the criteria are met.

60.1.3—Specimen Drawing for Dialysis Patients

(Rev. 1, 10-01-03)

A3 3644.1, PR 2711.1, B3-4270.2, PUB-29 322

See the Medicare Benefit Policy Manual, Chapter 11, for a description of laboratory services included in the composite rate.

Independent laboratories and independent dialysis facilities with the appropriate clinical laboratory certification in accordance with CLIA may be paid for ESRD clinical laboratory tests that are separately billable. The laboratories and independent dialysis facilities are paid for separately billable clinical laboratory tests according to the Medicare laboratory fee schedule for independent laboratories. Independent dialysis facilities billing for separately billable laboratory tests that they perform must submit claims to the FI. Independent laboratories must bill the carrier.

Hospital-based laboratories providing laboratory service to hospital dialysis patients of the hospital's dialysis facility are paid in accordance with the outpatient laboratory provisions. However, where the hospital laboratory does tests for an independent dialysis facility or for another hospital's facility, the nonpatient billing provisions apply (see §20.1).

Clinical laboratory tests can be performed individually or in pre-determined groups on automated profile equipment. A specimen collection fee determined by CMS (as of this writing, up to $3.00) will be allowed only in the following circumstances:

- Drawing a blood sample through venipuncture (i.e., inserting into a vein a needle with a syringe or vacutainer to draw the specimen).
- Collecting a urine sample by catheterization.

Special rules apply when such services are furnished to dialysis patients. The specimen collection fee is not separately payable for y patients dialyzed in the facility or for patients dialyzed at home under reimbursement Method I. Payment for this service is included under the ESRD composite rate, regardless of whether the laboratory test itself is included in the composite rate or is separately billable.

Fees for taking specimens from home dialysis patients, who have elected reimbursement Method II may be paid separately, provided all other criteria for payment are met. Also, fees for taking specimens in the hospital setting, but outside of the dialysis unit, for use in performing laboratory tests not included in the ESRD composite rate may be paid separately.

60.1.4—Coding Requirements for Specimen Collection

(Rev. 1, 10-01-03)

The following HCPCS codes and terminology must be used:

- G0001—Routine venipuncture for collection of specimen(s).
- P9615—Catheterization for collection of specimen(s).

The allowed amount for specimen collection in each of the above circumstances is included in the laboratory fee schedule distributed annually by CMS.

60.2—Travel Allowance

(Rev. 1584, Issued: 09-05-08, Effective: 07-01-08, Implementation: 10-06-08)

HO-437, A3-3628.F, B3-5114.1K; PM-AB-99-49

In addition to a specimen collection fee allowed under §60.1, Medicare, under Part B, covers a specimen collection fee and travel allowance for a laboratory technician to draw a specimen from either a nursing home patient or homebound patient under §1833(h)(3) of the Act and payment is made based on the clinical laboratory fee schedule. The travel allowance is intended to cover the estimated travel costs of collecting a specimen and to reflect the technician's salary and travel costs.

The additional allowance can be made only where a specimen collection fee is also payable, i.e., no travel allowance is made where the technician merely performs a messenger service to pick up a specimen drawn by a physician or nursing home personnel. The travel allowance may not be paid to a physician unless the trip to the home, or to the nursing home was solely for the purpose of drawing a specimen. Otherwise travel costs are considered to be associated with the other purposes of the trip.

The travel allowance is not distributed by CMS. Instead, the carrier must calculate the travel allowance for each claim using the following rules for the particular Code. The following HCPCS codes are used for travel allowances:

Per Mile Travel Allowance (P9603)

- The minimum "per mile travel allowance" is $1.035. The per mile travel allowance is to be used in situations where the average trip to patients' homes is longer than 20 miles round trip, and is to be pro-rated in situations where specimens are drawn or picked up from non-Medicare patients in the same trip.—one way, in connection with medically necessary laboratory specimen collection drawn from homebound or nursing home bound patient; pro-rated miles actually traveled (carrier allowance on per mile basis); or
- The per mile allowance was computed using the Federal mileage rate plus an additional 44 cents a mile to cover the technician's time and travel costs. Contractors have the option of establishing a higher per mile rate in excess of the minimum ($1.035 a mile in cy 2000) if local conditions warrant it. The minimum mileage rate will be reviewed and updated in conjunction with the clinical lab fee schedule as needed. At no time will the laboratory be allowed to bill for more miles than are reasonable or for miles not actually traveled by the laboratory technician.

Example 1: In CY 2000, a laboratory technician travels 60 miles round trip from a lab in a city to a remote rural location, and back to the lab to draw a single Medicare patient's blood. The total reimbursement would be $62.10 (60 miles × $1.035 a mile), plus the specimen collection fee of $3.00.

Example 2: In CY 2000, a laboratory technician travels 40 miles from the lab to a Medicare patient's home to draw blood, and then travels an additional 10 miles to a non-Medicare patient's home and then travels 30 miles to return to the lab. The total miles traveled would be 80 miles. The claim submitted would be for one half of the miles traveled or $41.40 (40 × $1.035), plus the specimen collection fee of $3.00.

Flat Rate (P9604)

The CMS will pay a minimum of $9.55 one way flat rate travel allowance. The flat rate travel allowance is to be used in areas where average trips are less than 20 miles round trip. The flat rate travel fee is to be pro-rated for more than one blood drawn at the same address, and for stops at the homes of Medicare and non-Medicare patients. The laboratory does the pro-ration when the claim is submitted based on the number of patients seen on that trip. The specimen collection fee will be paid for each patient encounter.

This rate is based on an assumption that a trip is an average of 15 minutes and up to 10 miles one way. It uses the Federal mileage rate and a laboratory technician's time of $17.66 an hour, including overhead. Contractors have the option of establishing a flat rate in excess of the minimum of $9.55, if local conditions warrant it. The minimum national flat rate will be reviewed and updated in conjunction with the clinical laboratory fee schedule, as necessitated by adjustments in the Federal travel allowance and salaries.

The claimant identifies round trip travel by use of the LR modifier

Example 3: A laboratory technician travels from the laboratory to a single Medicare patient's home and returns to the laboratory without making any other stops. The flat rate would be calculated as follows: 2 × $9.55 for a total trip reimbursement of $19.10, plus the specimen collection fee.

Example 4: A laboratory technician travels from the laboratory to the homes of five patients to draw blood, four of the patients are Medicare patients and one is not. An additional flat rate would be charged to cover the 5 stops and the return trip to the lab (6 × $9.55 = $57.30). Each of the claims submitted would be for $11.46 ($57.30/5 = $11.46). Since one of the patients is non-Medicare, four claims would be submitted for $11.46 each, plus the specimen collection fee for each.

Example 5: A laboratory technician travels from a laboratory to a nursing home and draws blood from 5 patients and returns to the laboratory. Four of the patients are on Medicare and one is not. The $9.55 flat rate is multiplied by two to cover the return trip to the laboratory (2 × $9.55 = $19.10) and then divided by five (1/5 of $19.10 = $3.82). Since one of the patients is non-Medicare, four claims would be submitted for $3.82 each, plus the specimen collection fee.

If a carrier determines that it results in equitable payment, the carrier may extend the former payment allowances for additional travel (such as to a distant rural nursing home) to all circumstances where travel is required. This might be appropriate, for example, if the carrier's former payment allowance was on a per mile basis. Otherwise, it should establish an appropriate allowance and inform the suppliers in its service area. If a carrier decides to establish a new allowance, one method is to consider developing a travel allowance consisting of:

- The current Federal mileage allowance for operating personal automobiles, plus a personnel allowance per mile to cover personnel costs based upon an estimate of average hourly wages and average driving speed.

Carriers must prorate travel allowance amounts claimed by suppliers by the number of patients (including Medicare and non-Medicare patients) from whom specimens were drawn on a given trip.

The carrier may determine that payment in addition to the routine travel allowance determined under this section is appropriate if:

- the patient from whom the specimen must be collected is in a nursing home or is homebound; and
- the clinical laboratory tests are needed on an emergency basis outside the general business hours of the laboratory making the collection.

110.4—Carrier Contacts With Independent Clinical Laboratories

(Rev. 1, 10-01-03)

B3-2070.1.F

An important role of the carrier is as a communicant of necessary information to independent clinical laboratories. Failure to inform independent laboratories of Medicare regulations and claims processing procedures may have an adverse effect on prosecution of laboratories suspected of fraudulent activities with respect to tests performed by, or billed on behalf of, independent laboratories. United States Attorneys often must prosecute under a handicap or may refuse to prosecute cases where there is no evidence that a laboratory has been specifically informed of Medicare regulations and claims processing procedures.

To assure that laboratories are aware of Medicare regulations and carrier's policy, notification must be sent to independent laboratories when any changes are made in coverage policy or claims processing procedures. Additionally, to completely document efforts to fully inform independent laboratories of Medicare policy and the laboratory's responsibilities, previously issued newsletters should be periodically re-issued to remind laboratories of existing requirements.

Some items which should be discussed are the requirements to have the same charges for Medicare and private patients, to document fully the medical necessity for collection of specimens from a skilled nursing facility or a beneficiary's home, and, in cases when a laboratory service is referred from one independent laboratory to another independent laboratory, to identify the laboratory actually performing the test.

Additionally, when carrier professional relations representatives make personal contacts with particular laboratories, they should prepare and retain reports of contact indicating dates, persons present, and issues discussed.

100-04 Chapter 17

80.1—Oral Cancer Drugs

(Rev. 1, 10-01-03)

A3 3660.13, SNF 536.1

Effective January 1, 1994, oral self administered versions of covered injectable cancer drugs furnished may be paid if other coverage requirements are met. To be covered the drug must have had the same active ingredient as the injectable drug. Effective January 1, 1999, this coverage was expanded to include FDA approved Prodrugs used as anticancer drugs. A Prodrug may have a different chemical composition than the injectable drug but body metabolizing of the Prodrug results in the same chemical composition in the body.

80.1.1—HCPCS Service Coding for Oral Cancer Drugs

(Rev. 1, 10-01-03)

The following codes may be used for drugs other than Prodrugs, when covered:

Generic/Chemical Name	How Supplied	HCPCS
Busulfan	2 mg/ORAL	J8510
Capecitabine	150mg/ORAL	J8520
Capecitabine	500mg/ORAL	J8521
Methotrexate	2.5 mg/ORAL	J8610
Cyclophosphamide *	25 mg/ORAL	J8530
Cyclophosphamide * (Treat 50 mg. as 2 units	50 mg/ORAL	J8530
Etoposide	50 mg/ORAL	J8560
Melphalan	2 mg/ORAL	J8600
Prescription Drug chemotherapeutic NOC	ORAL	J8999

Each tablet or capsule is equal to one unit, except for 50 mg./ORAL of cyclophosphamide (J8530), which is shown as 2 units. The 25m and 50 mg share the same code.

NOTE: HIPAA requires that drug claims submitted to DMERCs be identified by NDC.

80.1.2—HCPCS and NDC Reporting for Prodrugs

(Rev. 136, 04-09-04)

FI claims

For oral anti-cancer Prodrugs HCPCS code J8999 is reported with revenue code 0636.

DMERC claims

The supplier reports the NDC code on the claim. The DMERC converts the NDC code to a "WW" HCPCS code for CWF. As new "WW" codes are established for oral anticancer drugs they will be communicated in a Recurring Update Notification.

80.3.1—Requirements for Billing FI for Immunosuppressive Drugs

(Rev. 1, 10-01-03)

Hospitals not subject to OPPS bill on a Form CMS-1450 with bill type 12x (hospital inpatient Part B) or l3x (hospital outpatient) as appropriate. For claims with dates of service prior to April 1, 2000, providers report the following entries:

- Occurrence code 36 and date in FL 32-35;
- Revenue code 0250 in FL 42; and
- Narrative description in FL 43.

For claims with dates of service on or after April 1, 2000, hospitals report

- Occurrence code 36 and date in FL 32-35;
- Revenue code 0636 in FL 42;
- HCPCS code of the immunosuppressive drug in FL 44; and
- Number of units in FL 46 (the number of units billed must accurately reflect the definition of one unit of service in each code narrative. E.g.: If fifty 10-mg. Prednisone tablets are dispensed, the hospital bills J7506, 100 units (1 unit of J7506 = 5 mg.).

The hospital completes the remaining items in accordance with regular billing instructions.

100-04 Chapter 18

90—Diabetes Screening

(Rev. 457, Issued: 01-28-05, Effective: 04-01-05, Implementation: 04-04-05)

90.1—HCPCS Coding for Diabetes Screening

(Rev. 457, Issued: 01-28-05, Effective: 04-01-05, Implementation: 04-04-05)

The following HCPCS codes are to be billed for diabetes screening:

82947 – Glucose, quantitative, blood (except reagent strip)
82950 – post-glucose dose (includes glucose)
82951 – tolerance test (GTT), three specimens (includes glucose)

90.2—Carrier Billing Requirements

(Rev. 457, Issued: 01-28-05, Effective: 04-01-05, Implementation: 04-04-05)

Effective for dates of service January 1, 2005 and later, carriers shall recognize the above HCPCS codes for diabetes screening.

Carriers shall pay for diabetes screening once every 12 months for a beneficiary that is not pre-diabetic. Carriers shall pay for diabetes screening at a frequency of once every 6 months for a beneficiary that meets the definition of pre-diabetes.

A claim that is submitted for diabetes screening by a physician or supplier for a beneficiary that does not meet the definition of pre-diabetes shall be submitted in the following manner:

The line item shall contain 82947, 82950 or 82951 with a diagnosis code of V77.1 reported in the header.

90.2.1—Modifier Requirements for Pre-diabetes

(Rev. 457, Issued: 01-28-05, Effective: 04-01-05, Implementation: 04-04-05)

A claim that is submitted for diabetes screening and the beneficiary meets the definition of pre-diabetes shall be submitted in the following manner:

The line item shall contain 82497, 82950 or 82951 with a diagnosis code of V77.1 reported in the header. In addition, modifier "TS" (follow-up service) – shall be reported on the line item.

90.3—Fiscal Intermediary (FI) Billing Requirements

(Rev. 457, Issued: 01-28-05, Effective: 04-01-05, Implementation: 04-04-05)

Effective for dates of service January 1, 2005 and later, FIs shall recognize the above HCPCS codes for diabetes screening.

FIs shall pay for diabetes screening once every 12 months for a beneficiary that is not pre-diabetic. FIs shall pay for diabetes screening at a frequency of once every 6 months for a beneficiary that meets the definition of pre-diabetes.

A claim that is submitted for diabetes screening by a physician or supplier for a beneficiary that does not meet the definition of pre-diabetes shall be submitted in the following manner:

The line item shall contain 82947, 82950 or 82951 with a diagnosis code of V77.1.

90.3.1—Modifier Requirements for Pre-diabetes

(Rev. 457, Issued: 01-28-05, Effective: 04-01-05, Implementation: 04-04-05)

A claim that is submitted for diabetes screening and the beneficiary meets the definition of pre-diabetes shall be submitted in the following manner:

The line item shall contain 82497, 82950 or 82951 with a diagnosis code of V77.1. In addition, modifier "TS" (follow-up service) – shall be reported on the line item.

90.4—Diagnosis Code Reporting

(Rev. 457, Issued: 01-28-05, Effective: 04-01-05, Implementation: 04-04-05)

A claim that is submitted for diabetes screening shall include the diagnosis code V77.1.

90.5—Medicare Summary Notices

(Rev. 457, Issued: 01-28-05, Effective: 04-01-05, Implementation: 04-04-05)

When denying claims for diabetes screening based upon a CWF reject for 82947, 82950 or 82951 reported with diagnosis code V77.1, contractors shall use MSN 18.4, "This service is being denied because it has not been 6 months since your last examination of this kind." (See chapter 30 section 40.3.6.4(c) for additional information on ABN's.)

90.6—Remittance Advice Remark Codes

(Rev. 457, Issued: 01-28-05, Effective: 04-01-05, Implementation: 04-04-05)

Contractors shall use the appropriate remittance advice notice that appropriately explains the denial of payment.

90.7—Claims Adjustment Reason Codes

(Rev. 457, Issued: 01-28-05, Effective: 04-01-05, Implementation: 04-04-05)

Contractors shall use the appropriate claims adjustment reason code such as 119 "Benefit maximum for this time period or occurrence has been reached."

100-04 Chapter 20

30.6—Oxygen and Oxygen Equipment

(Rev. 1, 10-01-03)

For oxygen and oxygen equipment, contractors pay a monthly fee schedule amount per beneficiary. Unless otherwise noted below, the fee covers equipment, contents and supplies. Payment is not made for purchases of this type of equipment.

When an inpatient is not entitled to Part A, payment may not be made under Part B for DME or oxygen provided in a hospital or SNF. (See the Medicare Benefit Policy Manual, Chapter 15) Also, for outpatients using equipment or receiving oxygen in the hospital or SNF and not taking the equipment or oxygen system home, the fee schedule does not apply.

There are a number of billing considerations for oxygen claims. The chart in §130.6 indicates what amounts are payable under which situations.

30.6.1—Adjustments to Monthly Oxygen Fee

(Rev. 1, 10-01-03)

If the prescribed amount of oxygen is less than 1 liter per minute, the fee schedule amount for stationary oxygen rental is reduced by 50 percent.

The fee schedule amount for stationary oxygen equipment is increased under the following conditions. If both conditions apply, contractors use the higher of either of the following add-ons. Contractors may not pay both add-ons:

a. Volume Adjustment - If the prescribed amount of oxygen for stationary equipment exceeds 4 liters per minute, the fee schedule amount for stationary oxygen rental is increased by 50 percent. If the prescribed liter flow for stationary oxygen is different than for portable or different for rest and exercise, contractors use the prescribed amount for stationary systems and for patients at rest. If the prescribed liter flow is different for day and night use, contractors use the average of the two rates.

b. Portable Add-on - If portable oxygen is prescribed, the fee schedule amount for portable equipment is added to the fee schedule amount for stationary oxygen rental.

30.6.2—Purchased Oxygen Equipment

(Rev. 1, 10-01-03)

Contractors may not pay for oxygen equipment that is purchased on or after June 1, 1989.

30.6.3—Contents Only Fee

(Rev. 1, 10-01-03)

Where the beneficiary owns stationary liquid or gaseous oxygen equipment, the contractor pays the monthly oxygen contents fee. For owned oxygen concentrators, however, contractors do not pay a contents fee.

Where the beneficiary either owns a concentrator or does not own or rent a stationary gaseous or liquid oxygen system and has either rented or purchased a portable system, contractors pay the portable oxygen contents fee.

30.6.4—DMEPOS Clinical Trials and Demonstrations

(Rev. 961, Issued: 05-26-06; Effective: 03-20-06; Implementation: 10-03-06)

The definition of the QR modifier is "item or service has been provided in a Medicare specified study." When this modifier is attached to a HCPCS code, it generally means the service is part of a CMS related clinical trial, demonstration or study.

- The DMERCs shall recognize the "QR" modifier when associated with an oxygen home therapy clinical trial identified by CMS and sponsored by the National Heart, Lung & Blood Institute. DMERCs shall pay these claims if the patient's arterial oxygen partial measurements are from 56 to 65 mmHg, or whose oxygen saturation is at or above 89%.

The definition of condition code 30 is "qualified clinical trial." When this condition code is reported on a claim, it generally means the service is part of a CMS related clinical trial, demonstration or study.

The RHHIs shall recognize condition code 30, accompanied by ICD-9-CM diagnosis code V70.7 in the second diagnosis code position, when associated with an oxygen home therapy clinical trial identified by CMS and sponsored by the National Heart, Lung & Blood Institute. RHHIs shall pay these claims if the patient's arterial oxygen partial measurements are from 56 to 65 mmHg, or whose oxygen saturation is at or above 89%.

40.1—General

(Rev. 1, 10-01-03)

B3-5102.2.G, B3-5102.3

Contractors pay for maintenance and servicing of purchased equipment in the following classes:

- inexpensive or frequently purchased,
- customized items, other prosthetic and orthotic devices, and
- capped rental items purchased in accordance with §30.5.2 or §30.5.3.

They do not pay for maintenance and servicing of purchased items that require frequent and substantial servicing, or oxygen equipment. (Maintenance and servicing may be paid for purchased items in these two classes if they were purchased prior to June 1, 1989). Reasonable and necessary charges include only those made for parts and labor that are not otherwise covered under a manufacturer's or supplier's warranty. Contractors pay on a lump-sum, as needed basis based on

their individual consideration for each item. Payment may not be made for maintenance and servicing of rented equipment other than maintenance and servicing for PEN pumps (under the conditions of §40.3) or the maintenance and servicing fee established for capped rental items in §40.2.

Servicing of equipment that a beneficiary is purchasing or already owns is covered when necessary to make the equipment serviceable. The service charge may include the use of "loaner" equipment where this is required. If the expense for servicing exceeds the estimated expense of purchasing or renting another item of equipment for the remaining period of medical need, no payment can be made for the amount of the excess. Contractors investigate and deny cases suggesting malicious damage, culpable neglect or wrongful disposition of equipment as discussed in BPM Chapter 15 where they determine that it is unreasonable to make program payment under the circumstances. Such cases are referred to the program integrity specialist in the RO.

100.2—Certificates of Medical Necessity (CMN)

(Rev. 1, 10-01-03)

B3-3312

For certain items or services billed to the DME Regional Carrier (DMERC), the supplier must receive a signed Certificate of Medical Necessity (CMN) from the treating physician. CMNs are not required for the same items when billed by HHAs to RHHIs. Instead, the items must be included in the physician's signed orders on the home health plan of care. See the Medicare Program Integrity Manual, Chapter 6.

The FI will inform other providers (see §01 for definition pf provider) of documentation requirements.

Contractors may ask for supporting documentation beyond a CMN.

Refer to the local DMERC Web site described in §10 for downloadable copies of CMN forms.

See the Medicare Program Integrity Manual, Chapter 5, for specific Medicare policies and instructions on the following topics:

- Requirements for supplier retention of original CMNs
- CMN formats, paper and electronic
- List of currently approved CMNs and items requiring CMNs
- Supplier requirements for submitting CMNs
- Requirements for CMNs to also serve as a physician's order
- Civil monetary penalties for violation of CMN requirements
- Supplier requirements for completing portions of CMNs
- Physician requirements for completing portions of CMNs

100.2.1—Completion of Certificate of Medical Necessity Forms

(Rev. 1, 10-01-03)

1. SECTION A: (This may be completed by supplier.)
   a. Certification Type/Date - If this is an initial certification for this patient, the date (MM/DD/YY) is indicated in the space marked "INITIAL". If this is a revised certifi-

cation (to be completed when the physician changes the order, based on the patient's changing clinical needs), the initial date is indicated in the space marked "INITIAL", and the revision date is indicated in the space marked "REVISED". If this is a recertification, the initial date is indicated in the space marked "INITIAL", and the recertification date is indicated in the space marked "RECERTIFICATION". Whether a REVISED or RECERTIFIED CMN is submitted, the INITIAL date as well as the REVISED or RECERTIFICATION date is always furnished.

b. Patient Information - This indicates the patient's name, permanent legal address, telephone number, and his/her health insurance claim number (HICN) as it appears on his/her Medicare card and on the claim form.

c. Supplier Information - This indicates the name of the company (supplier name), address, telephone number, and the Medicare supplier number assigned by the National Supplier Clearinghouse (NSC).

d. Place of Service - This indicates the place in which the item is being used, i.e., patient's home is 12, skilled nursing facility (SNF) is 31, or end stage renal disease (ESRD) facility is 65. See chapter 23 for place of service codes.

e. Facility Name - This indicates the name and complete address of the facility, if the place of service is a facility.

f. HCPCS Codes - This is a list of all HCPCS procedure codes for items ordered that require a CMN. Procedure codes that do not require certification are not listed on the CMN.

g. Patient Date of Birth (DOB), Height, Weight, and Sex - This indicates patient's DOB (MM/DD/YY), height in inches, weight in pounds, and sex (male or female).

h. Physician Name and Address - This indicates the treating physician's name and complete mailing address.

i. UPIN - This indicates the treating physician's unique physician identification number (UPIN).

j. Physician's Telephone Number - This indicates the telephone number where the treating physician can be contacted (preferably where records would be accessible pertaining to this patient) if additional information is needed.

2. SECTION B: (This may not be completed by the supplier. While this section may be completed by a non-physician clinician, or a physician employee, it must be reviewed by the treating physician. Contractors publish this requirement about section B in their bulletins at least annually.)

a. Estimated Length of Need - This indicates the estimated length of need (the length of time (in months) the physician expects the patient to require use of the ordered item). If the treating physician expects that the patient will require the item for the duration of his/her life, 99 is entered. For recertification and revision CMNs, the cumulative length of need (the total length of time in months from the initial date of need) is entered.

b. Diagnosis Codes - Listed in the first space is the ICD-9 code that represents the primary reason for ordering this item. Additional ICD-9 codes that would further describe the medical need for the item (up to 3 codes) are also listed. A given CMN may have more than one item billed, and for each item, the primary reason for ordering may be different. For example, a CMN is submitted for a manual wheelchair (K0001) and elevating leg rests (K0195). The primary reason for K0001 is stroke, and the primary reason for K0195 is edema.

c. Question Section - This section is used to gather clinical information regarding the patient's condition, the need for the DME, and supplies.

d. Name of Person Answering Section B Questions - If a clinical professional other than the treating physician (e.g., home health nurse, physical therapist, dietician, or a physician employee) answers the questions in section B, he/she must print his/her name, give his/her professional title, and the name of his/her employer, where indicated. If the treating physician answered the questions, this space may be left blank.

3. SECTION C: (This is completed by the supplier.)
a. Narrative Description of Equipment and Cost - The supplier indicates (1) a narrative description of the item(s) ordered, as well as all options, accessories, supplies, and drugs; (2) the supplier's charge for each item, option, accessory, supply, and drug; and (3) the Medicare fee schedule allowance for each item, option, accessory, supply, or drug, if applicable.

4. SECTION D: (This is completed by the treating physician.)
a. Physician Attestation - The treating physician's signature certifies the CMN that he/she is reviewing includes sections A, B, C, and D, the answers in section B are correct, and the self-identifying information in section A is correct.

b. Physician Signature and Date - After completion and/or review by the treating physician of sections A, B, and C, the treating physician must sign and date the CMN in section D, verifying the attestation appearing in this section. The treating physician's signature also certifies the items ordered are medically necessary for this patient. Signature and date stamps are not acceptable.

Certifications and recertifications may not be altered by "whiting out" or "pasting over" and entering new data. Such claims are denied and suppliers that show a pattern of altering CMNs are identified for educational contact and/or audit.

Also suppliers who have questionable utilization or billing practices or who are under sanction are considered for audit.

100.2.2—Evidence of Medical Necessity for Parenteral and Enteral Nutrition (PEN) Therapy

(Rev. 1, 10-01-03)

B3-3324, B3-4450

The PEN coverage is determined by information provided by the treating physician and the PEN supplier. A completed certification of medical necessity (CMN) must accompany and support initial claims for PEN to establish whether coverage criteria are met and to ensure that the PEN therapy provided is consistent with the attending or ordering physician's prescription. Contractors ensure that the CMN contains pertinent information from the treating physician. Uniform specific medical data facilitate the review and promote consistency in coverage determinations and timelier claims processing.

The medical and prescription information on a PEN CMN can be most appropriately completed by the treating physician or from information in the patient's records by an employee of the physician for the physician's review and signature. Although PEN suppliers sometimes may assist in providing the PEN services, they cannot complete the CMN since they do not have the same access to patient information needed to properly enter medical or prescription information. Contractors use appropriate professional relations issuances, training sessions, and meetings to ensure that all persons and PEN suppliers are aware of this limitation of their role.

When properly completed, the PEN CMN includes the elements of a prescription as well as other data needed to determine whether Medicare coverage is possible. This practice will facilitate prompt delivery of PEN services and timely submittal of the related claim.

100-04 Chapter 32

70—Billing Requirements for Islet Cell Transplantation for Beneficiaries in a National Institutes of Health (NIH) Clinical Trial

(Rev. 986, Issued: 06-16-06, Effective: 05-01-06, Implementation: 07-31-06)

For services performed on or after October 1, 2004, Medicare will cover islet cell transplantation for patients with Type I diabetes who are participating in an NIH sponsored clinical trial. See Pub 100-04 (National Coverage Determinations Manual) section 260.3.1 for complete coverage policy.

The islet cell transplant may be done alone or in combination with a kidney transplant. Islet recipients will also need immunosuppressant therapy to prevent rejection of the transplanted islet cells. Routine follow-up care will be necessary for each trial patient. See Pub 100-04, section 310 for further guidance relative to routine care. All other uses for islet cell services will remain non-covered.

70.1—Healthcare Common Procedure Coding System (HCPCS) Codes for Carriers

(Rev. 261, Issued: 07-30-04, Effective: 10-01-04, Implementation: 10-04-04)

G0341: Percutaneous islet cell transplant, includes portal vein catheterization and infusion

Short Descriptor: Percutaneous islet cell trans

Type of Service: 2

G0342: Laparoscopy for islet cell transplant, includes portal vein catheterization and infusion

Short Descriptor: Laparoscopy islet cell trans

Type of Service: 2

G0343: Laparotomy for islet cell transplant, includes portal vein catheterization and infusion

Short Descriptor: Laparotomy islet cell transp

Type of Service: 2

70.2—Applicable Modifier for Islet Cell Transplant Claims for Carriers

(Rev. 986, Issued: 06-16-06, Effective: 05-01-06, Implementation: 07-31-06)

Carriers shall instruct physicians to bill using the above procedure code(s) with modifier QR (Item or service provided in a Medicare-specified study) for all claims for islet cell transplantation and routine follow-up care related to this service.

70.3—Special Billing and Payment Requirements for Carriers

(Rev. 261, Issued: 07-30-04, Effective: 10-01-04, Implementation: 10-04-04)

Payment and pricing information will be on the October 2004 update of the Medicare Physician Fee Schedule Database (MPFSDB). Pay for islet cell transplants on the basis of the MPFS. Deductible and coinsurance apply for fee-for-service beneficiaries.

70.4—Special Billing and Payment Requirements for Intermediaries

(Rev. 1192, Issued: 03-02-07, Effective: 10-01-04, Implementation: 04-02-07)

This procedure (ICD-9-CM procedure code 52.85-heterotransplantation of islet cells of pancreas) is covered for the clinical trial in an inpatient hospital setting. The applicable TOB is 11X. A secondary diagnoses (diagnoses positions 2 – 9) of V70.7 (examination of participant or control in clinical research) must be present along with condition code 30 (qualifying clinical trial). V70.7 and condition code 30 alerts the claims processing system that this is a clinical trial. The procedure is paid under inpatient prospective payment system for hospitals with patients in the trial. Deductible and coinsurance apply for fee-forservice beneficiaries.

Inpatient hospitals participating in this trial are entitled to an add-on payment of $18,848.00 for islet isolation services. This amount is in addition to the final IPPS payment made to the hospital. Should two infusions occur during the same hospital stay, Medicare will pay for two add-ons for isolation of the islet cells, but never for more than two add-ons for a hospital stay.

Inpatient hospitals shall report charges for organ acquisition in Revenue Code 0810, 0811, 0812, 0813, or 0819. This includes charges for the pre-transplant items and services related to the acquisition and delivery of the pancreatic islet cell transplants. As is Medicare's policy with other organ transplants, Medicare contractors deduct acquisition charges prior to processing through the IPPS Pricer. Pancreata procured for islet cell transplant are not included in the prospective payment. They are paid on a reasonable cost basis. This is a pass-through cost for which interim payments may be made.

Effective for services on or after May 1, 2006, contractors shall accept the QR modifier for islet cell transplantation follow up care when performed in an outpatient department of a hospital when the transplant was done in conjunction with an NIH-sponsored clinical trial, and when billed on type of bill 13X or 85X.

All other normal inpatient billing practices apply.

70.5—Special Billing and Payment Requirements Medicare Advantage (MA) Beneficiaries

(Rev. 261, Issued: 07-30-04, Effective: 10-01-04, Implementation: 10-04-04)

CMS will make payment directly on a fee-for service basis for the routine costs of pancreatic islet cell transplants as well as transplantation and appropriate related items and services, for MA beneficiaries participating in an NIH-sponsored clinical trial. MA organizations will not be liable for payment for routine costs of this new clinical trial until MA payments can be appropriately adjusted to take into account the cost of this national coverage decision. Medicare contractors shall make payment on behalf of MA organizations directly to providers of these islet cell transplants in accordance with Medicare payment rules, except that beneficiaries are not responsible for the Part A and Part B deductibles. MA enrollees will be liable for any applicable coinsurance amounts MA organizations have in place for clinical trial benefits.

100-04 Chapter 32

100 – Billing Requirements for Expanded Coverage of Cochlear Implantation

(Rev. 601, Issued: 07-01-05; Effective: 04-04-05; Implementation: 07-25-05)

Effective for dates of services on and after April 4, 2005, the Centers for Medicare & Medicaid Services (CMS) has expanded the coverage for cochlear implantation to cover moderate-to-profound hearing loss in individuals with hearing test scores equal to or less than 40% correct in the best aided listening condition on tape-recorded tests of open-set sentence recognition and who demonstrate limited benefit from amplification. (See Publication 100-03, chapter 1, section 50.3, for specific coverage criteria).

In addition CMS is covering cochlear implantation for individuals with open-set sentence recognition test scores of greater than 40% to less than or equal to 60% correct but only when the provider is participating in, and patients are enrolled in, either:

- A Food and Drug Administration (FDA)-approved category B investigational device exemption (IDE) clinical trial; or
- A trial under the CMS clinical trial policy (see Pub. 100-03, section 310.1); or

A prospective, controlled comparative trial approved by CMS as consistent with the evidentiary requirements for national coverage analyses and meeting specific quality standards.

100-08 Chapter 5

5.2.3—Detailed Written Orders

(Rev. 242: Issued: 02-22-08; Effective/Implementation Dates: 03-01-08)

Detailed written orders are required for all transactions involving DMEPOS. Detailed written orders may take the form of a photocopy, facsimile image, electronically maintained, or original "pen-and-ink" document. (See chapter 3, section 3.4.1.1.B.)

All orders must clearly specify the start date of the order.

For items that are dispensed based on a verbal order, the supplier must obtain a written order that meets the requirements of this section.

If the written order is for supplies that will be provided on a periodic basis, the written order should include appropriate information on the quantity used, frequency of change, and duration of need. (For example, an order for surgical dressings might specify one 4 x 4 hydrocolloid dressing that is changed 1-2 times per week for 1 month or until the ulcer heals.)

The written order must be sufficiently detailed, including all options or additional features that will be separately billed or that will require an upgraded code. The description can be either a narrative description (e.g., lightweight wheelchair base) or a brand name/model number.

If the supply is a drug, the order must specify the name of the drug, concentration (if applicable), dosage, frequency of administration, and duration of infusion (if applicable).

Someone other than the physician may complete the detailed description of the item. However, the treating physician must review the detailed description and personally sign and date the order to indicate agreement.

The supplier must have a detailed written order prior to submitting a claim. For items listed in chapter 5 section 5.2.3.1, the detailed written order must be obtained prior to delivery. If a supplier does not have a faxed, photocopied, electronic or pen and ink signed detailed written order in their records before they submit a claim to Medicare (i.e., if there is no order or only a verbal order), the claim will be denied. If the claim is for an item for which an order is required by statute (e.g., therapeutic shoes for diabetics, oral anticancer drugs, oral antiemetic drugs which are a replacement for intravenous antiemetic drugs), the claim will be denied as not meeting the benefit category and is therefore not appealable by the supplier (see Pub.. 100-4, chapter 29, §10, 30.3, 60 for more information on appeals). For all other items, (except those listed in section 5.2.3.1) if the supplier does not have an order that has been both signed and dated by the treating physician before billing the Medicare program, the item will be denied as not reasonable and necessary.

Medical necessity information (e.g., an ICD-9-CM diagnosis code, narrative description of the patient's condition, abilities, limitations) is NOT in itself considered to be part of the order although it may be put on the same document as the order.

In other sections of this chapter, the term "order" or "written order" means "detailed written order" unless otherwise specified.

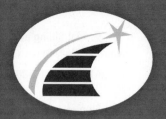

Trust Carol J. Buck and Elsevier for the
resources you need at *each step* of your coding career!

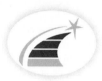
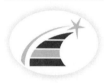
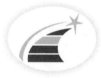
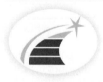
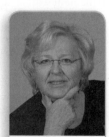